Cardiology
1986

Cardiology
1986

WILLIAM C. ROBERTS, MD, Editor
Chief, Pathology Branch
National Heart, Lung, and Blood Institute
National Institutes of Health, Bethesda, Maryland, and
Clinical Professor of Pathology and Medicine (Cardiology)
Georgetown University, Washington, D. C.
Editor-in-Chief, The American Journal of Cardiology

DEAN T. MASON, MD
Physician-in-Chief
Western Heart Institute
St. Mary's Hospital and Medical Center
San Francisco, California
Editor-in-Chief, American Heart Journal

CHARLES E. RACKLEY, MD
Chairman, Department of Medicine
Anton and Margaret Fuisz
Professor of Medicine
Georgetown University Medical Center
Washington, D. C.

JAMES T. WILLERSON, MD
Professor of Medicine
Chief, Division of Cardiology
Department of Medicine
University of Texas Health Science Center
Dallas, Texas

THOMAS P. GRAHAM, JR, MD
Professor of Pediatrics
Chief, Division of Pediatric Cardiology
Department of Pediatrics
Vanderbilt University
Nashville, Tennessee

ALBERT D. PACIFICO, MD
Professor and Director
Division of Cardiothoracic Surgery
University of Alabama Medical Center
Birmingham, Alabama

ROBERT B. KARP, MD
Chief, Cardiac Surgery Section
Department of Surgery
University of Chicago Medical Center
Chicago, Illinois

Contents

1. Coronary Artery Disease   1

DETECTION   1

Value of Family History of CAD   1

Value of Echo   1

Value of Valsalva Maneuver   2

Value of Logistic Regression Analysis or Probability Analysis of Multiple Noninvasive Tests   2

Value of Signal-Averaged Late Potentials   3

Value of Exercise Testing   4

Value of Radionuclide Studies   9

Angiographic Status of the Coronary Arteries in Symptomatic CAD ≤30 Years of Age   13

Meaning of Coronary Collaterals   13

Usefulness of Transstenotic Coronary Pressure Gradient   14

Coronary Ectasia and/or Aneurysm   16

PROGNOSIS   16

Based on Initial Manifestation of Myocardial Ischemia   16

Based on Leukocyte Count   19

Based on Exercise Thallium-201 Scintigraphy   19

Based on Jeopardy Score   21

Based on Ventricular Late Potentials   22

PROGRESSION OF CORONARY NARROWING   23

RISK FACTORS—GENERAL   24

BLOOD LIPIDS   25

Consensus Development Conference on the Value of Lowering Blood Cholesterol   25

Lipid Research Clinic Prevalence Study 27

New Cholesterol Education Program 28

Blood Lipids in China 29

Low-Density Lipoprotein Receptor Gene 29

Triglycerides 29

Levels in Patients Having Coronary Angiography 31

In the Nephrotic Syndrome 33

Effect of Obesity 33

Effect of Exercise 34

Effect of Coffee Drinking 34

Effect of Alcohol 35

Effect of Malignancy 35

Healthy and Harmful Diets 35

Treatment 39

Nathan Pritikin, Ph.D. 40

Review 41

CIGARETTE SMOKING 41

PHYSICAL ACTIVITY AND FITNESS 42

OBESITY 44

COFFEE DRINKING 45

ALCOHOL DRINKING 46

ESTROGEN 46

HOMOCYSTINURIA 47

PROSTAGLANDINS and PLATELET INHIBITORS 47

SILENT MYOCARDIAL ISCHEMIA 49

ANGINA PECTORIS 50

Relation of Chest Pain to Anxiety and Depression 50

Relation of Chest Pain to Degree of Myocardial Ischemia 50

Variation in Exercise Tolerance 53

Relation of Exercise ST/HR Slope to LV Function and Degree of Coronary Narrowing 53

Dipyridamole—Echo Test   54

Coronary Angiographic Findings   54

Coronary Hemodynamic Responses   55

Coronary Air Embolism -vs.- Coronary Spasm   55

Thromoxane A_2 Production   56

Pacing Induced   56

Significance of Coronary Arterial Adventitial Inflammation   58

Effect of Antianginal Therapy on Exercise Test   58

Relation of Time of Medical Training to Type of Therapy Prescribed   58

Buccal and Oral Nitrates   59

Transdermal Glyceryl Trinitrate   62

Molsidomine   63

Labetalol   64

Diltiazem   64

Nifedipine   66

Nicardipine   67

Nisoldipine   67

Combined Beta Blocker Plus Calcium Channel Blocker   67

Comparison of Nitrates and Calcium Channel Blocker   70

Aspirin and/or Sulfinpyrazone   70

Captopril   71

Coenzyme Q_{10}   71

Amiodarone   72

Therapeutic Review   72

VARIANT ANGINA PECTORIS   72

Effect of Hyperventilation and Cold Pressor Test   72

Frequency of Ventricular Ectopic Activity   73

Echo Findings   74

Coronary Colaterals   77

Diltiazem Therapy   77

Percutaneous Transluminal Coronary Angioplasty   77

PERCUTANEOUS TRANSLUMINIAL CORONARY 78
ANGIOPLASTY

   Creatine Release Afterward 78

   ECG Changes During PTCA 78

   Effect on LV Regional Function and/or Diastolic Filling 79

   On Myocardial Perfusion 80

   Distal Coronary Perfusion During Balloon Dilation 80

   Relation of Occlusion Pressure to Collaterals 81

   Nitroglycerin During PTCA 81

   Diltiazem After PTCA 81

   Results 82

   Of Totally Occluded Coronary Artery 85

   Of LM Coronary Artery 87

   Of Multiple Coronary Arteries 87

   For Unstable Angina Pectoris 88

   With Previous Coronary Thrombosis 89

   Restenosis After Successful PTCA 89

   Effect of Intimal Dissection 90

   Producing Acute Coronary Occlusion 91

CORONARY ARTERY BYPASS GRAFTING 91

   Factors Determining Long-Term Survival 91

   For Nonfatal Cardiac Arrest 91

   In Persons ≥65 Years of Age 92

   Effect on LV Function 93

   Results With Reduced LV Function Preoperatively 95

   Effect on Exercise-Induced Ventricular Arrhythmias 96

   Fate of Preoperative Defect on Exercise Thallium Imaging 96

   Effect of Platelet-Inhibiting Drugs on Graft Patency 97

   Effect of Exercise Training Postoperatively 98

   Results with Endarterectomy 98

   More Than One Operation 98

   Internal Mammary Artery -vs- Saphenous Vein as Conduit 99

   Arrhythmias Postoperatively 99

   Unstable Angina Pectoris and/or AMI Postoperatively 99

Effect on Hospital Readmissions 100

Pericardial Effusion Postoperatively 101

Frequency of Stroke Postoperatively 101

Adrenal Gland Function Postoperatively 101

Frequency of Narrowings in Unused Saphenous Veins 103

COMPARISON OF PTCA WITH CABG 103

2. **Acute Myocardial Infarction and its Consequences** **115**

GENERAL TOPICS 115

Time of Onset of Chest Pain 115

Creatine Kinase 116

Criteria for Diagnosis 116

In Cigarette-Smoking Women 117

In Elderly Individuals 117

Silent Infarction 117

Late After CABG 118

Quantitation of Infarct Size 119

Coronary Collaterals 120

LV Function 121

Relation of Type A Behavior to Survival 122

Coagulation Problems 122

ECG Observations 124

Echo Observations 125

RNA Observations 126

Comparison of Echo and Radionuclide Studies 127

Magnetic Resonance Imaging 128

Indications for Coronary Angiography After Infarction 128

Relation to Angina Pectoris 128

Outcome 129

Frequency and Outcome in a Large Employed Population 130

COMPLICATIONS 131

Recurrence 131

RV Infarction and/or Dysfunction 132

Atrial Fibrillation   135

Pericardial Effusion   135

LV Thrombi   135

LV Aneurysm   136

Rupture of LV Free Wall or Ventricular Septum   138

Rupture of Papillary Muscle   139

PROGNOSTIC INDEXES   139

Creatine Kinase Level   139

Type A Score   141

Initial ECG   141

ECG S-T Segment Depression   141

LV Thrombi   142

Location of Infarction   145

LV Ejection Fraction   145

Infarct Extension   146

Exercise Testing   147

Echocardiography   149

Radionuclide Angiography   149

Ventricular Arrhythmias   150

Programmed Ventricular Stimulation   153

TREATMENT   156

Morphine   156

Lidocaine   156

Digitalis   157

Anticoagulants   159

Dobutamine or Nitroprusside   159

Beta Blockers   159

Calcium Channel Blocker   164

Intracoronary Thrombolysis   165

Intravenous Thrombolysis   171

Intracoronary -vs- Intravenous Thrombolysis   178

PTCA With or Without Thrombolysis   179

Coronary Artery Bypass Grafting   180

At Home -vs- Group Rehabilitation   180

Exercise   180

3. Arrhythmias, Conduction Disturbances, and Cardiac Arrest   191

ARRHYTHMIAS IN HEALTHY INDIVIDUALS   191

ATRIAL FIBRILLATION/FLUTTER   192

In Infants and Children   192

Lone   193

Alcohol Related   194

Diltiazem Treatment   194

Amiodarone Treatment   195

SUPRAVENTRICULAR TACHYCARDIA WITH OR WITHOUT   195
SHORT P-R INTERVAL SYNDROMES

Natural History   195

Caused by Theophylline   196

Arrhythmias Produced by Antitachycardia Pacing   196

Transesophageal Atrial Pacing   196

Adenosine   197

Amiodarone   197

Propafenone   198

Verapamil   198

Esmolol -vs- Propranolol   199

Surgical Ablation   199

VENTRICULAR ARRHYTHMIAS   201

Diagnosis   201

Relation to Psychologic Factors   202

Overdose of Tricyclic Antidepressant Drug   202

Spontaneous Variability   203

Reproducibility of Responses to Programmed Electrical   204
Stimulation

Significance of Induction of Ventricular Arrhythmias By   205
Programmed Electrical Stimulation

Comparison of Holter Monitoring to Electrophysiologic   209
Study

Antiarrhythmic Drug Efficacy—General   209

Arrhythmogenicity of Antiarrhythmic Agents   209

Amiodarone   211

Bepridil   214

Encainide   215

Flecainide   215

Mexiletine   217

Lorcainide and Norlorcainide   218

Procainamide   220

N-Acetylprocainamide   221

Propafenone   221

Quinidine   222

Sotalol   224

Tocainide   225

Verapamil   225

Danger of Cardioversion With Therapeutic Serum Digoxin Levels   226

Antitachycardia Pacemaker   226

LV Endocardial Resection   227

CARDIAC ARREST   229

In Persons ≤21 Years of Age   229

Nonfatal Cardiac Arrest Out of Hospital   229

Ambulatory ECG Recordings at Time of Fatal Cardiac Arrest   231

Usefulness of Prehospital Cardiopulmonary Resuscitation   231

During Anesthesia   232

SYNCOPE   232

LONG Q-T INTERVAL SYNDROME   235

BUNDLE BRANCH BLOCK   236

ATRIOVENTRICULAR BLOCK   237

PACEMAKERS AND CARDIOVERTERS   238

Guidelines For Their Use   238

Sinus Node Dysfunction in Person ≤40 Years of Age   239

External Noninvasive Temporary Cardiac Pacing 240

Reviews and Related Topics 240

4. Systemic Hypertension 249

GENERAL TOPICS 249

Atrial Natriuretic Peptide 249

Effect of Cigarette Smoking 250

Effect of Alcohol 250

Relation to Blood Lead 252

Effect of Snoring 252

Sleep Apnea Syndrome 252

Osler's Maneuver and Pseudohypertension 252

Hypertensive Hypertrophic Cardiomyopathy in the Elderly 253

Effect on RV Wall Thickness 253

LV Diastolic Function 254

In Pregnancy 254

TREATMENT 254

Nondrug Means 254

Diuretics 257

Beta Blocker 258

Angiotensin Converting Enzyme Inhibitor 260

Nitroglycerin or Nitroprusside for Postoperative Hypertension 261

Major Clinical Trials 262

Calcium Channel Blocker 270

5. Valvular Heart Disease 273

MITRAL VALVE PROLAPSE 273

Long-Term Follow-up 273

With Ruptured Chordae Tendineae 273

With Infective Endocarditis 274

In Drug Addicts 275

Secondary to RV Enlargement 275

Relation to LV Size in the Marfan Syndrome   276

With Atrial Flutter   276

With Wolff-Parkinson-White Syndrome   276

Ventricular Arrhythmias   277

Safety of Labor and Delivery   277

Sickle-Cell Anemia   277

Hyperthyroidism   278

Operative Therapy   278

MITRAL REGURGITATION   279

Forward EF   279

Ventricular Arrhythmias   279

Secondary to Ruptured Chordae Tendineae   280

MITRAL STENOSIS   281

Effects of Atenolol on Exercise Capacity   281

Percutaneous Catheter Mitral Commissurotomy   281

Open Mitral Valve Reconstruction   281

MITRAL ANULAR CALCIUM   282

AORTIC VALVE STENOSIS   283

Morphologic Features of Operatively Excised Valves   283

Determining Severity by Echo   284

Usefulness of Echo in Predicting Proper Prosthetic Valve   288
    Size

H-V Conduction   288

Coronary Luminal Diameter   289

Significance of Angina as Predictor of Degree of Coronary   290
    Arterial Narrowing

AORTIC REGURGITATION   290

Idiopathic Etiology   290

Ankylosing Spondylitis and Variants   291

ECG Findings   291

E-Point Septal Separation   292

LV End-Systolic Dimension   293

Impact of Preoperative LV Function on Operative Result   295

Exercise EF Response   296

INFECTIVE ENDOCARDITIS   298

TRICUSPID VALVE DISEASE   300

MISCELLANEOUS TOPICS   301

    Morphologic Features of Operatively Excised Mitral   301
        Valves

    Normal Aortic Valve Anatomy   301

    The Heart in the Carcinoid Syndrome   303

    Echo Findings in Families with the Marfan Syndrome   303

    Evaluating Mitral Valve Operations by Echo   305

CARDIAC VALVE REPLACEMENT   305

    Determinants of Mortality after AVR   305

    Evaluation of MVR   306

    MVR Plus CABG   306

    St. Jude Medical Prosthesis   306

    Porcine Bioprosthesis   307

    Ionescu-Shiley Bioprosthesis   307

    Doppler Echo Evaluation of Prosthetic and Biopros-   308
        thetic Cardiac Valves

    Treatment of Right-Sided Cardiac Failure After MVR   308

    Anatomic Analysis of Prosthetic and Bioprosthetic Failure 309

    Prosthetic Valve Endocarditis   309

6. Myocardial Heart Disease   313

IDIOPATHIC DILATED CARDIOMYOPATHY   313

    Endomyocardial Biopsy in Infants and Children   313

    Relation to Acute Myocarditis   313

    Correlation of Myocardial Ultrastructural Findings to   314
        Myocardial Function

    Prevalence in 2 Regions in England   314

    Familial Aggregation   314

    Effect of Valsalva Maneuver   315

    Prognosis   316

    Effects of Digoxin   317

    Effects of Hydralazine   317

Metoprolol Therapy — 318

Nifedipine — 319

HYPERTROPHIC CARDIOMYOPATHY — 320

Myocardial Ischemia — 320

Doppler Flow Observations — 320

Diastolic Abnormalities — 321

Magnetic Resonance Imaging — 322

Comparison of Ventricular Emptying With and Without Outflow Pressure Gradient — 322

Anesthetic Risk for Noncardiac Surgery — 323

"Apical" Variety — 324

Frequency of Epicardial CAD — 324

Amiodarone — 325

Nifedipine — 325

Verapamil — 326

CARDIAC AMYLOIDOSIS — 326

ASSOCIATION WITH A CONDITION AFFECTING PRIMARILY A NONCARDIAC STRUCTURE(S) — 327

Myotonic Muscular Dystrophy — 327

Thalassemia Major — 327

7. Congenital Heart Disease — 331

ATRIAL SEPTAL DEFECT — 331

Transatrial Velocity by Doppler Echo — 331

Spontaneous Closure in Infancy — 331

ATRIOVENTRICULAR CANAL DEFECT — 332

Effect of Down's Syndrome on Management — 332

Left Atrioventricular Valve Replacement — 332

VENTRICULAR SEPTAL DEFECT — 333

Standardized Echo Nomenclature — 333

Localization by Superimposed Doppler and Cross-Sectional Echo — 333

Isolated in Adults 335

With Aneurysm of the Membraneous Ventricular Septum 335

Pulmonary Arterial Development in Infants 338

PULMONIC VALVE STENOSIS 338

PULMONIC VALVE ATRESIA 338

TETRALOGY OF FALLOT 340

With Absent Pulmonic Valve 340

Operative Repair 341

Electrophysiologic Findings After Operative Repair 343

COMPLETE TRANSPOSITION OF THE GREAT ARTERIES 343

Tricuspid Valve Abnormalities 343

Ventricular Function After Corrective Operations 344

*Results of Mustard-type Venous Switch and Insertion of
  Conduit From LV to PA* 344

Arrhythmias After the Mustard Procedure 345

Arterial Switch Operation 345

LEFT VENTRICULAR OUTFLOW OBSTRUCTION 346

Aortic Valve Stenosis 346

Subaortic Stenosis 346

AORTIC ISTHMIC COARCTATION REPAIR 347

MISCELLANEOUS TOPICS IN PEDIATRIC CARDIOLOGY 351

The Newborn Transitional Circulation 351

Aortic Valve Regurgitation and Nonimmune Hydrops 351

Congenital Heart Disease in Offspring of Affected Parents 351

*Absent Right Superior Vena Cava and Conduction Tissue
  Abnormalities* 352

Straddling AV Valve 352

Criss-Cross Heart 352

*LV Mechanics in Combined AS and Aortic Isthmic
  Coarctation* 353

Combined Subaortic Stenosis and VSD 353

Doppler PA Pressure Estimate   353

LV Function Before and After the Fontan Operation for   354
    Tricuspid Valve Atresia

MISCELLANEOUS TOPICS IN PEDIATRIC CARDIAC SURGERY   354

Blalock-Taussig Shunt   354

Repair of Congenital Pulmonary Venous Stenosis   354

Repair of Total Anomalous Pulmonary Venous Connection   355
    to Right Superior Vena Cava

Prostaglandin E_1 in Ductus-Dependent Neonates   355

Normothermic Caval Inflow Occlusion   355

Cavopulmonary Shunt   356

Intracardiac Repair Without Blood Transfusion   356

Results of Operations for Ebstein's Anomaly   357

Repair of Double-Orifice Mitral Valve   357

Repair of Discordant AV Connection   358

Baffle Obstruction After the Mustard Operation   358

Operations for Double-Outlet Right Ventricle   359

Arterial Switch for TGA and for Double-Outlet Right   359
    Ventricle

Assessment of Ventricular Function After Fontan Procedure   360

Permanent Pacing After Fontan Procedure   360

Repair of Truncus Arteriosus   361

Repair of Single Ventricle With Subaortic Stenosis   362

8. Congestive Heart Failure   367

GENERAL TOPICS   367

Mechanism of Fatigue   367

Associated Ventricular Arrhythmias   367

With Intact Systolic LV Function   368

Responses to Exercise   368

TREATMENT   371

Amrinone   371

Captopril and Enalapril   371

Captopril -vs- Isosorbide Dinitrate   377

Dopamine -vs- Enalaprilat   377

Fenoldopam   377

Milrinone   378

MDL 17,043   378

Captopril -vs- Milrinone   380

Nifedipine   380

Salbutamol   381

Sublingual Nitroglycerin   381

Transdermal Nitroglycerin   381

DIGITALIS AND WILLIAM WITHERING   382

9. Miscellaneous Topics   387

PERICARDIAL HEART DISEASE   387

Primary Acute Pericardial Disease   387

Magnetic Resonance Imaging in Constriction   388

Echo-Guided Pericardiocentesis   388

Pericardiectomy for Constriction   388

CARDIOVASCULAR EFFECTS OF EXERCISE   389

Athletic Heart Syndrome   389

Cardiovascular Evaluation of the Athlete   390

Runners   390

Swimmers and Weight Lifters   391

Endurance Training   391

Endurance Athletes   392

KAWASAKI DISEASE   392

Features of Coronary Disease   392

Ventricular Function   392

Salicylate Treatment   393

Aortocoronary Bypass Grafting   394

TAKAYASU'S ARTERITIS   394

CARDIOVASCULAR FINDINGS IN THE ELDERLY 395

 Intensity of Cardiac Sounds 395

 ECG Findings 395

 Ventricular Function 395

ECHO STUDIES 396

 Determining LV Mass and Volume 396

 In Obesity 396

 In Anorexia Nervosa 396

 In Habitual Alcoholics With and Without Hepatic Cirrhosis 397

 In Systemic Lupus Erythematosus 397

 Detecting Incomplete Mitral Leaflet Closure 398

 Review of Doppler Echocardiography 398

CARDIAC CATHETERIZATION 398

 As an Outpatient 398

 Return of Transseptal Approach 399

 Fick -vs- Indicator Dilution for Cardiac Output 399

PHARMACOLOGIC TOPICS 399

 Caffeine 399

 Alcohol 400

 Platelets, Prostaglandins, and Stress 401

 Calcium Channel Blockers—A Review 401

PRIMARY PULMONARY HYPERTENSION 401

 Morphologic Findings 401

 Spontaneous Hemodynamic Variability 402

 Therapy 402

CARDIOVASCULAR SURGICAL TOPICS 403

 Routine Preoperative Exercise Testing Before Major Noncardiac Surgery 403

 Therapy of Mediastinitis 404

CARDIAC AND/OR PULMONARY TRANSPLANTATION 404

UNCATEGORIZABLE   407

Asymptomatic Myocardial Ischemia in Diabetes Mellitus   407

Cardiac Problems in Pregnancy—Review   407

The King of Hearts   407

Pulmonary Veno-Occlusive Disease   408

Articles in USA Cardiology Journals in 1984   409

Preface

Cardiology 1986 is the sixth book to be published in this series. It contains summaries of 771 articles, all published in 1985. A total of 28 medical journals (Table I) were examined and at least 1, and usually many articles, were summarized from each of these journals. The number of articles summarized by each of the 7 authors is summarized in Table II. All of Mason's submissions were from *The American Heart Journal*; Rackley's from *Circulation*, and Willerson's from *The Journal of the American College of Cardiology*. Karp's and Pacifico's summaries were from articles published in surgical journals. The contributions of Graham and Roberts were from a variety of medical journals. The summaries from each contributor were submitted to me, organized into the various sections in each of the 9 chapters, and each summary was copyedited by me.

TABLE I. *Journals containing articles summarized in Cardiology 1986*

1. American Heart Journal
2. American Journal of Cardiology
3. American Journal of Medicine
4. Annals of Internal Medicine
5. Annals of Thoracic Surgery
6. Archives of Internal Medicine
7. Archives of Pathology and Laboratory Medicine
8. Atherosclerosis
9. British Heart Journal
10. British Medical Journal
11. Catheterization and Cardiovascular Diagnosis
12. Chest
13. Circulation
14. European Heart Journal
15. Heart and Vessels
16. Human Pathology
17. International Journal of Cardiology
18. Journal of American College of Cardiology
19. Journal of the American Medical Association
20. Journal of Arteriosclerosis
21. Journal of Thoracic & Cardiovascular Surgery
22. Lancet
23. Mayo Clinic Proceedings
24. Medicine
25. New England Journal of Medicine
26. Pediatric Cardiology
27. Progress in Cardiovascular Diseases
28. Science

TABLE II.   CARDIOLOGY 1986

AUTHOR	CHAPTER NUMBER									TOTALS
	1	2	3	4	5	6	7	8	9	
WCR	117	94	71	38	40	17	3	12	36	428 (55.51%)
DTM	32	9	23	7	6	0	3	8	6	94 (12.19%)
CER	21	21	10	0	6	9	2	7	7	83 (10.77%)
JTW	25	17	15	2	5	2	0	9	2	77 (9.99%)
TPG, Jr	0	0	5	1	0	0	25	0	2	33 (4.28%)
ADP	0	0	0	0	0	0	33	0	0	33 (4.28%)
RBK	8	0	1	1	11	0	0	0	2	23 (2.98%)
TOTALS	203	141	125	49	68	28	66	36	55	771 (100%)

A book of this type is made possible because of unselfish contributions from several individuals, none of whom are rewarded by authorship. I am enormously grateful to Marjorie Hadsell for typing perfectly the 428 summaries contributed by me, to Margaret M. M. Moore for organizing the figures and tables for photography, to Esther Bergman for typing the detailed table of contents, to Leslie Silvernail, Marcia Sheridan, Debra Lezama, Laurie Christian, Joy Phillips, Sue Long, and Mary Sawallisch also for typing many of the summaries. Jennifer Granger managed to carry the 30-pound package of edited summaries, reference cards, figures and tables from Bethesda to New York. Herbert V. Paureiss, Jr., efficiently coordinated the publishing of the book in New York.

WILLIAM C. ROBERTS, MD
EDITOR

Coronary Artery Disease

DETECTION

Value of family history of CAD

Conroy and associates[1] from Dublin, Ireland, examined the importance of a positive family history as a primary risk factor for CAD. Of 792 consecutive men aged <60 years who survived a first episode of unstable angina pectoris or AMI, 326 had a negative family history, 298 a positive history, and 168 a family history that could not be established with certainty. There was no significant difference in the distribution of the 3 primary coronary risk factors—cigarette smoking, systemic hypertension, and hypercholesterolemia—between those with and without a positive family history. The 133 subjects with a positive family history of premature CAD (occurrence in near relatives <60 years of age) were significantly younger than those with a negative family history. It was concluded that there is little evidence to confirm a positive family history as an important independent risk factor for CAD, although there may be familial aggregation of subjects with a high susceptibility to the effects of the 3 primary risk factors.

Value of echocardiography

To evaluate the usefulness of echo-defined regional wall motion abnormalities (RWMA) in detecting CAD in patients with LV dysfunction and a normal-sized or dilated left ventricle, 103 patients were studied by 2-D echo and cardiac catheterization by Medina and colleagues[2] from Philadelphia, Pennsylvania. In 60 patients (group I) who had LV dysfunction and a dilated left ventricle by echo (patients with dilated cardiomyopathy [DC]), RWMA were detected in 44 patients and 38 (86%) of them had significant CAD, usually 2- or 3-vessel obstruction; of the 16 patients with DC and diffuse LV hypokinesis, 8 had evidence of CAD. Thus, the presence of RWMA by 2D echo had an 83% sensitivity, a 57% specificity, and a 77% predictive accuracy in detecting CAD in patients with DC and thus in distinguishing ischemic from idiopathic DC. In 43 patients with LV dysfunction but normal LV size (group II), the sensitivity, specificity, and predictive accuracy of RWMA in detecting significant CAD was 95, 100, and 95%, respectively. It was concluded that the detection of RWMA by 2D echo was highly suggestive of significant CAD in patients with LV dysfunction and normal-sized or dilated left ventricle.

In a study carried out by Ren and associates[3] from Philadelphia, Pennsylvania, regional LV endocardial motion and wall thickening were quantitatively assessed in 9 normal subjects and in 21 patients with CAD using 2-D echo and a computerized light pen system. Eight equal sections of a cross-sectional image from parasternal short-axis, apical 4- and 2-chamber views were used for measuring sector area difference of endocardial motion and wall thickness between end-diastole and end-systole. In 13 patients with anterior wall motion abnormalities, area difference of wall thickening found by 2D echo was abnormal in 12 of 13 patients, and only in 6 of 13 patients by endocardial motion. In 10 patients with dyskinetic regions in apex or anterior wall, dyskinesia by wall thickening was found in all patients, but only in 6 of 10 by endocardial motion. Thus, wall thickening assessed by 2D echo is a more sensitive technique than analysis of endocardial motion in evaluating RWMA in patients with CAD.

Value of Valsalva maneuver

Labovitz and associates[4] from St. Louis, Missouri, determined the effects of the Valsalva maneuver on global and regional LV function by performing single-plane left ventriculograms in the 30° right anterior oblique projection in 50 patients during normal breath holding and during the late strain phase of the Valsalva maneuver: 31 patients had significant CAD (>70% luminal diameter narrowing in a major coronary artery). Ventriculograms were analyzed for determination of EF and end-diastolic and end-systolic volumes. Regional wall motion was analyzed by a chord method of calculating segmental fractional shortening. EF increased significantly in the entire group of patients (62 ± 16–70 ± 19%), whereas both end-diastolic (105 ± 33–88 ± 34 ml) and end-systolic volumes (43 ± 29–30 ± 29 ml) showed striking reductions with Valsalva maneuver. Patients without CAD usually had global augmentation in LV function, and those with CAD often had only segmental improvement. This augmentation appeared to be dependent on the patency of the supplying coronary artery.

Value of logistic regression analysis or probability analysis of multiple noninvasive tests

Melin and coinvestigators[5] from Brussels, Belgium, used conditional probability analysis for the diagnosis of CAD in 93 infarct-free women presenting with chest pain. Another group of 42 consecutive female patients was prospectively analyzed. For this latter group, the physician had access to the pretest and post-test probability of CAD before coronary angiography. All 135 women underwent stress ECG, thallium scintigraphy, and coronary angiography. The pretest and post-test probabilities of CAD were derived from a computerized Bayesian algorithm. Probability estimates were calculated by the following hypothetical strategies: S0, in which history, including risk factors, was considered; S1, in which history and stress ECG results were considered; S2, in which history and stress ECG and stress thallium scintigraphic results were considered; and S3, in which history and stress ECG results were used, but in which stress scintigraphic results were considered only if the poststress probability of CAD was between 10 and 90%. The strategies were compared with respect to accuracy with the coronary angiogram as the standard. For both groups of women, S2 and S3 were found to be the most accurate in predicting the presence or absence of CAD. However, it was found with use of S3 that more than one-third of the thallium scintigrams could have been avoided without loss of accuracy. It was also found that diagnostic catheterization performed to exclude CAD as a diagnosis could have been avoided in half of the patients without loss of accuracy. Studies in the prospective group of 42 women confirmed that S2 and S3 had the best diagnostic accuracy. The investigators also observed a high prevalence of angiographically documented CAD in this group (48 -vs- 26% in the first group of 93 women). In this prospectively studied group, there was a smaller proportion of patients with a low probability estimate of CAD. These results suggest that the treating physician's prior knowledge of probability estimates reduced the number of unnecessary diagnostic coronary angiographic procedures performed.

The incremental diagnostic yield of clinical data, exercise ECG, stress thallium scintigraphy, and cardiac fluoroscopy to predict coronary and multivessel disease was assessed in 171 symptomatic men by means of multiple logistic regression analyses in an investigation carried out by Hung and associates[6] from Montreal, Canada, and St. Louis, Missouri. When clinical variables alone were analyzed, chest pain type and age were predictive of CAD, whereas chest pain type, age, a family history of CAD before age 55 years, and abnormal ST-T wave changes on the rest ECG were predictive of multivessel CAD. The percentage of patients correctly classified by cardiac fluoroscopy (presence or absence of coronary artery calcium), exercise ECG, and thallium scintigraphy was 9, 25, and 50%, respectively, greater than for clinical variables, when the presence or absence of CAD was the outcome, and 13, 25, and 29%, respectively, when multivessel CAD was studied; 5% of patients were misclassified. When the 37 clinical and noninvasive test variables were analyzed jointly, the most significant variable predictive of CAD was an abnormal thallium scan and for multivessel CAD, the amount of exercise performed. The data from this study confirm previous reports that optimal diagnostic efficacy is obtained when noninvasive tests are ordered sequentially. In symptomatic men, cardiac fluoroscopy is an ineffective test when compared with exercise ECG and thallium scintigraphy.

Value of signal-averaged late potentials

LV dysfunction has been suggested as a cause of late potentials on the signal averaged ECG of patients with CAD. Pollak and colleagues[7] from Atlanta, Georgia, compared the average surface ECG with angiographic findings in 57 patients with CAD and LV dysfunction: 16 patients had sustained VT and 41 had no documented arrhythmia. These 2 patient groups were comparable with respect to age, mean EF, and wall motion score. Late potentials, defined as voltage <25 μv in the last 40 msec of the filtered QRS complex, were found in 10 of 16 patients with VT and in 6 of 41 patients without arrhythmia. Late potentials were independent of EF, wall motion score, or presence of dyskinesis in both groups. There was no correlation between the total filtered QRS duration and EF or wall motion score in either patient group. In patients with CAD, late potentials are associated with VT but are independent of global or regional LV function.

Value of exercise testing

A computer-derived treadmill exercise score that quantifies the ECG response to exercise has been reported to have a high sensitivity (87%) and specificity (92%) in patients with a high prevalence of CAD. To test its accuracy in young, asymptomatic men with a low prevalence of CAD, Hollenberg and associates[8] from 4 different medical centers evaluated the responses of 377 military officers (mean age, 37 years) by 2 independent methods. According to standard ECG criteria, 45 of the subjects (12%) had positive tests, whereas the treadmill exercise score indicated that only 3 (<1%) had positive tests. Since 2 of these 3 had LV hypertrophy and met only the criteria for the latter without associated CAD, the treadmill exercise score predicted that only 1 of 377 subjects would have clinically important CAD. Coronary arteriography, performed in 10 persons with the most positive scores on standard treadmill tests and the highest scores for risk factors, showed that 9 subjects did not have CAD and that 1 had single-vessel CAD (the same subject who the treadmill score predicted would have mild CAD). The treadmill exercise score appears to improve the diagnostic specificity of exercise ECG and may be more useful than values on standard stress tests in screening asymptomatic populations for CAD.

This article was followed by an editorial by Sheffield entitled, "Another Perfect Treadmill Test?"[9]

Braat and associates[10] from Maastricht, The Netherlands, utilized lead V_4R during exercise testing to predict proximal stenosis of the right coronary artery in 107 patients. A Bruce exercise test with simultaneous recordings of leads I, II, V_4R, V_1, V_4, and V_6 was followed by coronary arteriography. All patients were evaluated for the absence or presence of ST-segment deviation of ≥ 1 mm in lead V_4R. Seven of the 14 patients without AMI and with significant proximal stenosis in the right coronary artery developed ST-segment deviation of ≥ 1 mm in lead V_4R during exercise. Similar findings occurred in 11 of 18 patients with healed inferior AMI and proximal occlusion of the right coronary artery. None of the 53 patients without significant proximal stenosis of the right coronary artery had ST-segment changes in lead V_4R with exercise. Thus, exercise-related ST-segment depression in lead V_4R had a sensitivity of 56%, a specificity of 96%, and a predictive accuracy of 84% in identifying proximal stenosis in the right coronary artery. These data suggest that recording lead V_4R may be of value in predicting or excluding proximal stenosis in the right coronary artery during exercise testing.

The Multiple Risk Factor Intervention Trial (MRFIT),[11] a CAD primary prevention trial, examined the effect on the CAD mortality rate of a special intervention (SI) program to reduce blood cholesterol level, diastolic BP, and cigarette smoking in 35–57 year old men. Half of the 12,866 participants were randomly assigned to usual care (UC) in the community. During 6–8 years of follow-up, the CAD mortality rate was 7% lower in the SI than in the UC group, a nonsignificant difference. An *a priori* subgroup hypothesis proposed that men with a normal ECG response to a heart rate (HR) limited exercise test would have particular benefit from intervention. An abnormal response, defined as an ST-depression integral measured by computer greater than a predetermined voltage time cutpoint, was observed in 12.5% of the men at baseline and was associated with a 3-fold elevation in risk of CAD death within the UC group. In the subgroup with a normal exercise ECG response, there was no significant difference in the CAD mortality rate (16 and 14/1,000, respectively) for SI and UC men. In contrast, there was a 57% lower rate among men in the SI group with an abnormal test result compared with men in the UC group (22.2 -vs- 51.8/1,000). The relative risks (SI/UC) in these 2 strata were significantly different. These findings suggest that men with elevated risk factors who have an abnormal exercise text response may benefit substantially from risk factor reduction.

The exercise ECG has relatively poor specificity and predictive accuracy for 3-vessel CAD when conventional diagnostic criteria are used. ECG evaluation, however, using linear regression analysis of the HR-related change in ST-segment depression (ST/HR slope) is reported to distinguish accurately patients with from those without CAD and to separate accurately patients with 1-, 2-, and 3-vessel CAD. To assess the applicability of this method and to compare it with conventional interpretation, Okin and associates[12] from New York City retrospectively evaluated 50 patients in whom exercise ECG and coronary cineangiography had been performed for suspected CAD using a modified ST/HR slope analysis limited to leads V_5, V_6, and aVF. Eighteen patients had 3-vessel, 22 had 2-vessel, 6 had 1-vessel CAD, and 4 had no CAD. Standard ECG criteria ($\geq$1 mm of horizontal or downsloping ST depression) identified 3-vessel CAD with a sensitivity of 78%, specificity of 56%, and positive predictive value of only 50%. Peak ST/HR slope criteria ($\geq$6.0 μV/beat/min) identified 3-vessel CAD with a sensitivity of 78%, specificity of 97%, and positive predictive value of 93%. The overall test accuracy using measured peak ST/HR slope was 90%, compared with 64% for standard ST-depression criteria. In conclusion, analysis of the peak ST/HR slope can greatly improve the diagnostic accuracy of exercise ECG and further prospective study of this method is indicated.

Does 2 mm ST depression induced by exercise have the same clinical significance in a patient with a 30 mm R wave as a patient with a 10 mm R wave in the same monitored lead? To answer this question Hollenberg and associates[13] from San Francisco, California, compared exercise responses of 85 patients by 2 quantitative methods of assessing myocardial ischemia. A computer-derived treadmill exercise score, based largely on the characteristics of exercise-induced ST-segment depression, was compared with a thallium exercise score. Both scores correlated well over a wide range of values. Then, the treadmill exercise score was corrected (by adjusting the magnitude of the ST depression to a standardized R-wave amplitude of 12 mm in V_5 and 8 mm in aVF) to determine if this would improve its correlation with the thallium exercise score. The patients were separated into 2 groups by R-wave amplitude: 53 had an R_{V5} of 9–17 mm and 32 had an R_{V5} <9 or >17 mm. Correction of the treadmill exercise score for R-wave amplitude did not change the slope and intercepts of the regression line for patients with an R_{V5} amplitude of 9–17 mm, but did for those with an R_{V5} amplitude <9 or >17 mm. In this latter group, R-wave correction changed the regression line from one that differed significantly from that of patients with less extreme R_{V5} voltage to one that was indistinguishable from it. Correction of the treadmill exercise score also increased the correlation coefficient from 0.54 to 0.68 in this group. In several patients an abnormal score became normal when it was corrected for R-wave voltage. This corrected score was consistent with the coronary arteriographic findings, the lack of symptoms, and the good exercise tolerance. Thus, as judged independently by a thallium exercise score, the degree of exercise-induced ST depression is influenced by R-wave amplitude, and if not normalized to a standard voltage, may either exaggerate or underestimate the degree of exercise-induced myocardial ischemia.

Tzivoni and associates[14] from Jerusalem, Israel, performed a Bruce protocol treadmill exercise test during which an ECG was recorded simultaneously with a 2-channel Holter recorder with bipolar V_3- and V_5-like leads and by conventional 12-lead system in 144 patients, 95 of whom were referred for coronary arteriography: 68 patients had no ST depression on either the Holter or the 12-lead ECG during the exercise test, and 70 patients had ischemic changes by both methods; thus, in 138 of the 144 patients (96%), the results of the 2 tests were concordant. The severity of ST depression, as judged by the HR at which ischemic changes were first noted and the maximal ST depression observed, were similar on both recording systems. The Holter system identified 6 of the 7 patients whose ischemic changes were confined to the inferior wall on the 12-lead ECG. The addition of the V_3 lead as a second ischemic lead increased the ischemia detection by 10%. In 95 patients who also underwent coronary arteriography, the sensitivity of the Holter system during exercise in detecting significant CAD was 81% and that of 12-lead ECG was 84%, the specificity was 85% for both and the positive predictive value was 91% for both. Thus, the 2-channel Holter recording system with bipolar V_3- and V_5-like leads was as accurate as the 12-lead system in detecting ischemic changes during exercise and proved that ambulatory monitoring system can reliably reproduce ST segment.

Akhras and associates[15] from London, England, performed maximal treadmill stress testing and coronary angiography in 102 consecutive patients with a history of chest pain or recent AMI. The diastolic BP response was evaluated independently of ST-segment change and systolic BP. In the presence of a normal systolic BP response an increase in diastolic BP of 15 mmHg on at least 2 determinations during the same stage of exercise was considered abnormal. In 99 patients an accurate diastolic reading was possible. Of these, 61 had a normal diastolic BP response; in 25 the ST segment was ischemic, and 7 had 3-vessel CAD. Thirty-eight patients had an abnormal diastolic BP response and 27 of them had an ischemic ST response. Of the 11 with a negative ST response for ischemia, 1 had LM CAD; 7, 3-vessel CAD, and 3, 2-vessel CAD. Patients with an abnormal diastolic response had greater ST depression with more angina at a reduced workload than those with a normal diastolic response (Fig. 1-1). In patients with chest pain, an abnormal increase in diastolic BP on exercise reflected severe CAD. Although no false positives occurred in this study, there was an appreciable number of false negatives (sensitivity 46%) in both patients with chest pain and those with infarction. An abnormal diastolic response therefore represents a useful additional diagnostic indicator of CAD when the ST-segment response is normal or borderline. When the diastolic BP becomes increased with or without ST changes, the likelihood of severe CAD is increased.

Ho and associates[16] from Perth, Australia, carried out maximal treadmill testing in 50 patients with angiographically documented CAD in the presence and absence of β-adrenergic blockade. The results were related to the extent of CAD and interpreted relative to the clinical value of exercise testing. Maximal heart rate and systolic BP were significantly lower during treatment with β-blocking drugs. The average exercise duration was 1.3 ± 1.9 minutes greater, regardless of coronary anatomy. Of the 20 subjects with 3-vessel or LM CAD (severe CAD), 8 patients completed 3 stages (9 minutes) of exercise during treatment; only 4 did so without treatment. Angina was significantly more often the limiting symptom with severe CAD, and this association was abolished by β-blockade; 1 of 20 with severe CAD completed 3 stages of

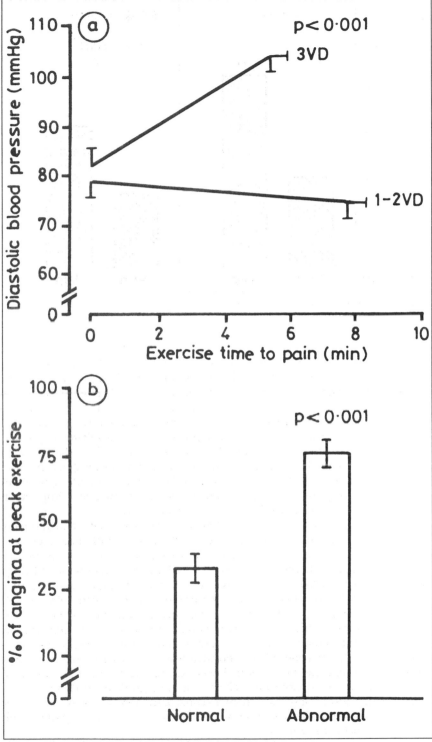

Fig. 1-1. Exercise time to pain (a) and percentage of angina (b) occurring at peak exercise in patients with normal and abnormal diastolic BP response to exercise. VD = vessel disease. Reproduced with permission from Akhras et al.[15]

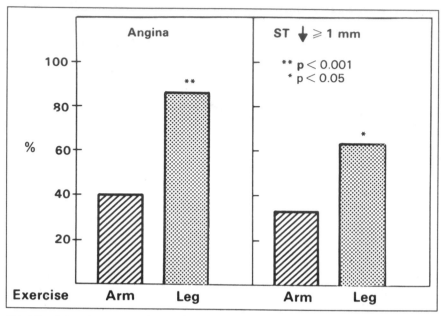

Fig. 1-2.   Ischemic responses to exercise.

exercise and was not limited by angina without β-blocking treatment, whereas 7 had these features during β-blockade therapy. Maximal ST-segment depression was not related to the extent of CAD with or without therapy. β-blockade suppressed the occurrence of ST depression, or delayed its appearance by an average of 2.0 ± 2.3 minutes and reduced its severity by 0.5 ± 0.9 mm. All tests in which ST depression was completely suppressed were associated with inadequate HR response, regarded as diagnostically inconclusive rather than negative. However, during β-blocking treatment, 14 tests (28%) were inconclusive. It was concluded that β-blockade significantly obscures the diagnostic interpretation of exercise testing and impairs the ability to select subjects likely to have extensive CAD.

Balady and associates[17] from Boston, Massachusetts, determined the sensitivity of arm exercise in detecting CAD in 30 patients with angina pectoris. They performed both arm ergometry and treadmill testing before coronary angiography. All patients had at least 70% diameter reduction in ≥1 major coronary artery. Ischemic ST depression (≥1 mm) or angina occurred more frequently (86%, 26 patients) with leg exercise than with arm exercise (40%, 12 patients) (Fig. 1-2). There was no significant difference in peak HR-BP product achieved with either test, although the peak oxygen consumption was significantly greater during leg exercise than during arm exercise (18 -vs- 13 ml/kg/min). For concordantly positive tests, the oxygen consumption at onset of ischemia was significantly lower during arm testing than during leg testing (12 -vs- 17 ml/kg/min). There was no significant difference in HR during either test at onset of ischemia. Thus, arm exercise testing is a reasonable, but not equivalent, alternative to leg exercise testing in patients who cannot perform leg exercise.

Sagiv and associates[18] from Madison, Wisconsin, studied cardiovascular and LV responses to upright handgrip and deadlift in 10 normal men and in 14 men with documented CAD who were in a supervised exercise program (Fig. 1-3). Handgrip and deadlift were each performed at 30% maximal

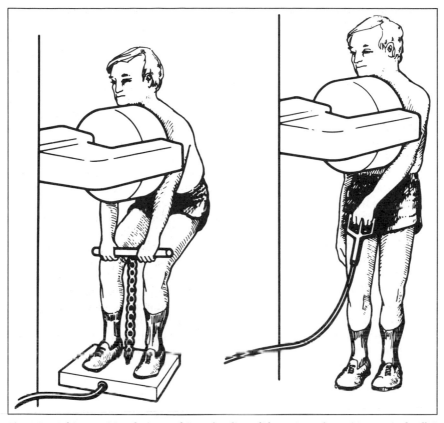

Fig. 1-3. Subject position during multigated radionuclide angiography and isometric deadlift (left) and isometric handgrip (right).

effort for 3 minutes. LV technetium-99m multigated radionuclide angiograms, ECG, and BP were measured during the final 60 seconds. CAD patients had a significantly lower LVEF at rest (41%) than normal subjects (57%). Both groups showed equal and significant increases in HR and systolic and diastolic BP during handgrip and deadlift. These responses were all significantly greater in both groups during deadlift. No significant changes in LVEF occurred in either group during handgrip of deadlift. LV wall motion abnormalities were present in 9 of 14 CAD patients at rest and increased with handgrip (11 men) and deadlift (13 men). No LV abnormalities occurred in normal subjects. These data indicate cardiovascular responses are similar in normal and exercise-trained CAD patients during upright submaximal isometric exercise using small or large muscle groups. Radionuclide measurements of global LV function remain stable in both groups during similar conditions of increased systolic BP afterload. However, LV wall motion abnormalities are aggravated in CAD patients during isometric exercise.

Value of radionuclide studies

Brown and associates[19] from Boston, Massachusetts, examined the incidence and causes of abnormal thallium-201 (^{201}Tl) myocardial perfusion studies in the absence of significant CAD. The study group consisted of 100 consecutive patients undergoing exercise ^{201}Tl testing and coronary angiography who were found to have maximal coronary artery diameter narrowing of <50%. Maximal coronary stenosis ranged from 0–40%. The independent and relative influences of patient clinical, exercise, and angiographic data were assessed by logistic regression analysis. Significant predictors of a positive stress ^{201}Tl test result were: 1) percent maximal coronary stenosis, 2) propranolol use, 3) interaction of propranolol use and percent maximal stenosis, and 4) stress-induced chest pain. No other patient variable had a significant influence. Positive ^{201}Tl test results were more common in patients with 21–40% maximal stenosis (59%) than in patients with 0–20% maximal stenosis (27%). Among patients with 21–40% stenosis, a positive test response was more common when 85% of maximal predicted heart rate was achieved (75%) than when it was not (40%). Of 16 nonapical perfusion defects seen in patients with 21–40% maximal stenosis, 14 were in the territory that corresponded with such a coronary stenosis. Patients taking propranolol were more likely to have a positive ^{201}Tl test result (45%) than patients not taking propranolol (22%). [201]Tl perfusion defects were more frequent when typical angina pectoris was elicited than when atypical chest pain developed. The high frequency of ^{201}Tl defects associated with 21–40% stenoses and the close correlation of such defects with myocardial territory supplied by these stenoses suggests that such coronary lesions may have true hemodynamic impact, especially at high levels of stress. The high incidence of positive ^{201}Tl studies in patients taking propranolol suggests that an attempt be made to wean patients off β-blocker treatment before ^{201}Tl exercise testing.

Kalff and associates[20] from Melbourne, Australia, tested the hypothesis that the results of stress ^{201}Tl myocardial perfusion scans are related to the mean transstenotic pressure gradient of coronary stenoses independent of the percent luminal narrowing by angiography. The 22 patients (20 men, 2 women, aged 30–62 years) had no previous AMI. Each had a symptom-limited, erect bicycle ^{201}Tl test off antianginal therapy, shortly before PTCA for isolated LAD coronary artery stenosis. All 4 patients with ≥90% diameter narrowing had positive ^{201}Tl responses, and the mean gradient was 72 ± 11 mmHg. Among the 18 patients with <90% diameter narrowing, the mean gradient was higher in the 11 with a positive [201]Tl (63 ± 15 mmHg) than in the 7 with a negative [201]Tl (33 ± 20 mmHg), but their percent narrowing did not differ significantly (72 ± 14 -vs- 66 ± 19%). Multiple regression analysis showed that the presence of a ^{201}Tl defect was a strong and percent narrowing a weak independent predictor for gradient. When the mean gradient was normalized for the prestenotic pressure, both percent narrowing and ^{201}Tl defects were significant independent predictors. Other variables, including age, location and length of stenosis, exercise ECG ST-segment changes, hemodynamics, workload, and chest pain, were not significant independent predictors of gradient. Therefore, ^{201}Tl adds valid information on the hemodynamic significance of a stenosis independent of percent luminal diameter narrowing; this may be of most value when percent narrowing is less than 90% and the clinical significance of a coronary stenosis is uncertain.

Kaul and associates[21] from Boston, Massachusetts, compared the relative value of exercise ECG and computer analyzed ^{201}Tl imaging in 124 patients with 1-vessel CAD. Of these, 78 had LAD, 32, right, and 14, LC CAD. In patients with no previous AMI, thallium imaging was more sensitive than the ECG (78 -vs- 64%), but in patients with previous AMI, sensitivity was similar. Further thallium imaging was more sensitive only in LAD and LC CAD. Redistribution was compared with ST-segment depression as a marker of ischemia. Only in patients with prior AMI (76 -vs- 44%) and only in LC and right CAD did redistribution occur more often than ST depression. Thallium imaging was more accurate in localizing stenoses than the ECG, but did not always correctly predict coronary anatomy. Septal thallium defects were associated with LAD disease in 84%, inferior defects with right CAD in 40%, and posterolateral lesion defects with LC CAD in 22%. The results indicate the overall superiority of thallium imaging in 1-vessel CAD compared with exercise ECG; however, there is a wide spectrum of extent and location of perfusion defects associated with each coronary artery. Thallium imaging complements coronary angiography by demonstrating the functional impact of CAD on myocardial perfusion.

To evaluate the severity of CAD in patients with peripheral vascular disease requiring operation, Boucher and associates[22] from Boston, Massachusetts, performed preoperative dipyridamole-thallium imaging in 54 stable patients with suspected CAD. Of the 54 patients, 48 had pheripheral vascular surgery as scheduled without coronary angiography, of whom 8 (17%) had postoperative cardiac ischemic events. The occurrence of these 8 cardiac events could not have been predicted preoperatively by any clinical factors but did correlate with the presence of thallium redistribution. Eight of 16 patients with thallium redistribution had cardiac events, whereas there were no such events in 32 patients whose thallium scan either was normal or showed only persistent defects. Six other patients also had thallium redistribution but underwent coronary angiography before vascular surgery. All had severe multivessel CAD, and 4 underwent CABG followed by uncomplicated peripheral vascular surgery. These data suggest that patients without thallium redistribution are at a low risk for postoperative ischemic events and may proceed to have vascular surgery. Patients with redistribution have a high incidence of postoperative ischemic events and should be considered for preoperative coronary angiography and CABG in an effort to avoid postoperative myocardial ischemia and to improve survival. Dipyridamole-thallium imaging is superior to clinical assessment and is safer and less expensive than coronary angiography for the determination of cardiac risk.

O'Hara and associates[23] from Middlesex, UK, performed coronary angiography and thallium imaging in 103 patients and the results were analyzed by Bayesian principles to assess the usefulness of semiquantitative stress thallium imaging for predicting the presence or absence of multivessel CAD. Significant CAD was found in 80 patients, of whom 77 had abnormal thallium scans (sensitivity 96%). Thallium images were normal in 15 of 23 patients with no significant disease (specificity 65%). Multiple thallium segmental defects were found to be 90% sensitive and 65% specific for multivessel CAD and were present in 80% of patients with LM CAD and in 93% of patients with 3-vessel CAD. A single thallium defect or normal scan excluded multivessel, LM, and 3-vessel CAD with 81, 94, and 91% predictive accuracy, respectively. By Bayesian analysis, the predictive accuracy for excluding multivessel CAD was >90% in patients with a pretest probability of multivessel CAD of ≤40%. Coronary arteriography to exclude multivessel CAD is therefore unnecessary in a high proportion of patients with known or suspected CAD.

Port and associates[24] from Milwaukee, Wisconsin, compared the ability of exercise ^{201}Tl perfusion imaging and RNA to detect physiologic alterations consistent with the presence of significant 1-vessel CAD in 46 patients with a significant occlusion (≥70% luminal diameter obstruction) of only 1 major coronary artery and no prior AMI. Exercise ECG was abnormal in 24 of the patients (52%). Quantitative planar ^{201}Tl images were abnormal in 42 patients (91%) and quantitative analyses of the tomographic thallium-201 images were abnormal in 41 patients (89%). An exercise EF of <0.56 or a new wall motion abnormality was seen in 30 patients (65%). The results were similar for the right (n = 11) and LAD (n = 28) coronary arteries, but all tests but the planar ^{201}Tl imaging showed a lower sensitivity for isolated LC CAD (n = 7). Specificity of the test was 72, 83, 89, and 72% for ECG, planar, thallium imaging, tomographic thallium imaging, and RNA, respectively. Thus, these data suggest that exercise ^{201}Tl perfusion imaging is a sensitive noninvasive test for the diagnosis of significant CAD.

In a study carried out by Reisman and associates[25] from Los Angeles, California, to determine the angiographic correlates of the severe stress ^{201}Tl defect, data from 44 consecutive patients with this finding undergoing both exercise thallium scintigraphy and cardiac catheterization were reviewed. A severe stress thallium defect was defined as a reduction in myocardial thallium uptake immediately after exercise so that thallium activity in that segment was close to background activity. In each patient, myocardial segments were assigned to 1 of 2 regions: anterior (including the septal and anterior walls) or posterior (including inferior, posterolateral, and posteroinferior walls). Each patient could have a maximum of 2 regions with a severe stress defect. Each severe defect region was analyzed for ventriculographic evidence (akinesis/dyskinesis) of infarction and presence of critical (≥90%) coronary stenosis of the corresponding artery. Fifty defect regions were identified: 18 were reversible and 32 were nonreversible. A critical coronary stenosis was associated with 16 (89%) of 18 reversible defects and with 28 (88%) of 32 nonreversible defects. Although 21 (66%) of 32 nonreversible defects had ventriculographic evidence of infarction, only 2 (11%) of 18 reversible defects had evidence. These data indicate that: 1) severe stress thallium defects are virtually indicative of critical (≥90%) coronary stenosis; 2) when nonreversible, such defects are usually associated with ventriculographic evidence of prior infarction; and 3) importantly, severe stress thallium defects are frequently reversible and not associated with infarction, but still indicate critical coronary stenosis.

Corbett and coworkers[26] from Dallas, Texas, compared planar and tomographic RNA to evaluate global and segmental ventricular function. Gated blood pool tomograms were acquired over 180° at 15 frames/cardiac cycle during the initial 90% of the cardiac cycle. Tomographic ventriculography showed an increased sensitivity for detecting LV segments supplied by significantly narrowed coronary arteries (97 -vs- 74%) without any loss in specificity. Compared with both planar RNA and contrast ventriculography, tomographic RNA detected more noninfarcted LV segments supplied by stenosed coronary arteries (81 -vs- 39 and 32%, respectively). Tomographic RNA measurements of LV volumes and EF showed close correlations with angiographic and planar radionuclide determinations. These data suggest that gated blood pool tomography is a sensitive method for evaluating segmental wall motion and an accurate method for the measurement of global LV volumes and EF.

Schwarzberg and colleagues[27] from New York City studied 10 normal subjects, 16 patients undergoing cardiac catheterization for unstable angina or nontransmural AMI, and normal LVEF and wall motion, and 10 patients with healed AMI and regional dyssynergy to determine whether peak regional acceleration images obtained from gated blood pool scans might be used to identify regional ventricular dysfunction noninvasively. The second derivative of the time-activity curve of each pixel generated and the maximal systolic value of the derivative for each pixel was displayed as a functional image (peak regional acceleration). Anterior and left anterior oblique views were evaluated for abnormalities and the presence and location of defects correlated with coronary anatomy. Scans from the 10 normal subjects were used to establish the normal range for regional second derivative values. In all 10 patients with healed transmural AMI, both gated blood pool scans and second derivative images showed regional abnormalities. Regional abnormalities were present in the second derivative images in the distribution of 17 of the 20 coronary arteries with >50% diameter stenosis; there were no regional abnormalities in the distribution of 7 of the 8 arteries with <50% stenoses. Moreover, regional second derivative image abnormalities were present in 15 of 16 patients with unstable angina and normal wall motion and global LVEF. These patients demonstrated regional abnormalities on second derivative images in the distribution of 19 of the 23 coronary arteries with significant stenoses and no regional abnormalities in the distribution of 21 of 23 coronary arteries without significant stenoses. These data provide optimism for the possibility that time derivative functional images derived from gated blood pool scintigraphy at rest may improve sensitivity for detecting regional ventricular dysfunction noninvasively.

Angiographic status of the coronary arteries in symptomatic CAD ≤30 years of age

Underwood and associates[28] from Cleveland, Ohio, identified 100 persons (88 men) aged ≤30 years with angiographically proved obstructive CAD. The men were compared by age and date of catheterization with a matched control group with angiographically normal coronary arteries. Significant risk factors were cigarette smoking and familial CAD manifested by age <50 years. Serum cholesterol values were significantly higher in the CAD group, but in most (54%) were still <250 mg/dl. Arteriography showed a spectrum of CAD: 1-vessel in 57, 2-vessel in 21, and 3-vessel in 22. One patient had significant LM CAD. Follow-up was obtained for all of the 94 subjects. One-year mortality was 3% and 5-year mortality was 20% (Fig. 1-4). The causes of death were predominantly cardiac: AMI in 10 patients, CHF in 2, and cardiac arrest in 6; 3 patients died of noncardiac causes.

Meaning of coronary collaterals

Elayda and associates[29] from Houston, Texas, reviewed the coronary arteriograms and left ventriculograms of 202 consecutive patients with ≥1 narrowing >75% in diameter in ≥1 major coronary artery. In 127 patients (63%), at least 1 major branch was totally occluded. Collateral circulation was seen in 125 of these 127 patients (190 of 192 totally occluded arteries). Of the 75 patients without total occlusion, only 2 with 99% (or near total) occlusion had demonstrable collateral circulation (2 of 208 arteries). In no patient with 75–98% diameter narrowing was collateral circulation demonstrated (0–164 arteries). An analysis was made of the relation between LV segmental wall motion and the quality of collateral circulation in 190 totally occluded arteries among 125 patients. Of 126 arteries with good collateral circulation, LV contraction was normal in 21%, hypokinetic in 48%, and akinetic/dyskinetic in 29%. Of 64 arteries with poor collateral circulation, LV contraction was normal in 23%, hypokinetic in 55%, and akinetic/dyskinetic in 20%. There was no statistically significant difference between the effect of good or poor collateral circulation on LV function. These data indicate that

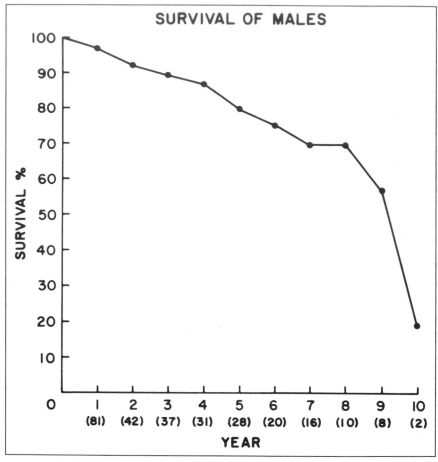

Fig. 1-4. Actuarial survival curve of the young American patients. Patients were treated as dropouts in the middle of the year if surgery was performed. The numbers in parentheses indicate the number of patients at risk at the beginning of the year. The 7 foreign patients were not followed. Actuarial survival was 57% at 10 years.

collateral circulation cannot be seen angiographically unless there is total or near total occlusion, and that the presence of collateral circulation does not correlate with LV wall motion abnormalities, that is, akinetic area, despite good collateral flow or normal wall motion despite absent or poor collateral flow.

Usefulness of transstenotic coronary pressure gradient

To evaluate during cardiac catheterization what constitutes a physiologically significant obstruction to blood flow in the human coronary artery, Wijns and coworkers[30] from Rotterdam, The Netherlands, performed computer-based quantitative analysis of coronary angiograms on 31 patients with isolated disease of the proximal LAD coronary artery. A curvilinear relation was found between the pressure gradient across the stenosis (normalized for the mean aortic pressure) and the residual minimal area of obstruction (after subtraction the area of the angioplasty catheter). The relation was best fitted by the equation: normalized mean pressure gradient =

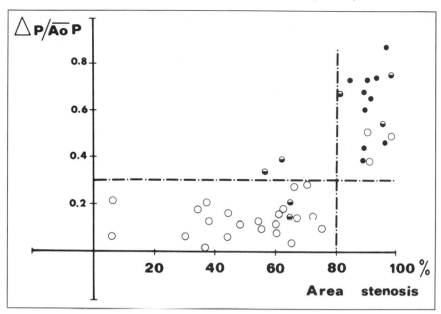

Fig. 1-5. The relation among mean normalized pressure gradients, percent area stenosis, and the results of thallium scintigraphy are shown. Open circles = patients with normal scintigrams (group I, n = 25); half filled circles = patients with abnormal thallium but normal exercise tests (group II, n = 7); filled circles = patients with abnormal thallium and exercise tests (group III, n = 10). Reproduced with permission from Wijns et al.[30]

a + b · log (obstruction area), r = 0.74. Thus, measurement of the percent area of stenosis (cutoff 80%) and of the transstenotic pressure gradient (cutoff 0.30) obtained at rest correctly predicted the occurrence of thallium perfusion defects induced by exercise in 83% of the patients (Fig. 1-5).

A difficult problem in coronary arteriography is the assessment of the hemodynamic significance of stenoses that appear angiographically to be of only moderate severity (25–75% diameter narrowing). This is particularly important in patients who may be candidates for invasive therapy, such as PTCA or CABG. To determine the significance of such narrowings, Ganz and associates[31] from Boston, Massachusetts, measured transstenotic coronary pressure gradients in 15 patients with angiographically moderate stenoses. For comparison, similar measurements were made in 17 patients with severe stenoses (>75% diameter narrowing) being considered for PTCA (Table 1-1). The transstenotic pressure gradients were measured with a 2.0 F polyvinyl chloride catheter cleared of microbubbles of air by flushing with carbon dioxide and degassed saline solution and attached to a low volume displacement transducer for optimal frequency response. Mean transstenotic pressure gradients >10 mmHg at rest or >20 mmHg under conditions of high coronary blood flow, as induced by Renografin 76, appeared to be associated with objective evidence of myocardial ischemia and symptomatic relief from PTCA (Fig. 1-6). Smaller pressure gradients occurred in patients whose symptoms probably were not ischemic in nature. Transstenotic pressure gradient determination performed at the time of diagnostic catheterization may provide assistance in clinical decision making in selected patients with angiographically moderate stenoses.

TABLE 1-1. *Clinical profile, angiographic and transstenotic coronary pressure gradients in patients with angiographically moderate stenoses*

PATIENT	CORONARY ARTERY	% DIAMETER STENOSIS	ΔP(mmHg) BASAL	ΔP(mmHg) RENOGRAFIN	CHEST PAIN
1	LAD	55	20	27	+ +
2	LAD	60	30	—	+ +
3	LAD	60	11	23	+ +
4	LAD	65	13	34	+ +
5	LAD	70	26	37	+ +
6	LAD	70	18	36	+ +
7	LAD	75	16	34	+ +
8	Right	30	6	17	0
9	LM	30	0	0	+
10	Right	45	0	10	+ +
11	LAD	50	5	21	0
12	Right	60	6	12	+
13	LAD	60	5	12	+
14	LAD	65	6	10	+
15	LAD	70	0	0	+

+ +=typical angina pectoris; +=atypical anginal pain; 0 = absent.

Coronary ectasia and/or aneurysm

The prevalence of coronary aneurysmal dilation without coronary stenosis is rare, and the clinical course of such an entity is unknown. Rath and colleagues[32] from Tel Hashomer, Israel, reported on 5 adults, 4 men and 1 woman, with such an anatomic finding. The age range was 44–60 years. In 4 patients, the aneurysmal dilations involved multiple coronary sites. The clinical course in all 5 patients was suggestive of myocardial ischemia. Despite no obstructive disease, 2 patients developed transient ischemic ECG changes accompanied by chest pain, and 2 others had ischemic exercise RNA. In time (3–15 months), all 5 patients developed AMI and recatheterization revealed complete occlusion of a previously nonstenosed aneurysmal artery. Thus, prevention of thrombus formation is recommended for this condition.

Hartnell and associates[33] from Harefield, UK, assessed the clinical significance of coronary artery ectasia in 4,993 consecutive patients having coronary angiography. Of the 4,993 patients, 1,598 had normal coronary angiograms and 96 had minor narrowings (<50% diameter reduction) and 3,299 had significant narrowings (>50% diameter reduction) of at least 1 major coronary artery. Coronary artery ectasia occurred in 70 patients, 12 of whom had minor narrowings and 4, no narrowings. Coronary ectasia was not related to the development of aortic aneurysm and did not effect outcome, results of CABG, or symptoms.

PROGNOSIS

Based on initial manifestation of myocardial ischemia

Elveback and Connolly[34] from Rochester, Minnesota, reviewed cases in whom a diagnosis of classic angina pectoris or AMI was the initial manifesta-

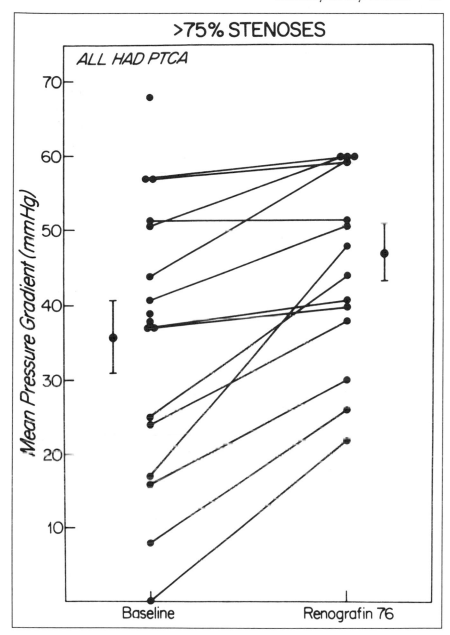

Fig. 1-6. Mean transstenotic coronary pressure gradients in 17 patients with angiographically severe stenosis. The gradients are shown basally (n = 17) and after injection of Renografin 76 (n = 14). Values are mean ± SEM.

tion of CAD during 1960 through 1979 in 2,027 residents of Rochester. Angina was the first manifestation of CAD in 1,014 residents and AMI was the initial manifestation in 1,013 residents (Figs. 1-7 and 1-8). In the angina cohort, about 50% were men and of them 20% were ≥70 years of age. The women on average were 6 years older than the men, and 43% were ≥70 years. In this cohort, the 5-year survival rate increased from 77% in the 1960s to 87% in the 1970s. The 5-year net survivorship free of an AMI increased from 76 to 85% during that same time. In the AMI cohort, the 5-year death

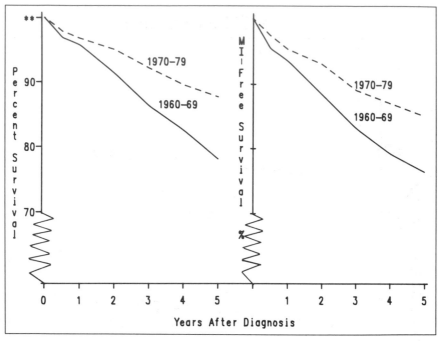

Fig. 1-7. Left: survivorship of patients with angina diagnosed in the 1960s (n = 431) and angina diagnosed in the 1970s (n = 583). Right: Net survivorship free of AMI in the cohort of patients who had angina as the initial manifestation of CAD. In this analysis, the history of a patient who died without having had an AMI was censored at the time of death. Reproduced with permission from Elveback and Connolly.[34]

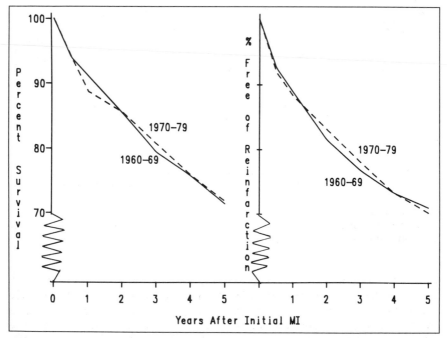

Fig. 1-8. Left: long-term survival of 30-day survivors of an AMI as the initial manifestation of CAD during the periods 1960–1969 (n = 431) and 1970–1979 (n = 582). Right: Net survivorship free of reinfarction for this cohort during the 2 decades of the study. Reproduced with permission from Elveback and Connolly.[34]

rate among the 30-day survivors of AMI was the same during both decades of the study. The age-adjusted reinfarction rate per 100 person-years at risk during the first 5 years of follow-up decreased slightly among men and increased among women; thus, it remained essentially unchanged overall. Although the case fatality rate in the AMI cohort declined sharply from the 1960s to the 1970s, the long-term prognosis of the 30-day survivors of an AMI did not improve.

Based on leukocyte count

Grimm and associates[35] of the Multiple Risk Factor Intervention Trial Research Group assessed the relation of white blood cell (WBC) count to fatal and nonfatal CAD incidence and all-cause and cancer mortality in a subset of participants in the Multiple Risk Factor Intervention Trial (MRFIT). For this group of 6,222 middle aged men, total WBC count was found to be strongly and significantly related to risk of CAD, independent of smoking status. Change in WBC count from baseline to the annual examination just before the CAD event was found to be a significant and independent predictor of CAD risk. For each decrease in WBC count of $1,000/mm^3$ the risk for CAD death decreased 14%, controlling for baseline WBC count and other CAD risk factors (smoking, cholesterol level, diastolic BP). The WBC count was strongly related cross-sectionally to cigarette smoking and smoking status as indicated by serum thiocyanate concentration. Smokers on average had a WBC count of $7,750/mm^3$ compared with $6,080/mm^3$ for nonsmokers. The WBC count was also significantly associated with cancer death, independent of reported smoking and serum thiocyanate levels.

Based on exercise thallium-201 scintigraphy

The usefulness of exercise thallium-201 (^{201}Tl) imaging to evaluate patients with suspected CAD is well established. However, a far-reaching use of the method is in risk stratification. Iskandrian and colleagues[36] from Philadelphia, Pennsylvania, examined the prognostic value of exercise ^{201}Tl imaging in 743 patients with suspected or known CAD. Exercise images in each of 3 projections were divided into 3 segments and each segment was assessed qualitatively and quantitatively as to the presence and nature of perfusion defects (fixed or reversible). There were 20 cardiac events at a mean follow-up of 13 months (range, 1–66); 8 patients had cardiac deaths (sudden or nonsudden) and 12 patients had nonfatal AMI. Univariate survival analysis revealed that the number of perfusion defects (Fig. 1-9), the presence of abnormal images, a history of previous AMI, and the presence of Q-wave AMI were important predictors of subsequent cardiac events. Multivariate survival analysis showed that once the number of perfusion defects was selected no other variable provided additional significant independent information about the risk of major cardiac events. Actuarial life-table analysis showed that patients with ≥3 perfusion defects had significantly worse prognosis than patients with no defects or <3 perfusion defects. Thus, exercise thallium imaging is useful in risk stratification; the extent of exercise-related perfusion defects identifies a group of patients at high risk for future events.

Pamelia and associates[37] from Charlottesville, Virginia, determined the prognostic value of a normal exercise ^{201}Tl scintigram by quantitative criteria in 349 patients with chest pain. Follow-up was obtained in 345 patients (99%) from 8–45 months (mean, 34 ± 7). Of these, 60% were men, 26% had typical angina, 21% had chest pain during exercise testing, 29% were unable to achieve 85% or more of maximal predicted heart rate, and in 9% ischemic

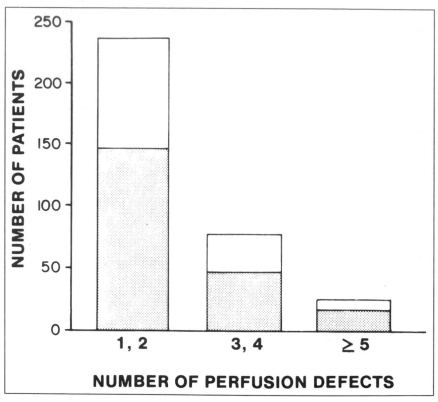

Fig. 1-9. Distribution of fixed and reversible perfusion defects in the patients with abnormal images. Stipled area represents patients with reversible defects and entire bar represents patients with either fixed or reversible defects. Patients with reversible defects may have other segments with normal perfusion or showing fixed defects. Reproduced with permission from Iskandrian et al.[36]

ST depression ($\geq$1.0 mm) developed during exercise. At the time of exercise testing, 45% of patients were taking nitrates and 38% were receiving a β-blocking drug. During the follow-up period, there were 5 cardiac deaths (0.51%/year), of which 2 were sudden, 6 patients had a nonfatal AMI (0.61%/year). Two of the 5 patients who died and 1 who had AMI had angiographically normal coronary arteries. The event rate was significantly higher in patients referred for early catheterization (5 of 53; 9%) compared with the rate for those not undergoing early angiography (6 of 298; 2%). However, the event rate was similar in those who underwent catheterization with angiographically normal coronary arteries and in those who had significant CAD. Patients with chest pain and normal ^{201}Tl scintigrams who had a cardiac event were not predominantly of the male sex, nor did they have a higher prevalence of typical angina, exercise-induced ST-segment depression, or an inability to achieve $\geq$85% of maximal predicted heart rate normalized for age, compared with those who had no cardiac events. Four other patients (1.1%) subsequently underwent CABG. At follow-up, 34% of patients were taking nitrates, 29% were receiving a β-blocking drug and 54% had persistence of chest pain. In conclusion, patients with chest pain and normal ^{201}Tl exercise scintigrams have a low cardiac death and nonfatal AMI rate (1.1%/year), which is comparable to that reported for patients with chest pain and angiographically normal coronary arteries.

Wackers and associates[38] from Burlington, Vermont, and New Haven, Connecticut, evaluated the prognostic significance of normal quantitative planar ^{201}Tl stress scintigraphy in patients with chest pain syndromes. The prevalence of cardiac events during follow-up was related to the pretest likelihood of CAD determined on the basis of symptoms, age, sex, and stress ECG. Of 344 patients with adequate ^{201}Tl stress scintigrams evaluated, 95 had normal studies by quantitative analysis. During a mean follow-up period of 22 ± 3 months, no patient died. Three patients (3%) had a cardiac event; 2 of these had a nonfatal AMI 8 and 22 months after stress scintigraphy, and 1 patient had PTCA 6 months after stress scintigraphy because of persisting angina. Three patients were lost to follow-up. Thus, these data indicate that patients with chest pain and normal findings on quantitative ^{201}Tl scintigraphy have an excellent prognosis. The risk of major cardiac events is approximately 1%/year in these individuals.

Based on jeopardy score

Califf and colleagues[39] from Durham, North Carolina, and Boston, Massachusetts, determined the prognostic value of a coronary artery jeopardy score in 462 consecutive nonsurgically treated patients with significant CAD, but without significant LM coronary stenosis. The jeopardy score developed estimated the amount of myocardium at risk on the basis of the specific location of coronary arterial narrowings. Patients with a previous AMI had higher jeopardy scores based on a lower LVEF. The 5-year survival was 97% in patients with a jeopardy score of 2, and 95, 85, 78, 75, and 56, for patients with jeopardy scores of 4, 6, 8, 10, and 12, respectively (Figs. 1-10 and 1-11, Table 1-2). Multivariate analysis utilized the jeopardy score and number of narrowed arteries and indicated that the jeopardy score contained the most

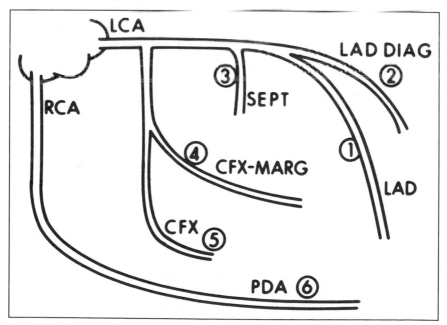

Fig. 1-10. Diagram of coronary artery tree demonstrating the 6 segments counted in the jeopardy score. CFX = LC; CFX-MARG = major marginal branch of the LC; LAD DIAG = major diagonal branch of the LAD; LCA = LM; PDA = posterior descending coronary artery; RCA = right coronary artery; SEPT = major septal perforating artery. Reproduced with permission from Califf et al.[39]

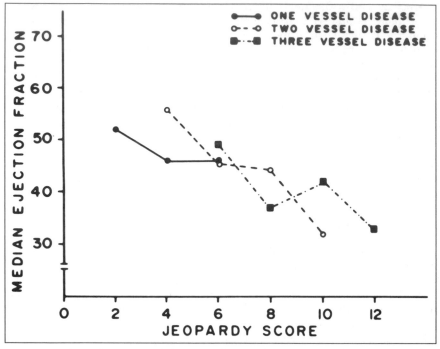

Fig. 1-11. Relation between jeopardy score and LVEF when patients with a previous AMI are grouped by number of diseased vessels. Reproduced with permission from Califf et al.[39]

important prognostic information. The number of narrowed arteries added no prognostic information to the jeopardy score. However, the LVEF was more closely related to prognosis than the jeopardy score (Fig. 1-12). In addition, the degree of stenosis in each coronary artery, especially the LAD coronary artery, added prognostic information to the jeopardy score. Thus, these data indicate that a jeopardy score may be used to describe coronary anatomy and provide useful prognostic information in patients with CAD. In addition, other variables, including LV function and the degree of LAD coronary artery stenosis, add important prognostic information in such patients.

Based on ventricular late potentials

By means of high-gain ECG and signal-averaging techniques, Zimmerman and associates[40] from Geneva, Switzerland, determined the prevalence

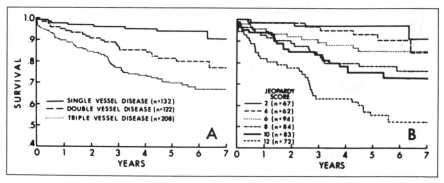

Fig. 1-12. Survival stratified by number of diseased vessels (A) and by jeopardy score (B). Reproduced with permission from Califf et al.[39]

TABLE 1-2. *Relative prognostic importance of invasive and noninvasive patient characteristics.* *Reproduced with permission from Califf et al.[39]*

	CHI-SQUARE	P
Left ventricular ejection fraction	18.9	<0.0001
Peripheral vascular disease	8.9	0.003
Characterization of angina (progressive versus stable; frequency; nocturnal; preinfarction)	5.4	0.02
Noninvasive indicators of myocardial damage (S_3 gallop, cardiomegaly, previous AMI by history or ECG, ST-T wave abnormality on ECG)	5.0	0.03
Luminal diameter narrowing of left anterior descending artery	4.2	0.04
Age	<3.84	>0.05
Sex	<3.84	>0.05
Mitral insufficiency	<3.84	>0.05
Left ventricular end-diastolic pressure	<3.84	>0.05

*The jeopardy score adds a chi-square value of 5.4 when considered jointly with the other characteristics listed above. Number of diseased vessels adds no additional prognostic information to the variables in this table.

and prognostic significance of ventricular late potentials (VLPs) in CAD. No VLPs were detected in normal subjects (n = 25) or in patients with various noncoronary cardiopathies with sustained VT or VF (n = 10). Among 92 CAD patients, VLPs were apparent in 35% (32 of 92) at the beginning of the study. The prevalence of VLPs increased to 48% (19 of 40) in the presence of LV aneurysm and to 82% (14 of 17) in the presence of a history of previous sustained VT/VF. To determine the prognostic significance of VLPs, a prospective analysis was conducted during a mean of 7.4 months (range, 1–22). During the follow-up period, 11 patients (12%) presented with an episode of sustained VT/VF, and 6 of them died from documented VT/VF. Three other patients died from cardiogenic shock. An episode of sustained VT/VF occurred in 31% (10 of 32) of the patients with VLPs -vs- 2% (1 of 58) of the patients without VLPs (p <0.001), and 6 patients with VLPs died from sustained VT/VF -vs- none in the group of patients without VLPs (p <0.01). This VLP-related increase in arrhythmic risk was still present in the particular subgroup of patients with a history of previous sustained VT/VF (n = 17) and in patients with LV aneurysm (n = 40). The risk of developing sustained VT/VF also was influenced by the length of the VLP and by a low mean EF. For predicting sudden arrhythmic death, VLP detection had a high sensitivity (6 of 6 patients), a specificity of 69%, and a predictive value of 19%; for predicting sustained VT/VF, VLP detection had a sensitivity of 90%, a specificity of 72%, and a predictive value of 31%. It was concluded that VLPs are frequent in CAD, that they are mainly associated with the presence of LV aneurysm, and that their presence increases the risk of sustained VT/VF and sudden arrhythmic death in CAD.

PROGRESSION OF CORONARY NARROWING

Moise and associates[41] from Montreal, Canada, performed a study to identify the subset of patients with normal or minimal (≤49% narrowing) stenoses of the coronary arteries. Data were collected from 51 patients with normal coronary arteries (20 patients), all with minimal narrowing (31 patients) on a first angiogram. All patients underwent repeat coronary angiography 4–120 months (mean, 52) later because of persistent chest pain. Three classic lifestyle-related risk factors (systemic hypertension, cigarette smoking status, and hypercholesterolemia) were noted; the number of diseased segments on the first angiogram was counted according to a 15-segment coding system. Progression of CAD required the consensus of 3 observers on a ≥30% decrease in luminal diameter. Progression was recorded in 16 of 31 patients with minimal CAD and in 3 of 20 patients with normal coronary arteries. By multivariate logistic regression, progression was predicted by number of diseased segments, age, smoking status, and initial cholesterol level. Using the probability computed by the logistic model, we could separate the 51 patients in groups with low (0–18), medium (9 of 23) and high (10 of 10) risk of progression. Thus, patients with normal or minimally narrowed coronary arteries at angiography form a heterogenous population, including both normal or borderline subjects and patients with CAD in its early stage. The latter condition was associated with presence of risk factors and to the angiographic extent of the disease.

RISK FACTORS—GENERAL

Klatsky and associates[42] from Oakland, California, studied data about coffee habits and total serum cholesterol in 42,627 white men and women who underwent health examinations between 1978 and 1981. There was a clear association of drinking more coffee to higher levels of total serum cholesterol in both men and women (Table 1-3). Significant increments of total serum cholesterol were found among persons whose average intake was <1 cup of coffee per day compared with nondrinkers of coffee. More than a third of the coffee-associated increment in cholesterol in men and about half of the

TABLE 1-3. *Adjusted mean levels of serum total cholesterol* in 22,187 white men and 25,424 white women according to coffee and tea consumption.*

	TOTAL CHOLESTEROL (MG/DL) (% OF PERSONS IN CATEGORY)			
	COFFEE		TEA	
CUPS/DAY	MEN	WOMEN	MEN	WOMEN
None	216.3	219.6	220.9	222.3
(reference)	(17.4)	(19.0)	(57.0)	(45.7)
< 1	219.5†	222.6†	218.8†	222.1
	(10.3)	(10.0)	(26.8)	(31.0)
1–3	222.3‡	224.0‡	219.6	222.4
	(48.9)	(51.6)	(14.2)	(19.8)
4–6	224.4‡	224.8‡	225.2	223.1
	(17.8)	(15.0)	(1.6)	(2.7)
> 6	225.9‡	225.4‡	223.8	226.4
	(5.6)	(4.4)	(0.4)	(0.8)

*Controlled for age and Quetelet's adiposity index as continuous variables and, categorically, for cigarette smoking (never smoked, exsmoker, smoked <1 pack/day, ≥1 pack/day), alcohol use (9 categories), marital status (4 categories), educational attainment (5 categories), and birthplace (United States or foreign).
†p <0.01 -vs- levels in noncoffee drinkers; ‡p <0.001 -vs- levels in noncoffee drinkers.

coffee-associated increment in women occurred among those users of small amounts of coffee. In contrast, no consistent relation of tea used to total serum cholesterol was present.

Miettinen and associates[43] from Helsinki and Espoo, Finland, in a 5-year multifactorial primary prevention trial of vascular diseases, hyperlipidemias, systemic hypertension, cigarette smoking, obesity, and abnormal glucose tolerance of the high-risk test group (n = 612 men) were treated with dietetic-hygienic measures and hypolipidemic (mainly probucol and clofibrate) and antihypertensive (mainly diuretic and β-blockers) agents. A matched high-risk control group (n = 610) and a low-risk control group (n = 593) were not treated. The program markedly improved the risk factor status, yet the 5-year coronary incidence tended to be higher in the intervention group than in the control group (3.1 -vs- 1.5%), whereas the stroke incidence was significantly reduced (1.3 -vs- 0%). The coronary events tended to be accumulated in subgroups treated with β-blocking agents or clofibrate, but there were few in those receiving probucol or diuretics. Thus, the intervention program significantly reduced development of stroke, but the occurrence of cardiac events was not prevented. Possible adverse drug effects offsetting the probable benefit of improved risk profile are not excluded.

BLOOD LIPIDS

Consensus development conference on the value of lowering blood cholesterol

A consensus development conference on lowering blood cholesterol to prevent heart disease was held December 10–12, 1984, and the consensus panel considered the evidence and agreed on answers to the following questions[44]: 1) Is the relation between blood cholesterol levels and CAD causal? 2) Will reduction of blood cholesterol levels help prevent CAD? 3) Under what circumstances and at what level of blood cholesterol should dietary or drug treatment be started? 4) Should an attempt be made to reduce the blood cholesterol levels of the general population? 5) What research direction should be pursued regarding the relation between blood cholesterol and CAD? The panel's conclusions were the following: Elevation of blood cholesterol levels is a major cause of CAD. It has been established beyond a reasonable doubt that lowering definitely elevated blood cholesterol levels (specifically, blood levels of LDL cholesterol) will reduce the risk of heart attacks caused by CAD. This has been demonstrated most conclusively in men with elevated blood cholesterol levels, but much evidence justifies the conclusion that similar protection will be afforded to women with elevated levels. After careful review of genetic, experimental, epidemiologic, and clinical trial evidence, the conference recommended treatment of individuals with blood cholesterol levels above the 75th percentile (upper 25% of values). Furthermore, the conference was persuaded that the blood cholesterol levels of most Americans are undesirably high, in large part because of high dietary intake of calories, saturated fat, and cholesterol. In countries with diets lower in these constituents, blood cholesterol levels are lower and CAD is less common. There is no doubt that appropriate changes in the diet will reduce blood cholesterol levels. Epidemiologic data and more than a dozen clinical trials allow with reasonable assurance the prediction that such a measure

TABLE 1-4. *Values for selecting adults at moderate and high risk requiring treatment. Reproduced with permission from Consensus Conference.*[44]

AGE (YR)	MODERATE RISK (MG/DL; mM)	HIGH RISK (MG/DL; mM)
20–29	>200 (5.17)	>220 (5.69)
30–39	<220 (5.69)	>240 (6.21)
≥40	>240 (6.21)	>260 (6.72)

will afford significant protection against CAD. For these reasons, the panel recommended the following:

1. Individuals with high-risk blood cholesterol levels (values above the 90th percentile) should be treated intensively by dietary means under the guidance of a physician, dietitian, or other health professional; if response to diet was inadequate, appropriate drugs should be added to the treatment regimen (Table 1-4). Guidelines for children were somewhat different, as discussed later.

2. Adults with moderate-risk blood cholesterol levels (values between the 75th and 90th percentiles) should be treated intensively by dietary means, especially if additional risk factors were present (Table 1-4). Only a small proportion should require drug treatment.

3. All Americans (except children <2 years of age) should be advised to adopt a diet that reduces total dietary fat intake from the current level of about 40% of total calories to 30% of total calories, reduces saturated fat intake to <10% of total calories, increases polyunsaturated fat intake but to no more than 10% of total calories, and reduces daily cholesterol intake to 250–300 mg or less.

4. Intake of total calories should be reduced, if necessary, to correct obesity and adjusted to maintain ideal body weight. A program of regular moderate level exercise will be helpful in this connection.

5. In persons with elevated blood cholesterol levels, special attention should be given to the management of other risk factors (systemic hypertension, cigarette smoking, diabetes mellitus, and physical inactivity).

6. New and expanded programs should be planned and initiated soon to educate physicians, other health professionals, and the public to the significance of elevated blood cholesterol levels and the importance of treating them.

7. The food industry should be encouraged to continue and intensify efforts to develop and market foods that will make it easier for persons to adhere to the recommended diets, and school food services and restaurants should serve meals consistent with these dietary recommendations.

8. Food labeling should include the specific sources of fat, total fat, saturated and polyunsaturated fat, and cholesterol content and other nutritional information. The public should be educated on how to use this information to achieve dietary aims.

9. All physicians should be encouraged to include, whenever possible, a blood cholesterol measurement on every adult patient when that patient is first seen. To ensure reliability of data, the panel recommended steps to improve and standardize methods for cholesterol measurement in clinical laboratories.

10. Further research should be encouraged to compare the effectiveness and safety of currently recommended diets with those of alternative diets; to

study human behavior as it related to food choices and adherence to diets; to develop more effective, better-tolerated, safer, and more economical drugs for lowering blood cholesterol levels; to assess the effectiveness of medical and surgical treatment of high blood cholesterol levels in patients with established clinical CAD; to develop more precise and sensitive noninvasive artery imaging methods; and to apply basic cell and molecular biology to increase the understanding of lipoprotein metabolism (particularly the role of HDL as a protective factor) and artery wall metabolism as they relate to CAD.

11. Plans should be developed that will permit assessment of the impact of the changes recommended as implementation proceeds and provide the basis for changes when and where appropriate.

This article was followed by a "Commentary on the Published Results of the Lipid Research Clinic's Coronary Primary Prevention Trial" by Kronmal[45] and also by an editorial by Rahimtoola.[46] Kronmal's summary of the outcome of the Lipid Research Clinic's Coronary Primary Prevention Trial and its justifiable conclusions is as follows: "The life table-determined event rate for the primary end point at seven years of follow-up was 7% in the cholestyramine group and 8.6% in the placebo group, a difference of 1.6 percentage points. This difference does not reach statistical significance at the .01 one-sided test level ($z = 1.92$). However, this difference is significant at the .05 level with a one-sided test. Mortality from all causes was 3.7% in the placebo group and 3.6% in the cholestyramine group (71 v 68 deaths). This difference is not statistically significant.

"Analysis of the data on the basis of actual declines in levels of total cholesterol and LDL-C levels separately for the cholestyramine-treated group and for the placebo group indicates a highly statistically significant benefit associated with reductions in both total cholesterol and LDL-C levels in the cholestyramine group, but no significant beneficial effects of reductions in the placebo (diet alone) group.

"It is reasonable to conclude from these results that a combination of diet and cholestyramine results in a small but real reduction in the rate of CHD end points as compared with the use of placebo plus diet in the control group. This result is reinforced by the observational data analysis focusing on the cholestyramine group alone and relating the degree of total levels of cholesterol and LDL-C lowering to the resultant primary end-point reductions. It is disappointing, however, that there was no difference in overall mortality between the 2 groups."

This study was also followed by an interesting letter to the editor by Adams from Dunedin, New Zealand.[47]

Lipid research clinic prevalence study

Green and colleagues[48] from Bethesda, Maryland, analyzed the distribution of the ratios of plasma HDL cholesterol (HDL-C) to total cholesterol (TC) and of HDL-C to LDL cholesterol in 6,900 white and 495 black examinees >4 years old. Measurements were obtained during the visit 2 survey of the Lipid Research Clinics Program Prevalence Study, and corresponded to a 15% random sample of 60,502 participants screened during the visit 1 survey. Apparent in these cross-sectional data was a consistent age-related decline in the ratio of HDL-C/TC for white male participants, from a mean of 0.36 in the age group 5–9 years to a mean of 0.21 in the age group 50–54 years. Thereafter, the mean ratio increased slightly. In white women not using gonadal hormones, the age-related decline in the ratio was evident only starting at the age group 35–39 years, from which it declined from 0.33–0.26 in the age group 55–59 years. White women using gonadal hormones showed minor age-related changes in the HDL-C/TC ratio, varying around a mean of 0.30. The number of blacks examined was low and thus the racial comparisons must be interpreted with caution. For each gender, age-related trends were similar in black and white study participants. Black men had a higher percentage of TC carried as HDL-C than white men in all age groups examined. Black women had a higher percentage of TC in HDL-C than white women only at <20 years of age; in the adult range no appreciable differences were seen. The ratio HDL-C/TC correlated highly with ratio HDL-C/LDL-C (>0.92 for all groups) and the former may be a more conveniently surrogate for the latter. Thus, the ratio HDL-C/TC has the advantage of summarizing complex associations into a single numerical approximation.

New cholesterol education program

Lenfant, the Director of the National Heart, Lung and Blood Institute (NHLBI), called attention to the launching of a new NHLBI-sponsored program called the National Cholesterol Education Program.[49] This program follows the highly successful NHLBI-sponsored national high BP education program that was initiated after the Veterans Administration clinical trial showed the benefit of treating patients with moderate and severe systemic hypertension. The cholesterol program followed another clinical trial, the Lipid Research Clinics Coronary Primary Prevention Trial (LRC CPPT) which provided the most impressive evidence to date that lowering elevated blood cholesterol levels lowers the incidence of heart disease. Results of a survey conducted in 1983—before the release of the findings of the LRC CPPT— showed that physicians regarded elevated blood cholesterol as less of a disease threat than either cigarette smoking or systemic hypertension (Table 1-5). The survey also showed that the cardiologist was more aggressive than the internist or family or general practitioner in initiating both dietary and drug therapy for hypercholesterolemia. On the average, the cardiologist initiated drug therapy at blood total cholesterol levels of 260–399 mg/dl, whereas a quarter of all physicians surveyed initiated drug therapy only at levels >400 mg/dl. When the lay public was asked in this 1983 survey whether or not they had ever had their BP checked, only 2% surveyed said "no." In contrast, when asked the same question about blood cholesterol, 65% said "no." Thus, a major initial thrust of the cholesterol effort must be to urge the public to have their blood cholesterol levels checked and to understand the implications of their cholesterol reading.

A new publication, *Cholesterol Counts*, can be obtained by writing to: PIRB, NHLBI, Bethesda, MD 20892. Among its initial activities, the National

TABLE 1-5. *Preventive actions affecting CAD.* Reproduced with permission from Lenfant.[49]*

RISK FACTOR REDUCTION	PHYSICIANS (%)	PUBLIC (%)
Smoking	88	85
Blood pressure	75	82
High blood cholesterol	39	64
High fat food		66
High cholesterol food	28†	62

*Response to poll conducted before LRC CPPT.
†Physicians were asked to consider these foods as 1 risk factor.

Cholesterol Education Program is encouraging a "physician first" approach that urges physicians to check their own blood lipid levels and to do an assessment of their own knowledge and practice regarding blood cholesterol. It is hoped that increased self-awareness and, when necessary, self-treatment will enhance the physician's ability to counsel and manage patients with high blood cholesterol. The national program is also addressing the problems faced by physicians in measuring blood cholesterol. Physicians must be able to rely on accurate readings from commercial clinical laboratory tests, which, unfortunately, are poorly standardized. At this time there is a new technology aimed at developing equipment and methods for quick, relatively inexpensive, and accurate blood cholesterol readings. This technology provides the opportunity for the practitioner to give the patient appropriate counseling during his visit as opposed to waiting days for a laboratory report. Early indications are that these new finger-stick devices are testing well on total cholesterol measurements. This equipment is expected to be affordable for office-based practitioners. The new cholesterol education effort is not only based on a solid scientific foundation but it is also subject to periodic scientific reassessment. As newer evidence is analyzed, priorities and strategies may be modified.

Blood lipids in China

Kesteloot and associates[50] from Beijing, People's Republic of China, and Leuven, Belgium, measured serum cholesterol and HDL cholesterol levels in an urban and a rural population of the People's Republic of China (Fig. 1-13) and compared the values obtained with those obtained in Belgium and in the Republic of Korea using the same measuring methods. Total cholesterol levels were markedly lower in the People's Republic of China than in Belgium and generally lower than in Korea, both in male and female patients. The differences in HDL cholesterol levels, however, among the 3 populations were small in males and only significantly high in Belgium in the age classes below 34 years. In women of all age groups, HDL cholesterol values were significantly higher in Belgium than in China and Korea. Total cholesterol levels <100 mg/dl were found in the People's Republic of China in about 2% of the participants.

Low-density lipoprotein receptor gene

Sudhof and associates[51] from Dallas, Texas, (associates include Joseph L. Goldstein and Michael S. Brown, recent recipients of the Nobel Prize for Medicine) reported the exon organization of the gene for the human LDL receptor, a classic example of a cell-surfaced protein that mediates endocytosis through coated pits (Fig. 1-14). The investigators found a close correlation between functional domains in the LDL receptor protein and the exon-intron organization of the gene. This article is an example of the complexity of the present research on cholesterol metabolism and it is mentioned here simply to call attention to the extent of the basic cholesterol research now being performed.

Triglycerides

Few studies have simultaneously examined the relation of triglyceride levels with a wide variety of potential covariates. Thus, Cowan and associates[52] from several medical centers designed a study to assess in a large, free-living population the association of fasting plasma triglyceride values

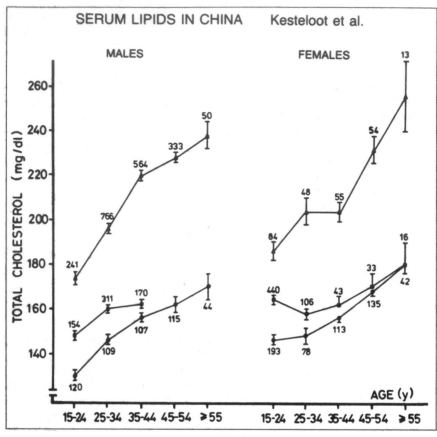

Fig. 1-13. Total cholesterol values (mean ± SEM) by age groups. Numbers of participants in each age class are also indicated. Triangle = Belgium; circle = People's Republic of China; squares = Korea. Reproduced with permission from Kesteloot et al.[50]

with selected demographic, behavioral, biochemical, and dietary measures. These analyses were done using data obtained from 5,189 white men and women aged 20–69 years who participated in the Lipid Research Clinics Program Prevalence Study. Of the 8 nondietary factors examined, age, Quetelet index, fasting plasma glucose, and cigarette smoking were strongly, positively associated with triglycerides in men and in women not using gonadal hormones (Fig. 1-15). Among women using oral contraceptives or estrogens, only Quetelet index and cigarette smoking were significantly related to triglyceride values. Physical activity was inversely associated and use of diuretic medications was positively related to triglycerides only in men. Results of analyses of triglycerides and 6 selected dietary measures varied by age, sex, and hormone use subgroups. Although none of the dietary variables showed consistent associations with triglycerides across all of the subgroups, triglycerides tended to be inversely associated with total calories/kg of body weight and the percentage of calories as dietary fat.

Certain primary hypertriglyceridemias cause abnormalities in lipoproteins that may predispose to CAD. Vega and Grundy[53] from Dallas, Texas, examined metabolism of LDL cholesterol in 11 men with both hypertriglyceridemia and CAD and compared them with that of controls. The LDL turnover was measured during placebo and gemfibrozil therapy. With placebo,

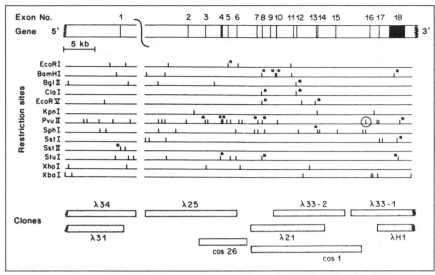

Fig. 1-14. Map of the human LDL receptor gene. The gene is shown in the 5′–3′ orientation at the top of the diagram and is shown to scale. Exons are denoted by filled areas, introns by open areas. The regions encompassed by genomic DNA inserts in the 7 bacteriophage λ and 2 cosmid clones are indicated at the bottom. Cleavage sites for 13 selected restriction endonucleases are shown. *=sites present in the cDNA. The encircled Pvu II site is polymorphic in human populations. The diagonal line between exons 1 and 2 represents a gap of unknown size not present in any of the genomic clones. Additional cleavage sites for the restriction enzymes shown may be present in this gap and in intron 6. The λ clones were isolated from 1.2×10^7 plaques of a human genomic bacteriophage λ library. Cos I was isolated from 6×10^6 colonies of a human cosmid library. Cos 26 was isolated from 0.9×10^6 colonies of a human cosmid library. The libraries were screened with ^{32}P-labeled probes derived from human LDL receptor cDNA, pLDLR-2. Probes were isotopically labeled by nick translation or hexanucleotide priming, and screening was carried out with standard procedures. Positive clones were plaque-purified or isolated as single colonies. Thirty fragments of the 9 genomic clones were subcloned into pBR322 and characterized by restriction endonuclease digestion, Southern blotting, and DNA sequencing of exon-intron junctions. The restriction map was verified by comparing overlapping and independently isolated genomic clones and by Southern blotting analysis of genomic DNA isolated from normal subjects. Reproduced with permission from Sudhof et al.[51]

LDL cholesterol level usually was normal, but production and fractional clearance of LDL were high. The LDL composition also was abnormal. Gemfibrozil reduced triglycerides, lowered production and fractional clearance of LDL, and normalized LDL composition. The LDL cholesterol level usually increased, but generally not to abnormally high levels. Therefore normalization of LDL metabolism and marked reduction of triglycerides by gemfibrozil suggest benefit to hypertriglyceridemic patients who are at high risk for CAD. However, when LDL cholesterol level increases excessively, gemfibrozil may not be sufficient therapy.

Levels in patients having coronary angiography

Breier and associates[54] from Innsbruck, Austria, investigated 89 consecutive men for whom coronary angiography had been performed because of suspected CAD and measured their plasma lipids, lipoproteins, postheparin lipoprotein lipase (LPL), and some hormones that influence LPL. The severity of CAD was expressed by the coronary score. CAD correlated with total

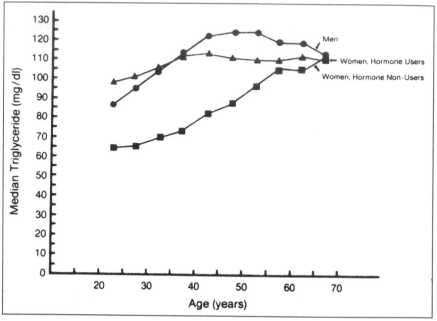

Fig. 1-15. Age-specific median plasma triglyceride values in white men (●) and women (▲) and not using (■) gonadal hormones. Reproduced with permission from Cowan et al.[52]

plasma cholesterol, LDL cholesterol, HDL cholesterol, and HDL$_2$. Additionally, there was a strong negative correlation between coronary score and LPL, and a positive correlation between coronary score and plasma triglycerides and VLDL. The impairment of LPL activity correlated with increased VLDL and decreased HDL cholesterol. The extent of CAD, thus, is strongly influenced by an LPL deficit. LPL activity correlated with plasma testosterone. Evidence was presented that low plasma testosterone may be partly responsible for the low LPL and HDL cholesterol.

Recent studies suggest that apolipoproteins and subfractions of HDL cholesterol may be better predictors of atherosclerotic CAD than are plasma cholesterol and total HDL cholesterol. To examine this hypothesis, Schmidt and associates[55] from Washington, D.C., measured plasma cholesterol and triglyceride, LDL cholesterol, HDL cholesterol and its subfractions 2 and 3, apolipoprotein A-1, the apolipoprotein B of LDL cholesterol, the ratio of apolipoprotein E$_{II}$ to E$_{III}$, and ratios of several of these variables in 126 patients who underwent coronary angiography for suspected CAD. Mean values of many of these variables differed significantly between the men with CAD and the men without significant CAD, when controlled for age, use of β-blockers and diuretic drugs (Fig. 1-16). Using multivariate logistic regression analysis, the only variable that made a significant independent contribution in predicting CAD in men was the ratio of HDL cholesterol to plasma total cholesterol. The mean of this ratio was 0.17 ± 0.01 in the men with CAD and 0.23 ± 0.02 in the male controls. All men with ratios of <0.15 mg/dl had significant CAD, defined as ≥50% luminal diameter narrowing of ≥1 major coronary artery. No measurement was a significant univariate or multivariate predictor of CAD in women, but the power to detect such predictors was reduced because of small group sizes. In conclusion, the ratio of HDL cholesterol to plasma cholesterol may be superior to many of the more recently described lipoprotein- and apolipoprotein-derived predictors of CAD.

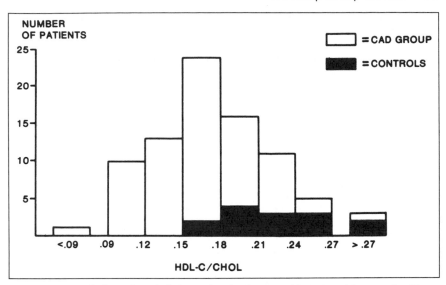

Fig. 1-16. HDL cholesterol/total cholesterol ratios in men with CAD and in control subjects. Reproduced with permission from Schmidt et al.[55]

In the nephrotic syndrome

Although hyperlipidemia is a common feature of the nephrotic syndrome, the distribution of cholesterol among the plasma lipoproteins and the mechanism of the enhanced hepatic synthesis of lipoprotein lipids are not well understood. Appel and associates[56] from New York City studied the distribution of cholesterol among the plasma lipoproteins and the relation between total cholesterol and plasma albumin concentration, oncotic pressure, and viscosity in 20 consecutive adult patients with uncomplicated nephrotic syndrome. The total plasma cholesterol (mean ± SD, 302 ± 100 mg/dl [8 ± 3 mmol/L]) and LDL cholesterol concentrations (215 ± 89 mg/dl [5.6 ± 2.3 mmol/L]) were elevated in most patients, but the HDL cholesterol level was normal or low (46 ± 18 mg/dl [1.2 ± 0.5 mmol/L]) in 95% of the patients. Thus, many hypercholesterolemic patients with unremitting nephrotic syndrome may be at increased risk for CAD. A significant inverse correlation was found between the plasma total cholesterol concentration and both the plasma albumin concentration and the plasma oncotic pressure, but not the plasma viscosity. Enhanced hepatic synthesis of lipoprotein lipids may be stimulated by a decreased plasma albumin concentration or oncotic pressure but does not appear to be due to changes in plasma viscosity.

Effect of obesity

Freedman and associates[57] from New Orleans, Louisiana, assessed relations between increases in triceps skin-fold thickness and changes in levels of serum lipids and lipoproteins in early life by examining 1,598 five–12 year olds 5 years after an initial examination. Significant positive correlations, controlled for age, were observed between changes in triceps skin-fold and changes in levels of serum total cholesterol, serum triglycerides, and LDL and VLDL cholesterol. Inverse associations between changes in triceps skin-fold and HDL cholesterol were weaker, but also statistically significant. Although females showed the largest increases in triceps skin-fold, most associations were stronger in males. Increases in estimated percentage body fat and ponderal index (kg/m^3) were highly associated with changes in triceps skin-fold, but showed slightly different associations with the serum lipids and lipoproteins. Results show that increases in obesity in youth are accompanied by an increasingly atherogenic lipoprotein profile.

Effect of exercise

Merians and associates[58] from Stanford, California, and Cleveland, Ohio, investigated the relation of exercise and oral contraceptive use to plasma lipids and lipoproteins in a cross-sectional study designed to compare lipid levels in 96 exercising and nonexercising women (aged 26–35 years) who did or did not use oral contraceptives. Exercisers had significantly lower plasma triglyceride concentrations and LDL/HDL ratios than nonexercisers after adjustment for differences in pill-type distribution between groups. Women using progestin-dominant pills had significantly lower plasma triglyceride and HDL concentrations and significantly higher LDL/HDL ratios compared with women using estrogen/progestin-balanced pills. As body fat was significantly associated with both pill type and physical activity, it is unclear how much of these lipoprotein differences were due to body fat, exercise, or pill use. Regular physical activity together with reduced body fat partially compensated for plasma lipoprotein differences associated with oral contraceptive use.

Tran and Weltman[59] from Boulder, Colorado, and Charlottesville, Virginia, analyzed, using meta-analysis, 95 studies conducted between September 1955 and October 1983 measuring changes in human serum lipid and lipoprotein levels in response to exercise training. Change in body weight during exercise training may confound observed serum lipid and lipoprotein level changes; thus, data from these studies were partitioned into those in which subjects gained, maintained, or lost body weight. Results showed differential changes in cholesterol, triglyceride, LDL cholesterol, HDL cholesterol, and cholestrol-HDL cholesterol levels in the 3 body weight categories. When body weight did not change, cholesterol and LDL-cholesterol levels decreased significantly (7.3 mg/dl and 3.3 mg/dl, respectively). When body weight decreased, cholesterol and LDL cholesterol levels also decreased significantly (13 mg/dl and 11 mg/dl, respectively). However, with body weight increase, cholesterol and LDL cholesterol levels increased by 2.9 mg/dl and 3.0 mg/dl, respectively. These results suggest that reductions in cholesterol and LDL cholesterol levels were greatest when exercise training was combined with body weight losses.

Effect of coffee drinking

Williams and associates[60] from Stanford, California, and Seattle, Washington, studied coffee intake from 3-day diet records in association with plasma lipoprotein concentrations in a cross-sectional sample of 77 men aged 30–55 years to determine the significance and form of their interrelations. The number of cups consumed per day correlated positively with levels of apolipoprotein and became more strongly correlated when adjusted for age, cigarette use, adiposity, aerobic capacity, nutrient intake, and stress. Coffee intake also correlated with total cholesterol and LDL cholesterol levels when adjusted for these confounding factors. Graphic analyses revealed that plasma concentrations of apolipoprotein B and LDL cholesterol were unrelated to intake of up to 2 cups of coffee per day and positively associated with intake exceeding 2–3 cups. These results suggest that male heavy coffee drinkers have lipoprotein profiles suggestive of increased cardiovascular disease risk, although the causality remains to be determined.

Effect of alcohol

High serum concentrations of apolipoprotein (Apo) A-1 are associated with a decreased risk of CAD. To study the effect of alcohol intake on serum Apo A-1 and A-2 concentrations, Camargo and associates[61] from Palo Alto, California, and Seattle, Washington, randomized 24 healthy male drinkers (38 ± 14 ml of ethanol per day) into treatment in control groups after a 3-week baseline. The treatment group abstained from all intake of alcohol for 6 weeks after randomization and then reverted to the usual level of intake for a 5-week period. The control group continued its usual level of drinking throughout the trial. The concentrations of Apo A-1 and A-2 of abstainers decreased significantly compared with the corresponding changes in controls. After drinking was resumed, Apo A-1 and A-2 concentrations were significantly increased in the treatment group compared with the corresponding changes in the control group. These results suggest that the association between moderate alcohol intake and reduced risk of CAD may be mediated in part by increased levels of serum Apo A-1 or A-2, or both.

Effect of malignancy

Several epidemiologic studies have shown an increased risk of death from cancer in subjects with low plasma cholesterol levels. Thus, hypocholesterolemia may be a predisposing factor to cancer development, or it may be secondary to malignant disease. The latter hypothesis is supported by 2 studies in which the inverse relation between plasma cholesterol and risk of death from cancer disappeared after patients with cancer detected within 2 years after cholesterol determination were excluded. In 1930 it was noted that patients with leukemia commonly had hypocholesterolemia. Subsequently, a number of studies in patients with different newly diagnosed malignant diseases had a high frequency of hypocholesterolemia unrelated to nutritional status. Vitols and associates[62] from Stokholm, Sweden, examined 59 patients with acute leukemia to see if hypocholesterolemia, which is commonly found in acute leukemia, was due to the high LDL receptor activity of leukemic cells. LDL receptor activity was found to be inversely correlated with plasma cholesterol concentration. Patients with both a high LDL receptor activity per cell and a high white blood cell count had the lowest cholesterol concentrations. During chemotherapy, cholesterol levels increased concomitantly with the disappearance from the peripheral blood of leukemic cells. Hypocholesterolemia in leukemia and other neoplastic disorders may be due to increased LDL receptor activity in the malignant cells. This high uptake and degradation of LDL by malignant cells could be utilized to target neoplastic cells with LDL bound chemotherapeutic agents.

Healthy and harmful diets

The low death rate from CAD among the Greenland Eskimos has been ascribed to their high fish consumption. Kromhout and associates[63] from Leiden, The Netherlands, therefore decided to investigate the relation between fish consumption and CAD in a group of men in Zutphen, The Netherlands. Information about the fish consumption of 852 middle-aged men without CAD was collected in 1960 by a careful dietary history obtained from the participants and their wives. During 20 years of follow-up, 78 men died

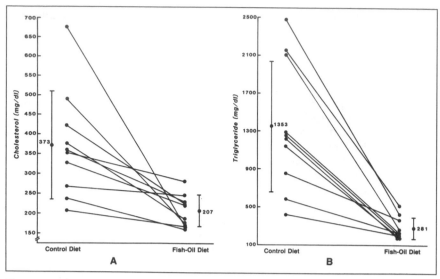

Fig. 1-17. Changes in levels of plasma cholesterol (A) and triglyceride (B) in 10 patients with the type V phenotype (control -vs- fish oil diet). To convert cholesterol and triglyceride values from mg/dl to mM/L, multiply by 0.026 and 0.0113, respectively. The mean change was −1,072 mg/dl (p <0.001) for triglyceride and −166 mg/dl (p <0.01) for cholesterol. Reproduced with permission from Phillipson et al.[64]

from CAD. An inverse dose-response relation was observed between fish consumption in 1960 and death from CAD during 20 years of follow-up. This relation persisted after multiple logistic regression analyses. Mortality from CAD was >50% lower among those who consumed at least 30 g/day of fish than among those who did not eat fish. It was concluded that the consumption of as little as 1 or 2 fish dishes per week may be of preventive value in relation to CAD.

Phillipson and associates[64] from Portland, Oregon, examined the effects of fish oil in 20 hypertriglyceridemic patients: 10 with type II hyperlipidemia and 10 with type V. These patients were put on 3 diets differing primarily in fatty acid consumption and fat content. The control diet contained a fatty acid mixture typical of a low fat therapeutic diet (ratio of polyunsaturated to saturated fat, 1.4), the fish oil diet contained omega-3 fatty acids, and the vegetable oil diet was rich in the omega-6 fatty acid, linoleic acid. Each diet was followed for 4 weeks. In the type 11b group, the fish oil diet led to decreases in both plasma cholesterol (−27%) and triglyceride (−64%) compared with the control diet (Fig. 1-17). VLDL was also reduced markedly. The vegetable oil diet had much less effect. With fish oil, the type V group had marked decreases in total cholesterol and triglyceride levels (−45 and −79%, respectively). VLDL levels were dramatically lowered, as were apolipoprotein E levels. The vegetable oil diet (unlike the fish oil diet) produced a rapid and significant increase in plasma triglyceride levels. The researchers concluded that fish oils and fish may be useful components of diets for the treatment of hypertriglyceridemia.

This article was followed by an editorial by Glomset entitled "Fish, Fatty Acids, and Human Health."[65]

The observation by Kromhout and colleagues[63] that consumption of fish was inversely associated with the risk of coronary death among men in Zutphen, The Netherlands, prompted Shekelle and associates[66] from 4 different medical centers to investigate this question in the Western Electric Study. The

TABLE 1-6. *Twenty-five-year risk of death, by amount of fish consumed, among middle-aged men who were free of CAD at entry. Reproduced with permission from Kromhout et al.*[63]

		DEATHS BY CAUSE								
FISH CONSUMPTION (G/DAY)	# MEN AT RISK	CAD		OTHER CVR DISEASES*		MALIGNANT NEOPLASMS		OTHER CAUSES		TOTAL DEATHS	
		#	%	#	%	#	%	#	%	#	%
0	205	42	20.5	15	7.3	13	6.3	14	6.8	84	41.0
1–17	686	128	18.7	39	5.7	72	10.5	25	3.6	264	38.5
18–34	779	121	15.5	31	4.0	78	10.0	38	4.9	268	34.4
>35	261	34	13.0	16	6.1	27	10.3	14	5.4	91	34.9
Total	1931	325	16.8	101	5.2	190	9.8	91	4.7	707	36.6
p value for trend		0.008		0.264		0.318		0.965		0.051	

*CVR = cardiovascular-renal.

lipid composition of the diet in that study was associated with the serum cholesterol concentration and the risk of coronary death in this cohort of middle-aged men employed by the Western Electric Company in Chicago during 1957. The new results (Table 1-6) support the observation of Kromhout and colleagues. Consumption of fish at entry was inversely associated in a graded manner with the 25-year risk of death from CAD and from all causes combined; it was not associated with death from other cardiovascular-renal diseases, from malignant neoplasms, or from other causes combined. Consumption of fish, furthermore, was not significantly associated cross-sectionally at entry with any of the major coronary risk factors—age, BP, serum cholesterol, and cigarette smoking—or with the body mass index, evidence of existing disease of a major organ system, the intake of dietary cholesterol, or the percentage of calories from saturated and monounsaturated fatty acids.

Vollset and associates[67] from Haukeland Sykehus, Norway, stimulated by the Kromhout and colleagues' report carried out new analyses of 11,000 men among 17,000 respondents to a postal dietary survey in Norway, who 3 years before the dietary survey had reported their smoking habits and selected cardiovascular symptoms. These new analyses were stratified on the basis of age, urban or rural status, region, and smoking habits. The follow-up covered 14 years through 1981 and only deaths before age 80 were considered. For all 2,587 deaths analyzed, the distributions of observed and expected numbers of events did not indicate any association between fish intake and total mortality. The same conclusion applies to the 967 deaths from CAD. These results do not support the hypothesis that persons with a high intake of fish are less susceptible to death from CAD.

Curb and Reed[68] of the Honolulu Heart Program also explored the relation of reported fish consumption to total and fatal CAD over a 12-year follow-up of 6,615 Japanese men without prevalent athrosclerotic disease. At the baseline examination, 2 kinds of dietary information were obtained to determine fish consumption: the usual frequency of eating fish and the amount of fish consumed during the previous 24 hours. Slightly <50% of the men eating fish ate it ≥2 times a week. Data from the 24-hour dietary recall revealed fish consumption on 44% of the records, ranging from 28–476 g in 24 hours. The apparent trends were not statistically significant in either analysis. The small number of cases in the "almost never" category of fish consumption should be taken into account when interpreting these data. Thus, although the dietary data collected by either the food frequency method or the 24-hour recall method have their limitations, the lack of significant trends despite the large number of subjects tends to discount a relation between fish consumption and CAD in this Japanese population. These researchers commented that the fish consumption in their population was significantly lower than that in a comparable sample of Japanese persons studied by the same methods and at the same time in Japan.

In a prospective epidemiologic study of 1,001 middle-aged men, aged 30–69 years, Kushi and associates[69] from Boston, Massachusetts, and Dublin, Ireland, examined the relation between dietary information collected approximately 20 years ago and subsequent mortality from CAD. The men were initially enrolled in 3 cohorts: men born and living in Ireland, those born in Ireland who had emigrated to Boston, and those born in the Boston area of Irish immigrants. There were no differences in mortality from CAD among the 3 cohorts. In within-population analyses, those who died of CAD had higher Keys and modified Hegsted dietary scores than did those who did not (a high score indicates a high intake of saturated fatty acids and cholesterol and a relatively low intake of polyunsaturated fatty acids). These associations were significant after adjustment for other risk factors for CAD. Fiber intake and a vegetable foods score, which increased with increased intake of fiber, vegetable protein, and starch, were lower among those who died from CAD, although not significantly so after adjustment for other risk factors. A higher Keys score carried an increased risk of CAD (relative risk, 1.60), and a higher fiber intake carried a decreased risk (relative risk, 0.57). Overall, these results tend to support the hypothesis that diet is related, albeit weakly, to the development of CAD.

This article was followed by an editorial by Blankenhorn entitled, "Two New Diet-Heart Studies."[70]

Macfarlane[71] from Iowa City, Iowa, commented on the report by Kushi and associates on the results of the Ireland-Boston diet-heart study. Macfarlane indicated that the daily consumption of various fats as expressed in the Kushi et al report was expressed and analyzed in terms of the subjects caloric intake (e.g., as mg/100 kcal). The use of this unjustified "correction" of the raw data that also was used in the Western Electric study reported in 1981 is unfortunate according to Macfarlane because it is now clearly established that men who subsequently have CAD consume about 10% fewer calories on average than those without subsequent disease, presumably reflecting the more sedentary lifestyle of the first group. This correction led Kushi and associates to report that the Irish consumed less cholesterol than the Bostonians, whereas in absolute terms they consumed more because of the higher caloric consumption. Macfarlane included a table that presents some of the data from Kushi's Table 4 concerning the dietary habits of the men who subsequently died of CAD and those who did not. In Macfarlane's table the data was recalculated with the inappropriate correction removed. About two-thirds of the reported difference between the 2 groups is actually attributable to the difference in caloric intake and has nothing to do with cholesterol. Similarly the men who died from CAD had actually consumed less saturated fat, not more, as Kushi and colleagues claimed.

Kushi and associates[72], in their response to Macfarlane's letter, indicated that it is precisely because the total consumption of nutrients is correlated with total energy intake that an adjustment was made for dietary kilocalories. Indeed, they argued that energy intake is largely determined by the level of physical activity, body size, and possibly some metabolic processes. Although adjustment of dietary constituents for energy may not deal adequately with these sources of a confounding effect, Kushi and associates believe it is inferentially more correct to make such an adjustment. Clearly, valid inferences that can be made from their study refer to dietary variables as a proportion of energy. They further argued that it is largely from investigations of dietary fats as a proportion of energy that it is possible to recommend alterations in the pattern of fat consumption. Nearly all dietary recommendations have uniformly suggested decreases in total fat and saturated fatty acids as a percentage of kilocalories rather than in absolute amount consumed. Kushi and associates concluded that despite the known limitations of methods for dietary assessment, prospective studies increasingly demonstrated that CAD is related to diet.

Arntzenius and associates[73] from Leiden, The Netherlands, studied the relation between diet, serum lipoproteins, and the progression of coronary narrowing in 39 patients with stable angina pectoris in whom coronary arteriography had shown at least 1 artery with 50% diameter reduction before intervention. Intervention consisted of a 2-year vegetarian diet that had a ratio of polyunsaturated to saturated fatty acids of at least 2 and that contained <100 mg/day of cholesterol. Dietary changes were associated with a significant increase in linoleic acid content of cholesteryl esters and a significant lowering of body weight, systolic BP, serum total cholesterol, and the ratio of total to HDL cholesterol. Angiographic examination was performed after 24 months; angiograms were assessed visually and by computer-assisted image analysis. Both types of assessment indicated progression of disease in 21 of 39 patients but no increased narrowing in 18. Increased coronary narrowing correlated with total to HDL cholesterol but not with BP, smoking status, alcohol intake, weight, or drug treatment. Disease progression was significant in patients who had values for total to HDL cholesterol that were higher than the median (>6.9) throughout the trial or who initially had higher values (>6.9) that were significantly lowered by dietary intervention.

Sacks and associates[74] from Boston and Framingham, Massachusetts, studied in 75 adult lactovegetarians living in the northeastern United States the influence of dairy products in the diet on plasma levels of total, LDL, and HDL cholesterol. Dairy products were the major sources of dietary saturated fat and cholesterol. The plasma total cholesterol level was positively correlated with dietary saturated fat and dietary cholesterol and inversely correlated with the ratio of polyunsaturated to saturated fats in the diet. Correlations between the LDL cholesterol level and the nutrients were similar to those of the TC level. The HDL cholesterol level was not significantly related to any nutrients in the diet. The cholesterol levels of the lactovegetarians were compared with those of strict vegetarians. Lactovegetarians had 24% higher LDL cholesterol levels and 7% higher HDL cholesterol levels than strict vegetarians. Analysis within and among vegetarian populations suggests that ingestion of fatty dairy products increases the LDL cholesterol level on a percentage basis about 3 times more than it increases the HDL cholesterol level.

Treatment

Recent prospective clinical trials have established that cholesterol reduction in patients with elevated (upper 90%) concentrations of LDL reduces the incidence of AMI and sudden coronary death. Because the level of protection from these cardiovascular sequelae is directly related to the degree of LDL reduction, combination therapy using different hypolipidemic agents have been used in patients with type II hyperlipoproteinemia (HLP). Neomycin is as effective as cholestyramine in reducing LDL levels and combination neomycin-niacin treatment normalizes the plasma lipoproteins in 92% of patients with type II HLP. Because neomycin could theoretically ameliorate some of the gastrointestinal side effects of cholestyramine in addition to further affecting cholesterol levels, Hoeg and associates[75] from Bethesda, Maryland, assessed in 18 patients with type II HLP in a 9-month clinical trial the effects of combination cholestyramine-neomycin treatment on the plasma lipoprotein levels. Compared with diet only treatment, cholestyramine reduced total and LDL cholesterol levels by 77 mg/dl (22%) and 78 mg/dl (31%), respectively. In addition to relieving cholestyramine-induced constipation, neomycin further reduced the total cholesterol level by 20 mg/dl (6%). However, this further reduction in total cholesterol concentration was the result of a decrease in the concentration of HDL cholesterol. These findings indicate that combination therapy does not have an additive LDL cholesterol-lowering effect and that neomycin and cholestyramine is not a useful drug combination. In addition, these results illustrate the importance of determining that HDL cholesterol concentration to interpret fully the effects of hypolipidemic treatment.

Abnormalities in plasma lipids are a recognized side effect of isotretinoin therapy for nodulocystic acne. Bershad and associates[76] from New York City studied 60 patients during 20 weeks of isotretinoin therapy to measure changes in plasma lipids and lipoproteins. Both men and women had significant increases in mean plasma levels of total cholesterol and LDL cholesterol and decreases in mean levels of HDL cholesterol. Mean triglyceride levels increased in men and women, with maximum mean increases of 46 and 52 mg/dl, respectively. The maximum level was reached by 4 weeks of therapy in men but not until the 12th week in women. Nine of 53 patients (17%) completing 20 weeks of isotretinoin therapy acquired hypertriglyceridemia with values of 200–600 mg/dl. There was no significant changes in mean levels of lipoprotein lipase or hepatic triglyceride lipase. Plasma lipid and lipoprotein levels returned to baseline by 8 weeks after discontinuation of the drug. Thus, if sustained over a long period, these changes would predict an increased risk of cardiovascular disease.

Nathan Pritikin, Ph.D.

Nathan Pritikin died in February 1985 at the age of 69 years and Hubbard and associates[77] from Albany, New York, and Santa Monica, California, reported the clinical and autopsy findings in this man who had such an enormous impact on CAD in the United States. When 42 years old (February 1958), a diagnosis of asymptomatic coronary insufficiency was made in Pritikin after a comprehensive medical evaluation. On a Master's 2-step test, while Pritikin's heart rate was 98 beats/minute (56% of the age-predicted maximum), ECG showed a 2 mm horizontal ST-segment depression in leads 2, aVF, and V_5 and a 1.5 mm ST depression in lead V_3. A similar positive Master's test also was present in December 1959. His fasting total serum cholesterol when Pritikin was 39 years old (December 1955) was 280 mg/dl, and at that time he started modifying his diet. By age 42, he had formulated and began to follow the Pritikin high complex carbohydrate, low fat, low cholesterol diet. His total serum cholesterol thereafter progressively decreased from 280 to 94 mg/dl. Specifically, at age 39 (February 1955) his total serum cholesterol was 280, at age 42 (February 1958), it was 210; by July

1958, 162; by September 1958, 122; by August 1959, 155; by July 1960, 120; by December 1963, 102 mg/dl. Thus, by age 47 (December 1963) his total serum cholesterol had reached a level where it remained for the remainder of his life. In March 1966, his total cholesterol was 119; in September 1968, 118; in January 1969, 112; in November 1984, 94 mg/dl. Pritiken led a vigorous life and until late 1984 he ran several kilometers daily. In 1958, Pritiken had a malignant lymphoma, most closely resembling well-differentiated lymphocytic lymphoma with macroglobulinemia. Intermittent chemotherapy provided control for 7 years. In 1980, a splenectomy was performed, and in 1984 and 1985 several experimental agents were tried. Anemia became worse during his last months and he died after several complications of therapy in February 1985.

The necropsy revealed lymphoma in partial remission and several findings referable to treatment. His heart weighed 380 g. The coronary arteries in their entirety were widely patent. A few yellow flat streaks were observed on the intimal lining of the coronary arteries, but there were no raised plaques and no clots were found in the coronary arteries. The myocardial walls were free of foci of fibrosis and necrosis. Several systemic arteries showed some yellow flat streaks on their intimal surface, but no elevated plaques were present and none of the lumens of the arteries were narrowed. Thus, at age 69 years, his coronary arteries and other systemic arteries were virtually free of athrosclerotic plaques. Mrs. Nathan Pritiken granted permission for the clinical and necropsy findings in her husband to be reported.

I (WCR) talked to the pathologist, Dr. Hubbard, 2 days after Pritiken's death. I learned that Dr. Pritiken had entered the Albany, New York, hospital under an assumed name and at the time of autopsy the pathologist did not know that he was doing an autopsy on Dr. Pritiken. Dr. Hubbard was assisted by a resident in pathology and remarked to the resident that the coronary arteries and aorta and arteries arising from the aorta were the cleanest he had ever seen in a man 69 years of age. No samples of the heart or other arteries were retained. The day after the autopsy, the pathologist became aware that the person in whom he had done the necropsy was, indeed, Nathan Pritiken.

Review

Schaefer and Levy[78] from Bethesda, Maryland, reviewed lipoprotein metabolism, their approach to the patient with lipoprotein disorders, the various types of lipoprotein disorders and appropriate therapy for the disorders (Tables 1-7 and 1-8).

CIGARETTE SMOKING

Cigarette smoking is an established risk factor for the occurrence of cardiovascular events and mortality. Whether recent smoking history or total life consumption best represents the increased risk due to smoking has not been previously established. Weintraub and associates[79] from Philadelphia, Pennsylvania, used a stepwise logistic regression analysis to determine the relative contributions of these factors to the risk of having significant CAD in 1,349 patients who underwent cardiac catheterization. Six risk factors were analyzed: total pack-years, current packs smoked per day, age, gender, family history, and symptomatic status. The results of this analysis showed that total pack-years, but not current packs per day, is a significant independent

TABLE 1-7. *Normal plasma lipid and lipoprotein-cholesterol concentrations.** Reproduced with permission from Schaefer and Levy.[78]

AGE (yr)	PLASMA CHOLESTEROL (MG/DL)			PLASMA TRIGLYCERIDE (MG/DL)			VLDL CHOLESTEROL (MG/DL)			LDL CHOLESTEROL (MG/DL)			HDL CHOLESTEROL (MG/DL)		
	10[+]	50	90	10	50	90	10	50	90	10	50	90	10	50	90
Males															
0–4	125	151	186	33	51	84	—	—	—	—	—	—	—	—	—
5–9	130	159	191	33	51	85	2	7	15	69	90	117	42	54	70
10–14	127	155	190	37	59	102	2	9	18	72	94	122	40	55	71
15–19	120	146	183	43	69	120	3	12	23	68	93	123	34	46	59
20–24	130	165	204	50	86	165	5	12	24	73	101	138	32	45	57
25–29	143	178	227	54	95	199	6	15	31	75	116	157	32	44	58
30–34	148	190	239	58	104	213	8	18	36	88	124	166	32	45	59
35–39	157	197	249	62	113	251	7	19	46	92	131	176	31	43	58
40–44	163	203	250	64	122	248	8	21	43	98	135	173	31	43	60
45–49	169	210	258	68	124	253	8	20	40	106	141	186	33	45	60
50–54	169	210	261	68	124	250	10	23	49	102	143	185	31	44	58
55–59	167	212	262	67	119	235	6	19	39	103	145	191	31	46	64
60–64	171	210	259	68	119	235	4	16	35	106	143	188	34	49	69
65–69	170	210	258	64	112	208	3	16	40	104	146	199	33	49	74
>70	162	205	252	67	111	212	3	15	31	100	142	182	33	48	70
Females															
0–4	120	156	189	38	59	96	—	—	—	—	—	—	—	—	—
5–9	134	163	195	36	55	90	1	9	19	73	98	125	38	52	67
10–14	131	158	190	44	70	114	3	10	20	73	94	126	40	52	64
15–19	126	154	190	44	66	107	4	11	20	67	93	127	38	51	68
20–24	130	160	203	41	64	112	3	10	22	62	98	136	37	50	68
25–29	136	168	209	42	65	116	4	11	22	73	103	141	40	55	73
30–34	139	172	213	44	69	123	2	9	20	76	108	142	40	55	71
35–39	147	182	225	46	73	137	3	13	26	81	116	161	38	52	74
40–44	154	191	235	51	82	155	5	12	26	89	120	164	39	55	78
45–49	161	199	247	53	87	171	4	14	32	90	127	173	39	56	78
50–54	172	215	268	59	97	186	4	14	32	102	141	192	40	59	77
55–59	183	228	282	63	106	204	4	18	40	103	148	204	39	58	82
60–64	186	228	280	64	105	202	3	13	30	105	151	201	43	60	85
65–69	183	229	280	66	112	204	3	15	36	104	156	208	38	60	79
>70	180	226	278	69	111	204	0	13	34	107	146	189	37	60	82

*Data are from Lipid Research Clinics population studies in the United States and Canada for white males and females (nonusers of sex hormone).[1] All subjects are tested in the fasting state. Values in the lowest 5th percentile and highest 95th percentile for all age and sex groups (mg/dl) are; cholesterol, 112–303; triglyceride, 29–327; VLDL cholesterol, 0–62; LDL cholesterol, 60–234; and HDL cholesterol, 27–91. To convert cholesterol and triglyceride values to millimoles per liter, multiply by 0.02586 and 0.01129, respectively. Dashes indicate that no data are available because there were fewer than 100 subjects in a cell.
[+]Percentile.

risk factor for the development of CAD. This was true in every age group up to but not older than age 70 years. Although the overall risk was lower in younger patients and in patients with less typical symptoms of angina, the relative risk in cigarette smokers relative to pack-years was consistently greater. The risk of total life consumption of cigarettes is thus greater than has heretofore been realized, particularly in persons who would otherwise be categorized as low risk.

PHYSICAL ACTIVITY AND FITNESS

The epidemiologic evidence linking physical inactivity to occurrence of CAD is substantial but inconclusive. Favorable effects of training on cardiovascular risk factors have been demonstrated, but it is not well established that ordinary levels of physical activity are important determinants of the

TABLE 1-8. *Plasma lipid and lipoprotein-cholesterol concentrations in dyslipidemic subjects. Reproduced with permission from Schaefer and Levy.*[78]

	PLASMA* (MG/DL)		CHOLESTEROL* (MG/DL)			RATIOS[†]		
	CHOLESTEROL	TRIGLYCERIDE	VLDL	LDL	HDL	C/TG	LDL/HDL	VLDL/TG
Hyperlipoproteinemic subjects								
Type I (n = 12)	324 ± 57	3316 ± 677	285 ± 57	22 ± 2	17 ± 2	0.10	1.29	0.09
Type II (n = 454)	354 ± 4	135 ± 4	24 ± 1	286 ± 9	44 ± 1	2.62	6.50	0.18
Type III (n = 66)	441 ± 54	694 ± 60	292 ± 19	111 ± 7	38 ± 2	0.64	2.92	0.42
Type IV (n = 299)	251 ± 4	438 ± 24	78 ± 4	132 ± 2	37 ± 1	0.57	3.57	0.18
Type V (n = 95)	373 ± 19	2071 ± 213	274 ± 22	72 ± 4	27 ± 1	0.18	2.67	0.13
Hypolipoproteinemic subjects								
Abetalipo- proteinemia (n = 4)	41 ± 4	20 ± 3	1 ± 0	2 ± 1	38 ± 2	2.05	0.05	0.05
Tangier disease (n = 11)	65 ± 4	200 ± 31	21 ± 4	42 ± 13	2 ± 1	0.33	21.00	0.11
Familial hypoalpha- lipopro- teinemia (n = 6)	165 ± 9	113 ± 8	24 ± 2	115 ± 10	26 ± 2	1.46	4.42	0.21

*Values are means ±SEM. VLDL represents the 1.006 g/ml supernatant fraction and therefore includes chylomicrons when present and VLDL. To convert cholesterol and triglyceride values to mM/L, multiply by 0.02586 and 0.01129, respectively.
[†]C/TG = the ratio of plasma cholesterol to plasma triglyceride; LDL/HDL, LDL cholesterol to HDL cholesterol; and VLDL/TG, VLDL cholesterol to plasma triglyceride. Normal C/TG, LDL/HDL, and VLDL/TG ratios are 2.17, 2.46, and 0.18, respectively.

major cardiovascular risk factors. Kannel and associates[80] from Boston, Massachusetts, and Dallas, Texas, prospectively collected epidemiologic data on overall mortality, cardiovascular mortality, and coronary mortality and found that all 3 were inversely related to the level of physical activity in men. For men but not women, the effect persisted when other risk factors were taken into account. For stroke, occlusive peripheral arterial disease, and cardiac failure, significant inverse relations to activity were not consistently demonstrated. A number of correlates of physical fitness, including adiposity, vital capacity, and heart rate, appeared to be useful surrogates for assessment of physical activity. Risk of cardiovascular mortality was related to each of these objective measures and mounted precipitously in those with multiple abnormalities of these possibly sedentary traits (Fig. 1-18). Lack of exercise appeared to predispose to lethal coronary attacks; a direct causal relation was uncertain, although dose related. Associations were modest and not entirely consistent among different studies; the possibility of self-selection was observed. Experimental evidence in animals has been neither strong nor consistent. Controlled trials have been uninterpretable because of confounding with other health behaviors and dropouts related to poor health. Better, more objective, practical, quantitative measures of activity and fitness distinct from each other are needed. It was concluded that it remains unclarified as to whether benefits of exercise require attainment of a trained state, since moderate exercise appears to be beneficial. Thus, it seems un-

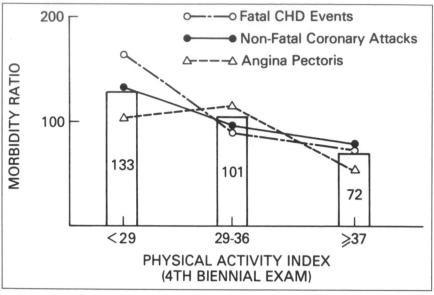

Fig. 1-18. Risk of CAD by physical activity status in a 10-year follow-up of men aged 35–69 years in the Framingham study. Reproduced with permission from Kannel et al.[80]

likely that exercise programs can make as great an impact on cardiovascular disease incidence as control of major risk factors. Physical exercise and conditioning appear best included in a comprehensive program of multiple risk factor intervention.

In a study by Sullivan and associates[81] from San Diego, California, of 156 patients with stable CAD randomized to either an exercise intervention group or a control group, 41 had complete gas analysis data. Continuous gas exchange data, including the ventilatory threshold, and selected heart rates, were determined initially and at 1 year. The mean attendance for the exercise group was 2.2 ± 0.7 days a week at an intensity of 60 ± 9% of estimated peak oxygen uptake for 1 year of the study. Statistically significant differences were observed between the exercise group (n = 19) and the control group (n = 22) for peak oxygen uptake (L/min), total treadmill time, and supine rest and submaximal heart rates after 1 year. The most remarkable change was a 16% increase in treadmill time. There was no difference between groups for the ventilatory threshold expressed either as an absolute oxygen uptake or as a percentage of peak oxygen uptake at 1 year. There was a significant correlation between the absolute change in peak oxygen uptake and the absolute change in the ventilatory threshold. These results indicate that a moderate exercise program is inadequate to alter the ventilatory threshold in CAD patients and that changes in ventilatory threshold do not explain the increase in treadmill time that usually occurs.

OBESITY

To resolve questions relating to the health implications of obesity, the Office of Medical Applications of Research of the National Institutes of Health, the National Institute of Arthritis, Diabetes and Digestive and Kidney

Diseases, and the National Heart, Lung and Blood Institute convened a consensus development conference on the health implications of obesity in February 1985.[82] After 1.5 days of presentation by experts in the field, a consensus panel representing the professional fields of nutrition, nutritional biochemistry and metabolism, endocrinology, internal medicine, gastroenterology, epidemiology, biostatistics, psychiatry, pediatrics, and family medicine and including medical literature and public representation considered the evidence and agreed on answers to the following questions: What is obesity? What is the evidence that obesity has adverse effects on health? What is the evidence that obesity affects longevity? What are the appropriate uses and limitations of existing height-weight tables? For what medical conditions can weight reduction be recommended? What should be the directions of future research in this area? Only these questions were addressed. Extremely important issues relating to obesity, such as prevention, treatment (including exercise), the impact on society, and the special relation of obesity to lower socioeconomic status, were not addressed. The evidence is now overwhelming that obesity, defined as excessive storage of energy in the form of fat, has adverse effects on health and longevity. Obesity is clearly associated with systemic hypertension, hypercholesterolemia, noninsulin-dependent diabetes mellitus, and excess of certain cancers and other medical problems. Height and weight tables based on mortality data or the body mass index are helpful measures to determine the presence of obesity and the need for treatment. Thirty-four million adult Americans have a body mass index >28 (men) or 27 (women); at this level of obesity, which is very close to a weight increase of 20% above desirable, treatment is strongly advised. When diabetes, hypertension, or a family history for these diseases is present, treatment will lead to benefits even when lesser degrees of obesity are present. Obesity research efforts should be directed toward elucidation of biologic markers; factors regulating the regional distribution of fat; studies of energy regulation; and studies using the techniques of anthropology, psychiatry, and the social sciences.

COFFEE DRINKING

It has been estimated that 82% of persons >18 years of age in the United States consume an average of 186 mg/day of caffeine in coffee, tea, cola beverages, and over-the-counter prescriptions. Although a limited amount of data on the arrhythmogenicity of caffeine is available, its effect on exercise-induced angina pectoris is unknown. Accordingly, Piters and associates[83] from Irvine, California, studied the effects of coffee on exercise-induced angina in 17 men with CAD using a double-blind treadmill protocol. Ingestion of either 1 or 2 cups of caffeinated coffee increased the exercise duration until onset of angina (8 and 12%, respectively), whereas decaffeinated coffee had no effect. The extent of ST-segment depression and the heart rate-BP product at angina were similar after drinking caffeinated and decaffeinated coffee. Exercise duration until 0.1 mV of ST-segment depression, and the heart rate, BP, and double product at angina and at 0.1 mV of ST-segment depression were similar after drinking caffeinated or decaffeinated coffee. The mean serum caffeine levels (±SD) after ingestion of 1 and 2 cups of caffeinated coffee were 1.97 ± 1.0 and 3.89 ± 1.6 μg/ml, respectively. The acute ingestion of 1–2 cups of caffeinated coffee had no deleterious effect on exercise-induced angina pectoris in patients with CAD.

ALCOHOL DRINKING

In a study performed by Colditz and associates[84] from Boston, Massachusetts, the association between moderate alcohol intake and subsequent cardiovascular mortality during a 5-year period was examined among 1,271 Massachusetts residents ≥66 years of age. Alcohol intake was calculated in g/day and the cohort was divided into abstainers (n = 450) and drinkers of 0.1–8.9 g/day (n = 40), 9–34 g/day (n = 232), and >34 g/day (n = 39). Compared with abstainers, the age-adjusted relative risk of death from CAD among those consuming 0.1–8.9 g/day was 0.3 (95% confidence limits 0.1–0.7), 9–34 g/day was 0.7 (0.3–1.7), and >34 g/day was 1.2 (0.3–4.8). After controlling for age, sex, cigarette smoking, and cholesterol intake using Cox regression analysis, when compared with abstainers those consuming <9 g/day had a significantly lowered risk of death from CAD, odds ratio 0.3 (0.1–0.7).

ESTROGEN

Stampfer and associates[85] from Boston, Massachusetts, surveyed 121,964 female nurses aged 30–55 years with questionnaires beginning in 1976 to see if there was a possible role of postmenopausal estrogen use to frequency of CAD. Information on hormone use and other potential risk factors was updated and the incidence of CAD was asserted through additional questionnaires in 1978 and 1980 with a 93% follow-up. Endpoints were documented by medical records. During 105,786 person-years of observation among 32,217 postmenopausal women who were initially free of CAD, 90 women had either nonfatal AMI (65 cases) or fatal CAD (25 cases). Compared with the risk in women who had never used postmenopausal hormones, the age-adjusted relative risk of CAD in those who had ever used them was 0.5, and the risk in current users was 0.3. The relative risks were similar for fatal and nonfatal disease and were unaltered after adjustment for cigarette smoking, systemic hypertension, diabetes mellitus, high cholesterol levels, a parental history of AMI, past use of oral contraceptives, and obesity. These data support the hypothesis that the postmenopausal use of estrogen reduces the risk of severe CAD.

Wilson and associates[86] from Framingham, Massachusetts, and Bethesda, Maryland, studied the effect of estrogen use on morbidity from cardiovascular disease in 1,234 postmenopausal women aged 50–83 years participating in the Framingham Heart Study's 12th biennial examination (index examination). The medication history recorded at biennial examinations 8 through 12 was used to classify the degree of estrogen exposure before 8 years of observation for cardiovascular morbidity and mortality. Despite a favorable cardiovascular risk profile and control for the major known risk factors for heart disease, women reporting postmenopausal estrogen use at ≥1 examination had >50% elevated risk of cardiovascular morbidity and more than a 2-fold risk for cerebrovascular disease after the index examination. Increased rates for AMI were observed among estrogen users who smoked cigarettes. Conversely, among nonsmokers, estrogen use was associated only with an increased incidence of stroke. No benefits from estrogen use were observed in the study group; in particular, mortality from all causes and from cardiovascular disease did not differ for estrogen users and nonusers.

These 2 estrogen articles were followed by an editorial by Bailar[87] entitled, "When Research Results Are in Conflict." Thus, the articles by Stampfer and by Wilson and their coworkers come to completely different conclusions. Bailar pointed out that the studies differ in many technical details. Bailar concluded that he could not tell from the present evidence whether estrogen or hormones add to the risk of various cardiovascular diseases, diminished the risk, or leave it unchanged. He simply concluded that more research was needed.

HOMOCYSTINURIA

Premature atherosclerosis and thromboembolic events are well-known complications of homozygous homocystinuria due to cystathionine synthase deficiency. It is unknown whether heterozygosity for hemocystinuria predisposes to premature vascular disease. Boers and associates[88] from 3 different medical centers explored the frequency of excessive homocysteine accumulation after standardized methionine loading in 75 patients presenting with clinical signs of ischemic disease before the age of 50 years: 25 with occlusive peripheral arterial disease, 25 with occlusive cerebrovascular disease, and 25 with AMI. In 7 patients in each of the first 2 groups but in none of the third group, heterozygosity for homocystinuria was established on the basis of pathologic homocysteinemia after methionine loading and cystathionine synthase deficiency in skin fibroblast cultures. Because the frequency of heterozygosity for homocystinuria in the normal population is 1 in 70 at the most, the investigators concluded that this condition predisposes to the development of premature occlusive arterial disease, causing intermittent claudication, renovascular hypertension, and ischemic cerebrovascular disease.

This article was followed by an editorial by Mudd entitled, "Vascular Disease and Homocysteine Metabolism."[89]

PROSTAGLANDINS AND PLATELET INHIBITORS

Despite numerous studies on the antithrombotic efficacy of aspirin, controversy remains over the optimal dosage. Since aspirin influences other systems that protect against thrombosis as well as inhibiting platelet function, Weksler and coworkers[90] from New York City investigated possible cumulative effects of low dose aspirin on vascular production of prostacyclin (PGI_2) in patients with documented atherosclerotic cardiovascular disease. Candidates for CABG ingested 20 mg of aspirin daily during the week before surgery, and platelet aggregation, platelet formation of thromboxane A_2 (TXA_2), aortic and saphenous vein production of PGI_2, and hemostatic status were measured at the time of the CABG. Low dose aspirin markedly inhibited platelet aggregation responses and reduced TXA_2 generation by >90%, effects similar to those observed with much higher doses of aspirin. Both aortic and saphenous vein production of PGI_2 were inhibited by 50% compared with PGI_2 produced by vascular tissues of control subjects who received no aspirin preoperatively. Blood loss at surgery was not significantly increased by preoperative low dose aspirin as measured by chest tube drainage (754 ml in aspirin-treated subjects -vs- 645 ml in control subjects), hematocrit nadir, or transfusions postoperatively. Endothelial recovery from aspirin-induced inhibition of PGI_2 formation was complete at 24 hours after the last dose, suggesting that cyclooxygenase turnover in endothelium may be more rapid than that in vascular smooth muscle. These findings indicate that preoperative low dose aspirin can inhibit platelet function without augmenting perioperative blood loss and that partial inhibition of PGI_2 formation by blood vessels accompanies even very low doses of aspirin. The investigators further add that the rapid recovery of PGI_2 synthetic capacity by vascular endothelium may permit use of a relatively selective antiplatelet schedule of low dose aspirin administration.

Platelet activation and the oxygenated metabolites of arachidonic acid have been implicated in the events surrounding vascular occlusion of the coronary circulation. The potent platelet inhibitory and vasodilator properties of PGI_2 suggest that levels of this substance may be of relevance to drug action and pathologic processes in the coronary vascular bed. Laboratory and clinical attempts to estimate the coronary secretion rate of PGI_2 have relied on measurements of metabolites obtained via cardiac catheter, usually as an adjunct to coronary angiography. To test the hypothesis that such procedures might themselves perturb endogenous biosynthesis of PGI_2, Roy and colleagues[91] from Nashville, Tennessee, used mass spectrometry to measure levels of 6-keto-prostaglandin $F_{1\alpha}$ ($PGF_{1\alpha}$) across the coronary vascular bed and to assess the excretion of a major urinary metabolite, 2,3-dinor-6-keto-$PGF_{1\alpha}$ (PGI-M), in patients undergoing cardiac catheterization. PGI-M increased variably during catheterization with angiography and remained elevated 2–4 hours after initiation of the procedure. Coronary catheterization without angiography also stimulated metabolic excretion, possibly reflecting catheter-induced vascular trauma. The direct effect of radiocontrast media on vascular release of PGI_2 was indicated by increased PGI-M excretion in healthy volunteers administered intravenous radiocontrast and by studies of the canine coronary artery and jugular vein in vitro. Measurement of plasma 6-keto-$PGF_{1\alpha}$ after left-sided heart catheterization showed that levels in aortic and coronary sinus blood were increased compared with peripheral venous levels determined before the procedure. Aortic and coronary sinus concentrations of 6-keto-$PGF_{1\alpha}$ both increased markedly in 1 of the 5 patients after injection of radiocontrast material, but an aortic coronary sinus gradient of 6-keto-$PGF_{1\alpha}$ was undetectable before or after angiography. Thus, these investigators concluded that these results indicate cardiac catheterization and angiography are associated with an increase in PGI_2 formation in vivo, and such procedure-related artifacts may obscure detection of PGI_2 production within the coronary bed.

Since adenosine is formed in the hearts of experimental animals during hypoxia or ischemia, this vasodilating metabolite has been proposed as a major link that couples the coronary flow rate to the metabolic state of the heart. Edlund and coinvestigators[92] from Huddinge, Sweden, studied the cardiac release of adenosine and PGI_2 in patients with CAD and assessed coronary vascular resistance before and after inhibition of synthesis. In 48 patients with CAD, arterial and coronary sinus blood samples were taken at rest, during atrial pacing to angina, and after pacing. Levels of purines were determined by high performance liquid chromatography and the PGI_2 metabolite 6-keto-PGF_{1a} was measured with radioimmunoassay. Coronary sinus blood flow was determined with retrograde continuous thermodilution before and after oral administration of indomethacin, aspirin, naproxen, or ibuprofen. Atrial pacing induced myocardial ischemia, as evidenced by typical chest pain and arrested lactate extraction. Adenosine was extracted at rest, but during ischemia there was a significant release of its metabolite hypoxanthine, indicating increased myocardial breakdown of high energy adenine nucleotides. Arterial and coronary sinus concentrations of 6-keto-$PGF_{1\alpha}$ were low, and no significant differences between them were found. After administration of the PG-synthesis inhibitor indomethacin, coronary vascular resistance was elevated, as was the coronary oxygen extraction. The 3 other PG synthesis inhibitors (aspirin, naproxen, and ibuprofen) did not induce any change in coronary vascular resistance or in the cardiac extraction of oxygen. On the basis of these data, the investigators suggest that in patients with CAD, cardiac ischemia results in increased myocardial production and release of purines, cardiac ischemia does not elicit any detectable increase in coronary production of PGI_2, and the increased coronary resistance induced by indomethacin does not reflect the involvement of locally performed prostaglandin in the maintenance of coronary flow but is rather a direct effect of the drug.

Elevated levels of beta-thromboglobulin (BTG) reflecting enhanced platelet aggregation have been reported in patients with AMI. Similarily, patients with AMI often present high levels of fibrinopeptide A (FPA), a reliable index of fibrin formation in vivo. Controversy has persisted as to whether FPA is elevated in patients with CAD without AMI. Gallino and coworkers[93] from Bern, Switzerland, measured FPA concentrations in plasma and in 24-hour urine specimens as well as BTG in plasma in 17 patients with severe angina pectoris, including both stable and unstable angina, and in 19 patients with AMI. Patients with unstable angina had plasma FPA and BTG levels of 5.2 and 91 ng/ml, respectively. Corresponding concentrations of FPA in the 24-hour urine specimens were 8.2 μg/24 hours. These values were similar to those obtained in patients with AMI and higher than the corresponding levels in patients with stable angina and in normal subjects. Thus, the similarity of the platelet and coagulation findings in patients with unstable angina and in those with AMI supports the hypothesis that coronary thrombosis may play a major role in the pathogenesis of AMI.

SILENT MYOCARDIAL ISCHEMIA

Von Arnim and associates[94] from Munich, West Germany, studied the frequency of transient ischemic ST-segment changes in 296 consecutive patients with CAD in the hospital for coronary angiography. Each patient underwent 2-channel, frequency modulated ambulatory monitoring for 24 hours. During this time, 56 episodes of transient ST elevation and 165 of ST depression with a horizontal deviation of $\geq$1 mm lasting $\geq$1 minute were found in 70 patients (24%) (Fig. 1-19). Only 34% of episodes were associated with pain. The duration of the episode, the heart rate at the beginning of the episode, or the extent of ST deviation were not related to the occurrence of pain (Figs. 1-20, 1-21). Episodes of ST elevation were of significantly shorter duration, occurred significantly more often during the early morning, and at significantly lower heart rates than episodes of ST depression. The considerable overlap between the characteristics of episodes of ST elevation and ST depression suggests that in many instances a combination of factors is responsible for transient ischemic ST-segment changes.

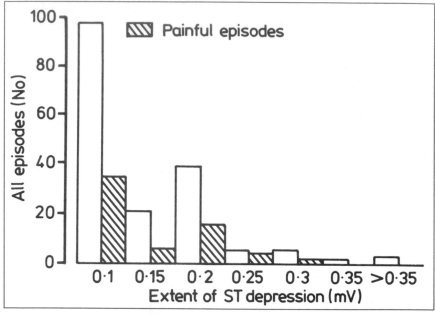

Fig. 1-19.   Number of episodes of ST depression and extent of ST depression. The proportion of painful episodes is not significantly greater with deeper ST depression (≥0.2 mV). Reproduced with permission from Arnim et al.[94]

ANGINA PECTORIS

Relation of chest pain to anxiety and depression

Channer and associates[95] from Bristol, UK, measured anxiety and depression in 87 consecutive patients (65 men and 22 women) with chest pain before diagnostic exercise treadmill testing. Chest pain was assessed as typical or atypical of angina by an independent observer. Fifty exercise tests were positive; 37 were negative (including 19 submaximal). Patients with negative tests had significantly higher scores for anxiety and higher depression scores than those with positive tests; 12% of patients with positive tests were women compared with 43% with negative tests. Twenty-seven patients (73%) with negative tests had atypical pain compared with 6 (12%) with positive tests. Depressed patients walked for a significantly shorter time. The probability of a negative test in patients without anxiety or depression who had typical pain was 8% in men and 32% in women; the probability of a negative test in patients who were both anxious and depressed and had atypical pain was 97% in men and 99% in women. Diagnostic exercise testing in patients with both affective symptoms and atypical chest pain may be unhelpful, misleading, and uneconomical.

Relation of chest pain to degree of myocardial ischemia

Because therapeutic decisions in patients with angina pectoris are usually based on the reported frequency of exertional and rest pain, the relations

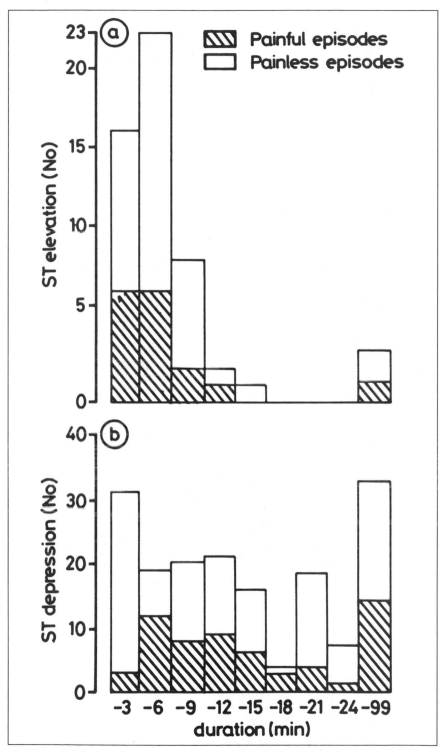

Fig. 1-20.   Number of episodes of ST elevation (a) and ST depression (b) by duration of episode (<10 minutes or ≥10 minutes). There were more short episodes with ST elevation (p <0.001). The proportion of painful episodes is not significantly greater with longer episodes (>10 minutes). Reproduced with permission from Arnim et al.[94]

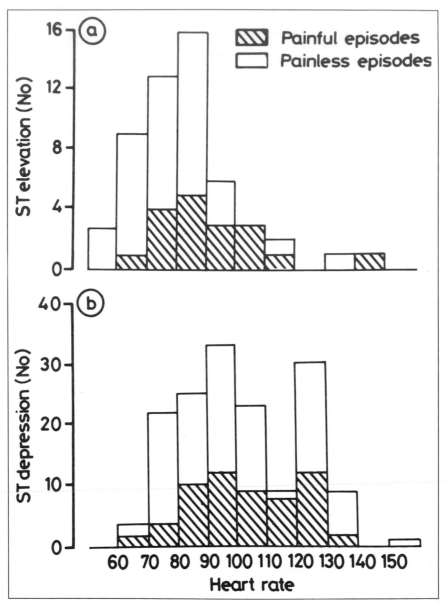

Fig. 1-21. Number of episodes of ST elevation (a) and ST depression (b) by heart rate at which ischemia became apparent. Most episodes with ST elevation occurred at heart rates >90 beats/minute. Reproduced with permission from Arnim et al.[94]

between the historical frequency of chest pain and objective evidence of myocardial ischemia during normal activity were investigated by Quyyumi and associates[96] from London, UK, in 100 patients by 48-hour ambulatory ST-segment monitoring. Of these 100 consecutive patients with chest pain, 91 had typical pain and 9 some atypical features. Twenty-six patients had normal coronary arteries and 52 of the 74 with significant CAD had ambulatory ST-segment changes. There was no relation between the frequency of reported exertional or rest pain and the severity of CAD or the frequency of daytime or nocturnal ST-segment changes. Twelve patients had nocturnal ST-segment changes and 4 had nocturnal angina. Most patients had both painful and painless episodes of ST-segment changes, but a substantial number had either painless or painful episodes only. These differences were not related to the severity of CAD. Chest pain after the onset of ST-segment change was perceived with wide interpatient and intrapatient variability. Thus, the frequency of pain is a poor indicator of the frequency of significant cardiac ischemia. Individual differences in the perception of pain may be more important.

Variation in exercise tolerance

Waters and coworkers[97] from Montreal, Canada, evaluated the frequency and mechanism of variable threshold angina in 28 patients with stable effort angina and exercise-induced ST-segment depression. In each patient, treadmill exercise tests were performed at 8 AM on 4 days within a 2-week period and on 1 of these days, 3 additional tests at 9 AM, 11 AM, and 4 PM were obtained. During the test, the time to 1 mm ST depression increased from 277 ± 172 seconds on day 1 to 319 ± 186 seconds on day 2, 352 ± 213 seconds on day 3, and 356 ± 207 seconds on day 4. The rate-BP product at 1 mm ST-segment depression remained constant. In addition, time to 1 mm ST depression increased from 333 ± 197 seconds at 8 AM to 371 ± 201 seconds at 9 AM and to 401 ± 207 seconds at 11 AM and decreased to 371 ± 189 seconds at 4 PM. Rate-BP products at 1 mm ST-segment depression remained constant. Among these patients, the SD for time to 1 mm ST depression, estimated as a percent of the mean for each patient's 7 tests and then averaged for the entire group, was 22 ± 11%. However, the SD for heart rate-BP products at 1 mm ST-segment depression was significantly less (8.4 ± 2.8%). These data suggest considerable variation in exercise tolerance in patients with effort angina, even when the double product at the onset of ischemia remains relatively constant. The variation is frequent enough that it would not appear to be explained solely on the basis of variations in coronary vasculature tone.

Relation of exercise ST/HR slope to LV function and degree of coronary narrowing

A rate-related change in ST-segment depression with exercise (ST/HR slope) of ≥6.0 μV/beat/min has been proposed as an active predictor of 3-vessel CAD. To assess the accuracy and functional correlates of this method further, Kligfield and associates[98] from New York City compared exercise ECGs with radionuclide rest and exercise LVEF and angiography in 35 patients with stable angina. The ST/HR slope was significantly increased in patients with 3-vessel CAD. An ST/HR slope of ≥6.0 identified 3-vessel CAD with a sensitivity of 89% and specificity of 88%. The predictive value for 3-vessel CAD was 73% owing to the presence of 3 false positive slopes. The patients from whom these slopes were derived had functionally severe 2-vessel CAD, with an average decrease in exercise LVEF of 13%. Two of these 3 had additional LM CAD and the third had unsuspected additional AR. For the entire group, the exercise ST/HR slope was linearly related to the exercise change in LVEF. Mean exercise change in LVEF for stable angina patients with ST/HR slopes of ≥4.5 was significantly different from that for patients with lower ST/HR slopes (−12 ± 1 -vs- +2 ± 2%). Thus, the ST/HR slope is both sensitive and specific for the identification of 3-vessel CAD, and high ST/HR slopes in patients with less extensive anatomic disease may predict functionally severe ischemia.

Dipyridamole-echocardiography test

Picano and associates[99] from Pisa, Italy, assessed the clinical feasibility and usefulness of dipyridamole infusion for the detection of CAD by using 2-D echo and 12-lead ECG monitoring. Dipyridamole infusion (0.14 mg/kg/min for 4 minutes) was performed in 66 consecutive patients with effort chest pain and in 9 control subjects. Among the 28 patients with positive dipyridamole-echo test responses, 18 had diagnostic ECG changes (ST-segment depression on anterolateral leads), but these changes were unrelated to the site of asynergy. The dipyridamole-echo test had an overall sensitivity of 56% and specificity of 100% for the presence of CAD. Exercise stress testing had an overall sensitivity of 62% and a specificity of 80%. Thus, the dipyridamole-echo test, which is feasible in essentially all patients with good basal echoes, has a lower overall sensitivity in detecting CAD than exercise stress testing but a higher specificity, detects the site of apparent ischemia as identified by regional asynergy more precisely than exercise testing, and can unmask ECG silent effort ischemia.

Coronary angiographic findings

Ambrose and associates[100] from New York City studied the coronary angiographic morphology in patients with unstable angina pectoris, attempting to provide further insight into mechanisms responsible for angina. The morphology of coronary artery lesions was qualitatively assessed at angiography in 110 patients with either stable or unstable angina. Each obstruction reducing the luminal diameter of the artery by ≥50% was categorized into 1 of the following morphologic groups: concentric (symmetric narrowing), type I eccentric (asymmetric narrowing with smooth borders and a broad neck), type II eccentric (asymmetric with a narrow neck or irregular borders or both), and multiple irregular coronary narrowings in series. Among these patients, type II eccentric lesions were more frequent in the 63 patients with unstable angina pectoris (Table 1-9). Concentric and type I eccentric lesions were seen more frequently in the 47 patients with stable angina pectoris. These data suggest that type II eccentric lesions are frequent in patients with unstable angina pectoris. These lesions may represent ruptured atherosclerotic plaques or partially occlusive thrombi.

Bresnahan and associates[101] from Rochester, Minnesota, studied patients with unstable angina pectoris to determine the frequency of coronary thrombi. Coronary angiograms of 268 consecutive patients undergoing diagnostic angiography were examined for intracoronary thrombus. Among

TABLE 1-9. *Angiographic morphology of coronary artery obstructions ≥50% and <100% in all 110 patients. Reproduced with permission from Ambrose et al.[100]*

	STABLE ANGINA PECTORIS (n = 47)	UNSTABLE ANGINA PECTORIS (n = 63)
# of vessels	55	92
Concentric	26 (47%)†	24 (26%)
Type I eccentric	19 (35%)*	16 (17%)
Type II eccentric	4 (7%)	50 (54%)‡
Multiple irregularities	6 (11%)*	2 (2%)

*p <0.05, †p <0.01, ‡p <0.001 by Student's *t* test.

these patients, 29 (11%) had angiographic evidence of coronary artery thrombi. Among the 29 patients with presumed thrombi, 24 (83%) had unstable angina before angiography. The remaining 5 patients with presumed thrombi had a transmural AMI 3–18 months before cardiac catheterization. In 21 patients, the presumed thrombus was distal to a significant stenosis; in 8, it was proximal to or at the site of a significant stenosis. Coronary artery thrombi were identified in 24 (36%) of 67 patients with unstable angina compared with only 5 (2.5%) of 201 patients with stable angina pectoris.

Capone and associates[102] from Philadelphia, Pennsylvania, surveyed angiograms of 119 patients with unstable angina who had rest pain within 14 days of angiography and 35 patients with stable angina. Patients with unstable angina were subgrouped according to how recent angina at rest was at the time of angiography. Group I consisted of 44 patients in whom rest pain occurred within 24 hours before angiography. The 75 patients in group II had angina at rest between 1 and 14 days before angiography. Patients in group II had stable angina. The angiographic criterion for intracoronary thrombus was an intraluminal filling defect, surrounded by contrast medium on 3 sides, located just distal to or within a coronary stenosis, as assessed by each of 2 independent observers blinded to the nature of the anginal syndrome and its temporal proximity. Intracoronary thrombi were found in 44 (37%) of 119 patients with unstable angina and 0 of 35 patients with stable angina. Intracoronary thrombi were found in 23 of 44 patients (52%) in group I and 21 of 75 (28%) in group II. Thus, intracoronary thrombi were common in patients with unstable angina who had active symptoms. They were less frequent in patients with recently unstable angina whose symptoms were well controlled, and absent in patients with stable angina.

Coronary hemodynamic responses

MacDonald and associates[103] from Gainesville, Florida, evaluated the mechanisms of spontaneous angina pectoris during cardiac catheterization in 13 patients who had angina occurring without provocation at rest. LV and systemic hemodynamics, coronary venous flows (thermodilution technique), ECG, and coronary angiograms were recorded before and during spontaneous angina. Angiography during spontaneous angina showed that 5 patients had coronary spasm (group I) and 8 patients did not (group II). In group II there was a preponderance of multivessel CAD. LV end-diastolic pressure increased in all patients in both groups during spontaneous angina. In group I, 4 patients had transient ST elevation and 1 patient had peaked T waves during angina. Transient ST depression occurred during spontaneous angina in all group II patients. Group I patients had decreased coronary sinus flow (4 of 5 patients) or decreased regional flow (5 of 5) during spontaneous angina. Coronary resistance and ratio of double product to coronary blood flow increased in all patients. In group II, coronary hemodynamic responses during spontaneous angina varied. Coronary venous flows, coronary resistance and ratio of double product to coronary blood flow showed no uniform pattern. Thus, patients with severe CAD can have spontaneous angina without angiographic findings of coronary spasm. After analysis of angiograms and coronary hemodynamics in these patients, no apparent uniform mechanism for spontaneous angina was found.

Coronary air embolism -vs- coronary spasm

Heupler and associates[104] from Cleveland, Ohio, described angiographic and ECG manifestations of coronary air embolism in 4 patients. All 4 had angina pectoris, 2 had ST elevation, 1 had ST depression, and 1 had no ECG change after the air embolus. Although the initial diagnosis in these 4 patients was coronary artery spasm, a subsequent ergonovine test response for coronary artery spasm was negative in the 3 patients in whom it was performed. The leading edge of contrast material that followed an air embolism stopped abruptly, appeared hazy and blunt, and pulsated back and forth. The air embolus produced temporary cessation of flow in the main artery and its branches. Initial injection of air during coronary angiography mimics coronary artery spasm by producing a syndrome characterized by angina, ischemic changes on the ECG, and delayed flow of contrast material. An initial air embolus may be differentiated from true coronary spasm by several distinct angiographic features.

Thromboxane A_2 production

In a study carried out by Serneri and colleagues[105] from Florence, Italy, thromboxane B_2 (TXB_2), the stable metabolite of thromboxane A_2 (TXA_2), was measured in the coronary sinus and in aortic blood before and after cold pressor test (CPT) in 21 patients with CAD (7 affected by stable effort angina and 14 by unstable angina) and in 12 patients without myocardial ischemia (control group) during coronary angiography. Aspirin (10 mg/kg intravenously) was administered before catheterization to prevent platelet and leukocyte TXA_2 formation. Control subjects and patients with effort angina had TXB_2 resting levels lower than unstable angina patients without a transcardiac gradient that, on the contrary, was found in unstable angina patients. Only in these patients CPT resulted in a significant TXB_2 increase more marked in the coronary sinus (from 50 ± 19–73 ± 35 pg/ml) than in the aorta (from 33 ± 17–43 ± 24 pg/ml) so that the transcardiac TXB_2 gradient significantly increased. In all but 2 unstable angina patients, TXB_2 elevation was not associated with a decrease of cardiac lactate extraction. The resting and CPT-induced TXB_2 gradients were unrelated to the presence and severity of coronary angiographic lesions. These results indicate that unstable angina patients show an abnormal cardiocoronary capacity to synthesize TXA_2, which seems not to be elicited by the occurrence of myocardial ischemia.

Pacing-induced

Sasayama and associates[106] Kyoto, Japan, studied mechanisms responsible for alterations in the diastolic properties of the LV during angina in 7 patients with CAD. Single-plane left ventriculograms were obtained using a high fidelity micromanometer-tipped catheter in both the resting state and immediately after rapid cardiac pacing. Typical angina pectoris developed with pacing stress in each patient. After atrial pacing, the LV end-diastolic pressure increased from 10 ± 3–21 ± 7 mmHg ($\pm$SD) irrespective of the changes in end-diastolic volume. The LVEF declined from 59 ± 10–$48 \pm 13\%$ ($p < 0.05$). In these studies, regional myocardial function was evaluated by a radial coordinate system with the origin at the center of gravity of the end-diastolic silhouette. Two representative radial grids for normal and ischemic segments were selected. In the normal segments, the end-diastolic length was increased by 15% and was associated with a 24% increase in stroke excursion with pacing stress. Increases in diastolic pressure were accompanied by similar increases in end-diastolic length, and the diastolic pressure-length relation moved up to a higher portion of the single curve. In the ischemic segment, the end-diastolic length remained unchanged in the postpacing beat, but segment shortening was significantly reduced. Diastolic pressure was higher for any given length and the pressure-length curve shifted upward with pacing-induced angina, suggesting intrinsic alterations in the function of the diastolic properties of the ischemic myocardium. Cellular mechanisms responsible for these changes in regional diastolic function during angina pectoris were not identified. These results confirm data presented by others that there are fundamental alterations in regional diastolic function and compliance that occur with myocardial ischemia.

McDaniel and associates[107] from Birmingham, Alabama, investigated the metabolic and mechanical effects of a solution of glucose-insulin-potassium (GIK) in 18 patients who underwent diagnostic cardiac catheterization for CAD. All patients were paced at a rate of approximately 140 beats/min before and after infusion of GIK. Basal and paced LV end-diastolic pressure, dP/dt, arterial substrate levels, and osmolarity were measured in all 18 patients. In 13 patients the cardiac index also was measured. GIK increased the blood sugar level to approximately 200 mg/dl and increased the serum osmolarity 9 mOsm. Pacing alone increased the cardiac index 4% and pacing with GIK increased the cardiac index 6%. Pacing before GIK augmented dP/dt (21%) and pacing with GIK increased it (30%). The metabolic changes noted included a shift in the respiratory quotient from 0.77–0.96 with GIK infusion. During GIK infusion, the myocardial oxygen consumption at rest increased from 17–22 ml/min (23%). Myocardial oxygen consumption during pacing was similar before and after GIK infusion. Before GIK infusion, nitrogen balance was slightly positive; after GIK infusion, it was negative with regard to the nitrogen-containing compounds measured. Thus, infusion of GIK at this concentration and rate alters myocardial carbohydrate, lipid, and nitrogen metabolism, with a significant increase in myocardial contraction.

Although systolic and diastolic dysfunction have been described during pacing-induced ischemia, the temporal sequence of systolic and diastolic impairment has not been established. Aroesty and coinvestigators[108] from Boston, Massachusetts, studied 22 patients with CAD by pacing at increasing heart rates with simultaneous hemodynamic monitoring, ECG recording, and radionuclide ventriculography. From synchronized LV pressure tracings and radionuclide volume curves, 3 sequential pressure-volume diagrams were constructed for each patient corresponding to baseline and intermediate and maximum pacing levels. Eleven patients (group I) had a nonischemic response to pacing tachycardia without chest pain, significant ECG changes, or significant increase in LV end-diastolic pressure (LVEDP) in the immediate postpacing period. These patients demonstrated a progressive decrease in LVEDP, end-diastolic volume, and end-systolic volume, no change in cardiac output or LVEF, and a progressive increase in LV diastolic peak filling rate and the end-systolic pressure to volume ratio. Pressure-volume diagrams shifted progressively leftward and slightly downward, suggesting both an increase in contractility and a mild increase in LV distensibility. The remaining 11 patients (group II) had an ischemic response to pacing tachycardia, with each patient having angina pectoris, demonstrating >1 mm ST-segment depression on the ECG, and had >5 mmHg increase in LVEDP immediately after pacing. LVEDP, end-diastolic volume, and end-systolic volume in these patients initially decreased and then subsequently increased during angina, with no change in cardiac output but a decrease in EF. LV peak diastolic filling rate and the LV end-systolic pressure to volume ratio both increased at the intermediate pacing rate but decreased at maximum pacing. Pressure-volume diagrams for these patients shifted leftward initially, then back to the right, during intermediate and peak pacing levels, often with an upward shift in the diastolic pressure to volume relationship. LVEDP in group II was significantly higher than that in group I at the intermediate pacing level, with no difference in end-diastolic or end-systolic volumes, suggesting decreased LV distensibility in these patients before the onset of systolic dysfunction at the maximum pacing level. The investigators concluded that an ischemic response to pacing tachycardia involved both systolic and diastolic dysfunction, with diastolic impairment often preceding systolic depression.

Significance of coronary arterial adventitial inflammation

Kohchi and coinvestigators[109] from Kitakyushu, Japan, quantitatively analyzed the adventitial inflammation of the coronary artery with intimal lesions in 12 patients who died from CAD and had had unstable angina at rest (group 1). After necropsy, the investigators examined epon-embedded cross-sections by light and electron microscopy, paying particular attention to the adventitia, and compared these results with those in 6 patients who had had angina but died of noncardiac causes (group 2) and those in 22 patients who did not have angina (group 3). Of the 132 segments from group 1 patients, 39 (30%) were narrowed 76–100% by atherosclerotic plaque (group 2, 27%; group 3, 1%), and 23 (17%) had occlusive thrombi. Of the 264 sections (2 from each segment) from group 1 that were examined, 98 (37%) (group 2, 15%; group 3, 9%) revealed clustered infiltrates of inflammatory cells in the adventitia, half of which were associated with vascular nerve involvement. These findings in adventitia may be related to the vasospastic component of unstable angina.

Effect of antianginal therapy on exercise test

Mukharji and associates[110] from Dallas, Texas, examined the effect of antianginal therapy on the incidence of an early positive exercise response as a screening tool for 3-vessel and LM CAD. Fifty-seven men with stable angina pectoris underwent bicycle ergometry before and after long-acting nitrate or calcium antagonist therapy was instituted. An early positive response was defined as signs of myocardial ischemia at low levels of myocardial and total body workload (corresponding to a workload of <300 kpm/min). Thirty-nine patients (68%) had an early positive response before therapy, compared with 14 (24%) after therapy. Of 24 patients undergoing coronary angiography, 12 had 3-vessel CAD (including 2 with LM), 5 had 2-vessel CAD, 6 had 1-vessel CAD, and 1 patient had no CAD. The sensitivity and specificity of an early positive response in predicting 3-vessel/LM CAD changed from 92 and 58% before to 42 and 75% after therapy. The positive and negative predictive values changed from 69 and 88% before to 63 and 63% after therapy. It was concluded that antianginal therapy reduces the value of an exercise test as a screening tool for 3-vessel/LM CAD.

Relation of time of medical training to type of therapy prescribed

Charap and associates[111] from New York City hypothesized that identifiable characteristics in a physician's background would influence the management of any condition. A vignette describing a patient with new-onset angina and a questionnaire ascertaining individual physician characteristics and management preferences were sent to attending physicians and house staff in the Department of Medicine at New York University School of Medicine.

Although physicians believed strongly that the patient had angina on the basis of the history, there was no consensus about managing the patient. The age of the physician was the single most important predictor of management, with the younger half of the sample more likely to hospitalize, less likely to prescribe nitroglycerin as a sole therapy, and more likely to prescribe β-blockers. The era in which a physician trains may determine practices that persist for a lifetime.

Buccal and oral nitrates

Parker and associates[112] from Kingston, Canada, studied 16 patients with chronic stable angina pectoris to compare the hemodynamic and antianginal effects of buccal nitroglycerin (NTG) in a dose of 3 mg administered 3 times daily and oral isosorbide dinitrate (ISDN) in a dose of 30 mg administered 4 times daily. Compared with placebo, both oral ISDN and buccal NTG treatment induced a decrease in systolic BP at rest over a 5-hour period during acute but not during sustained therapy. Neither buccal NTG nor oral ISDN modified the changes in systolic BP during exercise. Both treatment programs were associated with a higher exercise heart rate during acute therapy. During sustained treatment with buccal NTG, the heart rate during exercise remained greater than that during placebo throughout the 5-hour test period, but during treatment with oral ISDN, only the exercise heart rate at 1 hour was greater than that seen with placebo. Treadmill walking time to the onset of angina and to the development of moderate angina increased significantly during acute therapy with both buccal NTG and oral ISDN (Figs. 1-22 and 1-23). The clinical efficacy of buccal NTG was maintained after 2 weeks of 3 times daily therapy. In contrast, during 4 times daily therapy with oral ISDN, treadmill walking time was prolonged for only 1 hour after drug administration. This investigation indicates that tolerance develops during 4 times daily therapy with oral ISDN, but 3 times daily therapy with buccal NTG is not associated with diminished antianginal effects.

In an investigation carried out by Kaski and colleagues[113] from London, UK, exercise tolerance before and after sublingual ISDN, 10 mg, was assessed in 217 consecutive patients with stable angina, positive exercise test, and angiographically proved CAD. In 65 patients (30%), ISDN prevented exercise-induced ST-segment depression and/or increased exercise time to 1 mm ST-segment depression (≥ 3 minutes), despite the significantly higher ($\geq 25 \times 10^2$ increment) rate-BP product attained (increased coronary reserve). In 40 other patients, exercise test remained positive, and neither time to 1 mm ST-segment depression nor rate-BP product increased significantly (fixed coronary reserve). The remaining 106 patients had an intermediate response. To assess the mechanisms underlying the beneficial action of nitrates, these investigators further examined 13 patients with increased coronary reserve (group 1) and 5 with fixed coronary reserve (group 2) by the exercise response to ISDN and verapamil, the changes in LV volumes after ISDN and verapamil, the ECG response to intravenous ergonovine, and the changes in coronary stenosis severity after intravenous ergonovine and intracoronary nitrates. ISDN dramatically improved exercise capacity only in group 1 patients. It induced a significant reduction of LV volumes in both groups. Ergonovine provoked angina and ST-segment depression in 62% of group 1 patients and significantly increased the severity of their coronary stenoses. In all group 2 patients, ergonovine was negative, and no significant increase in stenosis severity was observed. Intracoronary nitrates reduced stenosis severity in group 1 (p <0.01) but not in group 2. These results suggest that in a large proportion of patients with chronic stable angina who dramatically

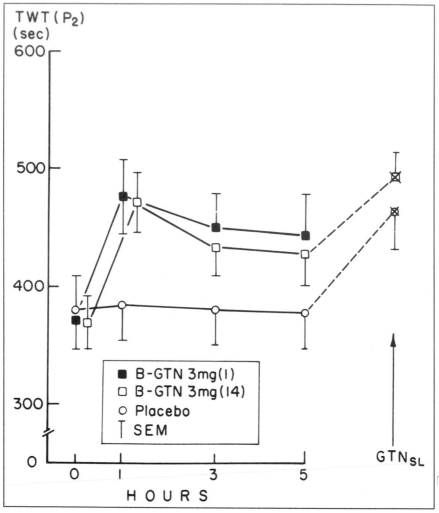

Fig. 1-22. Treadmill walking time (TWT) to the development of moderate angina (P_2) during placebo therapy, after the first dose of 3 mg of buccal NTG (■) and after the same dose on day 14 (□). The response to sublingual NTG (GTN_{SL}) is shown. Values represent mean ± SEM. TWT was significantly prolonged over placebo (p <0.01) at each testing time during acute and sustained therapy.

improve exercise capacity with sublingual nitrates, the beneficial effects of these drugs are due to an increase in coronary flow reserve rather than to a decreased myocardial oxygen demand.

Badger and associates[114] from Seattle, Washington, studied the response to sublingual ISDN in 10 men with suspected CAD who underwent coronary arteriography. A Swan-Ganz catheter was placed in the PA to record hemodynamic response. Diseased coronary segments were identified during routine Judkins selective coronary angiograms. Sublingual ISDN (5 or 10 mg) was then given with the catheters in place. Multiple sequential single-view coronary and pulmonary and systemic hemodynamic responses were recorded over 30 minutes after drug administration. At 30 minutes, there was a 53% reduction in PA wedge pressure and a 15% decrease in systemic and

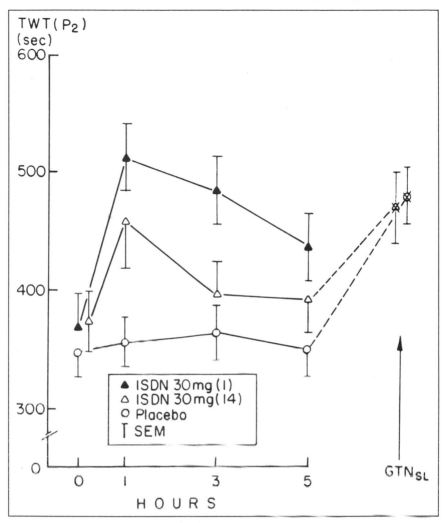

Fig. 1-23. Treadmill walking time (TWT) to the development of moderate angina (P_2) during placebo therapy, after the first dose of 30 mg of ISDN (▲) and after the same dose on day 14 (△). The response to sublingual NTG (GTN_{SL}) is shown. Values represent mean ± SEM. TWT was significantly prolonged over placebo (p <0.01) at each testing time during acute therapy. During sustained therapy, only the 1-hour value was > the placebo value (p <0.01).

pulmonary vascular resistance, with a net 13% decrease in cardiac output and 20% decrease in mean arterial pressure. Quantitative arteriography demonstrated substantial dilation of luminal cross-sectional area in both normal and diseased coronary arterial segments. Normal epicardial segments were grouped according to luminal area (1–4, 4–8, and >8 mm^2) and demonstrated maximal area dilation at 10 minutes of 55, 29, and 16%, respectively. Diseased epicardial segments (stenosis ≥50%) dilated 51% at 10 minutes. Calculated stenosis resistance decreased 40%. Diseased segments in small and middle-sized arteries (1–8 mm^2) were 4 times more reactive than those in larger arteries (>8 mm^2), with peak dilation of 77 -vs- 21% at 30 minutes. These responses occurred within 3 minutes after ISDN administration, peaked at 10 minutes, and persisted, unchanged, for the remaining 20 minutes. The response of epicardial arteries to ISDN is the maximum observed with any coronary vasodilating drug.

Transdermal glyceryl trinitrate

James and associates[115] from Bristol, UK, assessed the efficacy of a new transdermal preparation of glyceryl trinitrate in the 24-hour prophylaxis of angina and determined the duration of effect of a single patch application. Twelve men with chronic stable angina were studied in a randomized, placebo controlled, double-blind trial. By serial treadmill exercise testing, a therapeutic effect was shown at 3 hours; the exercise time to angina and to 1 mm ST-segment depression and the total exercise time were all significantly increased. At 24, 48, and 72 hours, however, no therapeutic effect was observed. Recent studies have shown a similar lack of effect at 24 hours for various forms of transdermal delivery systems. It was suggested that this lack of effect was due to the rapid onset of tolerance, probably as a result of the constancy of blood concentrations obtained by this method of administration.

Lin and Flaherty[116] from Baltimore, Maryland, examined the safety and efficacy of titrating a nitroglycerin (NTG) infusion to a fixed hemodynamic endpoint as initial therapy for patients admitted to a coronary care unit for medically refractory unstable angina, and to test the hypothesis that patients responding to the addition of intravenous (IV) NTG to their present antianginal regimen could be crossed over to NTG administered by a new transdermal delivery system. In 9 patients, the NTG infusion titrated upward at 3–10-minute intervals until a 10% reduction in mean arterial pressure was achieved. This titration schedule and hemodynamic endpoint proved safe and effective for controlling episodes of chest pain at rest in all 9 patients. Subsequently, this treatment strategy was tested in 17 consecutive patients with unstable angina treated in the coronary care unit during a 1-month period. In 10 of 15 successfully treated patients ischemia was the cause of chest pain, as documented by cardiac catheterization. No change was made in antianginal or vasoactive drugs during the period of IV NTG administration or during crossover to transdermal therapy. In this well-defined subgroup of patients with unstable angina, NTG infusion decreased the mean arterial pressure from 101 ± 18–87 ± 11 mmHg (mean ± SD), using an infusion rate of 84 ± 74 μg/min (range, 10–200). The mean duration of IV therapy was 36 ± 12 hours. In 4.8 ± 0.9 hours, all 10 patients were weaned off IV therapy and crossed over in a stepwise fashion to a mean dose of 23 ± 10 mg/24 hours of transdermal NTG patches (range, 5–40 mg/24 hours), while maintaining the mean arterial pressure reduction previously achieved after initiation of IV therapy (Fig. 1-24). Mean arterial pressure was 86 ± 11 mmHg with IV therapy immediately before crossover and was maintained at 83 ± 9 and 85 ± 11 mmHg 1 and 24 hours after crossover to transdermal NTG therapy, respectively. Two patients had episodes of chest pain during the first 24 hours of transdermal therapy. Both became pain free after upward titration of the transdermal dose by 10 mg/24 hours. Among these 10 patients, 7 had no further episodes of pain throughout the remainder of the hospitalization. One patient had a single episode of chest pain after transient interruption of transdermal NTG therapy and 1 patient had a single episode of pain after transient reduction in the transdermal dose. These results suggest that IV NTG, titrated to reduce mean arterial pressure by 10%, is safe and effective treatment for patients with unstable angina admitted to

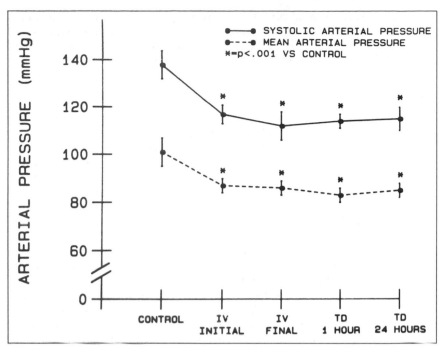

Fig. 1-24. Arterial pressure response to IV and transdermal (TD) NTG. Solid line = systolic pressure during control period before IV NTG. IV final = systolic pressure at the end of IV infusion just before beginning tapering; IV initial = systolic pressure after initial titration; TD 1 hour = systolic pressure 1 hour after crossover to the TD preparation; TD 24 hours = systolic pressure 24 hours after crossover.

a coronary care unit, and that the new transdermal NTG delivery systems can be used successfully to maintain the beneficial anti-ischemic effects initially achieved with IV NTG therapy.

Molsidomine

In studies carried out by Rudolph and Dirschinger[117] from Munich, West Germany, molsidomine, similar to nitrates, improved myocardial blood flow in hypoperfused, poststenotic myocardial regions, reduced LV pressure and volumes, and led to improvement in impaired regional wall motion. In patients with chronic, stable angina who underwent long-term treatment with 2 mg of molsidomine 3 times daily there were reductions in ST-segment depression of 45 and 9% at 1 and 3 hours after administration, respectively, and slight but statistically significant reductions in the rates of anginal attacks and nitrate consumption of 16 and 18%. Administration of 3 mg 3 times daily did not render more significant effects. Doubling the frequency of administration (2 mg 6 times daily) led to reductions in the rates of anginal attacks and nitrate consumption of 38 and 36%, respectively, and 4 mg led to a more marked reduction in ST-segment depression of 57%. With administration of 8 mg of sustained-release molsidomine, a prolonged anti-ischemic effect was documented with reductions in ST-segment depression of 74% at 1 hour and 31% at 8 hours after medication. In patients with CHF 1 hour after administration, 4 mg of molsidomine significantly reduced systolic and diastolic PA pressures of 25 and 30%, respectively. After 7 days of continuous treatment with 4 mg of molsidomine 4 times daily, comparable reductions in PA pressure were observed. Thus, molsidomine, in adequate dosages, elicits an unequivocal anti-ischemic and antianginal effect and a salutary reduction in LV filling pressure.

Labetalol

Quyyumi and associates[118] from London, England, investigated the effect of a combined α- and β-receptor antagonist, labetalol, in 10 patients with chronic stable angina pectoris. The optimal dose was determined during an initial dose titration when the patients were treated with 200, 400, and 600 mg (6 patients) of labetalol a day. The effective dose was then compared with placebo in a double-blind randomized study. The effects of the drug were monitored with anginal diaries, treadmill exercise testing, and 48-hour ambulatory ECG ST-segment monitoring. Plasma labetalol concentrations were measured during each treatment period. The mean effective antianginal dose of labetalol was 480 mg/day given by mouth twice a day. There was a dose-related reduction in daytime and nocturnal heart rate, the frequency of pain was significantly reduced by 41%, and exercise duration was significantly increased by 44% with labetalol when compared with placebo. The frequency and duration of the episodes of ST-segment depression were significantly reduced by 56 and 73%, respectively. Adverse effects resulted in a reduction of the dose of labetalol in 2 patients. Thus, labetalol is an effective agent in the treatment of angina pectoris.

Diltiazem

Although calcium-blocking agents have proved effective in the therapy of exertional and variant angina pectoris, the influence on LV function is complex and might affect abnormalities of systolic and diastolic function in patients with CAD. To assess the effect of diltiazem on LV systolic regional wall motion and diastolic function in patients with CAD, Dash and colleagues[119] from Hershey, Pennsylvania, performed biplane LV cineangiography before and after intravenous diltiazem in 22 patients. LV and RV pressures were measured by micromanometer-tipped catheters. Regional wall motion was assessed quantitatively with an area EF technique. Diltiazem decreased mean arterial pressure and heart rate and increased cardiac index and global EF. LV end-diastolic pressure increased 14% and LV end-systolic pressure to volume ratio exceeded 9%. Diltiazem decreased the time constant of LV relaxation by 14% despite lack of change in the LV diastolic pressure to volume relation in 16 patients. Diltiazem caused significant increase in area EF in 53% of hypokinetic areas supplied by narrowed coronary arteries compared with 13% of normokinetic areas supplied by narrowed arteries. Response of EF to diltiazem in areas supplied by normal coronary arteries was less than that in hypokinetic areas supplied by narrowed arteries. Thus, diltiazem improves regional wall motion abnormalities in patients with CAD and the improvement is associated with better LV relaxation but not with a change in the diastolic pressure to volume relations. Despite a mild negative inotropic effect, global indexes of LV systolic performance are favorably influenced by diltiazem.

Joyal and associates[120] from Gainesville, Florida, examined systemic and coronary hemodynamic effects of intravenous diltiazem, administered as a bolus of 250 μg/kg followed by an infusion of 1.4 μg/kg/min, in 14 patients with effort angina. There was no change in heart rate despite significant decreases in systolic, diastolic, and mean systemic pressures (13, 10, and 11%, respectively). The BP decrease was closely correlated with the initial BP. Neither LV end-diastolic pressure nor peak dP/dt changed significantly, but peripheral vascular resistance decreased 16% and stroke volume index increased 10%. The BP-heart rate product decreased 15%, but coronary blood flow was maintained as coronary resistance decreased 14%. Diltiazem increased regional coronary flow in some patients. Thus, intravenous diltiazem dilates coronary and systemic resistance vessels, without an increase in heart rate, favorably altering indexes of myocardial oxygen supply and demand.

To determine the systemic and coronary hemodynamic effects of diltiazem at rest and during pacing, Josephson and associates[121] from Los Angeles, California, administered diltiazem intravenously to 14 patients with stable angina pectoris undergoing coronary angiography before and after 0.17 mg/kg (n = 7) and 0.25 mg/kg (n = 7). Hemodynamic variables, metabolic measurements, and LVEF were obtained at rest and during coronary sinus pacing before and during diltiazem administration. Lactate production during control pacing turned into extraction after diltiazem. At rest, systemic resistance was reduced by 21% and mean arterial pressure by 12%; cardiac index increased from 2.4 ± 0.4–2.6 ± 0.4 L/min/m², with no significant change in heart rate. The mean PA pressure increased from 17 ± 2–19 ± 3 mmHg, but other hemodynamic variables were not affected. Diltiazem given during pacing reduced the mean aortic pressure (from 112 ± 15–104 ± 15 mmHg), but other hemodynamic variables were not affected significantly. LVEF decreased 16%, from 0.63 ± 0.9–0.53 ± 0.8 with coronary sinus pacing; when the pacing was performed after diltiazem administration, the 8% decrease in LVEF from 0.64 ± 0.09–0.59 ± 13 was less marked. Diltiazem had no significant effect on LVEF at rest. The overall data suggest that the ischemic manifestations of coronary sinus pacing are attenuated by diltiazem in doses of the drug that exert no significant depressant effect on LV function in patients with CAD.

To assess the long-term efficacy of diltiazem for angina pectoris, 8 patients with chronic stable exertional angina who were previously entered into a 4-month randomized, double-blind placebo controlled study, were investigated for an additional 12 months by Petru and associates[122] from San Antonio, Texas. The patients continued to take diltiazem, 360 mg/day, and underwent treadmill exercise testing after 10 and 16 months of therapy. A single-blind placebo week was introduced after 16 months and a treadmill test was performed at the end of this week. Diltiazem therapy continued to augment exercise duration until 0.1 mV of ST depression at 10 and 16 months compared with the final placebo period: 573 ± 133 seconds at 10 months; 565 ± 148 seconds at 16 months; -vs- 431 ± 151 seconds at final placebo. Also, the time to angina pectoris was prolonged on diltiazem by 181 seconds at 16 months and the total duration of exercise was increased by 101 seconds compared with placebo. In addition, angina frequency decreased from 17 ± 11 attacks/week on placebo to 0.6 ± 0.6 attacks/week during diltiazem therapy at 16 months. Two of the 8 patients had mild pedal edema, but no other adverse effects. Thus, diltiazem, 360 mg/day, can be an effective single agent for the long-term treatment of chronic stable angina pectoris.

Calcium-entry blocking drugs produce different effects on systemic and coronary hemodynamics and myocardial oxygen extraction. Kern and associates[123] from San Antonio, Texas, examined the effects on myocardial oxygen extraction, intravenous diltiazem (100 μg/kg bolus with a continuous 10 μg/kg/min infusion) in 11 CAD patients at rest and during controlled heart rates (100 ± 5 and 120 ± 5 beats/min). At rest, diltiazem decreased mean arterial pressure from 109 ± 13–99 ± 14 mmHg, increased heart rate from

64 ± 12–74 ± 14 beats/min, and decreased coronary sinus resistance (1.02 ± 0.41–0.87 ± 0.40 U). Myocardial oxygen extraction was significantly reduced, since coronary sinus oxygen content increased (6.0 ± 0.9–7.8 ± 1.2 ml/dl) and the arterial-coronary sinus oxygen difference decreased (12 ± 2–11 ± 2 ml/dl). Similar changes occurred with heart rate held constant. There were no significant changes in absolute coronary sinus blood flow, calculated myocardial oxygen consumption, or LV rate of pressure increase. Diltiazem decreased mean arterial pressure while reducing both myocardial oxygen extraction and coronary arterial resistance, suggesting that a principal mechanism of a beneficial effect on the coronary circulation appears to be an improvement in myocardial oxygen extraction relative to myocardial oxygen demand.

Nifedipine

Feldman and associates[124] from Gainesville, Florida, studied 13 patients with exercise-induced angina and proximal LAD occlusion in 11 and critical LAD narrowing in 2 to determine mechanisms responsible for the beneficial effects of nifedipine in relieving effort angina. Nifedipine was given bucally in a dose of 10 or 20 mg and 1 that decreased aortic pressure 5 mmHg or more. Nifedipine increased collateral flow as measured by regional thermo-dilution in only 3 patients, but consistently decreased coronary resistance in the LV anterior region. The anterior region myocardial oxygen consumption did not change significantly after nifedipine therapy. During atrial pacing stress, angina occurred in all patients before nifedipine and at the same or lower heart rate in 9 patients after nifedipine. Collateral flow and myocardial oxygen consumption were usually lower at the same heart rate that induced angina during control. Lactate metabolism usually was not improved after nifedipine during atrial pacing stress. Thus, these data indicate that nifedipine does not consistently alter pacing-induced angina, but it does maintain collateral flow even when aortic pressure decreases.

Boden and associates[125] from Providence, Rhode Island, observed paradoxical myocardial ischemia in 10 patients with refractory angina (7 receiving combined β-blocker and nitrate therapy and 3 receiving nitrate treatment alone) in whom nifedipine (mean dosage, 92 mg/day; range, 60–120 mg/day) induced a decrease in BP, angina pectoris (10 of 10 patients) and ischemic ECG changes (7 of 10 patients). These 10 patients, all of whom regularly reported angina within 20–30 minutes of nifedipine ingestion, were prospectively studied before and after usual nifedipine dose administration, while BP, heart rate, and ECG were recorded. Mean systolic BP fell from 109–94 mmHg after nifedipine; mean heart rate increased from 64–68 beats/minute; 7 patients developed transient ECG changes (5 with ST-T wave depression and 2 with ST-T wave elevation) during the hypotensive period. Thus, nifedipine may provoke angina and myocardial ischemia in certain patients with refractory angina pectoris receiving concomitant β-blocker and nitrate therapy.

White and associates[126] from Boston, Massachusetts, assessed in 14 patients with CAD the effects of oral nifedipine on LV diastolic function. The patients had symptoms despite therapy with β-blocking drugs and nitrates. Rest and gated radionuclide ventriculography was performed before and a mean of 13 days after the addition of oral nifedipine (80–120 mg/day) to baseline medication. EF did not increase in any patient during exercise. The addition of nifedipine slightly improved the LVEF response to exercise (control, 49 ± 8% rest -vs- 44 ± 9% exercise; nifedipine, 47 ± 6% -vs- 48 ± 8%). With nifedipine treatment, diastolic function improved, with a decrease in the time to peak filling rate (PFR) at rest (from 174 ± 34–152 ± 31 ms) and an increase in PFR with exercise (from 2.5 ± 0.6–3.4 ± 0.7 end-diastolic volume/s). Using the ratio of PFR:peak ejection rate as a variable, preferential improvement of diastolic over systolic function occurred during exercise (1.03 ± 0.29 baseline -vs- 1.4 ± 0.43 with nifedipine). Duration of exercise increased by a mean of 21% with nifedipine (from 454 ± 150–550 ± 159 seconds); all 14 patients were limited by angina pectoris at baseline, whereas only 5 patients were limited by angina pectoris after nifedipine treatment. This study shows that global LV diastolic function is improved by oral nifedipine treatment both at rest and during exercise in patients on maximally tolerated doses of β-blockers and nitrates, and is associated with improvement of symptoms and exercise tolerances.

Nicardipine

Gelman and associates[127] from Gainesville, Florida, assessed the anti-ischemic effects and safety of nicardipine in 17 patients with angina pectoris at rest and coronary arterial spasm in a randomized placebo controlled study over 8–13 weeks. Eleven patients previously had unsatisfactory results with long-acting nitrates or other calcium blockers. The average daily dosage of nicardipine for optimal angina relief was 89 mg (range, 40–160). During the double-blind phase, angina frequency decreased with nicardipine compared with placebo (mean, 0.47 -vs- 2.11 attacks/day). A similar decrease in nitroglycerin requirements occurred (0.51 -vs- 2.77 tablets/day). During placebo periods, 51 episodes of ischemic ST-segment shifts occurred during 482 hours of ambulatory ECG monitoring and 12 (24%) were associated with angina. During nicardipine treatment, only 15 episodes of ST-segment shifts occurred during 498 hours of monitoring. In 1 patient a burning skin rash developed; otherwise, the drug was generally well tolerated. Thus, nicardipine is effective and safe in preventing symptomatic and asymptomatic ischemia in patients with coronary spasm. It may be particularly beneficial in patients with unsatisfactory responses to other therapy.

Nisoldipine

Lam and coworkers[128] from St. Louis, Missouri, and Montreal, Canada, evaluated the influence of nisoldipine, a dihydropyridine slow-channel calcium blocker similar to nifedipine, given orally in altering stable effort angina in 12 patients. A double-blind, randomized, placebo controlled design was used. Improvement in stable angina pectoris was observed as early as 1 hour after 10 and 20 mg doses and persisted for 8 hours after the 20 mg dose, as was evident from an enhanced exercise tolerance. At 3 hours, the onset of exercise-induced ST-segment depression of ≥0.1 mV was increased by 62, 75, and 117 seconds with 5, 10, and 20 mg doses of nisoldipine, respectively, compared with placebo. In addition, the time to onset of angina also was significantly increased at each of these doses. The heart rate-BP product was significantly greater with nisoldipine than with placebo at the onset of ischemia and at peak exercise. Thus, these data indicate that nisoldipine is an effective antianginal agent with a rapid onset and sustained duration of effect in patients with chronic stable angina pectoris.

Combined beta blocker plus calcium channel blocker

Kenny and associates[129] from London, England, investigated the antianginal effects of diltiazem (180 mg/day) and propranolol (240 mg/day), alone and in combination, in 15 patients with effort-related angina in a double-blind placebo controlled crossover trial, with each period of treatment lasting 4 weeks. Patients performed a symptom-limited treadmill exercise test at the end of each period of treatment. Mean time to onset of angina was increased from 293 seconds when receiving placebo to 347 seconds when receiving diltiazem alone, to 350 seconds when receiving propranolol alone, and further to 421 seconds when receiving diltiazem and propranolol combined. Similar changes occurred in the duration of exercise testing and time to 1 mm ST-segment depression. The sum of ST-segment depression at peak exercise was reduced by both diltiazem and propranolol alone compared with placebo, and combination treatment produced a further significant improvement. Heart rate-BP product was significantly reduced at rest and at peak exercise after propranolol alone and combination treatment. The study clearly showed the superior value of diltiazem and propranolol combined in effort-related angina when compared with either drug used alone.

Théroux and associates[130] from Montreal, Canada, evaluated 100 consecutive patients hospitalized for unstable angina, excluding patients with Prinzmetal's variant angina. Patients were randomized within 24 hours of admission to treatment with diltiazem (50 patients) or propranolol (50 patients). Patients with prior CABG and those receiving a β-blocker at the time of hospital admission were excluded. LV function and the extent of CAD were similar in the 2 groups. The number of episodes of chest pain decreased from a mean of 0.75 ± 0.1 per patient per day to 0.26 ± 0.07 with diltiazem and 0.29 ± 0.1 with propranolol. After 1 month, 14 of the patients treated with diltiazem were symptom-free compared with 13 treated with propranolol. After 5 months (range, 1–15 months), 2 patients had died in each group and AMI had occurred in 5 patients treated with diltiazem and 4 treated with propranolol. CABG had been performed in 21 diltiazem- and 19 propranolol-treated patients. Only 15 patients were without symptoms, 9 who had received diltiazem and 6 treated with propranolol. These data suggest that diltiazem and propranolol have near equal efficacy in the treatment of unstable angina pectoris and that coronary artery spasm is probably not the main factor responsible for the development of unstable angina when patients with Prinzmetal's variant angina are excluded.

In an investigation by Braun and associates[131] from Tel-Aviv, Israel, to determine the comparative effectiveness and hemodynamic effects of long-term oral treatment with propranolol alone and combined with nifedipine in patients with stable angina, 20 patients with CAD were studied by equilibrium RNA. Measurements were performed at rest and during supine bicycle exercise before treatment, after 4 weeks on propranolol, 1 hour after institution of combined propranolol and nifedipine treatment, and after 4 weeks on the combined treatment. The reduction in exercise rate-BP product induced by the combination ($17 \pm 3 \times 10^3$) was significantly greater than that attained by propranolol alone ($19 \pm 3 \times 10^3$). In patients at rest, neither propranolol nor the combined therapy altered global LVEF. Without drugs and on propranolol, exercise LVEF decreased significantly. On the combined therapy, there was a significant improvement in exercise LVEF compared both with rest values and with exercise LVEF on propranolol. Exercise tolerance, expressed as total work load, significantly increased on propranolol and further increased on combined therapy. Thus, combined propranolol and nifedipine therapy in patients with stable angina proved to be hemodynamically superior to therapy with propranolol alone and safe even in patients with moderately depressed LV function.

Wolfe and associates[132] from Dallas, Texas, studied acute hemodynamic and electrophysiologic effects of intravenous propranolol in the presence and absence of oral diltiazem treatment. In 22 patients (11 men, 11 women; mean age, 50 years), 12 receiving diltiazem (mean, 243 mg/day; range, 180–360) and 10 not receiving diltiazem, hemodynamic and electrophysiologic variables were measured before and 5 minutes after intravenous propranolol (0.1 mg/kg). Cardiac index (by thermodilution) and LV peak dP/dt decreased and LV end-diastolic pressure increased similarly in both groups. Mean systemic arterial pressure was unchanged. Coronary sinus blood flow (by thermodilution) decreased slightly in patients receiving diltiazem and was unchanged in those not receiving it. Propranolol caused a similar reduction in heart rate and increase in atrio-His conduction in both groups. Thus, when intravenous propranolol is given to patients with normal or only mildly depressed LV systolic function, the hemodynamic and electrophysiologic effects are similar in those receiving and not receiving oral diltiazem.

Johnston and associates[133] from London, Canada, studied clinical and hemodynamic effects of propranolol, propranolol-verapamil, propranolol-nifedipine and propranolol-diltiazem in 19 patients with chronic exertional angina pectoris. A placebo-controlled, double-blind, randomized, crossover study design was used in which patients took each treatment for a 4-week period. The 3 combinations equally reduced the incidence of angina attacks and decreased ST-segment depression. LV hypokinesia during exercise was lessened and end-systolic volume during exercise decreased with all combinations. Because of a corresponding reduction of normokinetic segmental function, global EF during exercise remained unchanged. Heart size increased and the PR interval lengthened with propranolol-verapamil and propranolol-diltiazem compared with propranolol-nifedipine. The largest number of adverse clinical reactions occurred with propranolol-verapamil, whereas the fewest occurred with propranolol-diltiazem. Almost all patients preferred combined therapy over propranolol and many favored 1 combination over the others. In summary, when therapy with combined β- and calcium channel-blocking drugs is planned, propranolol-diltiazem should be considered the combination of first choice because of its low incidence of adverse clinical effects. In the presence of possible or definite abnormalities of AV nodal conduction or decreased LV function, propranolol-nifedipine should be considered. Although propranolol-verapamil is associated with frequent adverse reactions, a trial may be warranted if the other combinations are unsuccessful.

To compare a propranolol-verapamil with a propranolol-nifedipine combination in patients with severe angina pectoris of effort, Winniford and associates[134] from Dallas, Texas, studied 16 patients with ≥5 episodes/week of angina and a positive exercise tolerance test despite propranolol (229 ± 44 mg/day [range, 180–360]) maintained on this dose of propranolol and in addition received verapamil (360 mg/day) and nifedipine (60 mg/day) for 3 weeks each in a double-blind, randomized fashion. In comparison with propranolol alone, anginal frequency and nitroglycerin usage were reduced by propranolol-verapamil but not by propranolol-nifedipine. Exercise time (standard Bruce protocol) was similar for the 2 combinations (6.4 ± 2.0 minutes with propranolol-verapamil, 6.6 ± 2.1 minutes with propranolol-nifedipine, difference not significant), but the magnitude of ST-segment depression at peak exercise was less during propranolol-verapamil (0.03 ± 0.06 mV) than during propranolol alone (0.18 ± 0.07 mV) and propranolol-nifedipine (0.08 ± 0.07 mV). LVEF at rest was higher with propranolol-nifedipine (0.62 ± 0.10) than with propranolol-verapamil (0.58 ± 0.10), but neither differed from EF at rest with propranolol alone (0.59 ± 0.08). EF at peak exercise was similar during all 3 periods. In 2 patients, verapamil caused weakness, lightheadedness, and severe sinus bradycardia (40–48 beats/min), and the dosage was reduced (blindly) to 240 mg/day, with the alleviation of bradycardia and associated symptoms. Thus, in patients with severe angina of effort with propranolol alone, the addition of verapamil is more effective than the addition of nifedipine in reducing anginal frequency, nitroglycerin usage, and the magnitude of ECG response to exercise. Although both combinations are generally safe and well-tolerated, in an occasional patient symptomatic sinus bradycardia develops during therapy with propranolol-verapamil; therefore, this combination must be given carefully.

Comparison of nitrates and calcium channel blocker

Morse and Nesto[135] from San Diego, California, and Boston, Massachusetts, performed, on 27 patients with fixed CAD and stable angina pectoris, a double-blind crossover study of 2 combinations, nifedipine and propranolol and isosorbide dinitrate and propranolol, to determine the effects of both regimens on the frequency of angina and exercise tolerance by treadmill testing. In this study, the combination of nifedipine and propranolol was superior to isosorbide dinitrate and propranolol in reducing the number of anginal attacks, improving total exercise time, and increasing the time to onset of angina during exercise. Nitroglycerin consumption was reduced from control values during propranolol and nifedipine therapy, but there was no significant difference between nifidepine and propranolol and isosorbide dinitrate and propranolol therapy regarding the frequency of reduction in nitroglycerin consumption. The major beneficial effect of nifedipine coupled to propranolol appeared to be a reduction in afterload greater than that noted with isosorbide dinitrate coupled to propranolol. These data indicate that both propranolol and nifedipine and propranolol and isosorbide dinitrate are superior to propranolol alone in relieving symptoms of effort-related angina pectoris. However, the combination of nifedipine and propranolol appears more effective in reducing the incidence of angina and improving exercise capability.

Aspirin and/or sulfinpyrazone

Cairns and associates[136] from Hamilton, Toronto, and London, Canada, performed a randomized, double-blind, placebo controlled trial in 555 patients with unstable angina, all hospitalized in coronary care units. Patients received 1 of 4 possible treatment regimens: aspirin (325 mg 4 times daily), sulfinpyrazone (200 mg 4 times daily), both, or neither. They were entered into the trial within 8 days of hospitalization and were treated and followed for up to 2 years (mean, 18 months). The incidence of cardiac death and nonfatal AMI, considered together, was 8.6% in the groups given aspirin and 17% in the other groups, representing a risk reduction with aspirin of 51% (Fig. 1-25). The corresponding figures for either cardiac death alone or death from any cause were 3% in the groups given aspirin and 11.7% in the other groups, representing a risk reduction of 71%. Analysis by intention to treat yielded smaller risk reductions with aspirin of 30, 56, and 43% for the outcomes of cardiac death or nonfatal AMI, cardiac death alone, and all deaths, respectively. There was no observed benefit of sulfinpyrazone for any outcome event, and there was no evidence of an interaction between sulfinpyrazone and aspirin. Considered together with the results of a previous clinical trial, these findings provide strong evidence for a beneficial effect of aspirin in patients with unstable angina.

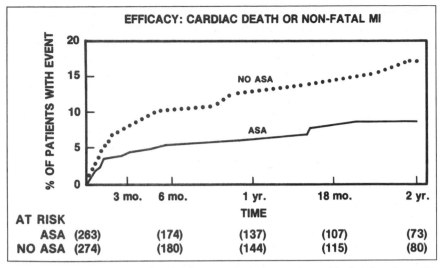

Fig. 1-25. Occurrence of cardiac death or nonfatal AMI in the aspirin (ASA) and no ASA groups. The graph is a life-table depiction of the cumulative risk and time of the first occurrence of an outcome event, according to ASA allocation. Numbers of patients at risk is indicated below graph. Reproduced with permission from Cairns et al.[136]

Captopril

Although vasodilators have been tried as antianginal agents, reflex increase in sympathetic tone produced by these drugs necessitate caution in patients with angina. Daly and coworkers[137] from Montreal, Canada, administered captopril to 14 patients with angina and systolic arterial pressures of >120 mmHg. Over the short term, captopril decreased arterial BP from 110–98 mmHg without increasing heart rate, arterial concentrations of epinephrine or norepinephrine, or transmyocardial norepinephrine balance. Captopril decreased average myocardial oxygen consumption from 9.7 8.2 ml/min. Given over the long term (5.5 months), captopril decreased the severity of angina from New York Heart Association classification 3.0 1.6. In the second part of the study, captopril was administered in a prospective, randomized, double-blind, placebo-controlled study to 21 patients with stable exercise-induced angina and systolic arterial pressures >120 mmHg. Captopril increased exercise time from 309–374 seconds without changing anginal threshold (rate-BP product 17 -vs- 17). These investigators concluded that captopril decreased mean arterial pressure without causing a reflex in myocardial sympathetic tone. By decreasing myocardial oxygen consumption, captopril may prove to be a useful adjunct to the antianginal drug regimens of patients with systolic arterial pressures >120 mmHg.

Coenzyme Q_{10}

Kamikawa and associates[138] from Hamamatsu, Japan, studied the effects of coenzyme Q_{10} (CoQ_{10}) on exercise performance in 12 patients with stable angina pectoris. The study involved a double-blind, placebo-controlled, randomized, crossover protocol, using multistage treadmill exercise tests. CoQ_{10} (150 mg/day in 3 daily doses) was administered orally for 4 weeks, tended to reduce anginal frequency from 5.3 ± 4.9–2.5 ± 3.3 attacks for 2 weeks and nitroglycerin consumption from 2.6 ± 2.8–1.3 ± 1.7 tablets for 2 weeks compared with patients receiving the placebo, but the reduction was not statistically significant. Exercise time increased from 345 ± 102 seconds with placebo to 406 ± 114 seconds during CoQ_{10} treatment. The time until 1 mm of ST-segment depression occurred increased from 196 ± 76 seconds with placebo to 284 ± 104 seconds during CoQ_{10} treatment. During the exercise test, ST-segment depression, heart rate and BP-rate product at the same and at the maximal workload showed no significant difference between patients after placebo and CoQ_{10} administration. The average CoQ_{10} plasma concentration increased from 0.95 ± 0.48–2.20 ± 0.98 μg/ml after CoQ_{10} treatment. This increase was significantly related to the increase in exercise duration. This study suggests that CoQ_{10} is a safe and promising treatment for angina pectoris.

Amiodarone

Pfisterer and associates[139] from Basel, Switzerland, compared the hemodynamic effects of short- and long-term administration of amiodarone in the same 10 patients with CAD and stable angina pectoris. Simultaneous right-sided heart catheterization and RNA were performed at rest and during exercise before therapy, after a 5-minute intravenous infusion of 7.5 mg/kg of amiodarone, and after 21 ± 4 days of amiodarone therapy given orally as 800 mg/day for 10 days, 400 mg/day for 7 days, and then 200 mg/day thereafter. The acute administration of amiodarone decreased LVEF, stroke index, and systolic BP, and increased heart rate, LV and RV filling pressures, and systemic vascular resistance. These hemodynamic effects were reversed after long-term therapy with all measured variables returning to control levels except for heart rate, which was decreased below control values, and RA pressure, which remained slightly elevated. Amiodarone serum levels decreased from 4.8 ± 1.8 after intravenous administration to 1.2 ± 0.6 mg/L after long-term therapy. Thus, these data indicate that the intravenous administration of amiodarone is associated with a negative inotropic effect. In contrast, oral administration of amiodarone long-term has less depressant influence on hemodynamics.

Therapeutic review

Shub and associates[140] from Rochester, Minnesota, superbly reviewed the proper medical therapy of patients with angina pectoris (Tables 1-10, 1-11, and 1-12).

VARIANT ANGINA PECTORIS

Effect of hyperventilation and cold pressor test

Coronary constriction at the site of atherosclerotic stenoses has been suggested to play an important role in modulating the frequency of symptoms in patients with exertional angina. To investigate whether stimuli triggering coronary constriction have similar effects in patients with exertional and variant angina, Crea and associates[141] from London, England, evaluated responses to hyperventilation and cold pressor test. Twenty patients with chronic exertional angina, positive exercise test results and CAD were compared with 14 patients with variant angina and ST-segment elevation during an ergonovine test. In patients with exertional angina, the cold pressor test

TABLE 1-10. *Effects of antianginal agents on indices of myocardial oxygen supply and demand.* Reproduced with permission from Shub et al.[140]

INDEX	NITRATES	β-ADRENERGIC BLOCKERS ISA† NO	ISA† YES	CARDIO-SELECTIVE NO	CARDIO-SELECTIVE YES	CALCIUM ENTRY BLOCKERS NIFEDIPINE	VERAPAMIL	DILTIAZEM
Supply								
Coronary resistance								
Vascular tone	↓↓	↑	0	↑	0↑	↓↓↓	↓↓↓	↓↓↓
Intramyocardial diastolic tension	↓↓↓	↑	0	↑	↑	↓↓	0↑	0
Coronary collateral circulation	↑	0	0	0	0	↑	0	↑
Duration of diastole	0 (↓)	↑↑↑	0↓	↑↑↑	↑↑↑	0↑(↓↓)	↑↑↑(↓)	↑↑(↓)
Demand								
Intramyocardial systolic tension								
Preload	↓↓↓	↑	0	↑	↑	↓0	↑0↓	0↓
Afterload (peripheral vascular resistance)	↓	↑	↑	↑↑	↑	↓↓	↓	↓
Contractility	0(↑)	↓↓↓	↓	↓↓↓	↓↓↓	↓(↑↑)‡	↓↓(↑)‡	↓(↑)‡
Heart rate	0(↑)	↓↓↓	0↓	↓↓↓	↓↓↓	0 (↑↑)	↓↓(↑)	↓↓(↑)

*↑ = increase; ↓ = decrease; 0 = little or no definite effect. Number of arrows represents relative intensity of effect. Symbols in parentheses indicate reflex-mediated effects.

†ISA = intrinsic sympathomimetic activity.

‡Effect of calcium entry blockers on LV contractility, as assessed in the intact animal model;[1] the net effect on LV performance is variable, being influenced by alterations in afterload, reflex cardiac stimulation, and the underlying state of the myocardium.

produced diagnostic ST-segment depression in 6 of 20 patients (30%) at levels of rate-BP product much lower than those during the exercise test; all patients had low effort tolerance and severe CAD. Hyperventilation produced diagnostic ST-segment depression in only 1 of 20 patients (5%). Conversely, in patients with variant angina, hyperventilation produced ST-segment elevation in 11 of 14 patients (78%) and cold pressor test produced elevation in only 2 of 14 (14%). Thus, coronary constriction can provoke myocardial ischemia not only in patients with variant angina, but also in some patients with exertional angina. Furthermore, the 2 groups of patients have a different susceptibility to stimuli known to produce coronary constriction.

Frequency of ventricular ectopic activity

Gabliani and associates[142] from Dallas, Texas, assessed the frequency of ventricular ectopic activity (ventricular bigeminy, couplets, or VT) during spontaneous variant angina, assessed the relation between ventricular ectopic activity and the severity and duration of ischemia, and evaluated the precise temporal relation between episodes of ischemia and ventricular ectopic activity. Fifteen ambulatory patients with variant angina (12 men, 3 women, aged 50 ± 8 years) had Holter monitoring for 24 hours/week for 10 months (total, 10,238 hours). Of 645 episodes of ST deviation, 79 (12%) had associated ectopic activity, almost all of which occurred in 3 patients. The 79

TABLE 1-11. *Dosages and selected pharmacologic properties of currently available β-blocking agents. Reproduced with permission from Shub et al.*[140]

DRUG GENERIC NAME (TRADE NAME)	USUAL DAILY ORAL DOSE (MG)		CARDIO-SELECTIVE	ISA*	LIPID SOLUBILITY	PLASMA HALF-LIFE (H)	PRIMARY ROUTE OF ELIMINATION
	RANGE	# DAILY DOSES					
Propranolol (Inderal)	160–480	2–4	No	No	High	3.2–6	Hepatic
Nadolol (Corgard)	40–320	1	No	No	Low	12–24	Renal and biliary (90% unchanged)
Timolol (Blocadren)	20–40	2	No	Mini-mal	Low to interme-diate	3–5	Hepatic and renal (20% unchanged)
Metoprolol (Lopressor)	100–200	2–3	Yes	No	Intermediate	3–4	Hepatic
Atenolol (Tenormin)	50–200	1	Yes	No	Low	6–9	Renal (<40% unchanged) and hepatic
Pindolol (Visken)	7.5–22.5	3	No	Yes	Intermediate	3–4	Renal (≈40% unchanged) and hepatic
Acebutolol (Sectral)	400–1,200	2–4	Yes	Yes	Low	4–6	Hepatic and renal
Labetalol† (Normodyne or Trandate)	300–1,200	3	No	(Yes)‡	Low to interme-diate	3–4	Hepatic

*ISA = intrinsic sympathomimetic activity.
†Labetalol possesses combined β-blocking and relatively mild α-blocking activity (β-blocking potency at least 4 times the α-blocking potency).
‡Partial agonism of β_2 receptors.

episodes of ST deviation with ectopic activity lasted 4.6 ± 3.3 minutes and averaged 0.16 ± 0.12 mV, whereas the 566 episodes of ST deviation without ectopy lasted 4.7 ± 6.1 minutes and averaged 0.17 ± 0.11 mV (NS in comparison to the 79 episodes with ectopy). Of 489 episodes of ST elevation, 72 (15%) were accompanied by ventricular ectopy; of 156 episodes of ST depression, only 7 (4.5%) had ectopy (Fig. 1-26). Of the 79 episodes of ventricular ectopy, almost all appeared during a period of increasing or maximal ST deviation, whereas only 2 appeared as ST deviation was resolving. Thus, in ambulatory patients with variant angina, ventricular ectopic activity occurs only in an occasional patient and in association with only about 10 to 20% of episodes of transient ST deviation; it occurs more often with transmural (ST elevation) than with subendocardial (ST depression) ischemia, but there is no clear relation between ectopy and the duration or magnitude of ST deviation; and ectopy almost always appears during the initial 2–3 minutes of ST deviation, at a time when its magnitude is increasing or maximal.

Echocardiographic findings

In patients with Prinzmetal angina, episodes of transient T-wave abnormalities are often documented in addition to the typical episodes of ST-segment elevation. As the interpretation of these minor ECG changes is still uncertain, Rovai and associates[143] from Pisa, Italy, investigated if transient T-wave abnormalities are associated with reversible ventricular asynergies, similar to episodes with ST elevation. An ECG lead and a 2-D echo projection,

TABLE 1-12. *Recommended drug therapy (calcium entry blocker versus β-blocker) in patients who have angina in conjunction with other medical conditions.* Reproduced with permission from Shub et al.[140]

CLINICAL CONDITION	RECOMMENDED DRUG (ALTERNATIVE DRUG)
Cardiac arrhythmias and conduction abnormalities	
Sinus bradycardia	Nifedipine
Sinus tachycardia (not due to cardiac failure)	β-blocker
Supraventricular tachycardia	Verapamil or β-blocker
Atrioventricular block	Nifedipine
Rapid atrial fibrillation (with digitalis)	Verapamil or β-blocker
Ventricular arrhythmias	β-blocker (±group 1 antiarrhythmic agent)
Left ventricular dysfunction	
Congestive heart failure	
Mild (LVEF ≥40%)	Nifedipine (verapamil, diltiazem, or β blockers cautiously)
Moderate to severe (LVEF <40%)	Nifedipine (cautiously, in combination with other therapy)
Left-sided valvular heart disease†	
Aortic stenosis (mild)‡	β-blocker
Aortic insufficiency	Nifedipine
Mitral regurgitation	Nifedipine
Mitral stenosis§	β-blocker
Miscellaneous medical conditions	
Systemic hypertension	β-blocker (calcium entry blockers)
Severe preexisting headaches	β-blocker (verapamil or diltiazem)
COPD with bronchospasm or asthma	Nifedipine, verapamil, or diltiazem (low-dose β₁-selective blocker or β-ISA)
Hyperthyroidism	β-blocker
Raynaud's syndrome	Nifedipine
Claudication	Nifedipine, verapamil, or diltiazem (low dose β₁-blocker or β-ISA)
Depression	Nifedipine, verapamil, or diltiazem
Neurasthenia or fatigue states	Nifedipine, verapamil, or diltiazem
Insulin-dependent diabetes mellitus	Nifedipine, verapamil, or diltiazem (low dose β₁-blocker or β ISA)

*β-ISA = β-blocker with intrinsic sympathomimetic activity, such as pindolol or acebutolol; COPD = chronic obstructive pulmonary disease.

†Surgical therapy should be considered for patients with severe valvular heart disease; β-blockers are not routinely used in patients with valvular heart disease and left ventricular failure.

‡Vasodilators may increase aortic valve gradient, and β-blockers can cause LV failure. Any of these drugs should be used with extreme caution in patients with severe aortic stenosis.

§If congestive heart failure (associated with normal LV function) occurs in a patient with angina, severe mitral stenosis, and rapid AF, a β-blocker (in combination with digitalis) may be used to decrease the heart rate.

which showed clear-cut changes during previous episodes of ST elevation, were simultaneously monitored in 5 patients with Prinzmetal angina for a total of 13 hours and 20 minutes. In all patients, the 30 episodes of ST elevation recorded were all accompanied by reversible ventricular asynergies. Furthermore, in 4 patients, 14 episodes of T-wave abnormalities (peaking, flattening, or the appearance of a diphasic T wave) were recorded. All T-wave abnormalities were associated with reversible asynergies. The mechanical impairment occurred in the same ventricular wall both during ST

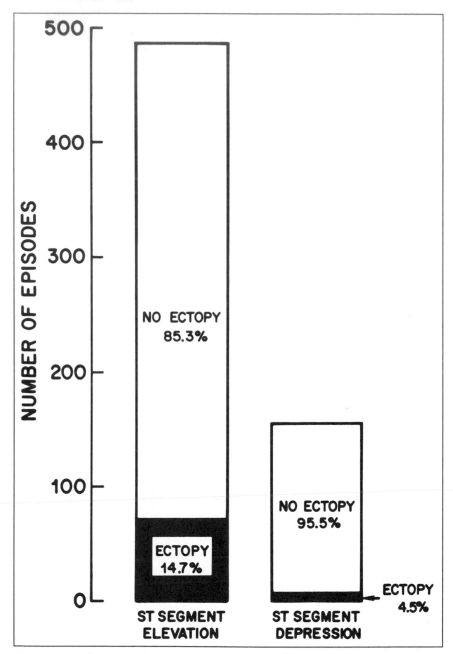

Fig. 1-26. Number of episodes of ST elevation (left) and depression (right) without (white) and with (black) ventricular ectopic activity, which occurred with 14.7% episodes of ST elevation but only 4.5% of episodes of ST depression (p < 0.001). Reproduced with permission from Gabliani et al.[142]

elevation and T-wave abnormalities. During T-wave abnormalities, the degree of mechanical impairment appeared less severe (hypokinesia in 12 and akinesia in 2 episodes) than during ST elevation (hypokinesia in 1, akinesia in 25, and dyskinesia in 4 episodes). The duration of asynergies was less during T-wave abnormalities (107 ± 76 s) than during ST elevation (169 ± 83 s). Chest pain was reported in 5 of 14 episodes of T-wave abnormalities (36%)

and in 20 of 30 (67%) episodes of ST elevation. An incomplete coronary spasm in 1 patient and an increase in LV filling pressure in another were documented during T-wave abnormality. In conclusion, in patients with Prinzmetal angina, minor T-wave abnormalities are accompanied by reversible ventricular asynergies, suggesting the ischemic nature of the phenomenon.

Coronary collaterals

In a study carried out by Matsuda and colleagues[144] from Yamaguchi, Japan, coronary angiography of both right and left coronary arteries, using the Sones technique, was performed during the attack of total spastic obstruction in 11 patients with clinically documented history of variant angina. No patient had >70% diameter stenosis by atherosclerosis in any coronary artery and none had a history of AMI. Total spastic obstruction occurred spontaneously in 3 of 11 patients, and was provoked by ergonovine maleate in 8 patients. Six patients had total spastic obstruction in the LAD coronary artery, 4 patients had total obstruction in the right coronary artery, and 1 patient had total obstruction in the LAD and right coronary arteries. In 7 of 11 patients, the coronary artery distal to the total spastic obstruction received collaterals from the nonspastic artery. The collaterals disappeared promptly when the spastic coronary artery was patent. These patients had ST-segment elevation during the attacks. In the remaining 4 patients, the spastic artery did not receive any collaterals from the nonspastic artery, associated with ST-segment elevation during the attacks. These findings suggest that the brief, repetitive total occlusion of the coronary artery may stimulate the enlargement of collaterals. These collaterals may not always function to prevent ischemia of the myocardium by ECG analysis.

Diltiazem therapy

Schroeder and associates[145] from Stanford, California, and Kansas City, Missouri, determined whether there is a rebound in anginal symptoms after abrupt withdrawal of calcium channel blocking agents in patients with Prinzmetal's variant angina abruptly withdrawn from diltiazem therapy. Values for daily frequency of angina between placebo periods after diltiazem therapy and after placebo were evaluated. No intergroup differences existed between mean changes in daily frequency of angina from baseline values on either treatment regimen. Furthermore, in 13 (28%) of 46 occurrences, when placebo followed placebo, daily frequency of angina exceeded baseline values in the immediate 3-day period after placebo compared with 17 (21%) of 80 occurrences when placebo followed diltiazem. There was no increased rebound occurrence of angina comparing high dose (240 mg/day) with low dose (120 mg/day) diltiazem therapy. No patient developed unstable angina pectoris or AMI after withdrawal of diltiazem or placebo. Thus, these data fail to suggest a rebound phenomenon in the frequency of angina after abrupt withdrawal of therapy with diltiazem in patients with Prinzmetal's angina.

Percutaneous transluminal coronary angioplasty

Corcos and colleagues[146] from Montreal, Canada, evaluated 268 patients receiving PTCA to determine the efficacy of this procedure in patients with variant angina. Twenty-one patients among the total of 268 patients had variant angina documented before angioplasty in 14 and after angioplasty in

7. All 21 patients had rest angina and 17 also had effort angina. Single-vessel CAD with 65–90% diameter stenosis was present in all patients and the LAD coronary artery was involved in all but 3 patients. PTCA was successful in 19 of the 21 patients (90%). Eight of the 19 patients remained symptom-free without coronary restenosis after successful angioplasty. In the remaining 11 patients, angina redeveloped within 4 months, usually in association with restenosis. Of the 9 patients with coronary restenosis, 6 had repeated angioplasty (5 successful procedures and 1 failure), 2 received medical therapy, and 1 had CABG. In patients in whom calcium blockers were discontinued soon after angioplasty, there was a high incidence of restenosis (8 of 10 successful attempts), but when calcium antagonists were continued for an average of 6 ± 4 months after angioplasty, the restenosis rate was low (3 of 14 successful attempts). The follow-up period was for a mean interval of 33 ± 13 months. One patient died and the remaining 20 patients (95%) were symptom-free. Among these 20 patients, 15 (75%) did not receive antianginal medications for >1 year, 2 received calcium blockers, and 3 had CABG performed. Repeat coronary arteriography at 14 ± 7 months after PTCA in the 17 patients without PTCA-related AMI or CABG had ≤50% coronary stenosis in 13 patients. These data suggest that PTCA is an alternative means of treating patients with variant angina pectoris and fixed coronary stenosis.

PERCUTANEOUS TRANSLUMINAL CORONARY ANGIOPLASTY

Creatine release afterward

In a study carried out by Oh and colleagues[147] from Rochester, Minnesota, after successful PTCA, 25 (20%) of 128 patients had elevation of creatine kinase (CK) MB isoenzyme. The increase was mild (mean, 9% MB with total CK of 179 U/liter). Three variables were significantly related to the enzyme elevation: chest pain, small branch vessel occlusion, and recent AMI. Of the patients with CK-MB elevation, 60% had chest pain and 32% had a small branch vessel occlusion during PTCA, compared with 11 and 8%, respectively, of the 103 patients without enzyme elevation. Of 16 patients with recent AMI 7 (44%) had release of CK-MB. Although mild enzyme elevation after successful PTCA is likely due to a small amount of myocardial necrosis, this phenomenon was not associated with increased cardiac morbidity or mortality. Therefore, release of CK-MB without other clinical evidence for AMI after successful PTCA does not in itself warrant longer hospitalization, and routine serial enzyme determinations are probably unnecessary.

ECG changes during PTCA

Brymer and coworkers[148] from Detroit, Michigan, evaluated the mechanism of ECG ST-segment changes during acute coronary occlusion in 28 consecutive patients with 1-vessel CAD undergoing PTCA. Patients were monitored continuously with a 6-lead ECG. Twenty-three patients had ST changes in the primary zone of occlusion, and 13 had additional ST changes in a remote zone. Ten of these 13 patients had unusually extensive arteries supplying the remote zone. The balloon occluded 2 adjacent normal arteries in 2 patients, and no coronary anatomic explanation was evident for the ECG changes in 1 patient. In 10 patients with striking primary zone ST changes, there were no remote changes. Seven patients had nonextensive primary zone arteries, and 3 had abundant collateral vessels. Five patients had no ECG changes in primary or remote zones, 4 had collateral vessels, and 1 had LV hypertrophy. These data indicate that remote ECG changes are most likely due to occlusion of unusually extensive coronary arteries and are not simply reciprocal alterations when they occur during PTCA.

Effect on LV regional function and/or diastolic filling

LV diastolic filling is impaired in many patients with CAD despite normal LV systolic function and is improved in many patients after PTCA. Bonow and coinvestigators[149] from Bethesda, Maryland, studied regional asynchrony by RNA in 26 patients with 1-vessel CAD before and after successful PTCA. Before PTCA all patients had normal EF at rest and normal qualitative LV regional wall motion by RNA and contrast angiography. Quantitative LV regional function was assessed by dividing the LV region into 20 sectors. Phase analysis was performed on each sector's time-activity curve, and the average intersector phase difference was used as an index of LV regional synchrony. Before PTCA, average intersector phase difference was increased compared with normal, which indicated asynchronous regional function. After PTCA, EF at rest was unchanged, but peak LV filling rate at rest increased from 2.5–3 end-diastolic volume/second and was associated with a decrease in average intersector phase difference from 6°–5.1°. Average intersector phase difference decreased in 16 of 21 patients in whom peak filling rate increased after PTCA, compared with 1 of 5 patients in whom peak filling rate was unchanged or decreased. Thus, improved global LV filling after PTCA was associated with more synchronous LV regional behavior. To identify the cause of regional asynchrony before PTCA, the investigators generated time-activity curves from each of 4 LV quadrants. The data indicated that the asynchrony was caused by regional variation in timing of diastolic rather than systolic events and that PTCA resulted in reduction in regional diastolic asynchrony. These data suggest that in many patients with CAD and normal LV systolic function, impaired global diastolic filling may result from asynchronous LV regional diastolic function, which is a reversible manifestation of myocardial ischemia or reduced coronary flow.

In an investigation carried out by Lewis and colleagues[150] from Houston, Texas, LV global and regional systolic function, ventricular volumes, and peak diastolic filling rate (PDFR) were studied in 30 patients with CAD, before and 2–5 days after PTCA, utilizing equilibrium RNA at rest and during exercise. At rest, the global EF was unchanged before (60 ± 9%) and after PTCA (62 ± 10%). During exercise, global EF increased from 59 ± 11% before to 67 ± 10 after PTCA. Twenty-two patients had abnormal EF response to exercise before -vs- 7 after PTCA. Improvements in exercise regional EF paralleled the changes in global EF. End-systolic volume was unchanged at rest but decreased significantly with exercise after PTCA (60 ± 36 ml before -vs- 49 ± 32 ml after PTCA). At rest, the PDFR was unchanged after PTCA. During exercise, PDFR increased from 2.1 ± 0.7 end diastolic volume (EDV)/s before to 2.5 ± 0.7 EDV/s after PTCA. It was concluded that in patients with CAD, successful PTCA improves global and regional systolic function during exercise. Diastolic function is improved during exercise, a fact not previously demonstrated.

On myocardial perfusion

Although coronary collaterals have been shown to influence ventricular function after thrombolytic therapy for AMI, techniques for accurately assessing coronary collateral flow have remained clinically difficult. To evaluate the effects of PTCA and intracoronary streptokinase (SK) on relative myocardial perfusion, Wahr and coinvestigators[151] from San Francisco administered technetium-99m and macroaggregated albumin (MAA) to the involved coronary artery before successful PTCA in 33 patients and before successful intracoronary infusion of SK in 8 patients and of In-MAA into the same artery after the intervention. In 10 patients who underwent PTCA, MAA was injected into the instrumented coronary artery. Computer-processed images were acquired in registry and compared. Similar scintigraphic studies were performed in 6 control patients and in 11 in whom planned interventions were not performed or were unsuccessful. Distribution of MAA also was compared with angiographic results and with the distribution of thallium-201 (^{201}Tl) on images obtained in patients at rest or on redistribution images obtained before and soon after intervention in 22 patients. In control patients and those studied after aborted or unsuccessful intervention, scintigraphic results showed excellent correlation with the angiographic anatomy and were without serial change. When MAA was injected into the uninvolved vessel, the scintigram revealed evidence of collateral perfusion with retraction of the perfusion zone from that of the involved coronary in 19 of 33 patients undergoing PTCA and in 3 of 8 of those receiving SK. When MAA was injected into the involved artery, a relative increase in perfusion was seen in 8 of 10 patients after PTCA. Although 30 patients had scintigraphic evidence of collateral vessels, only 10 patients had angiographic evidence of collateral circulation before intervention. The distribution of ^{201}Tl demonstrated little change in its global pattern, and regions previously supplied by collaterals were generally well perfused after intervention. Coronary collateral perfusion may be inapparent angiographically and regress rapidly after angioplasty or reperfusion. Native perfusion is generally and quickly restored after successful PTCA or SK infusion, which obviates the need for collaterals. Thus, after intervention, the distribution of total perfusion may not change, but its regional source may demonstrate beneficial alterations in shifting from collateral to native circulation.

Distal coronary perfusion during balloon dilation

Anderson and colleagues[152] from Atlanta, Georgia, perfused the coronary artery distal to an occluding angioplasty balloon in 34 patients undergoing PTCA. A randomized crossover study was employed using 2 exogenous substances as perfusates: lactated Ringer's solution and a fluorocarbon emulsion, Fluosol-DA 20%. Both substances are electrolyte solutions, but the Fluosol-DA will dissolve more oxygen than the Ringer's solution. During 2 attempted coronary artery occlusions of 90 seconds each, the investigators perfused through the central lumen (guidewire channel) of the PTCA catheter at 60 ml/minute. With Fluosol-DA perfusion the mean time to onset of angina after occlusion was delayed (41 ± 21 -vs- 33 ± 16 s), the mean duration of angina was shortened (77 ± 58 -vs- 92 ± 70 s), and the increase in the ST segment of the ECG was reduced (0.15 ± 0.24 -vs- 0.2 ± 0.23 mV) when compared with Ringer's solution perfusion. Balloon occlusion time was able to be extended with Fluosol-DA perfusion (71 ± 22 -vs- 59 ± 22 s). These results indicate that perfusion of the distal coronary artery is possible during PTCA and can reduce ischemia during a prolonged balloon occlusion time.

Relation of occlusion pressure to collaterals

Probst and associates[153] from Vienna, Austria, investigated the relation of the gradient across a coronary artery stenosis and the pressure distal to the stenosis after proximal occlusion during PTCA to the amount of angiographically estimated collateral circulation in 63 patients. All patients had 1-vessel CAD (54 LAD, 8 right, and 1 LC coronary artery). All patients had documented ischemia and PTCA was carried out within 4 weeks after the initial angiogram. The patients were separated into 4 groups: 0 = no collaterals (35 patients), +1 = just visible collaterals (8 patients), +2 = collaterals without reaching the contralateral vessel (10 patients), and +3 = filling of the contralateral vessel (10 patients). There was no difference in age among the 4 groups. There was a significant negative relation of the gradient -vs- the extent of collateral circulation, although the degree of stenosis increased significantly from group 0 to group +3. There was a significant positive relation of the occlusion pressure (in absolute terms and in percent of the proximal systolic pressure -vs- the extent of collateral circulation. There was a significantly smaller change of the occlusion if good collaterals were present. The occlusion pressure remained constant during 1 occlusion up to 40 seconds and was reproducible in 3 successive occlusions. In conclusion, the pressure distal to a coronary artery stenosis is mainly dependent on the severity of the stenosis and on the collateral flow. If anterograde flow is eliminated by proximal occlusion, the distal pressure is only dependent on the extent of collateral circulation.

Nitroglycerin during PTCA

Doorey and coworkers[154] from Heidelberg, West Germany, and Boston, Massachusetts, evaluated the efficacy of nitroglycerin in ameliorating ischemia associated with PTCA in 10 patients during inflation of an angioplasty balloon in the proximal LAD. Regional wall motion was assessed by LV angiography during a separate balloon inflation. Nitroglycerin (200 μg) was administered intravenously, and hemodynamic and ventriculographic assessments during balloon inflations were repeated. Balloon inflation caused an increase in LV end-diastolic pressure from 9 ± 2–19 ± 3 mmHg and in the time constant of LV relaxation, while also decreasing distal coronary artery perfusion pressure. Time to onset of angina was 29 ± 3 seconds and the time to ST-segment depression of ≥1 mm was 30 ± 3 seconds during the control inflation. Regional wall motion 30 seconds after onset of balloon inflation revealed marked hyperkinesia and akinesia in the anteroapical segments with graduated depression of inferior wall motion as well. With nitroglycerin administration, balloon inflation caused a smaller increase in LV end-diastolic pressure and the time constant of LV relaxation. Distal coronary artery pressure remained similar to that noted during standard balloon inflation, but the time to onset of angina and to 1-mm ST segment depression were substantially prolonged. Thus, nitroglycerin administration results in an attenuation or delay in the development of ischemia during balloon inflation associated with PTCA of LAD lesions.

Diltiazem after PTCA

A prospective randomized trial was carried out by Corcos and associates[155] from Montreal, Canada, in 92 patients who underwent successful

PTCA and had no evidence of coronary spasm before PTCA. All patients were premedicated with calcium antagonists and platelet inhibitors and received platelet inhibitors (aspirin and dipyridamole) for 6 months after PTCA. The diltiazem group (46 patients with 50 stenoses successfully dilated) received diltiazem, 90 mg 3 times a day by mouth for 3 months after PTCA; in the control group (46 patients, 53 stenoses), calcium antagonists were discontinued immediately after PTCA. All patients underwent a control angiogram 5–10 months after PTCA unless recurrence of angina dictated its need earlier. Baseline characteristics were similar in both groups, except for the number of diseased arteries with ≥70% luminal diameter narrowing, which was higher in the control group (1.2 ± 0.55 -vs- 0.9 ± 0.39 for the diltiazem group). In the diltiazem group, the degree of stenosis increased from 38 ± 15% immediately after PTCA to 42 ± 23% at repeat angiography 8.2 ± 4.8 months after PTCA and there were 7 restenoses. In the control group, the degree of stenosis increased from 37 ± 12–44 ± 23% at repeat angiography 8.3 ± 4.9 months after PTCA, and there were 10 restenoses (NS -vs- the diltiazem group). It was concluded that in patients without variant angina before PTCA, adjunction of diltiazem to platelet inhibitors does not decrease the incidence of restenosis. These data suggest that coronary spasm is not the major mechanism of restenosis.

Results

To evaluate the influence of gender on the outcome of PTCA, Cowley and colleagues[156] from Richmond, Virginia, analyzed data from the National Heart, Lung and Blood Institute (NHLBI) PTCA Registry. Early results were compared in 705 women and 2,374 men. Women were older and had more unstable angina and class 3 or 4 angina, whereas men had more multivessel CAD, prior CABG, and abnormal LV function. Women had a lower angiographic success rate, and a lower clinical success rate and had more complications. Overall frequency of major complications (death, AMI, emergency surgery) was not different. Women had a higher incidence of coronary dissection and a higher in-hospital mortality (1.8 -vs- 0.7%). PTCA-related mortality was nearly 6 times higher in women and mortality with emergency surgery was more than 5 times higher. Multivariate analysis indicated that female gender was an independent predictor for lower success and early mortality and was the only baseline predictor for PTCA-related mortality. The last results in 2,272 patients from centers with virtually complete follow-up of ≥1 year showed comparable or better results in women than men (Table 1-13). Men had higher rates of angiographic restenosis, repeat PTCA, additional revascularization, and cumulative mortality, and frequency of symptomatic improvement was similar to that in women. These NHLBI Registry data indicate that PTCA in women was associated with less favorable short-term outcome, lower initial success rate, and higher mortality rate than in men. However, longer-term results after PTCA were comparable or better in women, with similar symptomatic improvement, lower rates of restenosis, and improved survival compared with men.

Okada and associates[157] from Boston, Massachusetts, described their experience in the short- and long-term follow-up of clinical, angiographic, hemodynamic, perfusional, and functional effects of PTCA in 20 patients with single vessel LAD CAD. Exercise capacity in terms of peak workload, heart rate, and systolic BP all increased significantly 1 week after PTCA. All patients had some decrease in stenosis size and gradient. All patients except 1 had an improvement in functional class. Eight of 12 patients with an abnormal exercise ECG before PTCA had a normal ECG after the procedure.

TABLE 1-13. *Clinical results of PTCA. Reproduced with permission from Cowley et al.[156]*

	WOMEN (%)		MEN (%)
Angiographic success	60.3	B*	66.2
Clinical success	56.6	B	62.3
Mean % stenosis change	52.0		52.0
Unsuccessful result			
Inability to pass	25.2	A	21.8
(failure to cannulate)	(5.0)	A	(2.0)
Inability to dilate	8.4		7.2
Abrupt reclosure	2.6		2.9
Other failure	7.2		5.9
Intimal tear	16.5	A	10.7
Bypass surgery	30.0	A	24.2
Elective	23.5	A	17.6
Emergency	6.5		6.6

*Statistical comparisons: [A]$p < 0.05$; [B]$p < 0.01$.

Exercise thallium-201 (^{201}Tl) myocardial perfusion images obtained in all 20 patients before and 1 week after PTCA were analyzed using a new computer method designed to quantitate regional myocardial ^{201}Tl distribution, redistribution, and clearance rate. Significant improvement in ^{201}Tl activity was present in the anterior and septal segments of the LV 1 week after PTCA. This increase in ^{201}Tl uptake was associated with a significant reduction in the amount of ^{201}Tl redistribution between initial and delayed postexercise images in the same regions. ^{201}Tl clearance rate in the segments supplied by the dilated vessel also improved significantly. Abnormal ^{201}Tl lung uptake was seen in 17 patients before and in 4 patients after PTCA. Exercise EF response and septal wall motion also improved after PTCA of the LAD stenosis in all 17 patients who had exercise radionuclide ventriculography. Thus, improvement in clinical, angiographic, and hemodynamic factors as well as in global and regional myocardial perfusion and function occurs after PTCA for 1-vessel LAD CAD.

In 1979, the first report on PTCA comprised the results of such attempts in 50 patients; the trial was of primary success in 32 of these 50 patients. In a study by Hirzel and associates[158] from Zurich, Switzerland, 23 of the 32 primary success patients could be followed clinically for >5 years (62 ± 6 [SD] months). Repeat noninvasive laboratory data were available from 15 of the 23 patients and 11 of 15 were restudied by arteriography at the end of the observation period. In no patient was the procedure complicated by AMI; neither did such an event occur in any of them during the follow-up period. Early recurrence of the stenosis occurred in 5 of 32 (16%) patients, 2 of whom were again successfully treated by a second PTCA, while 3 were operated on as requested. Twenty-two of 23 (96%) patients remained free of angina throughout the entire follow-up period. Treadmill thallium scintigraphy tests were in close agreement with the clinical findings. Arteriography revealed an excellent lasting effect of PTCA in 8 of 11 reexamined patients, a slight renarrowing of the 3 stenoses treated by PTCA in 2 patients who showed general progression of atherosclerosis, and late recurrence of the dilated stenosis in 1 patient.

Bredlau and coworkers[159] from Atlanta, Georgia, prospectively recorded all in-hospital complications of the first 3,500 consecutive patients to undergo elective PTCA at Emory University Hospitals from July 14, 1980, to

August 28, 1984, by 3 operators. PTCA was attempted in 3,933 lesions, with a primary success rate of 91%. Multiple lesion PTCA was performed in 401 patients, and PTCA of 172 saphenous vein grafts was attempted. No complications were recorded in 3,116 (89%), isolated minor complications occurred in 241 (6.9%), and major complications (emergency surgery, AMI death) were observed in 145 (4.1%) (Fig. 1-27). Emergency CABG was performed in 96 patients (2.7%), with an AMI rate of 49% (47 of 96), a Q-wave AMI rate of 23% (22 of 96), and an emergency surgery mortality rate of 2% (2 of 96). Hospital discharge occurred within 2 weeks of attempted PTCA in 91% (87 of 96) of patients undergoing emergency CABG. The overall AMI rate was 2.7% (94 of 3,500). There were 2 nonsurgical deaths, giving a total mortality rate of 0.1% (4 of 3,500). Univariate and multivariate analysis of 3,099 patients undergoing single lesion PTCA identified 5 preprocedure predictors of major complications: multivessel CAD, lesion eccentricity, presence of calcium in the lesion, female gender, and lesion length. Unstable angina, duration of angina, lesion severity, previous CABG, and vein graft dilation were not associated with an increased incidence of major complications. The strongest predictor of a major complication was the procedural appearance of an intimal dissection. Intimal dissection was evident in 894 of 3,099 (29%) patients. Of these, 93 (10.4%) patients developed a major complication -vs- only 35 of 2,205 (1.6%) patients without evidence of an intimal dissection. Angiographic evidence of intimal dissection resulted in a 6.5-fold increase in the risk of a major complication. In conclusion, these results illustrate what can be expected when elective PTCA is performed with current techniques and good surgical and anesthetic support.

Three distinct periods in catheter design have been identified since the advent of PTCA in 1977. In the first period, PTCA was performed using a

Fig. 1-27. Comparison of major complication rates in the NHLBI Registry series and the Emory University Hospital (EUH) series. Reproduced with permission from Bredlau et al.[159]

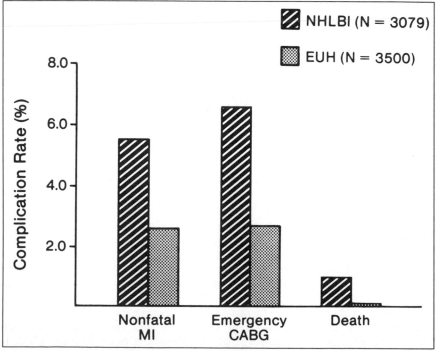

double-lumen balloon catheter that had a fixed, flexible guidewire at the tip. In the second period, an independent, steerable guidewire and the steerable catheter system were used. In the third period, low profile catheters were introduced. Anderson and associates[160] from Atlanta, Georgia, in 2,969 patients who had single-vessel PTCA of a native coronary artery separated the patients into the 3 groups according to the period during which PTCA was performed. Introduction of the steerable catheter system was accompanied by improvement in primary success rate in PTCA attempts on the right coronary artery (78 -vs- 88%) (Fig. 1-28). Introduction of a low profile catheter was accompanied by improved primary success in PTCA attempts on the LAD coronary artery (90 -vs- 94%). The percentage of PTCA attempts on the LAD decreased over the 3 periods (70–60–56%), whereas the percentage of attempts on the LC increased (7–12–16%) (Fig. 1-29). Before steerable and low profile catheters were used, there were significant differences in ability to reach and cross stenoses among the 3 major coronary arteries. These differences no longer exist. These results indicate that technical improvements and operator experience have made stenoses in all 3 major coronary arteries equally accessible to dilation catheters and that primary success rates and reasons for failure in these arteries are now similar.

Of totally occluded coronary artery

Serruys and associates[161] from Rotterdam, The Netherlands, had 49 patients among 652 consecutive patients referred for PTCA between September 1980 and March 1984 who had total or functional occlusion of the involved coronary artery. Total vessel occlusion was defined as absent anterograde filling beyond the lesion. Functional occlusion was defined as faint, late anterograde opacification of the distal segment in the absence of a discernible luminal continuity. In 39 patients, the total or functional occlusion represented a progression, without AMI, of a previously diagnosed stenotic lesion.

Fig. 1-28. Primary success rate in single-vessel PTCA of a native coronary artery—monthly data. A = end of learning curve; B = introduction of the steerable catheter system; C = introduction of the low profile catheter.

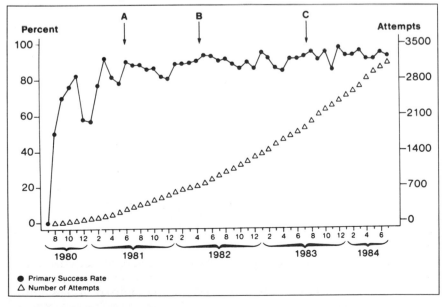

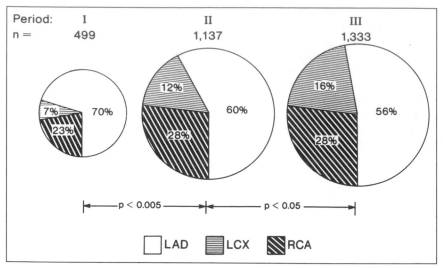

Fig. 1-29. Single-vessel PTCA attempts of a native coronary artery. LCX = LC; RCA = right coronary artery.

The maximal potential duration of occlusion was estimated to be ≤4 weeks in 21 patients, >4–8 weeks in 12, and >8 weeks in 16. Dilation of the occluded artery was attempted in the LAD coronary artery in 30 patients, in the right coronary artery in 8, in the LC coronary in 7 and in 4 jump grafts. For the whole group, PTCA was successful in 28 patients (57%). The primary success rate with the functionally occluded vessel (81%) was significantly higher than with the total occlusion (45%). In 33 patients with an occlusion estimated to be of ≤8 weeks, PTCA was successful in 65%. In the 16 patients with an occlusion estimated to be >8 weeks duration, dilation was successful in 44%. Of the 21 patients in whom PTCA was unsuccessful, 11 required surgery (1 urgent with persistent pain and ST elevation and 10 elective). Of the 28 patients in whom PTCA was successful, 10 patients had recurrence of symptoms during follow-up (1–42 months): 4 were kept on medical therapy, 3 had CABG, and 3 had repeat PTCA. After primary success, late angiographic studies obtained in 20 of 28 patients showed reocclusion in 8. In conclusion, elective PTCA of totally occluded coronary arteries is feasible, but the primary success rate is lower than that associated with conventional lesions. The long-term clinical results after successful PTCA are satisfactory (64%), but the incidence of reocclusion is higher (40%).

Kereiakes and colleagues[162] from Redwood City, California, studied 76 consecutive patients with total coronary artery occlusion to determine the efficacy of PTCA. PTCA was performed successfully in 53%, and the likelihood of successful PTCA was influenced by: a history of prior AMI in the distribution of the occluded arterial segment, a maximal duration of arterial occlusion of <20 weeks, and a length of nonvisualized arterial segment distal to the point of occlusion of <1.5 cm. In these studies, there were no deaths and no vascular perforations. Four patients had recurrent coronary occlusions within 24 hours and in 3 of these patients, the recurred occlusions were successfully treated with repeat PTCA. In 1 patient, emergent PTCA was performed. Embolic occlusion of the artery distal to the location of total coronary occlusion occurred in 4 of 40 successfully recanalized patients. Thus, 75% of patients having successful recanalization of an occluded coronary artery were improved symptomatically in a mean follow-up period of 7.3 months. These data indicate that PTCA may be utilized to reestablish perfusion in a totally occluded coronary artery, especially in patients with a history of prior AMI, a relatively brief duration of coronary occlusion, and a short nonvisualized occluded arterial segment.

Of LM coronary artery

PTCA for significant LM coronary artery narrowing has been sporadic and controversial. Stertzer and associates[163] from Daly City, California, and New York City performed PTCA in 19 patients who had severe narrowing of the LM coronary artery. PTCA was performed twice in 1 patient. Primary success occurred in 19 of the 20 patients (95%). Emergency CABG was performed in 1 patient (5%), and none died secondary to the PTCA procedure itself. In a follow-up period (mean, 41 months), 12 patients (63%) remained in satisfactory condition with no further need for an additional procedure; 7 patients (37%) ultimately had CABG. Thus, although CABG will remain the fundamental treatment of choice for LM coronary narrowing, this study indicates that PTCA may be utilized as the primary treatment for significant LM coronary narrowing.

Of multiple coronary arteries

Vandormael and associates[164] from St. Louis, Missouri, evaluated 135 patients to determine the safety and therapeutic benefit of multilesion PTCA. Sixty-six patients had a minimum of 6 months' follow-up evaluation. Among these patients, success from PTCA was defined as a successful dilation of the most critical coronary lesion or of all lesions attempted without major in-hospital complication. Success was obtained in 117 (87%) of 135 patients. Cardiac complications occurring in association with PTCA were relatively uncommon, but included prolonged angina in 5%, AMI in 3%, and emergency CABG in 4%. No patient died. Complete revascularization was possible with PTCA in 46% of 117 patients with a primary success. Among the 66 patients followed for 6 months, 80% had an uncomplicated course and required no further procedures; 90% had less severe angina pectoris after PTCA. Cardiac events, including the need for a second revascularization procedure, were more common in patients who had incomplete compared with complete revascularization (35% compared with 9%). Patients undergoing repeat cardiac catheterization at 5 months after PTCA (mean time) had restenosis in 18 of 22 symptomatic and 3 of 9 asymptomatic patients. Restenosis occurred at the site of a single dilation in 12 patients, at 2 sites in 8 patients, and at 3 sites in 1 patient. Thus, these data indicate that multilesion PTCA is a reasonable therapeutic option for selected patients with multivessel stenoses. Improvement in angina status may be expected even in patients with incomplete revascularization. However, in patients with incomplete revascularization, the need for a second revascularization procedure is relatively frequent.

Cowley and coworkers[165] from Richmond, Virginia, reviewed their experience with PTCA of multiple vessels to assess results. PTCA of multiple vessels was performed in 100 of the initial 500 patients (20%) who underwent PTCA at the Medical Center between July 1979 and August 1984; 89% had class 3 or 4 angina, and 66% had unstable angina. Two-thirds had severe stenosis of 2 vessels or major branches and one-third had 3-vessel CAD. One or more significant lesions were dilated in 2 vessels in 84 patients, in 3 vessels in 14, and in 4 vessels in 2. PTCA of 273 lesions (2.7/patient) was attempted (range, 2–8/patient) with angiographic success in 250 lesions (92%). Primary success (angiographic and clinical improvement) was achieved in 95 of 100 patients (95%); 84% in multiple vessels and 79% in all attempted lesions.

Complications occurred in 11 patients (11%); 4 patients (4%) underwent urgent CABG and 4 additional patients (4%) had AMI. Long-term results were assessed in 44 patients with primary success who had follow-up of >1 year (mean, 26 months) after multiple-vessel PTCA. Twenty-eight (64%) remain event-free and improved and 48% are event-free and asymptomatic. Clinical recurrence developed in 15 (34%); 4 had sustained improvement with repeat PTCA, 3 remain improved with medical therapy, and 8 (18%) have undergone CABG during follow-up. One patient developed late AMI, and no deaths have occurred in the follow-up cohort. Including repeat PTCA, 75% have maintained clinical success during follow-up and 82% remain improved without CABG. These follow-up results suggest that PTCA of multiple vessels is a safe and effective therapy in selected patients with multiple-vessel CAD.

Mata and associates[166] from Montreal, Canada, evaluated patients with double-vessel CAD undergoing PTCA. Of 769 patients who had PTCA between 1980 and 1984 at the Montreal Heart Institute, 74 had 2-vessel stenoses of ≥50% and underwent 2-vessel PTCA. In these patients, primary success was obtained for both stenoses in 63 patients (85%), for 1 lesion in 11 patients (15%), and for 137 of 148 coronary stenoses overall (93%). One patient had an AMI, but no other serious complications occurred. Among the 74 patients with 2-vessel stenoses, 15 had unstable angina, 14 had severe and limiting angina, and 32 had mild to moderate angina induced with effort. Only 2 patients were asymptomatic before PTCA. Six months after PTCA, 27 patients were asymptomatic, 27 had mild to moderate effort-induced angina, 5 had severe and restricting effort angina, and 2 had a new episode of unstable angina pectoris. In addition, 2 patients had an AMI and 1 had CABG during follow-up. Restenosis occurred in 30 (23%) of 132 segments studied at a mean of 5.5 ± 2.1 months after PTCA. Restenosis occurred in 1 vessel in 17 patients and in 2 vessels in 4 patients. Among the 34 patients with definite or probable angina, 50% had coronary restenosis. A stepwise logistic regression analysis, identified the following as predictors of restenosis: the angioplasty site, the degree of residual coronary arterial stenosis, whether the stenosis was calcified, and the balloon to artery diameter ratio. Thus, double-vessel PTCA can be performed in selected patients with excellent results except for a substantial risk of restenosis with time, the likelihood of which can be predicted on the basis of several angiographic variables.

For unstable angina pectoris

De Feyter and associates[167] from Rotterdam, The Netherlands, performed PTCA as an emergency procedure in 60 patients with unstable angina pectoris that was refractory to treatment with maximally tolerated doses of β-blockers, calcium channel blockers, and intravenous nitroglycerin. The initial success rate for PTCA occurred in 56 patients (93%). There were no deaths related to the procedure, although total occlusion occurred in 4 patients. Despite emergency CABG, all 4 patients had an AMI. All the patients were followed for at least 6 months. Late cardiac death occurred in 1 patient, whereas 8 had recurrent angina pectoris. No additional patients had AMI. Coronary restenosis occurred in 13 of 46 patients (28%) with initially successful PTCA who had repeat angiography. Improved cardiac functional status after sustained successful PTCA was demonstrated by an almost normal capacity on bicycle exercise testing in the absence of ischemia during thallium studies in 80%. The investigators concluded that emergency PTCA may be useful for treatment of selected patients with unstable angina pectoris who are unresponsive to intensive pharmacologic treatment.

With previous coronary thrombosis

Mabin and colleagues[168] from Rochester, Minnesota, analyzed the coronary angiograms from 238 consecutive patients undergoing PTCA at the Mayo Clinic to determine the presence of intracoronary thrombus before dilation. Patients with previously occluded vessels and those receiving streptokinase (SK) therapy were excluded from these analyses. Intracoronary thrombus before PTCA was found in 15 patients (6% of the total) and complete occlusion occurred in 11 (73% of the total) of these during or immediately after dilation. No patient had angiographic evidence of important coronary intimal dissection. However, among 223 patients in whom no intracoronary thrombus was present before dilation, complete occlusion occurred in 18 (8%), and in 12 it was associated with major intimal dissection. Thus, patients with coronary occlusion before PTCA had significantly higher risks of complete occlusion after the procedure (73 -vs- 8%, respectively). These data indicate that the presence of intracoronary thrombus identifies a group of patients at increased risk of developing complete occlusion during or after attempted PTCA.

Restenosis after successful PTCA

Wijns and associates[169] from Rotterdam, The Netherlands, prospectively evaluated the value of exercise testing and thallium scintigraphy in predicting recurrence of angina pectoris and restenosis after a primary successful PTCA. In 89 patients, a symptom-limited exercise ECG and thallium scintigraphy were performed 4 weeks after they had undergone successful PTCA. Thereafter, the patients were followed for 6.4 ± 2.5 months (mean ± SD) or until recurrence of angina. They all underwent a repeat coronary angiography at 6 months or earlier if symptoms recurred. PTCA was considered successful if the patients had no symptoms and if the stenosis was reduced to <50% of the luminal diameter. Restenosis was defined as an increase of the stenosis to >50% luminal diameter. The ability of the thallium scintigram (presence of a reversible defect) to predict recurrence of angina was 66 -vs- 38% for the exercise ECG (ST-segment depression or angina at peak workload). Restenosis was predicted in 74% of patients by thallium scintigraphy, but in only 50% of patients by the exercise ECG. Thus, thallium scintigraphy was highly predictive but the exercise ECG was not. These results suggest that restenosis had occurred to some extent already at 4 weeks after the PTCA in most patients in whom it was going to occur.

To evaluate the clinical status and restenosis rate after PTCA, Levine and associates[170] from Washington, D. C., studied 251 consecutive patients who had undergone a successful procedure from February 1979 to May 1983. Angiography was done routinely in 92 of the initial 100 consecutive patients in whom the procedure was successful (group I) 1–11 months (mean, 6) after PTCA. Restenosis occurred in 37 of 92 patients (40%); all but 2 (who had collateral flow to the restenosed vessel) had symptoms (Fig. 1-30). Conversely, 44 of 46 asymptomatic patients had no restenosis. The other 159 patients (group II) were followed up clinically, with angiography performed only if signs or symptoms of ischemia recurred. Restenosis suspected clinically and confirmed angiographically occurred in 35 of 92 patients (38%) in group I and 36 of 154 patients (23%) in group II. Of 251 patients with follow-up for ≥ 6 months, 109 patients (43%) became symptomatic. Of 109 symptomatic patients, 104 consented to coronary angiography; restenosis was found in 67%, progression of narrowing in other arteries occurred in 13%, and the remaining patients were presumed to have large or small vessel

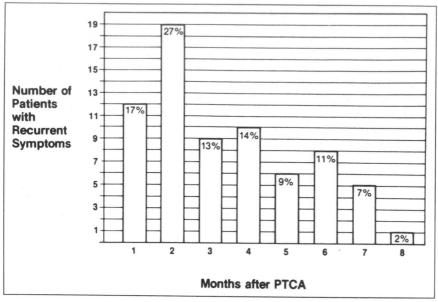

Fig. 1-30. Number of months after PTCA until the return of symptoms in 70 patients with restenosis. Most patients manifest symptoms by 3 months after PTCA, although some did not become symptomatic until 8 months later.

vasospasm. The mortality rate for the entire group was 0.8%. When repeat PTCA was applied to patients with restenosis, >80% improved at an average follow-up time of 21 months. Symptomatic restenosis may occur less often when higher balloon inflation pressures are used during PTCA.

Effect of intimal dissection

Stretching of the arterial wall and disruption of intima and media are thought to be the most important contributors in increasing the arterial lumen with PTCA. These processes are recognized arteriographically as an intimal tear or intimal dissection. Leimgruber and colleagues[171] from Atlanta, Georgia, studied 986 patients who underwent follow-up angiography after successful PTCA to determine the influence of uncomplicated intimal dissection on the restenosis rate. Angiographic evidence of intimal dissection after PTCA was present in 245 patients (25%). After a mean follow-up time of 17 ± 5 months, the restenosis rate in patients without intimal dissection was 30% compared with 24% with intimal dissection. Patients with available transstenotic pressure gradients were divided according to the hemodynamic result into 2 subgroups: those with final gradients at the conclusion of PTCA of ≤15 mm (n = 638) and those with gradients >15 mm (n = 244). Patients with intimal dissection had a significantly lower restenosis rate than patients without intimal dissection if the final gradient was ≤15 mmHg (19 -vs- 28%). If the final gradient was >15 mmHg, the presence or absence on intimal dissection had no significant influence on restenosis rate, which was 35 and 39%, respectively. These investigators concluded that an uncomplicated intimal dissection after a successful PTCA had no adverse influence on angiographic restenosis. An excellent angiographic long-term outcome can be expected if the intimal dissection is associated with a favorable hemodynamic result.

Producing acute coronary occlusion

Shiu and associates[172] from Birmingham, Leeds, and Sheffield, UK, described acute occlusion of the coronary artery undergoing PTCA in 20 (8%) of 240 patients having PTCA. The cause of the occlusion was dissection in 6, spasm in 7, thrombus in 4, and in 3 the mechanism could not be determined. Immediate reintroduction of a balloon dilation catheter was attempted in 10 patients and resulted in restoration of adequate coronary flow in 6. The remaining 14 patients underwent CABG.

CORONARY ARTERY BYPASS GRAFTING

Factors determining long-term survival

The Coronary Artery Surgery Study (CASS) has yielded important reports. Kaiser and colleagues[173] evaluated the effects of the severity of angina pectoris and the treatment method on survival of 4,209 patients in the CASS registry. This was a nonrandomized study and these patients met the criteria used in CASS randomized trial except for the degree of angina pectoris and the method of selection of treatment. The 5-year survival rate was ≥93% in patients with classes I and II angina and normal LV function regardless of the number of involved arteries narrowed or treatment received. Late survival of surgically treated patients with class III or IV angina and normal LV function was similar regardless of the number of arteries involved (≥92% at 5 years). Nonoperatively treated patients with classes III and IV angina pectoris and normal LV function had poor 5-year survival rates, lowest, 74% in patients with 3-vessel CAD. This difference also was observed in patients with abnormal LV function, 3-vessel CAD and classes III and IV angina: the 5-year survival rates were 82% for the operative group and 52% for the nonoperative group. These data confirm the importance of both clinical and anatomic factors in determining the prognosis of patients with CAD and indicate that CABG can improve late survival in patients with 3-vessel CAD and severe angina pectoris.

McCormick and associates[174] from Boston, Massachusetts, identified factors determining mortality and long-term survival among 3,311 patients who underwent surgical therapy for unstable angina. Overall mortality was 3.9% and no differences in operative mortality were found between patients with various subsets of unstable angina. Logistic regression analysis indicated that age, LV score, and presence of a LM stenosis and a left dominant circulation were related to operative mortality. The 7-year cumulative survival was 79%. The operative mortality of 3.9% is similar to that mentioned in previous reports of smaller populations of unstable angina patients and is slightly higher than the 2.3% surgical mortality for the entire CASS population of 6,176 patients undergoing isolated CABG. Long-term survival is decreased in patients with severe LV dysfunction, CHF, 3-vessel CAD, and cardiac enlargement on chest radiographs. Early survival was not influenced by whether the operation was deemed appropriate in the initial hospitalization during unstable angina or was deemed advisable at a delayed hospitalization.

For nonfatal cardiac arrest

Although CABG is beneficial to patients with severe CAD, its role in preventing the recurrence of prehospital cardiac arrest in patients is not clear. Tresch and colleagues[175] from Milwaukee, Wisconsin, reported on the long-term follow-up of 49 survivors of prehospital coronary arrest who had CABG. Before their prehospital cardiac arrest, 14% had a history of unstable angina. Coronary angiograms obtained after prehospital cardiac arrest showed that 71% of the patients had 3-vessel CAD and 6% had 1-vessel CAD. The mean LVEF was 45%. There were 4 postoperative deaths; 3 were caused by pump failure, and 1 was caused by refractory ventricular arrhythmias. After a maximum follow-up period of 102 months (mean, 55), there were 7 cardiac deaths, 5 of the patients died of recurrent VF, and 2 patient deaths were related to refractory CHF. Actuarial analyses of the 49 patients showed that the probability of survival at 6 months and 1, 2, 3, and 5 years was 92, 92, 89, 82, and 72%, respectively. After surgery, 35 of the 45 patients who were discharged from the hospital were asymptomatic, and 23 of the 32 patients who were employed when their prehospital cardiac arrest occurred returned to their employment.

In persons ≥65 years of age

Gersh and associates[176] in a multicenter study compared the results of CABG with those of medical therapy alone in 1,491 nonrandomized patients ≥65 years of age. Cumulative survival at 6 years (adjusted for major differences and important baseline characteristics) was 79% in the surgical group and 64% in the medical group (Fig. 1-31). At 5 years, chest pain was absent in 62% of the surgical group and 29% of the medical group. Analysis by the Cox proportional hazards model suggested an independent beneficial effect of surgery on survival. Patients were divided into risk quartiles on the basis of preoperative predictors of survival identified by the Cox model (Fig. 1-32).

Fig. 1-31.   Cumulative 6-year survival in surgical and medical groups for entire series. Adjusted for LV wall motion score, CHF score, number of diseased vessels, number of associated medical diseases, and age at baseline angiography. Log rank statistic = 36.485; p <0.0001. In 59 cases, the LV wall motion score could not be obtained. Reproduced with permission from Gersh et al.[176]

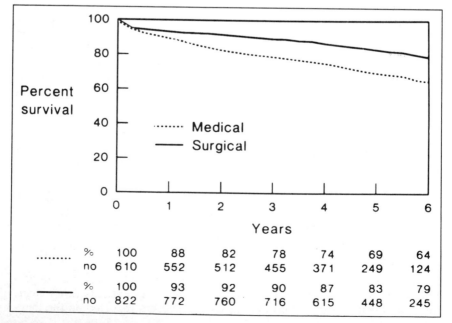

		0	1	2	3	4	5	6
....	%	100	88	82	78	74	69	64
	no	610	552	512	455	371	249	124
———	%	100	93	92	90	87	83	79
	no	822	772	760	716	615	448	245

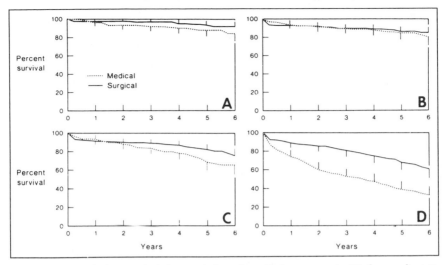

Fig. 1-32. Cumulative survival in surgical and medical groups, stratified according to prognostic quartile (in order of increasing risk). A: survival at 6 years in quartile I: medical, 84%; surgical 92%; p = 0.0203; log rank statistic = 5.387. B: survival at 6 years in quartile II: medical 81%; surgical, 86%; p = 0.4845; log rank statistic = 0.489. C: survival at 6 years in quartile III: medical, 66%; surgical, 76%; p = 0.0322; log rank statistic, 4.588. D: survival at 6 years in quartile IV: medical, 33%; surgical, 62%; p <0.0001; log rank statistic. 35.993. Reproduced with permission from Gersh et al.[176]

Surgical benefit was greatest in high risk patients (those in the 2 quartiles containing patients with the poorest prognosis). Among 234 low risk patients with mild angina, relatively good ventricular function, and no LM CAD, there was no survival difference between those treated medically and those treated surgically. The investigators concluded that in specific higher risk subsets of nonrandomized patients ≥65 years of age, CABG appeared to improve survival and symptoms in comparison with medical therapy alone. These conclusions must be tempered by consideration of the limitations of nonrandomized studies, particularly since patients in the 2 treatment groups differed substantially with regard to important baseline characteristics.

Kunis and associates[177] from New York City described 4 elderly patients with recurrent ischemia-mediated acute pulmonary edema that was refractory to anti-ischemic drug therapy. In each patient, CABG was performed for relief of symptoms and because of the grave prognosis associated with this syndrome. Three obtained prolonged relief of symptoms as a result of the operation. The important feature of their report was the demonstration that acute LV dysfunction, manifested as acute pulmonary edema, could be caused by transient myocardia ischemia.

Effect on LV function

Ren and associates[178] from Philadelphia, Pennsylvania, performed intraoperative 2-D echo in 15 patients during CABG and in 14 patients during AVR or MVR before and immediately after cardiopulmonary bypass by means of a 3.5 MHz transducer. LVEF and LV end-diastolic and end-systolic volumes were measured by a light pen system and biplane Simpson's rule from short axis and apical 2-chamber views. In 7 patients with CABG and new abnormal Q waves or >5% MB to total creatine kinase (CK) ratio postoperatively, the mean LVEF decreased significantly (from 52 ± 10–43 ± 12%). Patients undergoing MVR for MR showed a significant decrease in LVEF (from 63 ± 10–42 ± 23%) and LV end-diastolic volume (from 166 ± 34–147 ± 44 ml). Mean LVEF also decreased after AVR for AR (from 46 ± 16–26 ± 15%). Six patients with valve replacement and postoperative hypotension had the greatest decrease in intraoperative LVEF (from 50 ± 12–24 ± 10%). It was concluded that: 1) intraoperative 2-D echo can be used to assess immediate changes in LV function after CABG or valve replacement; 2) LVEF decreases significantly immediately after AVR for AR and MVR for MR; and 3) intraoperative 2-D echo may identify those patients who can benefit from inotropic support in the immediate postoperative period after valve replacement.

Carroll and coinvestigators[179] from Zurich, Switzerland, designed a study to investigate not only the degree to which complete revascularization alters hemodynamics, but also to contrast the postoperative results with those in a group of patients without significant CAD. LV systolic and diastolic functions were studied before and after CABG in 24 patients with stable angina who all had an excellent clinical response. From micromanometer LV pressure measurements and ventricular volumes, calculated from biplane cineangiograms, LV function at rest and during exercise before and after CABG was compared. Before CABG, all patients had exercise-induced ischemia with new asynergy, a decrease in EF from 57–49%, and an increase in LV end-diastolic pressure from 23—37 mmHg. Postoperative exercise produced no new asynergy and EF increased from 59–61%. LV end-diastolic pressure still increased from 17–22 mmHg. LV pressure decay during exercise was greatly improved after CABG and allowed maintenance of reduced early diastolic pressures. The early diastolic pressure nadir before CABG increased from 9–21 mmHg; the postoperative nadir was 5 mmHg at rest and 6 mmHg during exercise. All patients had an upward shift in the diastolic pressure-volume relation during preoperative exercise. After CABG, there was no upward shift in some patients and a much smaller shift in others. The postoperative increase in LV end-diastolic pressure was due to increased end-diastolic volume, not altered compliance. There was an increase in mean RA pressure during exercise either before or after surgery. These increases were variable, suggesting no consistent role of pericardial restrain during exercise. During postoperative exercise, early diastolic filling rates were greater than normal, reflecting the persistence of abnormally high atrial pressures for filling. As at preoperative study, late diastolic filling during exercise was restricted after CABG when compared with that in a control group. Thus, postoperatively patients undergoing CABG with a good clinical result showed significantly improved LV diastolic and systolic function. Persistent elevation of end-diastolic and atrial pressures and other abnormalities of diastolic function may reflect chronic structural changes and need to be taken into account when evaluating patients after CABG.

It is well established that CABG can reverse exercise-induced LV ischemic dysfunction, but the effects on resting ventricular performance are controversial. Rankin and coworkers[180] from Durham, North Carolina, studied 183 patients having CABG for CAD, and 166 underwent bypass graft arteriography an average of 7–14 days postoperatively. In 149, satisfactory preoperative and postoperative biplane left ventriculograms were obtained. Regional wall motion was assessed by the 100-segment method of Sheehan and Dodge, and a perioperative change in shortening >2 SD from normal variability over ≥20 adjacent segments was considered significant. Ninety-five patients had stable or progressive angina; 88 had medically refractory unstable angina; 37 had a preoperative LVEF <40%. Myocardial protection utilized crystalloid cardioplegia and topical hypothermia. Seven hundred ninety-eight grafts were performed (522 vein grafts and 276 internal mammary artery grafts). Thirteen patients had concomitant LV aneurysmectomy. Mortality was 2.2%, the over-all early graft patency was 96% (94% for vein grafts, 100% for mammary arteries). Only 1 patient had a decrement in regional wall motion and 51 patients (37%) had significant postoperative improvement (27 in the unsta-ble angina group and 24 in the stable angina group). In the patients with improved regional wall motion, EF increased by an average of 18%. EF also improved after aneurysmectomy and the increments seemed to result from both a reduction in end-diastolic volume and improved regional wall motion. Thus, reversible ischemic myocardial dysfunction appears to be common in the general population of patients undergoing CABG. Thus, 40% of patients with unstable angina and 34% of those with stable angina can be expected to have improved regional wall motion after successful revascularization. These excellent results reflect a 96% incidence of complete revascularization and a similarly high incidence of graft patency. They also reflect the current expec-tations for preservation of myocardial integrity using conventional cold crys-talloid cardioplegia.

Results with reduced LV function preoperatively

The Coronary Artery Surgery Study (CASS) was designed to compare medical and surgical treatment of selected patients with chronic, stable CAD. Passamani and associates[181] from multiple medical centers described findings in a subset of patients with reduced LV function. Of 780 patients randomly assigned to medical or surgical treatment, 160 had an EF >34% but <50% at baseline and these patients were followed an average of 7 years. Eighty-two patients were assigned to medical therapy and 78 to surgical therapy; the 2 groups were comparable at baseline with regard to prognosti-cally important variables. At 7 years, 84% of the patients in the surgical group were alive compared with 70% of the medical group (Fig. 1-33). Nearly half the patients with impaired ventricular function had 3-vessel CAD at entry; at 7 years, observed survival in this group was 88 and 65% to those assigned to surgical and medical treatment, respectively (Fig. 1-34). Survival of patients with single- or double-vessel CAD was similar in the 2 treatment groups (Fig. 1-34). The investigators concluded that patients with 3-vessel

Fig. 1-33. The 7-year cumulative survival rates for medical (M) and surgical (S) patients with EF <0.50 and single-vessel (p = 0.45), double-vessel (p = 0.4), or triple-vessel (p = 0.0094) disease. Reproduced with permission from Passamani et al.[181]

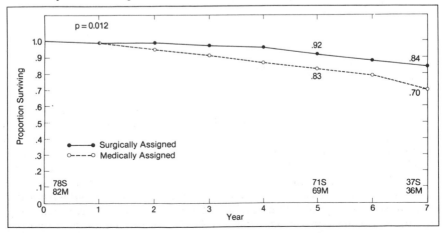

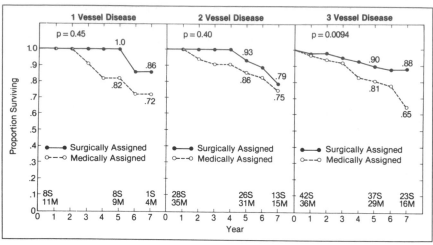

Fig. 1-34. The 7-year cumulative survival rates for medical (M) and surgical (S) patients with EF <0.50 (p = 0.012). Reproduced with permission from Passamani et al.[181]

CAD and an EF >34% but <50% appeared to have improved 7-year survival with elective CABG.

Effect on exercise-induced ventricular arrhythmias

Huikuri and associates[182] from Oulu, Finland, examined the effect of CABG on exercise-induced ventricular arrhythmias in 53 patients. A bicycle exercise test and an isometric handgrip exercise test were performed before and 3 months after CABG. Exercise-induced ventricular arrhythmias were detected preoperatively in 14 patients (26%), in 13 during the bicycle test and in 11 during the handgrip test, and in 18 patients (34%) after CABG. Thus, CABG had no significant effect on the occurrence of exercise-induced ventricular arrhythmias. Nine patients had new exercise-induced ventricular arrhythmis after CABG, 8 of whom had evidence of previous AMI, whereas only 8 of the 35 patients (23%) without postoperative ventricular arrhythmias had had a previous AMI. The rate of graft patency or improvement in exercise tolerance in patients with new postoperative arrhythmias did not differ from that in patients who did not have exercise-induced arrhythmias after CABG. The results confirm that CABG has no influence on the occurrence of ventricular arrhythmias induced by physical exercise. Patients with a previous AMI appear to be prone to new ventricular arrhythmias despite successful CABG.

Fate of preoperative defect on exercise thallium imaging

Persistent defects on serial thallium scans are commonly thought to represent fibrosis or scar. Such a pattern also may represent severe ischemia. Liu and colleagues[183] from Boston, Massachusetts, reviewed exercise thallium and resting gated blood pool scans in 52 patients before and after PTCA for single-vessel LAD CAD, and the fate of persistent defects after successful CABG. Persistent and transient defects were defined from the average scores of 3 observers. Ten patients with 16 myocardial segments with persistent defects were compared with another 11 patients with 20 myocardial segments with transient defects. After PTCA, 75% of the regions that had persistent defects and 85% of the regions that had transient defects were normal by visual assessment. In the persistent defect group, only regional wall motion on the resting gated blood pool scan before PTCA helped to distinguish those segments that would or would not revert to normal. It was concluded that regions of persistent defect on thallium scan often revert to normal after PTCA (75%), suggesting that persistent defects may represent hypoperfusion of viable myocardium and should not preclude consideration of an intervention.

Effect of platelet-inhibiting drugs on graft patency

Previous studies have revealed about 10% of all grafts used for CABG are occluded after the first or second weeks and 17 and 20% after 6 and 12 months, respectively. In patent grafts after 1 year, the occlusion rate varies from 2–4%. Since the platelet seems to be involved in several mechanisms that lead to thrombus formation, Brown and colleagues[184] from Seattle, Washington, designed a randomized, double-blind, risk-stratified study on the comparison of aspirin (ASA) plus dipyridamole (DP) and a placebo in a sufficiently large number of consecutive patients to investigate the hypothesis that inhibition of platelets would improve graft patency: 147 consecutive CABG patients were enrolled in a trial evaluating the effects on graft patency of 325 mg 3 times daily of ASA plus 75 mg three times daily DP or ASA alone; 127 patients (399 total grafts) underwent CABG, initiation of drug therapy 67 hours postoperatively, 5 clinic visits, and repeat angiography at 1 year. A statistical model was used to determine the effects of 28 different measured variables on graft patency and to adjust for these effects in determining the relation between antiplatelet therapy and graft occlusion. No patient-specific variable contributed significantly to the prediction of occlusion in either the placebo or the treated group. Six graft-specific variables (arterial diameter, severity of stenosis, graft flow, reactive hyperemia, presence or absence of collaterals, and graft type) did contribute and were included in the model; 21% of placebo-treated grafts became occluded. Compared with placebo, the relative risk of graft occlusion with ASA was 0.47; with ASA and DP, it was 0.50. This benefit was principally due to reduction of occlusion in the most common and presumably most important groups of grafts, those in which flow exceeded 40 ml/minute, or supplying arteries having luminal diameters >1.5 mm. Grafts lacking reactive hyperemia had a 32% occlusion rate in placebo-treated patients; relative risk of their occlusion averaged 0.26 with platelet-inhibiting therapy. Therapy is most effective if started on or before the second postoperative day. ASA and the combination of ASA and DP given after surgery were equally effective in maintaining graft patency. Thus, early postoperative ASA appears to be a simple, inexpensive, and effective form of therapy for most CABG patients and these investigators question the need for the addition of preoperative or postoperative DP to this ASA regimen.

Rajah and colleagues[185] from Leeds, England, confirmed the earlier (1982) Mayo Clinic results in a double-blind placebo-controlled, randomized trial involving 125 patients undergoing CABG. The patients received the perioperative regimen of 330 mg of ASA plus 75 mg of DP, beginning on the evening before operation, and continued postoperatively 3 times daily. In addition, all patients were given warfarin for 3 months. Repeat angiography was performed at 6 months in 103 patients. In the treatment group, 95 grafts were implanted in 48 patients, of which 87 were patent (92% patency rate). This figure compares with 88 grafts patent of 118 implanted in 55 patients in the placebo group (75% patency rate). Additionally, 40 of 48 patients in the treatment group (88%) had all grafts patent compared with 31 of 55 patients

(56%) in the placebo group. The intraoperative blood loss revealed no marked difference between the groups. The mean blood loss postoperatively was greater in the treatment group, but the difference did not reach statistical significance. Three patients (2 in the treatment group and 1 in the placebo group) were withdrawn because of gastric upset and headache.

Effect of exercise training postoperatively

Cardiac rehabilitation programs have been shown to improve exercise capacity, decrease symptoms, and improve psychologic well-being in patients with angina or previous AMI. Previous studies of cardiac rehabilitation in patients who have had CABG have been hampered by lack of sufficient numbers of patients, design problems, failure to consider patients with less successful surgery, and limitations in assessing results. Froelicher and associates[186] from Long Beach, California, recruited 53 male volunteers who had undergone CABG and randomized them to a medically supervised exercise program (n = 28) or to usual community care (n = 25). They were tested initially and at 1 year with exercise tests for thallium scintigraphy, maximal oxygen uptake, and electrocardiography. Approximately one-third of the patients had signs or symptoms of ischemia consistent with incomplete or unsuccessful revascularization. Over the year, there were 5 dropouts, but no major complications occurred. The exercisers attended an average of 82% of the sessions (3 times a week) and trained at 80% of their maximal heart rate. Both the exercisers with and those without angina had significant declines in submaximal and resting heart rate. There was a trend toward improved thallium scans in the exercised patients with angina.

Results with endarterectomy

Although endarterectomy to the right coronary artery has been used fairly frequently in patients with diffuse CAD, endarterectomy's role in the management of patients with disease in the left coronary system has not been defined. Qureshi and associates[187] from Middlesex, UK, analyzed a 10-year experience with 278 patients undergoing CABG who had additional endarterectomy to the left system. This constituted 28% of all patients undergoing CABG in their institution. Endarterectomy of the LAD was performed in 250 and of the LC in 75 patients. There were 11 (4%) early and 29 (10%) late deaths with an actuarial survival rate of 93% at 3 years and 80% at 6 years. Perioperative AMI occurred in 12% of patients; 243 grafts (75%) were restudied early with patency rates to the LAD equal 83% and to the LC, 75%; 81 grafts were restudied ≥1 year after CABG with a patency rate of 75%. The runoff of grafts to endarterectomized left coronary arteries was judged to be good in 76%, moderate in 14%, and poor in 10%. The investigators concluded that endarterectomy of the left coronary system is a worthwhile procedure. The saphenous vein graft patency was similar to that for nonendarterectomized arteries. The operative mortality is acceptable but the incidence of perioperative AMI is slightly higher than reported when endarterectomy was not done.

More than one operation

Pidgeon and associates[188] from London, England, retrospectively followed up 102 patients who had undergone a second CABG necessitated by persistence or recurrence of intractable angina pectoris. Operative mortality was 2%. During follow-up of the survivors (mean interval, 36 months) 5 died,

2 after further operation, and 5 underwent further surgery. Sixty-eight patients reported an improvement in symptoms, 57 of whom claimed to have little or no angina. Less favorable results were recorded for those patients with longer follow-up. No useful indicators of prognosis were identified. Obviously, it is best not to have to perform a second CABG. PTCA may have great usefulness in the situation of recurrence of clinical evidence of myocardial eschemia in patients who have 1 CABG. Of the 102 patients evaluated in the present study, 27 at the initial operation had received only 1 conduit; 39, only 2 conduits; 33, three, and 3, four conduits. Endarterectomy had been performed in 33 coronary arteries in 24 patients at the initial CABG.

Internal mammary artery -vs- saphenous vein as conduit

Lytle and colleagues[189] from Cleveland, Ohio, reported the results of serial arteriograms obtained in 501 patients after CABG. Arteriograms were done for various reasons, including suspected angina, interval AMI, and routine study to document graft status. The short-term patency (mean postoperative interval, 15 months) was compared with the long-term patency (mean postoperative interval, 88 months) for saphenous veins -vs- internal mammary artery grafts. At study one, 645 (82%) of 786 vein grafts were patent, 42 (5%) stenotic or irregular, and 99 (13%) occluded. Of 140 mammary artery grafts, 136 (97%) were patent, 2 (1.4%) stenotic and 2 (1.4%) occluded. Of the 645 vein grafts patent in study one, 357 (55%) remained patent in study two, 119 (18%) were stenotic or irregular, and 169 (26%) were occluded. Of 136 mammary artery grafts patent in study one, 130 (96%) were unchanged, 1 was stenotic, and 5 (4%) were occluded in study 2. Thus, serial arteriograms in this large group of patients demonstrate that within 5 years of operation mammary artery graft patency exceeded vein graft patency. Between 5 and 12 years after operation, the attrition rate of vein grafts greatly exceeded that of mammary artery grafts.

Arrhythmias postoperatively

Rubin and coworkers[190] from Valhalla, New York, evaluated the incidence, risk factors, and long-term prognosis of complex ventricular arrhythmias after CABG in 92 patients with normal LV function. Ventricular arrhythmias were documented by predischarge 24-hour ambulatory ECG monitoring; 43% of the patients had no or simple ventricular arrhythmias and 57% had complex ventricular arrhythmias. No risk factor identified patients at higher risk for complex ventricular arrhythmias. Patients were followed for a mean of 16 months. Those patients with complex ventricular arrhythmias did not have a higher incidence of sudden death, cardiac death, syncope, angina, AMI, or stroke. Thus, these data indicate that complex ventricular arrhythmias are relatively common after CABG; no obvious risk factor identifies high risk patients; complex ventricular arrhythmias after CABG do not necessarily indicate a poor prognosis in patients with normal LV function.

Unstable angina pectoris and/or AMI postoperatively

Effective therapy for patients with unstable angina or evolving AMI after CABG requires accurate delineation of the pathoanatomy and prompt intervention. Slysh and colleagues[191] from Philadelphia, Pennsylvania, performed cardiac catheterization in 10 consecutive patients: 4 with AMI and 6 with refractory unstable angina. All patients with AMI had completely thrombosed vein grafts supplying totally occluded native coronary arteries. In 3 patients with AMI occurring within 4 weeks of CABG, graft thrombosis was caused by venous valves in 2 patients and a suboptimal anastomosis in a third. The fourth patient sustained an AMI 7 years after CABG with atherosclerotic plaque rupture causing vein graft thrombosis. Therapy with intragraft streptokinase (SK) resulted in complete clearing of thrombus, pain relief, and control of injury current in all 4 patients. Rest angina with concomitant ST and T-wave changes occurred in 6 patients. In 2 patients symptoms occurred early (within 6 months), whereas angina developed 4–10 years after CABG in 4 patients. In the 2 patients with early recurrence of symptoms suboptimal anastomosis was found in 1, and the other patient had a venous valve in the vein graft in conjunction with a stenosis in the native coronary artery. In 3 of 4 patients with late recurrence of angina, symptoms developed as a result of atherosclerotic stenosis in their vein grafts; in the fourth patient an occluded graft was found to supply a stenosed native coronary artery. PTCA was successfully performed in all 6 patients. It was concluded that AMI and unstable angina occurring early after CABG are caused by graft thrombosis as a result of mechanical graft problems, that late events are caused by atherosclerotic stenosis and plaque rupture, and that interventional catheterization with SK and PTCA are effective therapy for patients with recurrent ischemia or AMI after CABG.

With the introduction of hypothermic potassium cardioplegia for cardiac surgery, marked reductions in perioperative mortality and the rate of Q-wave-associated AMI have been observed. No study has evaluated whether there has been an equally dramatic improvement in the incidence of postoperative AMI unassociated with Q-wave development. Force and coworkers[192] from Boston, Massachusetts, used a previously validated quantitative 2-D echo analytic algorithm to determine the incidence and severity of regional wall motion abnormalities (RWMA) and first-pass radionuclide ventriculography to assess deterioration in global LV function in 4 groups of patients: 1) 10 patients with peak postoperative creatine kinase (CK)-MB levels equal to or less than the mean value for patients undergoing CABG; 2) 10 patients with CK-MB levels between the mean and 1 SD above the mean; 3) 25 patients with peak CK-MB levels higher than 1 SD above the mean; and 4) 20 patients with new pathologic Q waves on the postoperative ECG. All patients had ECG without pathologic Q waves and normal wall motion and EF by contrast ventriculography before CABG. The incidence of postoperative RWMA by 2-D echo for groups 1–4 was 0, 20, 55, and 89%, respectively. Percent of abnormal LV segments, wall motion scores, and the deterioration in LVEF as assessed by radionuclide ventriculography were similar for patients with new RWMAs whether or not new Q waves developed. Thus, although the incidence of both Q-wave and no Q-wave perioperative AMI appears to have declined significantly with the use of cold potassium cardioplegia, the incidence of no Q-wave AMI remains high and in this study was calculated to be 3 times greater than the 4.5% incidence of Q-wave AMI. The impact of a no Q-wave AMI on LV function is significant and equal to that of a Q-wave AMI.

Effect on hospital readmissions

A neglected but important measure of early morbidity after CABG operations is rehospitalization. Stanton and associates[193] from 4 medical centers, conducted a study to collect data from all readmissions occurring within the first 6 postoperative months in 326 patients after CABG: 24% of them had readmissions. The most common categories of readmission discharge diagnoses were cardiac (57%), noncardiac (26%), and surgical sequelae (17%). Several factors from the initial hospitalization were identified as risk factors for rehospitalization: length of stay in intensive care unit after CABG, severe noncardiac complications, duration of preoperative cardiac symptoms, intra-aortic balloon insertion, and preoperative resting angina.

Pericardial effusion postoperatively

To assess the clinical importance of hemopericardium after CABG, serial blood pool scintigrams were performed randomly in 13 patients throughout the initial hours after CABG by Viquerat and associates[194] from San Francisco, California. Hemodynamics and chest tube drainage were monitored; and symptoms of postpericardiotomy syndrome were recorded for a mean of 7.4 months after CABG. Seven of the 13 patients had no scintigraphic evidence of bloody pericardial effusion. Six patients had scintigraphic evidence of bloody pericardial effusion; 3 of these effusions were small, localized posteriorly, and evident throughout the study. In 2 other patients, large collections of fluid (>100 ml) developed: in 1, increased mediastinal drainage required reoperation; the other patient remained stable although mediastinal drainage decreased. The sixth patient showed a moderate effusion (95 ml) that decreased without evident effusion or drainage when the last image was taken. Two patients (1 with evidence of a postoperative bloody effusion) had symptoms of postpericardiotomy syndrome in the follow-up period. This study reports the generally benign occurrence of bloody postoperative mediastinal effusions, the frequent accumulation of substantial amounts of undrained sanguineous fluid, and the lack of connection between the presence or amount of pericardial blood and the postpericardiotomy syndrome.

Frequency of stroke postoperatively

There has been a trend in recent years toward an increased incidence of cerebral vascular accidents after cardiopulmonary bypass for CAD. Gardner and colleagues[195] from Baltimore, Maryland, noted this trend and analyzed it in a group of patients having isolated CABG. From 1974–1983, 3,279 consecutive patients were reviewed. During that period, the risk of death decreased from 3.9–2.6%. The stroke rate decreased initially, but then increased from 0.57% in 1979 to 2.4% in 1983 (Fig. 1-35). The risk of stroke increased largely because of an increase in the mean age of patients undergoing CABG (Fig. 1-36). Risk factors significantly associated with the development of stroke in a univariant analysis included increased age, preexisting cerebral vascular disease, severe atherosclerosis of the ascending aorta, protracted cardiopulmonary bypass time, and severe perioperative hypotension. Variables not found to correlate with postoperative stroke included previous AMI, systemic hypertension, diabetes mellitus, lower extremity vascular disease, LV function, and intraoperative perfusion techniques.

Adrenal gland function postoperatively

Little is known about adrenocortical function after CABG in which moderate to deep hypothermia and cardiopulmonary bypass are used particularly with intraoperative steroid administration. Weiskopf and associates[196] from Los Angeles, California, determined immediately preoperative and 18-hour

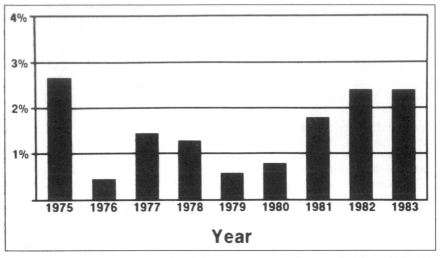

Fig. 1-35. Annual incidence of stroke after CABG at Johns Hopkins Hospital from 1975–1983. Between 1979 and 1983, the incidence of stroke increased from 0.57–2.39% (p <0.005). Reproduced with permission from Gardner et al.[195]

postoperative serum cortisol levels in 8 patients who received 1.0–1.5 g of methylprednisolone intravenously during CABG; postoperative serum cortisol (3 ± 1 μg/dl) levels were lower than preoperative levels (15 ± 3 μg/dl). To determine the possible cause of these findings, the effects of moderate to profound hypothermia and cardiopulmonary bypass on adrenocortical function were then investigated without the influence of intraoperative steroid administration. Serum cortisol and aldosterone levels and their response to adrenocorticotropic hormone (ACTH) were determined before CABG and at various postoperative intervals in 7 patients. Postoperative cortisol and aldo-

Fig. 1-36. The incidence of stroke after CABG at Johns Hopkins Hospital from 1974–1983 increased dramatically according to the age of the patient (p <0.001). The incidence of stroke was 0.42% for patients 41–50 years old, but increased to 7.14% for patients >75 years. Reproduced with permission from Gardner et al.[195]

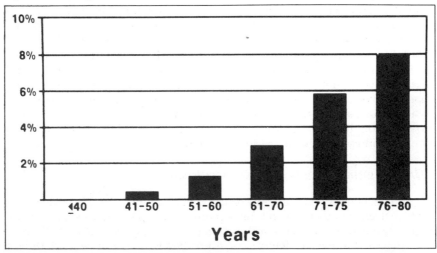

Coronary Artery Disease • 103

sterone levels increased markedly over their preoperative values, reaching a maximum at 6–12 hours (cortisol, 16 ± 8 -vs- 63 ± 23 μg/dl; aldosterone, 15 ± 5 -vs- 51 ± 22 ng/dl). Adrenal response to ACTH was normal preoperatively, during rewarming from hypothermia, and 18 hours and 7 days postoperatively. Thus, normal adrenal responsiveness occurs after CABG despite hypothermic cardiopulmonary bypass and the effects of anesthesia, and a single dose of methylprednisolone during CABG is associated with markedly lower serum cortisol levels and prevents the usual adrenal stress response to CABG for at least 18 hours postoperatively.

Frequency of narrowings in unused saphenous veins

To assess the status of a saphenous vein (SV) excised for CABG, Waller and Roberts[197] from Bethesda, Maryland, examined 3,394 cm of remnant SV from 402 patients who underwent CABG. The SV remnants were 0.5–52 cm long (mean, 8.4). They were sectioned into 5 mm long segments, and the resulting 6,788 5 mm segments were examined histologically: 5,896 (87%) were narrowed 0–25% in cross-sectional area by fibrous tissue; 853 (12.6%) were narrowed 26–50%; 23 (0.3%), 51–75%, and 16 (0.2%) segments were narrowed 76–100%. Of the 16 segments severely narrowed, 7 (44%) were nearly totally occluded by fibrous tissue. In 17 patients who died within 24 hours of CABG, similar degrees of luminal narrowing were observed in remnant segments and in utilized segments of SV. Thus, significant preexisting luminal narrowing of SV used for CABG is infrequent. The intimal fibrous thickening is variable within the same vein when each 5 mm long segment is analyzed; it is variable from vein to vein in the same patient, and it varies among patients.

COMPARISON OF PTCA WITH CABG

In an editorial by Mock and associates[198] from Rochester, Minnesota, a case was made for a randomized trial comparing PTCA with CABG with the logical primary endpoints being subjective degree of relief of angina pectoris as assessed by standardized angina history obtained by an independent observer and an objective evaluation of functional capacity, determined by an exercise ECG test, and RNA assessment of LV function at rest and during exercise, or both.

To evaluate the long-term improvement of coronary artery hemodynamics after revascularization by either CABG or PTCA, Bates and coinvestigators[199] from Ann Arbor, Michigan, measured regional coronary flow reserve (CFR) by digital computer analysis of 35 mm cine film, in 50 men undergoing cardiac catheterization. CFR in 12 atherosclerotic arteries before revascularization was 1.02. Mean CFR in 29 arteries of men with normal coronary arteriograms was significantly higher (2.59) than that of 16 atherosclerotic arteries of patients revascularized by CABG (2.02) or in 14 atherosclerotic arteries of those revascularized by PTCA (1.97). No difference in CFR between the CABG and PTCA groups was found and variables known to influence CFR were similar between groups. The equivalent and significant long-term improvement in coronary artery hemodynamics is provided by either CABG or PTCA.

Raft and associates[200] from Chapel Hill, North Carolina, compared life adaptation of 32 patients who had undergone PTCA with that of 15 patients who had CABG. Patients were matched for psychosocial, anatomic, and cardiac functions. Life adaptation was measured at 6 and 15 months after PTCA or CABG by the Psychosocial Adjustment to Illness Scale, a multidimensional instrument that evaluates change in 7 primary life domains. The overall scores for patients who had undergone PTCA were significantly better than the scores for those who had undergone CABG after 6 months, and this superior functioning continued after 15 months. After 6 months, patients who had undergone PTCA functioned better at work, in sexual performance, and with their families. The improvement in work functioning continued at 15 months, but the differences in sexual and family domains became nonsignificant.

Corbelli and associates[201] from Cleveland, Ohio, performed PTCA for 115 narrowings in 94 patients with angina pectoris and prior CABG at a mean of 60 months (range, 4–192) after CABG. Fifteen patients were in Canadian Cardiovascular Society functional class I, 32 were in class II, 31 were in class III, and 16 were in class IV. Patients were 37–76 years old (mean, 57). PTCA was successful (at least a 40% reduction in stenosis diameter and improvement in symptomatic status) in 83 patients (88%) and 103 (90%) lesions. Mean stenosis was reduced from $80 \pm 14\%–20 \pm 16\%$ (mean $\pm$ SD) and mean pressure gradient from $41 \pm 7–14 \pm 6$ mmHg. Seven patients had narrowings that could not be crossed for technical reasons and these patients underwent nonemergency CABG. Four patients required emergency CABG after PTCA; 1 patient subsequently died and 2 survived AMI. One patient had a femoral artery laceration, which required surgical repair. At a mean follow-up of 8 ± 4 months, 63 patients (76%) with initially successful results were free of angina or in improved condition. Of the remaining 20 patients, 18 consented to repeat coronary angiography. Four patients did not have restenosis. Of the 14 patients with documented restenosis, 5 underwent successful repeat PTCA, 5 had repeat CABG, and 4 were treated medically. Thus, when coronary anatomy is suitable, PTCA is an effective alternative to reoperation in symptomatic patients with prior CABG.

Killen and associates[202] from Kansas City, Kansas, reported their experience in patients undergoing CABG after PTCA. During a 4-year period, 286 patients had CABG: 73 had 1-vessel and 213 had multivessel CAD; 115 patients underwent CABG on an emergency basis. Indications for emergency CABG after PTCA were prolonged chest pain (79%), worsening of coronary artery obstruction (59%), "current of injury" (31%), cardiogenic shock (28%), and, in a lesser incidence, VF, coronary artery dissection, heart block, and cardiac arrest. The 286 patients had 2.1 anastomoses per patient with a 30-day mortality of 6.3% (18 patients). The incidence of AMI was 44 -vs- 4%; low cardiac output syndrome, 35 -vs- 7%, and operative death 11 -vs- 3% in the emergency and nonemergency groups, respectively. Other significant predictors of operative death were previous CABG (17 -vs- 5%), multivessel CAD (8 -vs- 1%), and preoperative cardiogenic shock (16 -vs- 3%). Approximately 3,000 PTCA procedures were performed at this group's institution during the period of study. The 115 emergency CABG procedures represented an incidence of 4% of all PTCA procedures. The overall survival in this series at 4 years postoperatively was 91%. The linearized annual mortality was 1.4%/year and the 4-year survival in the emergency and elective CABG groups was 86 and 95%, respectively. It is obvious that these results with CABG performed after failed PTCA can be influenced greatly by the type of patients selected for PTCA. Great care should be exercised in the inclusion of patients for PTCA with previous CABG, multivessel CAD, and other complex variants of CAD. When complications arise after PTCA, prompt undertaking of emergency CABG could perhaps decrease the incidence of AMI and death.

Kelly and coworkers[203] from Springfield, Illinois, evaluated a consecutive series of 78 patients having PTCA for 1-vessel CAD and 85 patients having 1-vessel CABG with a follow-up for 1 year. The intent of this study was to determine the cost of care per patient for each of these procedures. Days in the hospital and the cost for angiography and revascularization procedures were determined and the total cost of care for 12 months was calculated. Among these patients, PTCA was successful in 74%. However, CABG was ultimately needed in 23 of the 78 patients having PTCA because of initial failure in 26% and late restenosis in 18%. Although CABG was ultimately necessary in approximately 30% of these patients, the cost of care per patient was 43% lower for those having PTCA as an initial procedure for 1-vessel CAD.

References

1. CONROY RM, MULCAHY R, HICKEY N, DALY L: Is a family history of coronary heart disease an independent coronary risk factor? Br Heart J 1985 (Apr); 53:378–381.
2. MEDINA R, PANIDIS IP, MORGANROTH J, KOTLER MN, MINTZ GS: The value of echocardiographic regional wall motion abnormalities in detecting coronary artery disease in patients with or without a dilated left ventricle. Am Heart J 1985 (Apr); 109:799–803.
3. REN J-F, KOTLER MN, HAKKI A-H, PANIDIS IP, MINTZ GS, ROSS J: Quantitation of regional left ventricular function by two-dimensional echocardiography in normals and patients with coronary artery disease. Am Heart J 1985 (Sept); 110:552–560.
4. LABOVITZ AJ, DINCER B, MUDD G, AKER UT, KENNEDY HL: The effects of Valsalva maneuver on global and segmental left ventricular function in presence and absence of coronary artery disease. Am Heart J 1985 (Feb); 109:259–264.
5. MELIN JA, WIJNS W, VANBUTSELE RJ, ROBERT A, DE COSTER P, BRASSEUR LA, BECKERS C, DETRY JR: Alternative diagnostic strategies for coronary artery disease in women: demonstration of the usefulness and efficiency of probability analysis. Circulation 1985 (Mar); 71:535–542.
6. HUNG J, CHAITMAN BR, LAM J, LESPERANCE J, DUPRAS G, FINES P, CHERKAOUI O, ROBERT P, BOURASSA MG: A logistic regression analysis of multiple noninvasive tests for the prediction of the presence and extent of coronary artery disease in men. Am Heart J 1985 (Aug); 110:460–469.
7. POLLAK SJ, KERTES PJ, BREDLAU CE, WALTER PF: Influence of left ventricular function on signal averaged late potentials in patients with coronary artery disease with and without ventricular tachycardia. Am Heart J 1985 (Oct); 110:747–752.
8. HOLLENBERG M, ZOLTICK JM, GO M, YANEY SF, DANIELS W, DAVIS RC, BEDYNEK JL: Comparison of a quantitative treadmill exercise score with standard electrocardiographic criteria in screening asymptomatic young men for coronary artery disease. N Engl J Med 1985 (Sept 5); 313:600–606.
9. SHEFFIELD LT: Another perfect treadmill test? N Engl J Med 1985 (Sept 5); 313:633–635.
10. BRAAT SH, KINGMA H, BRUGADA P, WELLENS HJJ: Value of lead V_4R in exercise testing to predict proximal stenosis of the right coronary artery. J Am Coll Cardiol 1985 (June); 5:1308–1311.
11. MULTIPLE RISK FACTOR INTERVENTION TRIAL RESEARCH GROUP: Baseline rest electrocardiographic abnormalities, antihypertensive treatment, and mortality in the multiple risk factor intervention trial. Am J Cardiol 1985 (Jan 1); 55:16–24.
12. OKIN PM, KLIGFIELD P, AMEISEN O, GOLDBERG HL, BORER JS: Improved accuracy of the exercise electrocardiogram: identification of three-vessel coronary disease in stable angina pectoris by analysis of peak rate-related changes in ST segments. Am J Cardiol 1985 (Feb 1); 55:271–276.
13. HOLLENBERG M, GO M, MASSIE BM, WISNESKI JA, GERTZ EW: Influence of R-wave amplitude on exercise-induced ST depression: need for a "gain factor" correction when interpreting stress electrocardiograms. Am J Cardiol 1985 (July 1); 56:13–17.
14. TZIVONI D, BENHORIN J, GAVISH A, STERN S: Holter recording during treadmill testing in assessing myocardial ischemic changes. Am J Cardiol 1985 (Apr 15); 55:1200–1203.

15. AKHRAS F, UPWARD J, JACKSON G: Increased diastolic blood pressure response to exercise testing when coronary artery disease is suspected: an indication of severity. Br Heart J 1985 (June); 53:598–602.

16. HO SWG, McCOMISH MJ, TAYLOR RR: Effect of beta-adrenergic blockade on the results of exercise testing related to the extent of coronary artery disease. Am J Cardiol 1985 (Jan 1); 55:258–262.

17. BALADY GJ, WEINER DA, McCABE CH, RYAN TJ: Value of arm exercise testing in detecting coronary artery disease. Am J Cardiol 1985 (Jan 1); 55:37–39.

18. SAGIV M, HANSON P, BESOZZI MY, NAGLE F: Left ventricular responses to upright isometric handgrip and deadlift in men with coronary artery disease. Am J Cardiol 1985 (May 1); 55:1298–1302.

19. BROWN KA, OSBAKKEN M, BOUCHER CA, STRAUSS HW, POHOST GM, OKADA RD: Positive exercise thallium-201 test responses in patients with less than 50% maximal coronary stenosis: angiographic and clinical predictors. Am J Cardiol 1985 (Jan 1); 55:54–57.

20. KALFF V, KELLY MJ, SOWARD A, HARPER RW, CURRIE PJ, LIM YL, PITT A: Assessment of hemodynamic significance of isolated stenosis of the left anterior descending coronary artery using thallium-201 myocardial scintigraphy. Am J Cardiol 1985 (Feb 1); 55:342–346.

21. KAUL S, KIESS M, LIU P, GUINEY TE, POHOST GM, OKADA RD, BOUCHER CA: Comparison of exercise electrocardiography and quantitative thallium imaging for one-vessel coronary artery disease. Am J Cardiol 1985 (Aug 1); 56:257–261.

22. BOUCHER CA, BREWSTER DC, DARLING RC, OKADA RD, STRAUSS HW, POHOST GM: Determination of cardiac risk by dipyridamole-thallium imaging before peripheral vascular surgery. N Engl J Med 1985 (Feb 14); 312:389–394.

23. O'HARA MJ, LAHIRI A, WHITTINGTON JR, CRAWLEY JCW, RAFTERY EB: Detection of high risk coronary artery disease by thallium imaging. Br Heart J 1985 (June); 53:616–623.

24. PORT SC, OSHIMA M, RAY G, McNAMEE P, SCHMIDT DH: Assessment of single vessel coronary artery disease: results of exercise electrocardiography, thallium-201 myocardial perfusion imaging and radionuclide angiography. J Am Coll Cardiol 1985 (July); 6:75–83.

25. REISMAN S, BERMAN D, MADDAHI J, SWAN HJC: The severe stress thallium defect: an indicator of critical coronary stenosis. Am Heart J 1985 (July); 110:128–134.

26. CORBETT JR, JANSEN DE, LEWIS SE, GABLIANI GI, NICOD P, FILIPCHUK NG, REDISH GA, AKERS MS, WOLFE CL, RELLAS JS, PARKEY RW, WILLERSON JT: Tomographic gated blood pool radionuclide ventriculography: analysis of wall motion and left ventricular volumes in patients with coronary artery disease. J Am Coll Cardiol 1985 (Aug); 6:349–358.

27. SCHWARZBERG RJ, SELDIN DW, ALDERSON PO, JOHNSON LL: Peak regional acceleration: a method to identify subtle regional ventricular dysfunction from gated blood pool scans at rest in patients with coronary artery disease. J Am Coll Cardiol 1985 (Sept); 6:589–596.

28. UNDERWOOD DA, PROUDFIT WL, LIM J, MACMILLAN JP: Symptomatic coronary artery disease in patients aged 21 to 30 years. Am J Cardiol 1985 (Mar 1); 55:631–634.

29. ELAYDA MA, MATHUR VS, HALL RJ, MASSUMI GA, GARCIA E, DeCASTRO CM: Collateral circulation in coronary artery disease. Am J Cardiol 1985 (Jan 1); 55:58–60.

30. WIJNS W, SERRUYS PW, REIBER JHC, VAN DEN BRAND M, SIMMONS ML, KOOIJMAN CJ, BALAKUMARAN K, HUGENHOLTZ PG: Quantitative angiography of the left anterior descending coronary artery: correlations with pressure gradient and results of exercise thallium scintigraphy. Circulation 1985 (Feb); 71:273–279.

31. GANZ P, ABBEN R, FRIEDMAN PL, GARNIC JD, BARRY WH, LEVIN DC: Usefulness of transstenotic coronary pressure gradient measurements during diagnostic catheterization. Am J Cardiol (Apr 1); 55:910–914.

32. RATH S, HAR-ZAHAV Y, BATTLER A, AGRANAT O, ROTSTEIN Z, RABINOWITZ B, NEUFELD HN: Fate of nonobstructive aneurysmatic coronary artery disease: Angiographic and clinical follow-up report. Am Heart J 1985 (Apr); 109:785–791.

33. HARTNELL GG, PARNELL BM, PRIDIE RB: Coronary artery ectasia: its prevalence and clinical significance in 4993 patients. Br Heart J 1985 (Oct); 54:392–395.

34. ELVEBACK LR, CONNOLLY DC: Coronary heart disease in residents of Rochester, Minnesota. V. Prognosis of patients with coronary heart disease based on initial manifestation. Mayo Clin Proc 1985 (May); 60:305–311.

35. GRIMM RH, NEATON JD, LUDWIG W: Prognostic importance of the white blood cell count for coronary, cancer, and all-cause mortality. JAMA 1985 (Oct 11); 254:1932–1937.

36. ISKANDRIAN AS, HAKKI A-H, KANE-MARSCH S: Prognostic implications of exercise thallium-201 scintigraphy in patients with suspected or known coronary artery disease. Am Heart J 1985 (July); 110:135–143.

37. PAMELIA FX, GIBSON RS, WATSON DD, CRADDOCK GB, SIROWATKA J, BELLER GA: Prognosis with chest pain and normal thallium-201 exercise scintigrams. Am J Cardiol 1985 (Apr 1); 55:920–926.

38. WACKERS FJT, RUSSO DJ, RUSSO D, CLEMENTS JP: Prognostic significance of normal quantitative planar thallium-201 stress scintigraphy in patients with chest pain. J Am Coll Cardiol 1985 (July); 6:27–30.

39. CALIFF RM, PHILLIPS HR III, HINDMAN MC, MARK DB, LEE KL, BEHAR VS, JOHNSON RA, PRYOR DB, ROSATI RA, WAGNER GS, HARRELL FE JR: Prognostic value of a coronary artery jeopardy score. J Am Coll Cardiol 1985 (May); 5:1055–1063.

40. ZIMMERMAN M, ADAMEC R, SIMONIN P, RICHEZ J: Prognostic significance of ventricular late potentials in coronary artery disease. Am Heart J 1985 (Apr); 109:725–732.

41. MOISE A, THEROUX P, TAEYMANS Y, WATERS DD: Factors associated with progression of coronary artery disease in patients with normal or minimally narrowed coronary arteries. Am J Cardiol 1985 (July 1); 56:30–34.

42. KLATSKY AL, PETITTI DB, ARMSTRONG MA, FRIEDMAN GD: Coffee, tea and cholesterol. Am J Cardiol 1985 (Feb 15); 55:577–588.

43. MIETTINEN TA, HUTTUNEN JK, NAUKKARINEN V, STRANDBERG T, MATTILA S, KUMLIN T, SARNA S: Multifactorial primary prevention of cardiovascular diseases in middle-aged men: risk factor changes, incidence, and mortality. JAMA 1985 (Oct 18); 254:2097–2102.

44. CONSENSUS CONFERENCE: Lowering blood cholesterol to prevent heart disease. JAMA 1985 (Apr 12); 253:2080–2086.

45. KRONMAL RA: Commentary on the published results of the lipid research clinics coronary primary prevention trial. JAMA 1985 (Apr 12); 253:2091–2093.

46. RAHIMTOOLA SH: Cholesterol and coronary heart disease: a perspective (Editorial). JAMA 1985 (Apr 12); 253:2094–2095.

47. ADAMS D: Lowering cholesterol and the incidence of coronary heart disease (letter). JAMA 1985 (June 7); 253:3090.

48. GREEN MS, HEISS G, RIFKIND BM, COOPER GR, WILLIAMS OD, TYROLER HA: The ratio of plasma high-density lipoprotein cholesterol to total and low-density lipoprotein cholesterol: age-related changes and race and sex differences in selected North American populations. The Lipid Research Clinics Program Prevalence Study. Circulation 1985 (July); 72:93–104.

49. LENFANT C: New national cholesterol education program. Cardiovasc Med 1985 (Nov); 10:39–40.

50. KESTELOOT H, HUANG DX, YANG XS, CLAES J, ROSSENEU M, GEBOERS J, JOOSSENS JV: Serum lipids in the People's Republic of China: comparison of western and eastern populations. Arteriosclerosis 1985 (Sept/Oct); 5:427–433.

51. SUDHOF TC, GOLDSTEIN JL, BROWN MS, RUSSELL DW: The LDL receptor gene: a mosaic of exons shared with different proteins. Science 1985 (May 17); 228:815–824.

52. COWAN LD, WILCOSKY T, CRIQUI MH, BARRETT-CONNOR E, SUCHINDRAN CM, WALLACE R, LASKARZEWSKI P, WALDEN C: Demographic, behavioral, biochemical, and dietary correlates of plasma triglycerides: lipid research clinics program prevalence study. Arteriosclerosis 1985 (Sept/Oct); 5:466–480.

53. VEGA GL, GRUNDY SM: Gemfibrozil therapy in primary hypertriglyceridemia associated with coronary heart disease: effects on metabolism of low-density lipoproteins. JAMA 1985 (Apr 26); 253:2398–2403.

54. BREIER C, DREXEL H, LISCH HJ, MUHLBERGER V, HEROLD M, KNAPP E, BRAUNSTEINER H: Essential role of post-heparin lipoprotein lipase activity and of plasma testosterone in coronary artery disease. Lancet 1985 (June 1); 1:1242–1244.

55. SCHMIDT SB, WASSERMAN AG, MUESING RA, SCHLESSELMAN SE, LAROSA JC, ROSS AM: Lipoprotein and apolipoprotein levels in angiographically defined coronary atherosclerosis. Am J Cardiol 1985 (June 1); 55:1459–1462.

56. APPEL GB, BLUM CB, CHIEN S, KUNIS CL, APPEL AS: The hyperlipidemia of the nephrotic syndrome: relation to plasma albumin concentration, oncotic pressure, and viscosity. N Engl J Med 1985 (June 13); 312:1544–1548.

57. FREEDMAN DS, BURKE GL, HARSHA DW, SRINIVASAN SR, CRESANTA JL, WEBBER LS, BERENSON GS: Relationship of changes in obesity to serum lipid and lipoprotein changes in childhood and adolescence. JAMA 1985 (July 26); 254:515–520.

58. MERIANS DR, HASKELL WL, VRANIZAN KM, PHELPS J, WOODS PD, SUPERKO R: Relationship of exercise, oral contraceptive use, and body fat to concentrations of plasma lipids and lipoprotein cholesterol in young women. Am J Med 1985 (June); 78:913–919.

59. Tran ZV, Weltman A: Differential effects of exercise on serum lipid and lipoprotein levels seen with changes in body weight: A Meta-analysis. JAMA 1985 (Aug 16); 254:919–924.

60. Williams PT, Wood PD, Vranizan KM, Albers JJ, Garay SC, Taylor CB: Coffee intake and elevated cholesterol and apolipoprotein B levels in men. JAMA 1985 (Mar 8); 253:1407–1411.

61. Camargo CA, Williams PT, Vranizan KM, Albers JJ, Wood PD: The effect of moderate alcohol intake on serum apolipoproteins A-1 and A-2: a controlled study. JAMA 1985 (May 17); 253:2854–2857.

62. Vitols S, Bjorkholm M, Gahrton G, Peterson C: Hypocholesterolemia in malignancy due to elevated low-density-lipoprotein-receptor activity in tumor cells: evidence from studies in patients with leukemia. Lancet 1985 (Nov 23); 2:1150–1154.

63. Kromhout D, Bosschieter EB, Coulander CD: The inverse relation between fish consumption and 20-year mortality from coronary heart disease. N Engl J Med 1985 (May 9); 312:1205–1209.

64. Phillipson BE, Rothrock DW, Connor WE, Harris WS, Illingworth DR: Reduction of plasma lipids, lipoproteins, and apoproteins by dietary fish oils in patients with hypertriglyceridemia. N Engl J Med 1985 (May 9); 312:1210–1216.

65. Glomset JA: Fish, fatty acids, and human health. N Engl J Med 1985 (May 9); 312:1253–1254.

66. Shekelle RB, Missell L, Paul O, Shryock AM, Stamler J: Fish consumption and mortality from coronary heart disease. N Engl J Med 1985 (Sept 26); 313:820–821.

67. Vollset SE, Heuch I, Bjelke E: Fish consumption in mortality from coronary disease (letter). N Engl J Med 1985 (Sept 26); 313:621.

68. Curb JD, Reed DM: Letter to the Editor. N Engl J Med 1985 (Sept 26); 313:821.

69. Kushi LH, Lew RA, Stare FJ, Ellison RC, Lozy M, Bourke G, Daly L, Graham I, Hickey N, Mulcahy R, Kevaney J: Diet and 20-year mortality from coronary heart disease: The Ireland-Boston diet-heart study. N Engl J Med 1985 (Mar 28); 312:811–818.

70. Blankenhorn DH: Two new diet-heart studies. N Engl J Med 1985 (Mar 28); 312:851–852.

71. Macfarlane D: Letter to the editor. N Engl J Med 1985 (July 11); 313:118.

72. Kushi LH, Lozy M, Stare FJ, Lew RA, Ellison RC, Bourke G, Daly L, Hickey N, Mulcahy R, Graham I, Kevaney J: Letter to the editor. N Engl J Med 1985 (July 11); 313:119.

73. Arntzenius AC, Kromhout D, Barth JD, Reiber JHC, Bruschke VG, Buis B, Van Gent CM, Kempen-Voogd N, Strikwerda S, Van Der Velde EA: Diet, lipoproteins, and the progression of coronary atherosclerosis: the Leiden intervention trial. N Engl J Med 1985 (Mar 28); 312:805–811.

74. Sacks FM, Ornish D, Rosner B, McLanahan S, Castelli WP, Kass EH: Plasma lipoprotein levels in vegetarians: the effect of ingestion of fats from dairy products. JAMA 1985 (Sept 13); 254:1337–1341.

75. Hoeg JM, Maher MB, Bailey KR, Zech LA, Gregg RE, Sprecher DL, Brewer HB: Effects of combination cholestyramine-neomycin treatment on plasma lipoprotein concentrations in type II hyperlipoproteinemia. Am J Cardiol 1985 (May 1); 55:1282–1286.

76. Bershad S, Rubinstein A, Paterniti JR, Le NA, Poliak SC, Heller B, Ginsberg HN, Fleischmajer R, Brown WV: Changes in plasma lipids and lipoproteins during isotretinoin therapy for acne. N Engl J Med 1985 (Oct 10); 313:981–985.

77. Hubbard JD, Inkeles S, Barnard RJ: Nathan Pritikin's heart. N Engl J Med 1985 (July 4); 313:52.

78. Schaefer EJ, Levy RI: Pathogenesis and management of lipoprotein disorders. N Engl J Med 1985 (May 16); 312:1300–1310.

79. Weintraub WS, Klein LW, Seelaus PA, Agarwal JB, Helfant RH: Importance of total life consumption of cigarettes as a risk factor for coronary artery disease. Am J Cardiol 1985 (Mar 1); 55:669–672.

80. Kannel WB, Wilson P, Blair SN: Epidemiological assessment of the role of physical activity and fitness in development of cardiovascular disease. Am Heart J 1985 (Apr); 109:876–885.

81. Sullivan M, Ahnve S, Froelicher VF, Meyers J: The influence of exercise training on the ventilatory threshold of patients with coronary heart disease. Am Heart J 1985 (Mar); 109:458–463.

82. National Institutes of Health Consensus Development Conference Statement: Health implications of obesity. Ann Intern Med 1985 (July); 103:147–151.

83. Piters KM, Colombo A, Olson HG, Butman SM: Effect of coffee on exercise-induced angina

pectoris due to coronary artery disease in habitual coffee drinkers. Am J Cardiol 1985 (Feb 1); 55:277–280.

84. COLDITZ GA, BRANCH LG, LIPNICK RJ, WILLETT WC, ROSNER B, POSNER B, HENNEKENS CH: Moderate alcohol and decreased cardiovascular mortality in an elderly cohort. Am Heart J 1985 (Apr); 109:886–889.

85. STAMPFER MJ, WILLETT WC, COLDITZ GA, ROSNER B, SPEIZER FE, HENNEKENS CH: A prospective study of postmenopausal estrogen therapy and coronary heart disease. N Engl J Med 1985 (Oct 24); 313:1044–1049.

86. WILSON PWF, GARRISON RJ, CASTELLI WP: Postmenopausal estrogen use, cigarette smoking, and cardiovascular morbidity in women over 50: The Framingham Study. N Engl J Med 1985 (Oct 14); 313:1038–1043.

87. BAILAR JC: When research results are in conflict (Editorial). N Engl J Med 1985 (Oct 24); 313:1080–1081.

88. BOERS GHJ, SMALS AGH, TRIJBELS FJM, FOWLER B, BAKKEREN JAJM, SCHOONDERWALDT HC, KLEIJER WJ, KLOPPENBORG PWC: Heterozygosity for homocystinuria in premature peripheral and cerebral occlusive arterial disease. N Engl J Med 1985 (Sept 19); 313:709–715.

89. MUDD SH: Vascular disease and homocysteine metabolism. N Engl J Med 1985 (Sept 19); 313:751–753.

90. WEKSLER BB, TACK-GOLDMAN, SUBRAMANIAN VA, GAY WA: Cumulative inhibitory effect of low-dose aspirin on vascular prostacyclin and platelet thromboxane production in patients with atherosclerosis. Circulation 1985 (Feb); 71:332–340.

91. ROY L, KNAPP HR, ROBERTSON R, FITZGERALD GA: Endogenous biosynthesis of prostacyclin during cardiac catheterization and angiography in man. Circulation 1985 (Mar); 71:434–440.

92. EDLUND A, BERGLUND B, VAN DORNE D, KAIJSER L, NOWAK J, PATRONO C, SOLLEVI A, WENNMALM A: Coronary flow regulation in patients with ischemic heart disease: release of purines and prostacyclin and the effect of inhibitors of prostaglandin formation. Circulation 1985 (June); 71:1113–1120.

93. GALLINO A, HAEBERLI A, BAUR HR, STRAUB PW: Fibrin formation and platelet aggregation in patients with severe coronary artery disease: relationship with the degree of myocardial ischemia. Circulation 1985 (Jan); 72:27–30.

94. VON ARNIM T, HOFLING B, SCHREIBER M: Characteristics of episodes of ST elevation or ST depression during ambulatory monitoring in patients subsequently undergoing coronary angiography. Br Heart J 1985 (Nov); 54:484–488.

95. CHANNER KS, JAMES MA, PAPOUCHADO M, REES JR: Anxiety and depression in patients with chest pain referred for exercise testing. Lancet 1985 (Oct 12); 2:820–822.

96. QUYYUMI AA, WRIGHT CM, MOCKUS LJ, FOX KM: How important is a history of chest pain in determining the degree of ischemia in patients with angina pectoris? Br Heart J 1985 (July); 54:22–26.

97. WATERS DD, McCANS JL, CREAN PA: Serial exercise testing in patients with effort angina: variable tolerance, fixed threshold. J Am Coll Cardiol 1985 (Nov); 6:1011–1015.

98. KLIGFIELD P, OKIN PM, AMEISEN O, WALLIS J, BORER JS: Correlation of the exercise ST/HR slope with anatomic and radionuclide cineangiographic findings in stable angina pectoris. Am J Cardiol 1985 (Sept 1); 56:418–421.

99. PICANO E, DISTANTE A, MASINI M, MORALES MA, LATTANZI F, L'ABBATE A: Dipyridamole-echocardiography test in effort angina pectoris. Am J Cardiol 1985 (Sept 1); 56:452–456.

100. AMBROSE JA, WINTERS SL, STERN A, ENG A, TEICHHOLZ LE, GORLIN R, FUSTER V: Angiographic morphology and the pathogenesis of unstable angina pectoris. J Am Coll Cardiol 1985 (Mar); 5:609–616.

101. BRESNAHAN DR, DAVIS JL, HOLMES DR JR, SMITH HC: Angiographic occurrence and clinical correlates of intraluminal coronary artery thrombus: role of unstable angina. J Am Coll Cardiol 1985 (Aug); 6:285–289.

102. CAPONE G, WOLF NM, MEYER B, MEISTER SG: Frequency of intracoronary filling defects by angiography in angina pectoris at rest. Am J Cardiol 1985 (Sept 1); 56:403–406.

103. MacDONALD RG, FELDMAN RL, HILL JA, CONTI CR, PEPINE CJ: Coronary hemodynamic responses during spontaneous angina in patients with and patients without coronary artery spasm. Am J Cardiol 1985 (July 1); 56:41–46.

104. HEUPLER FA, FERRARIO CM, AVERILL DB, BOTT-SILVERMAN C: Initial coronary air embolus in the differential diagnosis of coronary artery spasm. Am J Cardiol 1985 (Mar 1); 55:657–661.

105. SERNERI GGN, GENSINI GF, ABBATE R, PRISCO D, ROGASI PG, LAUREANO R, CASOLO GC, FANTINI F,

Di Donato M, Dabizzi RP: Abnormal cardiocoronary thromboxane A$_2$ production in patients with unstable angina. Am Heart J 1985 (Apr); 109:732–738.

106. Sasayama S, Nonogi H, Miyazaki S, Sakurai T, Kawai C, Eiho S, Kuwahara M: Changes in diastolic properties of the regional myocardium during pacing-induced ischemia in human subjects. J Am Coll Cardiol 1985 (Mar); 5:599–606.

107. McDaniel HG, Rogers WJ, Russell RO, Rackley CE: Improved myocardial contractility with glucose-insulin-potassium infusion during pacing in coronary artery disease. Am J Cardiol 1985 (Apr 1); 55:932–936.

108. Aroesty JM, McKay RG, Heller GV, Royal HD, Als AV, Grossman W: Simultaneous assessment of left ventricular systolic and diastolic dysfunction during pacing-induced ischemia. Circulation 1985 (May); 71:889–900.

109. Kohchi K, Takebayashi S, Hiroki T, Nobuyoshi M: Significance of adventitial inflammation of the coronary artery in patients with unstable angina: results at autopsy. Circulation 1985 (Apr); 71:709–716.

110. Mukharji J, Kremers M, Lipscomb K, Blomqvist CG: Early positive exercise test and extensive coronary disease: effect of antianginal therapy. Am J Cardiol 1985 (Feb 1); 55:267–270.

111. Charap MH, Levin RI, Weinglass J: Physician choices in the treatment of angina pectoris. Am J Med 1985 (Oct); 79:461–466.

112. Parker JO, Vankoughnett KA, Farrell B: Comparison of buccal nitroglycerin and oral isosorbide dinitrate for nitrate tolerance in stable angina pectoris. Am J Cardiol 1985 (Nov 1); 56:724–728.

113. Kaski JC, Plaza LR, Meran DO, Araujo L, Chierchia S, Maseri A: Improved coronary supply: prevailing mechanism of action of nitrates in chronic stable angina. Am Heart J 1985 (July); 110:238–245.

114. Badger RS, Brown BG, Gallery CA, Bolson EL, Dodge HT: Coronary artery dilation and hemodynamic responses after isosorbide dinitrate therapy in patients with coronary artery disease. Am J Cardiol 1985 (Sept 1); 56:390–395.

115. James MA, Walker PR, Papouchado M, Wilkinson PR: Efficacy of transdermal glyceryl trinitrate in the treatment of chronic stable angina pectoris. Br Heart J 1985 (June); 53:631–635.

116. Lin SG, Flaherty JT: Crossover from intravenous to transdermal nitroglycerin therapy in unstable angina pectoris. Am J Cardiol 1985 (Nov 1); 56:742–748.

117. Rudolph W, Dirschinger J: Effectiveness of molsidomine in the long-term treatment of exertional angina pectoris and chronic congestive heart failure. Am Heart J 1985 (Mar); 109:670–674.

118. Quyyumi A, Wright C, Mockus L, Shackell M, Sutton GC, Fox KM: Effects of combined alpha and beta adrenoceptor blockade in patients with angina pectoris: a double blind study comparing labetalol with placebo. Br Heart J 1985 (Jan); 53:47–52.

119. Dash H, Copehaver GL, Ensminger S: Improvement in regional wall motion and left ventricular relaxation after administration of diltiazem in patients with coronary artery disease. Circulation 1985 (Aug); 72:353–363.

120. Joyal M, Cremer KF, Pieper JA, Feldman RL, Pepine CJ: Systemic, left ventricular and coronary hemodynamic effects of intravenous diltiazem in coronary artery disease. Am J Cardiol 1985 (Sept 1); 56:413–417.

121. Josephon MA, Hopkins J, Singh BN: Hemodynamic and metabolic effects of diltiazem during coronary sinus pacing with particular reference to left ventricular ejection fraction. Am J Cardiol 1985 (Feb 1); 55:286–290.

122. Petru MA, Crawford MH, Kennedy GT, Amon KW, O'Rourke RA: Long-term efficacy of high-dose diltiazem for chronic stable angina pectoris: 16-month serial studies with placebo controls. Am Heart J 1985 (Jan); 109:99–103.

123. Kern MJ, Walsh RA, Barr WK, Porter CB, O'Rourke RA: Improved myocardial oxygen utilization by diltiazem in CAD patients. Am Heart J 1985 (Nov); 110:986–990.

124. Feldman RL, Hill JA, Conti CR, Pepine CJ: Effect of nifedipine on coronary hemodynamics in patients with left anterior descending coronary occlusion. J Am Coll Cardiol 1985 (Feb); 5:318–325.

125. Boden WE, Korr KS, Bough EW: Nifedipine-induced hypotension and myocardial ischemia in refractory angina pectoris. JAMA 1985 (Feb 22); 253:1131–1135.

126. White HD, Polak JF, Wynne J, Holman BL, Antman EM, Nesto RW: Addition of nifedipine to maximal nitrate and beta-adrenoreceptor blocker therapy in coronary artery disease. Am J Cardiol 1985 (May 1); 55:1303–1307.

127. GELMAN JS, FELDMAN RL, SCOTT E, PEPINE CJ: Nicardipine for angina pectoris at rest and coronary arterial spasm. Am J Cardiol 1985 (Aug 1); 56:232–236.

128. LAM J, CHAITMAN BR, CREAN P, BLUM R, WATERS DD: A dose-ranging, placebo-controlled, double-blind trial of nisoldipine in effort angina: duration and extent of antianginal effects. J Am Coll Cardiol 1985 (Aug); 6:447–452.

129. KENNY J, KIFF P, HOLMES J, JEWITT DE: Beneficial effects of diltiazem and propranolol, alone and in combination, in patients with stable angina pectoris. Br Heart J 1985 (Jan); 53:43–46.

130. THÉROUX P, TAEYMANS Y, MORISSETTE D, BOSCH X, PELLETIER GB, WATERS DD: A randomized study comparing propranolol and diltiazem in the treatment of unstable angina. J Am Coll Cardiol 1985 (Mar); 5:717–722.

131. BRAUN S, TERDIMAN R, BERENFELD D, LANIADO S: Clinical and hemodynamic effects of combined propranolol and nifedipine therapy versus propranolol alone in patients with angina pectoris. Am Heart J 1985 (Mar); 109:478–485.

132. WOLFE CL, TILTON GD, HILLIS LD, ASHRAM NE, WINNIFORD MD: Acute hemodynamic and electrophysiologic effects of propranolol in patients receiving diltiazem. Am J Cardiol 1985 (July 1); 56:47–50.

133. JOHNSTON DL, LESOWAY R, HUMEN DP, KOSTUK WJ, MICKLE P: Clinical and hemodynamic evaluation of propranolol in combination with verapamil, nifedipine and diltiazem in exertional angina pectoris: a placebo-controlled, double-blind, randomized, crossover study. Am J Cardiol 1985 (Mar 1); 55:680–687.

134. WINNIFORD MD, FULTON KL, CORBETT JR, CROFT CH, HILLIS LD: Propranolol-verapamil versus propranolol-nifedipine in severe angina pectoris of effort: a randomized, double-blind, crossover study. Am J Cardiol 1985 (Feb 1); 55:281–285.

135. MORSE JR, NESTO RW: Double-blind crossover comparison of the antianginal effects of nifedipine and isosorbide dinitrate in patients with exertional angina receiving propranolol. J Am Coll Cardiol 1985 (Dec); 6:1395–1401.

136. CAIRNS JA, GENT M, SINGER J, FINNIE KJ, FROGGATT GM, HOLDER DA, JABLONSKY G, KOSTUK WJ, MELENDEZ LJ, MYERS MG, SACKETT DL, SEALEY BJ, TANSER PH: Aspirin, sulfinpyrazone, or both in unstable angina: results of a Canadian multicenter trial. N Engl J Med 1985 (Nov 28); 313:1369–1375.

137. DALY P, METTAUER B, ROULEAU J, COUSINEAU D, BURGESS JII: Lack of reflex increase in myocardial sympathetic tone after captopril: potential antianginal effect. Circulation 1985 (Feb); 71:317–325.

138. KAMIKAWA T, KOBAYASHI A, YAMASHITA T, HAYASHI H, YAMAZAKI N: Effects of coenzyme Q_{10} on exercise tolerance in chronic stable angina pectoris. Am J Cardiol 1985 (Aug 1); 56:247–251.

139. PFISTERER M, BURKART F, MÜLLER-BRAND J, KIOWSKI W: Important differences between short- and long-term hemodynamic effects of amiodarone in patients with chronic ischemic heart disease at rest and during ischemia-induced left ventricular dysfunction. J Am Coll Cardiol 1985 (May); 5:1205–1211.

140. SHUB C, VLIETSTRA RE, McGOON MD: Selection of optimal drug therapy for the patient with angina pectoris. Mayo Clin Proc 1985 (Aug); 60:539–548.

141. CREA F, DAVIES G, CHIERCHIA S, ROMEO F, BUGIARDINI R, KASKI JC, FREEDMAN B, MASERI A: Different susceptibility to myocardial ischemia provoked by hyperventilation and cold pressor test in exertional and variant angina pectoris. Am J Cardiol 1985 (July 1); 56:18–22.

142. GABLIANI GI, WINNIFORD MD, FULTON KL, JOHNSON SM, MAURITSON DR, HILLIS LD: Ventricular ectopic activity with spontaneous variant angina: frequency and relation to transient ST segment deviation. Am Heart J 1985 (July); 110:40–43.

143. ROVAI D, DISTANTE A, MOSCARELLI E, MORALES MA, PICANO E, PALOMBO C, L'ABBATE A: Transient myocardial ischemia with minimal electrocardiographic changes: an echocardiographic study in patients with Prinzmetal's angina. Am Heart J 1985 (Jan); 109:78–83.

144. MATSUDA Y, OGAWA H, MORITANI K, MATSUDA M, KATAYAMA K, FUJII T, KOHNO M, MIURA T, KOHTOKU S, KUSUKAWA R: Transient appearance of collaterals during vasospastic occlusion in patients without obstructive coronary atherosclerosis. Am Heart J 1985 (April); 109:759–763.

145. SCHROEDER JS, WALKER SD, SKALLAND L, HEMBERGER JA: Absence of rebound from diltiazem therapy in Prinzmetal's variant angina. J Am Coll Cardiol 1985 (July); 6:174–178.

146. CORCOS T, DAVID PR, BOURASSA MG, GUITERAS VAL P, ROBERT J, MATA LA, WATERS DD: Percutaneous transluminal coronary angioplasty for the treatment of variant angina. J Am Coll

Cardiol 1985 (May); 5:1046–1054.

147. OH JK, SHUB C, ILSTRUP DM, REEDER GS: Creatine kinase release after successful percutaneous transluminal coronary angioplasty. Am Heart J 1985 (June); 109:1225–1231.

148. BRYMER JF, KHAJA F, MARZILLI M, GOLDSTEIN S, ALBAN J: Ischemia at a distance during intermittent coronary artery occlusion: A coronary anatomic explanation. J Am Coll Cardiol 1985 (July); 6:41–45.

149. BONOW RO, VITALE DF, BACHARACH SL, FREDERICK TM, KENT KM, GREEN MV: Asynchronous left ventricular regional function and impaired global diastolic filling in patients with coronary artery disease: reversal after coronary angioplasty. Circulation 1985 (Feb); 71:297–307.

150. LEWIS JF, VERANI MS, POLINER LR, LEWIS JM, RAIZNER AE: Effects of transluminal coronary angioplasty on left ventricular systolic and diastolic function at rest and during exercise. Am Heart J 1985 (April); 109:792–798.

151. WAHR DW, PORTS TA, BOTVINICK EH, DAE M, SCHECHTMANN N, HUBERTY J, HATTNER RS, O'CONNELL JW, TURLEY K: The effects of coronary angioplasty and reperfusion on distribution of myocardial flow. Circulation 1985 (Aug); 72:334–343.

152. ANDERSON HV, LEIMGRUBER PP, ROUBIN GS, NELSON DL, GRUENTZIG AR: Distal coronary artery perfusion during percutaneous transluminal coronary angioplasty. Am Heart J 1985 (Oct); 110:720–726.

153. PROBST P, ZANGL W, PACHINGER O: Relation of coronary arterial occlusion pressure during percutaneous transluminal coronary angioplasty to presence of collaterals. Am J Cardiol 1985 (May 1); 55:1264–1269.

154. DOOREY AJ, MEHMEL HC, SCHWARZ FX, KÜBLER W: Amelioration by nitroglycerin of left ventricular ischemia induced by percutaneous transluminal coronary angioplasty: assessment by hemodynamic variables and left ventriculography. J Am Coll Cardiol 1985 (Aug); 6:267–274.

155. CORCOS T, DAVID PR, VAL PG, RENKIN J, DANGOISSE V, RAPOLD HG, BOURASSA MG: Failure of diltiazem to prevent restenosis after percutaneous transluminal coronary angioplasty. Am Heart J 1985 (May); 109:926–931.

156. COWLEY MJ, MULLIN SM, KELSEY SF, KENT KM, GRUENTZIG AR, DETRE KM, PASSAMANI ER: Sex differences in early and long-term results of coronary angioplasty in the NHLBI PTCA Registry. Circulation 1985 (Jan); 71:90–97.

157. OKADA RD, LIM YL, BOUCHER CA, POHOST GM, CHESLER DA, BLOCK PC: Clinical, angiographic, hemodynamic, perfusional and functional changes after one-vessel left anterior descending coronary angioplasty. Am J Cardiol 1985 (Feb 1); 55:347–356.

158. HIRZEL HO, EICHHORN P, KAPPENBERGER L, GANDER MP, SCHLUMPF M, GRUENTZIG AR: Percutaneous transluminal coronary angioplasty: late results at 5 years following intervention. Am Heart J 1985 (Mar); 109:575–581.

159. BREDLAU CE, ROUBIN GS, LEIMGRUBER PP, DOUGLAS JS, KING SB III, GREUNTZIG AR: In-hospital morbidity and mortality in patients undergoing elective coronary angioplasty. Circulation 1985 (Nov); 72:1044–1052.

160. ANDERSON HV, ROUBIN GS, LEIMGRUBER PP, DOUGLAS JS, KING SB, GRUENTZIG AR: Primary angiographic success rates of percutaneous transluminal coronary angioplasty. Am J Cardiol 1985 (Nov 1); 56:712–717.

161. SERRUYS PW, UMANS V, HEYNDRICKX GR, BRAND MVD, DEFEYTER PJ, WIJNS W, JASKI B, HUGENHOLTZ PG: Elective PTCA of totally occluded coronary arteries not associated with acute myocardial infarction; short-term and long-term results. Eur Heart J 1985 (Jan); 6:2–12.

162. KEREIAKES DJ, SELMON MR, McAULEY BJ, McAULEY DB, SHEEHAN DJ, SIMPSON JB: Angioplasty in total coronary artery occlusion: experience in 76 consecutive patients. J Am Coll Cardiol 1985 (Sept); 6:526–533.

163. STERTZER SH, MYLER RK, INSEL H, WALLSH E, ROSSI P: Percutaneous transluminal coronary angioplasty in left main stem coronary stenosis: a five-year appraisal. Int J Cardiol 1985 (Oct); 9:149–159.

164. VANDORMAEL MG, CHAITMAN BR, ISCHINGER T, AKER UT, HARPER M, HERNANDEZ J, DELIGONUL U, KENNEDY HL: Immediate and short-term benefit of multilesion coronary angioplasty: influence of degree of revascularization. J Am Coll Cardiol 1985 (Nov); 6:983–991.

165. COWLEY MH, VETROVEC GW, CISCIASCIO G, LEWIS SA, HIRSH PD, WOLFGANG TC: Coronary angioplasty of multiple vessels: short-term outcome and long-term results. Circulation 1985 (Dec); 72:1314–1320.

166. MATA LA, BOSCH X, DAVID PR, RAPOLD HJ, CORCOS T, BOURASSA MG: Clinical and angiographic

assessment 6 months after double vessel percutaneous coronary angioplasty. J Am Coll Cardiol 1985 (Dec); 6:1239–1244.

167. DE FEYTER PJ, SERRUYS PW, VAN DEN BRAND M, BALAKUMARAN K, MOCHTAR B, SOWARD AI, ARNOLD AER, HUGENHOLTZ PG: Emergency coronary angioplasty in refractory unstable angina. N Engl J Med 1985 (Aug 8); 313:342–346.

168. MABIN TA, HOLMES DR JR, SMITH HC, VLIETSTRA RE, BOVE AA, REEDER GS, CHESEBRO JH, BRESNAHAN JF, ORSZULAK TA: Intracoronary thrombus: role in coronary occlusion complicating percutaneous transluminal coronary angioplasty. J Am Coll Cardiol 1985 (Feb); 5:198–202.

169. WIJNS W, SERRUYS PW, REIBER JHC, FEYTER PJ, BRAND M, SIMOONS ML, HUGENHOLTZ PG, TIJSSEN JGP: Early detection of restenosis after successful percutaneous transluminal coronary angioplasty by exercise-redistribution thallium scintigraphy. Am J Cardiol 1985 (Feb 1); 55:357–361.

170. LEVINE S, EWELS CJ, ROSING DR, KENT KM: Coronary angioplasty: Clinical and angiographic follow-up. Am J Cardiol 1985 (Mar 1); 55:673–676.

171. LEIMGRUBER PP, ROUBIN GS, ANDERSON HV, BREDLAU CE, WHITWORTH HB, DOUGLAS JS, KING SB, GREUNTZIG AR: Influence of intimal dissection on restenosis after successful coronary angioplasty. Circulation 1985 (Sept); 72:530–535.

172. SHIU MF, SILVERTON NP, OAKLEY D, CUMBERLAND D: Acute coronary occlusion during percutaneous transluminal coronary angioplasty. Br Heart J 1985 (Aug); 54:129–133.

173. KAISER GC, DAVIS KB, FISHER LD, MYERS WO, FOSTER ED, PASSAMANI ER, GILLESPIE MJ: Survival following coronary artery bypass grafting in patients with severe angina pectoris (CASS). An observational study. J Thorac Cardiovasc Surg 1985 (Apr); 89:513–524.

174. MCCORMICK JR, SCHICK EC, MCCABE CH, KRONMAL RA, RYAN TJ: Determinants of operative mortality and long-term survival in patients with unstable angina. J Thorac Cardiovasc Surg 1985 (May); 89:683–688.

175. TRESCH DD, WETHERBEE JN, SIEGEL R, TROUP PJ, KEELAN MH JR, OLINGER GN, BROOKS HL: Long-term follow-up of survivors of prehospital sudden cardiac death treated with coronary bypass surgery. Am Heart J 1985 (Dec); 110:1139–1145.

176. GERSH BJ, KRONMAL RA, SCHAFF HV, FRYE RL, RYAN TJ, MOCK MB, MYERS WO, ATHEARN MW, GOSSELIN AJ, KAISER GC, BOURASSA MG, KILLIP T, PARTICIPANTS IN THE CORONARY ARTERY SURGERY STUDY: Comparison of coronary artery bypass surgery and medical therapy in patients 65 years of age or older: a nonrandomized study from the coronary artery surgery study (CASS) registry. N Engl J Med 1985 (July 25); 313:217–224.

177. KUNIS R, GREENBERG H, YEOH CB, GARFEIN OB, PEPE AJ, PINKERNELL BH, SHERRID MV, DWYER EM: Coronary revascularization for recurrent pulmonary edema in elderly patients with ischemic heart disease and preserved ventricular function. N Engl J Med 1985 (Nov 7); 313:1207–1210.

178. REN J-F, PANIDIS IP, KOTLER MN, MINTZ GS, GOEL I, ROSS J: Effect of coronary bypass surgery and valve replacement on left ventricular function: assessment by intraoperative two-dimensional echocardiography. Am Heart J 1985 (Feb); 109:281–289.

179. CARROLL JD, HESS OM, HIRZEL HO, TURINA M, KRAYENBUEHL HP: Left ventricular systolic and diastolic function in coronary artery disease: effects of revascularization on exercise-induced ischemia. Circulation 1985 (July) 72:119–129.

180. RANKIN J, NEWMAN G, MUHLBAIER L, BEHAR V, FEDOR J, SABISTON D: The effects of coronary revascularization on left ventricular function in ischemic heart disease. J Thorac Cardiovasc Surg 1985 (Dec); 90:818–832.

181. PASSAMANI E, DAVIS KB, GILLESPIE MJ, KILLIP T, CASS PRINCIPAL INVESTIGATORS AND ASSOCIATES: A randomized trial of coronary artery bypass surgery: survival of patients with a low ejection fraction. N Engl J Med 1985 (June 27); 312:1665–1671.

182. HUIKURI HV, KORHONEN UR, TAKKUNEN JT: Ventricular arrhythmias induced by dynamic and state exercise in relation to coronary artery bypass grafting. Am J Cardiol 1985 (Apr 1); 55:948–951.

183. LIU P, KIESS MC, OKADA RD, BLOCK PC, STRAUSS HW, POHOST GM, BOUCHER CA: The persistent effect on exercise thallium imaging and its fate after myocardial revascularization: does it represent scar or ischemia? Am Heart J 1985 (Nov); 110:996–1001.

184. BROWN BG, CUKINGNAN RA, DEROUEN T, GOEDE LV, WONG M, FEE HJ, ROTH JA, CAREY JS: Improved graft patency in patients treated with platelet-inhibiting therapy after coronary bypass surgery. Circulation 1985 (July); 72:138–146.

185. RAJAH SM, SALTER MCP, DONALDSON DR, RAO RS, BOYLE RM, PARTRIDGE JB, WATSON DA: Acetyl-

salicylic acid and dipyridamole improve the early patency of aorta-coronary bypass grafts. J Thorac Cardiovasc Surg 1985 (Sept); 90:373–377.

186. FROELICHER V, JENSEN D, SULLIVAN M: A randomized trial of the effects of exercise training after coronary artery bypass surgery. Arch Intern Med 1985 (Apr); 145:689–692.

187. QURESHI SA, HALIM MA, PILLAI R, SMITH P, YACOUB MH: Endarterectomy of the left coronary system. Analysis of a 10 year experience. J Thorac Cardiovasc Surg 1985 (June); 89:852–859.

188. PIDGEON J, BROOKS N, MAGEE P, PEPPER JR, STURRIDGE MF, WRIGHT JEC: Reoperation for angina after previous aortocoronary bypass surgery. Br Heart J 1985 (Mar); 53:269–275.

189. LYTLE BW, LOOP FD, COSGROVE DM, RATLIFF NB, EASLEY K, TAYLOR PC: Long-term (5–12 years) serial studies of internal mammary artery and saphenous vein coronary bypass grafts. J Thorac Cardiovasc Surg 1985 (Feb); 89:248–258.

190. RUBIN DA, NIEMINSKI KE, MONTEFERRANTE JC, MAGEE T, REED GE, HERMAN MV: Ventricular arrhythmias after coronary artery bypass graft surgery: incidence, risk factors and long-term prognosis. J Am Coll Cardiol 1985 (Aug); 6:307–310.

191. SLYSH S, GOLDBERG S, DERVAN JP, ZALEWSKI A: Unstable angina and evolving myocardial infarction following coronary bypass surgery: pathogenesis and treatment with interventional catheterization. Am Heart J 1985 (Apr); 109:744–752.

192. FORCE T, KEMPER AJ, BLOOMFIELD P, TOW DE, KHURI SF, JOSA M, PARISI AF: Non-Q wave perioperative myocardial infarction: assessment of the incidence and severity of regional dysfunction with quantitative two-dimensional echocardiography. Circulation 1985 (Oct); 72:781–789.

193. STANTON BA, JENKINS D, GOLDSTEIN RL, VANDER SALM TJ, KLEIN MD, AUCOIN RA: Hospital readmissions among survivors six months after myocardial revascularization. JAMA 1985 (June 28); 253:3568–3573.

194. VIQUERAT CE, HANSEN RM, BOTVINICK EH, DAE MW, WIENER-KRONISH JP, MATTHAY MA: Undrained bloody pericardial effusion in the early postoperative period after coronary bypass surgery: a prospective blood pool study. Am Heart J 1985 (Aug); 110:335–341.

195. GARDNER T, HORNEFFER P, MANOLIO T, PEARSON T, GOTT V, BAUMGARTNER W, BORKON A, WATKINS L, REITZ B: Stroke following coronary artery bypass grafting: a ten-year study. Ann Thorac Surg 1985 (Dec); 40:574–581.

196. WEISKOPF M, BRAUNSTEIN GD, BATEMAN TM, SOWERS JR, CONKLIN CM, MATLOFF JM, GRAY RJ: Adrenal function following coronary bypass surgery. Am Heart J 1985 (July); 110:71–76.

197. WALLER BF, ROBERTS WC: Remnant saphenous veins after aortocoronary bypass grafting: analysis of 3,394 centimeters of unused vein from 402 patients. Am J Cardiol 1985 (Jan 1); 55:65–71.

198. MOCK MB, REEDER GS, SCHAFF HV, HOLMES DR, VLIETSTRA RE, SMITH HC, GERSH BJ: Percutaneous transluminal coronary angioplasty versus coronary artery bypass: isn't it time for a randomized trial? N Engl J Med 1985 (Apr 4); 312:916–919.

199. BATES ER, AUERON FM, LEGRAND V, LEFREE MT, MANCINI GBJ, HODGSON JM, VOGEL RA: Comparative long-term effects of coronary artery bypass graft surgery and percutaneous transluminal coronary angioplasty on regional coronary flow reserve. Circulation 1985 (Oct); 72:833–839.

200. RAFT D, MCKEE DC, POPIO KA, HAGGERTY JJ: Life adaptation after percutaneous transluminal coronary angioplasty and coronary artery bypass grafting. Am J Cardiol 1985 (Sept 1); 56:395–398.

201. CORBELLI J, FRANCO I, HOLLMAN J, SIMPFENDORFER C, GALAN K: Percutaneous transluminal coronary angioplasty after previous coronary artery bypass surgery. Am J Cardiol 1985 (Sept 1); 56:398–401.

202. KILLEN DA, HAMAKER WR, REED WA: Coronary artery bypass following percutaneous transluminal coronary angioplasty. Ann Thorac Surg 1985 (Aug); 40:133–138.

203. KELLY ME, TAYLOR GJ, MOSES HW, MIKELL FL, DOVE JT, BATCHELDER JE, WELLONS HA JR, SCHNEIDER JA: Comparative cost of myocardial revascularization: percutaneous transluminal angioplasty and coronary artery bypass surgery. J Am Coll Cardiol 1985 (Jan); 5:16–20.

2

Acute Myocardial Infarction and Its Consequences

GENERAL TOPICS

Time of onset of chest pain

Thompson and associates[1] from Leeds, UK, studied the time of onset of chest pain in 1,000 patients admitted to a coronary care unit with AMI. Statistical analysis demonstrated an excess of infarcts with time of onset of chest pain at 7 am (14%) and at midnight (11%) with the remaining AMI population (75%) forming a background distribution over the other 22 hours.

To determine whether the onset of AMI occurs randomly throughout the day, Muller and associates[2] from several centers analyzed the time of onset of pain in 2,999 patients admitted with AMI. A marked circadian rhythm in the frequency of onset was detected, with a peak from 6 am to noon. In 703 patients, the time of the first elevation in the plasma creatine kinase (CK) MB level could be used to time the onset of AMI objectively. CK-MB-estimated timing confirmed the existence of a circadian rhythm, with a 3-fold increase in the frequency of onset of AMI at peak (9 am) compared with trough (11 pm) periods (Fig. 2-1). The circadian rhythm was not detected in patients receiving beta-adrenergic blocking agents before AMI but was present in those not receiving such therapy. If the rhythmic processes that drive the circadian rhythm of AMI onset can be identified, their modification may delay or prevent the occurrence of AMI.

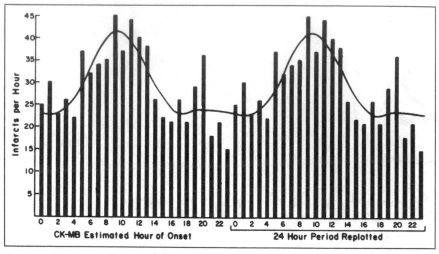

Fig. 2-1. The hourly frequency of onset of AMI as determined by the CK-MB method in 703 patients. The number of infarctions beginning during each of the 24 hours is plotted on the left. On the right, the identical data are plotted again to show the relation between the end and the beginning of the day. A 2-harmonic regression equation for the frequency of onset of AMI has been fitted to the data (curved line). A prominent circadian rhythm is present, with a primary peak incidence of infarction at 9 am and a secondary peak at 8 pm. Reproduced with permission from Muller et al.[2]

Creatine kinase

Ingwall and associates[3] from Boston, Massachusetts, measured creatine kinase (CK) activity, isoenzyme composition, and total creatine content in biopsy samples of LV myocardium from 34 adults in 4 groups: subjects with normal LV walls, patients with LV hypertrophy due to AS, patients with CAD without LV hypertrophy, and patients with CAD with LV hypertrophy due to AS. Compared with specimens of normal LV walls, those from all patients with LV hypertrophy had lower CK activity, higher CK-MB isoenzyme content and activity, and lower creatine content. Specimens from the patients without LV hypertrophy had normal CK activity, increased CK-MB isoenzyme content activity, and decreased total creatine content. The normal ventricles had almost no MB isoenzyme content or activity. These data suggest that changes in the CK system occur in both pressure overload hypertrophy and CAD. Patients with AMI who have mild or no preexisting fixed CAD or pressure overload hypertrophy would not be expected to have elevation of serum CK-MB.

Criteria for diagnosis

Turi and associates[4] from multiple medical centers compared methods for detecting AMI in a prospective study of 726 patients with pain presumed to be caused by ischemia that lasted >30 minutes and was associated with ECG changes (ST-segment deviation ≥0.1 mV or new Q waves or left BBB). Using creatine kinase (CK)-MB values of >12 IU/L as the standard criterion for detection of AMI, 639 patients (88%) were judged to have AMI. Total plasma CK values, technetium-99m stannous pyrophosphate images 48–72 hours after admission, and serial 12-lead ECGs over 10 days were analyzed by investigators blinded to other clinical and laboratory data. For detection of AMI, total CK, ECG, and pyrophosphate imaging were all highly accurate and sensitive (total CK accuracy was 97%, ECG, 92%, pyrophosphate, 88%;

total CK sensitivity was 98%, ECG, 96%, and pyrophosphate, 91%). However, both pyrophosphate and ECG were less specific than total CK (total CK specificity was 89%, pyrophosphate, 64%, and ECG, 59%). The sensitivity and accuracy of total CK and pyrophosphate for those patients with Q-wave development were slightly greater than for those in whom Q waves did not evolve. The ECG was less accurate and pyrophosphate was less specific in patients with prior AMI compared with those with initial AMI. Pyrophosphate failed to detect larger infarcts than either the ECG or total CK. Combined pyrophosphate and ECG criteria were more accurate than pyrophosphate or the ECG alone, and pyrophosphate was helpful in identifying infarcts considered "indeterminate" on the ECG. Although each method has certain limitations, individual and combined use of these diagnostic criteria represent powerful means for detecting AMI.

In cigarette smoking women

Rosenberg and associates[5] from Boston, Massachusetts, and Philadelphia, Pennsylvania, evaluated the modifying influence of individual risk factors on the relation between AMI and cigarette smoking in a case-controlled study of women <50 years of age. Data from 555 women who survived a first AMI were compared with 1,864 hospital control subjects of similar ages. The risk of AMI increased with the number of cigarettes smoked, both in the presence and absence of factors that predispose to AMI. The association was apparent at all ages, at all levels of total serum cholesterol and HDL cholesterol, and in the presence and absence of oral contraceptive use, systemic hypertension, diabetes mellitus, blood group A, tendency to type A behavior, and family history of AMI. The relative increase in risk was generally greater the lower the underlying predisposition to AMI. There was clear evidence that recent oral contraceptive use substantially augmented the increased risk for smokers, and hypercholesterolemia may have had the same effect.

In elderly individuals

The frequency of AMI increases rapidly after age 55 years in women and after age 45 years in men. Eighty-three of 237 women (35%) and 130 of 469 men (28%) with initial AMI in the Framingham Study had unrecognized AMI that was detected by ECG later. Aronow and associates[6] from New York City investigated the prevalence of unrecognized AMI detected by routine ECG in geriatric patients in a long-term health care facility. The patients included 353 women and 127 men, with a mean age of 82 ± 9 years (range, 64–100). An ECG was taken in these 480 patients at admission, when clinically indicated, and routinely every year. The ECGs were reviewed at the time the study was initiated without knowledge of the clinical history. Unrecognized Q-wave AMI detected by routine ECG occurred in 78 of the 480 patients (16%). Unrecognized non-Q-wave AMI would not have been detected in their study. Unrecognized Q-wave AMI not present on entry ECG was detected by serial ECGs in some patients. Of the 115 patients with either documented clinical history of AMI or current ECG evidence of Q-wave AMI, 78 (68%) had unrecognized AMI detected by routine ECG.

Silent infarction

The risk of unrecognized AMI in relation to hypertensive status was examined using 30-year-old follow-up of the Framingham cohort in an investigation by Kannel and associates[7] from Boston, Massachusetts, and Bethesda,

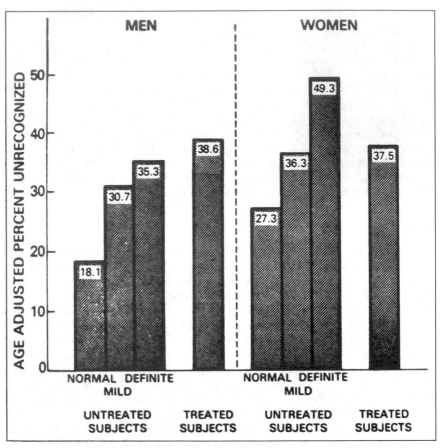

Fig. 2-2. Proportion of AMI unrecognized by sex and hypertensive status in a 30-year follow-up of Framingham cohort subjects free of CHD at examination. Differences for untreated men significant at p <0.01. Reproduced with permission from Kannel et al.[7]

Maryland. Of subjects who developed initial AMI, 130 of 469 men and 83 of 239 women had the AMI detected solely by routine biennial ECGs. The 10-year age-adjusted incidence of AMI among persons with definite systemic hypertension (≥160/95 mmHg) was more than twice that of normotensive persons (<140/90 mmHg). In subjects with no preexisting heart disease, the proportion of AMIs that were unrecognized significantly increased with the severity of systemic hypertension from 18% among normotensive men to 35% among men with definite hypertension; for women, this proportion increased from 27 to 49% (Fig. 2-2). Persons with hypertension are thus at an increased risk both for sustaining an AMI and for such an event to be unrecognized, despite presumably closer medical supervision. Given the similar prognoses for unrecognized and recognized AMI, routine ECG surveillance of hypertensive persons may be warranted. Early initiation of secondary preventive measures, including risk factor modification and use of β-blockers or other drugs may benefit hypertensive persons who experience unrecognized AMI.

Late after CABG

As the proportion of patients with CAD who have had CABG increases, the proportion of such patients among hospital admissions with AMI is also likely to increase. Crean and coworkers[8] from Montreal, Canada, compared infarct size and the angiographically determined cause of AMI in 52 control patients and in 52 consecutive patients with AMI at least 2 months after they had undergone CABG. Baseline characteristics were similar in both groups except for a higher incidence of preexisting Q waves in the post-CABG group. Indexes of myocardial infarct size were smaller in the post-CABG group compared with those in control patients: peak creatine kinase (CK) level (IU/L) was 1,113 -vs- 1,824, peak CK-MB level was 173 -vs- 272, peak summed ST-segment elevation (mm) was 3.5 -vs- 8.2, and QRS score on days 7–9 was 1.9 -vs- 4.3. Postinfarction LVEF was higher in the post-CABG group compared with that in control patients (53 -vs- 47%). The incidence of total occlusion of the artery to the infarct zone was smaller in the post-CABG and control patients (33 -vs- 27), as was the incidence of 1-, 2-, and 3-vessel CAD (artery plus graft). Collateral blood flow to the infarct zone was found in 27 post-CABG patients and in 23 control patients. The cause of AMI in post-CABG and control patients was a lesion in a major artery proximal to all branches in 7 -vs- 22, a lesion in a diagonal or marginal artery in 15 -vs- 4, and a lesion in a distal small vessel in 8 -vs- 1. In addition, 8 patients with graft and artery occlusion had an occluded native vessel before CABG. Thus, patients who have undergone previous CABG have smaller myocardial infarcts and better residual LV function due to the presence of less jeopardized myocardium lying distal to the infarct-producing lesion.

Quantitation of infarct size

Jansen and colleagues[9] from Dallas, Texas, used single-photon emission computed tomography (SPECT) with technetium-99m pyrophosphate (^{99m}Tc-PPi) to estimate infarct size in patients and compared the ^{99m}Tc-PPi SPECT measurements with similar measurements of infarct size obtained from the serial measurements of plasma creatine kinase (CK)-MB activity. Thirty-three patients with AMI and 16 control patients without AMI were evaluated. Eleven patients had transmural anterior AMI, 16 had transmural inferior AMI, and 6 had nontransmural AMI. SPECT was performed with a commercially available rotating gamma camera. Identical projection images of the distribution of ^{99m}Tc-PPi and the ungated cardiac blood pool were acquired sequentially over 180°. Reconstructed sections were color coded and superimposed for purposes of localization of the AMI. Areas of increased ^{99m}Tc-PPi uptake within the AMI was given a threshold of 65% of peak activity. The blood pool was given a threshold of 50% and subtracted to determine the endocardial border for the LV. The AMI ranged in size from 1–126 g equivalents CK-MB. The correlation of CK-MB, estimates of size of the AMI with size determined by SPECT was good. Close correlations were found between estimates of the size of the AMI in patients with anterior transmural AMI, with inferior transmural AMI, and with nontransmural (non-Q wave) AMI. These data suggest that SPECT measurements using ^{99m}Tc-PPi provide accurate estimates of AMI size in patients irrespective of the location of the MI.

Diabetic patients have a higher risk of death after a first AMI compared with nondiabetic patients. Rennert and associates[10] from Beer Sheva, Israel, designed a study to test the hypothesis that AMI size is larger in diabetic than in nondiabetic patients. AMI size was determined by the QRS scoring system that uses 12-ECG leads and R/S amplitude ratios. Of the 44 diabetic patients, 28 were treated by diet only, 12 were taking oral drugs, and 4 were taking insulin. The median QRS score was 6.0 in diabetic patients and 4.0 in the matched nondiabetic patients. Overall, the mean QRS score was significantly higher in diabetic patients than in patients in the comparison groups: 6.7 -vs- 4.9, respectively; mean difference was 1.8 ± 0.6. The difference was statistically significant for inferior wall AMI and of borderline statistical significance for anterior wall AMI. A statistically significant difference was found between diabetic and nondiabetic women but for men the difference was of borderline significance. No difference in QRS score was found between diabetic men and women. These findings suggest that diabetic patients have larger infarcts than do nondiabetic patients. These results may explain, at least in part, the higher mortality rate of diabetic patients with a first AMI compared with that of nondiabetic patients.

Coronary collaterals

Despite a large number of studies, the functional significance of coronary collateral vessels visualized at angiography remains controversial. Freedman and colleagues[11] from Sydney, Australia, selected patients with severe obstruction in only 1 major coronary artery so that the functional significance of collateral flow could be assessed without the interference of ischemia in another area or obstruction in the vessel supplying collaterals. They studied 121 patients with severe (≥80%) 1-vessel CAD, 64 with and 57 without Q-wave AMI. All patients underwent exercise thallium imaging and coronary angiography. On angiography, collateral flow was present in 85% of 74 occluded arteries, compared with only 17% of 47 arteries with subtotal obstruction. Collateral flow was not seen in arteries with lesions of <90% obstruction but was present in 100% of 29 occluded arteries in patients without Q-wave AMI, compared with only 76% of 45 occluded arteries with Q-wave AMI. Clinical variables did not correlate with collateral flow. Collateral flow did not prevent ischemia on exercise thallium imaging in patients without Q-wave AMI: 30 of 33 (91%) with collateral flow had reversible thallium defects, compared with 24 of 24 without collateral flow. In patients with Q-wave AMI, partially reversible exercise thallium defects were more common with flow to the area from either subtotal obstruction or collateral flow than with no flow from total occlusion. In patients with 1-vessel CAD, the presence of collateral flow is principally determined by coronary occlusion. Although collateral flow may protect from Q-wave AMI, it does not prevent exercise ischemia on thallium imaging.

Selzer and Rokeach[12] from San Francisco, California, evaluated the effects of total occlusion of the right coronary artery, a sole lesion, in an unselected series of 45 patients. Findings ranged from no detectable consequences to massive post-AMI LV scars. Patients were divided into 3 groups: Group I, those without clinical or ventriculographic evidence of AMI (10 patients); group II, those with clinical or angiographic evidence of nontransmural AMI (8 patients); group III, those with ECG evidence of transmural AMI (27 patients). The critical compensatory importance of collateral vessels was demonstrated by the difference between the presence of adequate collaterals in groups I and II (89%) -vs- 45% in group III, and by the fact that the 3 patients without demonstrable collaterals had the most extensive wall motion abnormalities. Four patients in group I had no clinical evidence of ischemic disease, occlusion being an incidental finding. The investigators concluded that the natural history of total occlusion of the right coronary artery depends largely on the function of collateral vessels.

To assess the change in angiographically visualized collaterals in evolving AMI, Nitzberg and associates[13] from Birmingham, Alabama, obtained coronary arteriograms from 53 patients 6.2 ± 0.2 hours after onset of AMI symptoms and compared the findings with follow-up angiograms obtained 14 ±

1 day later. Collaterals were graded according to intensity score and percent of distal infarct-related artery visualized. Collateral intensity score and the percent of distal infarct vessel visualized by collaterals at baseline were low, and there was a significant increase in both values at follow-up angiography. The group of 20 patients with occluded infarct vessels at follow-up study accounted for these increases. In 33 patients with patent infarct arteries at repeat angiography, collateral intensity score and percent of segment visualized were unchanged. Among the patients with occluded infarct vessels at baseline and subsequent improvement in LVEF, baseline collateral score, and percent of segment visualized were significantly greater than in patients in whom LVEF did not improve. Thus, in patients with evolving AMI, angiographically visible collaterals are not extensive within the early hours of AMI, the extent of collaterals on follow-up angiography may not be representative of that on the day of AMI, collaterals are considerably more common 2 weeks after AMI, especially in patients with occluded infarct arteries during follow-up, and collaterals present at the time of AMI are associated with improved LVEF at 2 weeks.

LV function

Cortina and colleagues[14] from Oviedo, Spain, and New York City evaluated the coronary anatomy, collateral circulation, and quantitative LV function in 39 patients who underwent angiography within 3 weeks of a first transmural AMI. This study correlated angiographic findings soon after AMI with clinical status before AMI. In the patients studied, the arteries supplying the infarct were occluded at the time of angiography. Patients without angina before AMI (group I) had fewer coronary obstructions than did patients with a long history of angina before AMI (group II) (1.5 ± 0.5 -vs- 2.5 ± 0.5, respectively), but poorer overall and regional LV function. These differences between patients in groups I and II were present irrespective of the location of the infarct. In addition, patients in group I had fewer collateral vessels supplying the infarct-related artery. Preservation of anterior wall motion in group II patients with anterior AMI was associated with collateral flow to the anterior wall and more distal obstruction of the LAD. Thus, there are often differences in coronary anatomy in patients with and without angina pectoris before AMI.

To characterize the changes in LVEF after AMI, Schwartz and coworkers[15] from Washington, D.C., compared radionuclide ventriculograms obtained acutely and 2 weeks after AMI in 40 patients. The patients underwent angiography within a mean of 4 hours and 2 minutes after the onset of symptoms of AMI and either received no therapy (32 patients who were control subjects in a thrombolysis trial) or did not have reperfusion (8 patients) despite receiving streptokinase (SK) infusions. In all 40 patients, the change in LVEF over the 2-week period was small. Patients were then grouped according to the presence or absence of residual flow on the angiograms. Residual flow was considered present in 21 patients, in 12 by virtue of subtotal occlusion of the artery supplying the area of infarct and in 9 because of well-developed coronary collaterals to the distal infarct artery. Mean change in EF for patients with residual flow was 7% -vs- -2% for patients without residual flow. Fourteen of 21 patients with residual flow had a spontaneous increase in EF of $>5\%$, compared with 2 of 19 (11%) patients without residual flow. Time to peak level of creatine kinase (CK) was significantly shorter in the residual flow group, and the peak level of CK was lower in these patients. Of patients with residual flow, those with subtotal occlusions had greater improvement in EF (10%) than those with collateral vessels

(3%). These investigators conclude that spontaneous improvement in LVEF is frequently observed in patients after AMI and that the presence of residual flow on angiograms obtained shortly after appearance of symptoms is predictive of subsequent improvement. Such findings must be considered when evaluating the results of nonrandomized AMI trials.

Despite the widespread use of thrombolytic agents, PTCA, and emergency CABG in AMI, systematic description of coronary anatomic findings during the early hours of AMI has not yet been reported. Stadius and coworkers[16] from Seattle, Washington, evaluated the relation among clinical variables, coronary anatomy, and LV function during the early hours of AMI from data acquired in the Western Washington Intracoronary Streptokinase Trial. All patients had symptoms and ECG changes typical of AMI. All data were obtained before treatment with SK. Mean time to catheterization was 4.1 hours after onset of symptoms. Coronary angiograms (n = 245) were analyzed for location of infarct-related occlusion and collateral flow to the infarct bed. LVEF and regional LV function were quantitated in 227; 62% of occlusions were in the most proximal segment of the involved coronary artery. Collateral circulation was seen in 42% overall, in 31% with LAD occlusion, and in 52% with right coronary artery occlusion. LVEF was lowest and regional function was most abnormal in the group with proximal LAD occlusion. Hyperkinesis was present in 32%; in those with hyperkinesis, hyperkinetic segment length was longest in those with right or circumflex occlusion. Multivariate analysis identified proximal LAD occlusion as the factor most closely associated with LVEF and with measures of LV regional hypofunction. The investigators concluded that AMI is usually caused by occlusion or subtotal occlusion in the most proximal portion of the involved coronary artery, collateral circulation is more frequent with right than with LAD occlusion, and location of the infarct-related occlusion is the most important determinant of global and regional LV function in the early hours of AMI.

Relation of type A behavior to survival

To ascertain the influence of personality factors on the cause of CAD, Case and associates[17] of the Multicenter Post Infarction Research Group measured type A behavior in 516 patients within 2 weeks of onset of AMI, using the Jenkins Activity Survey Questionnaire. Over a follow-up period of 1–3 years, there was no relation between the type A score and total mortality, cardiac mortality, time to death for nonsurvivors, LVEF, or duration of the stay in the coronary care unit. These negative findings were not changed by restricting the analyses to men <61 years of age or by comparing extreme score categories. The contributions of behavioral, demographic, and cardiac physiologic factors to post-AMI mortality also were evaluated by multivariate survivorship analyses. The physiologic factors were the only ones that contributed a significant and independent mortality risk; the type A score did not enter the survivorship model. Thus, no relation was found between type A behavior and the long-term outcome of AMI.

Coagulation problems

Since prostaglandin plasma levels are elevated in patients with transient myocardial ischemia, Friedrich and colleagues[18] from Berlin, West Germany, measured 6-keto-prostaglandin $F_{1\alpha}$ (6-keto-PGF$_{1\alpha}$) and thromboxane B_2 (TXB$_2$) in venous blood of 32 patients with AMI on the first, third, and seventh days. TXB$_2$ and 6-keto-PGF$_{1\alpha}$ levels in these patients (up to 117 ± 237 and 96 ± 105 pg/ml, mean ± SD, respectively) differed significantly from levels in normal control subjects (10 ± 12 and 4 ± 7 pg/ml, respectively). Prostaglandin values remained elevated from day 1 through day 7. In most patients, 6-keto-PGF$_{1\alpha}$ levels prevailed over those of TXB$_2$. In a subgroup having cardiac arrhythmias, the ratio of 6-keto-PGF$_{1\alpha}$ to TXB$_2$ was inverse. It was concluded that prostaglandin generation is increased for at least 7 days after AMI. A disturbed ratio of 6-keto-PGF$_{1\alpha}$ to TXB$_2$ in favor of the latter may be associated with cardiac arrhythmias in AMI.

Evidence continues to accumulate that platelets play an important role in the pathogenesis of acute ischemic heart disease. Mueller and associates[19] from New York City studied during AMI in 59 patients platelet activity in the peripheral circulation and across the ischemic/infarcting myocardial compartment, the locus of presumed platelet hyperactivity, and the effects of prostacyclin (PGI$_2$), a most potent antiplatelet agent and vasodilator. Twenty-two patients had arterial and coronary sinus catheters inserted and received intravenous infusion of PGI$_2$ for 90 minutes. In 15 patients with anterior AMI, transcardiac platelet function and response to PGI$_2$ were studied. Plasma levels of β-thromboglobulin (BTG) and of TXB$_2$, in vivo measures of platelet activity, were elevated 3- and 10-fold; 6-keto-PGF$_{1\alpha}$, the stable end product of PGI$_2$, was <10 pg/ml, reflecting a leftward shift of the TXB$_2$/PGI$_2$ ratio. Platelets circulating during AMI ("ischemic platelets") were hyperaggregable in response to adenosine diphosphate and relatively resistant to PGI$_2$ both in vivo and in vitro. Concentrations of platelet cyclic adenosine monophosphate (cAMP) and the cAMP response to PGI$_2$ were diminished. The platelet hyperreactivity, expressed by plasma BTG, platelet aggregation, and PGI$_2$-induced inhibition of aggregation, was most intense during infarct evolution and decreased with time. The increased platelet performance resulted in platelet fatigue, indicated by decreased contents of BTG of the ischemic platelet and decreased TXA$_2$ production in response to collagen. The ischemic platelet produced twice normal TXA$_2$ in response to arachidonic acid (stimulus and substrate), demonstrating a heightened metabolic capacity. TXA$_2$ was produced across the ischemic/infarcting compartment in 10 of 15 patients with anterior AMI. The antiplatelet effect of PGI$_2$ was greatly diminished. Thus, the data define an abnormal pattern of platelet behavior during AMI characterized by a proaggregatory environment, heightened platelet reactivity in both the peripheral and coronary circulation, and relative resistance to PGI$_2$.

Fibrinopeptide A (FPA) is a product of proteolysis by thrombin on fibrinogen. Elevation of FPA levels occurs in association with disorders such as disseminated intravascular coagulation, deep vein thrombosis, arterial thrombosis, and malignancies. To determine whether coronary thrombosis in vivo is reflected by elevation in levels of FPA in plasma, Eisenberg and coworkers[20] from St. Louis, Missouri, sequentially characterized plasma FPA levels associated in AMI in patients admitted to the cardiac care unit early after the onset of symptoms, in patients with transmural AMI admitted later, and in patients with nontransmural AMI. Studies also were performed in patients in whom the diagnosis of AMI was suspected but subsequently excluded. FPA values were significantly higher in patients with transmural AMI compared with those in patients with nontransmural AMI (42 -vs- 5 ng/ml) or with those in patients in whom AMI was subsequently excluded as a diagnosis (3.5 ng/ml). Elevations in FPA levels were greatest in patients with transmural AMI from whom samples were obtained within 10 hours after the onset of symptoms (39 patients) compared with 14 patients from whom samples were obtained initially >10 hours after the onset of symptoms (56 -vs- 5 ng/ml). In 30 of these 39 patients the level of FPA was >8 ng/ml, compared with only 2 of the 14 patients from whom initial samples were obtained >10 hours after the onset of symptoms. In patients admitted early after transmural AMI from whom samples were obtained sequentially, FPA values declined consistently during the 24-hour sampling period. These data suggest that an elevated FPA level appears to be a criterion of AMI.

ECG observations

Hoffman and Igarashi[21] from Los Angeles, California, prospectively evaluated 100 consecutive adult patients who presented to their emergency room and were triaged to the monitored unit during the hours 8:00 am to 8:00 pm with chest pain or what was considered by the triage nurse as a "chest pain equivalent" of typical neck, jaw, or arm pain. Emergency department physicians were asked to commit themselves to recommending either coronary care unit admission or some other disposition, both before and after evaluating current comparison ECG findings. They were also asked, before reviewing these results, whether they thought information gained from the ECG would have any affect on their decision. Despite wide expectation that ECG findings would affect decision-making, neither current nor comparison ECGs virtually ever altered the ultimate decision to admit or not. Faculty and house officers performed similarly in all regards, except insofar as attending physicians were less likely to expect ECG findings to help them in patients who were ultimately discharged. Thus, ECG findings are rarely if ever helpful in determining the need for admission to a coronary care unit in patients presenting to the emergency department with chest pain, and seem to have particularly little value in patients in whom AMI is considered clinically unlikely.

Lew and associates[22] from Los Angeles, California, studied 61 patients with inferior wall AMI and no evidence of prior AMI to determine which factors influenced the magnitude of precordial ST-segment depression. There was a significant but weak correlation between the magnitude of precordial ST-segment depression and the magnitude of inferior ST-segment elevation. In the 29 patients with evidence of concomitant RV involvement, precordial ST-segment depression was significantly smaller both in absolute terms (-1.3 ± 1.8 -vs- 2.8 ± 1.9 mm) and relative to the magnitude of inferior ST-segment elevation (ratio of -0.2 ± 1.0 -vs- -1.1 ± 0.5), whereas in the 15 patients with lateral ST-segment elevation (≥ 1 mm in lead V_6), precordial ST-segment depression was significantly greater both in absolute terms (-3.5 ± 2.3 -vs- -1.6 ± 1.7 mm) and relative to the magnitude of inferior ST-segment elevation (ratio of -1.1 ± 0.8 -vs- -0.5 ± 0.9). Consistent with these findings, the correlation between the magnitudes of precordial and inferior ST-segment deviations was considerably improved when only the 24 patients with neither evidence of RV involvement nor lateral ST-segment elevation were analyzed. These data suggest that in patients with inferior AMI, there is a reciprocal relation between precordial and inferior ST-segment deviations, which is distorted by concomitant RV involvement and by concomitant lateral LV wall involvement.

Tzivoni and associates[23] from Jerusalem, Israel, used RA pacing as a myocardial stress method in 137 consecutive patients recovering from a transmural AMI and the appearance of pacing-provoked ischemia before hospital discharge was correlated to the presence or absence of ST depression in the opposite wall during the initial 48 hours. Of the 137 patients, 83 (61%) had reciprocal changes; they were more common in inferior (87%) than in anterior (37%) AMI. Of 54 patients without reciprocal changes, only 5 (9%) had ST depression during predischarge pacing; of the 83 patients with reciprocal changes, 41 had pacing-induced ischemia and 42 did not, indicating that in half of this group the reciprocal changes represent ischemia of the opposite wall. In the other half of the group without ST depression during pacing, these changes may be a "mirror image" phenomenon. Follow-up showed that angina pectoris, positive treadmill test response 6 months later, or recurrent AMI, all consequences of impaired myocardial blood supply, were significantly more frequent in patients with reciprocal changes. This group could be further separated according to the results of RA pacing, because angina pectoris or recurrent AMI were infrequent among those with reciprocal changes and negative pacing responses but was frequent among those with reciprocal changes and positive pacing responses. Thus, reciprocal changes during AMI may be due to different mechanisms, ischemia and mirror image.

Levine[24] from Boston, Massachusetts, studied 53 patients with subendocardial AMI; all were elderly and the group was equally divided by sex. About half had >1 subendocardial AMI; the recurrences or extensions often involved adjacent areas. Six had fibrinous "pericarditis." This large study showed more widespread and severe coronary narrowing than earlier reports. Six patients had thrombi in the right coronary artery. Six had ECG evidence of concomitant anteroseptal and inferior AMI (Roesler-Dressler) and 12 had intraventricular block generally preceding high grade block or arrhythmias. At some time during the terminal hospitalization, 27 patients developed distinctive protracted RS-T depression or T-wave inversion: 24 were diagnosed on accepted criteria as transmural AMI but the diagnosis was sustained in only 4. Thus, neither the presence of changes in RS-T segment or T wave nor the absence of QRS changes are mandatory for the diagnosis of subendocardial AMI.

Gash and associates[25] from Philadelphia, Pennsylvania, retrospectively examined angiographic and ECG data in 55 symptomatic patients with non-Q-wave AMI. ST-T-wave patterns on admission were classified as either ischemic (transient ST elevation, persistent horizontal ST depression, or persistent T-wave inversion) or nonspecific. Eleven patients (20%) had normal or nearly normal coronary arteries; 10 patients (18%) had 1, 7 patients (13%) had 2, and 19 patients (35%) had 3-vessel CAD; 8 patients (15%) had LM disease. Six of the 11 with normal coronary arteries had ergonovine tests and all 6 were negative. Segmental LV wall motion abnormalities were commonly observed; however, diffuse LV wall motion abnormalities were present only among patients with 3-vessel and LM CAD. EF was <0.50 in 48% of patients with 3-vessel or LM CAD. Although ischemic ST-T wave patterns were more common among patients with significant CAD than among those with normal coronary arteries, neither the ST-T-wave pattern nor EF, alone or in combination, allowed confident separation of those with normal coronary arteries from those with significant CAD.

Echo observations

In a study performed by Arvan and Varat[26] from Pittsburgh, Pennsylvania, the initial 2-D echo and ECG of 50 consecutive patients with chest pain and a possible non-Q-wave AMI were compared to determine the value of echo in this type of AMI. The ECG markers for a non-Q-wave AMI were ≥0.15 mV ST-segment depression, ST-segment elevations with reciprocal ST-segment depression, and new symmetric deep T-wave changes compared with a recent preadmission ECG. The 2-D echo was considered positive for AMI if akinesia, dyskinesia, or severe hypokinesia was seen in ≥1 LV segment. The sensitivity, specificity, and predictive value of the 2-D echo compared with the ECG was 66 and 52%, respectively (sensitivity); 91 and 95%, respectively (specificity); and 91 and 94%, respectively (predictive value). Statistically, there were no differences in the proportion of patients who had a positive 2-D echo compared with the proportion of patients who had a positive ECG. The ECG and 2-D echo results were combined and the sensitivity increased to 76%, but the specificity decreased to 86%. AMI size was not significantly different in infarcted patients who had a positive echo (395 ± 125 IU/L) compared with those who had a negative echo (727 ± 187 IU/L).

Chandraratna and associates[27] from Los Angeles, California, evaluated the ability of a system developed in their laboratory to differentiate between AMI and healed myocardial infarction (HMI). Gated 2-D echo was performed in 10 patients with AMI (within 48 hours) and in 10 patients with HMI (>4 weeks). The 2-D echo images were digitized using a Datacube VG-120 videoframe digitizer and each digitized videoframe (320 × 240 matrix) was transmitted using a high speed serial data link to a second computer and stored on floppy disc. Five gated video frames of each patient were time averaged to give a smoothed digitized image. This image was displayed on high resolution color monitor connected to a color graphic subsystem. Sixty-four colors indicated pixel intensity. The exact pixel value at any given location was determined using a high resolution light pen. Color or pixel values were not significantly different between the area of AMI (pixel intensity 23 ± 3, mean ±SD) identified by a regional wall motion abnormality, and the adjacent normal muscle (23 ± 4). In each patient with HMI, an increase in color intensity and pixel value (43 ± 6) was seen in the area of infarction (area of regional wall motion abnormality) compared with adjacent normal muscle (23 ± 2). These preliminary data indicate that this technique enables differentiation between AMI and HMI.

RNA observations

Wahl and associates[28] from Philadelphia, Pennsylvania, examined the scintigraphic features of patients in Killip class I or II after AMI with relation to ECG changes. The 41 consecutively studied patients (23 men and 18 women) with first AMI were divided into 2 groups: group 1 (n = 25) had Q-wave AMI, and group 2 (n = 16) had non-Q-wave AMI. Rest thallium-201 myocardial scintigrams and RNA were obtained 10 days (mean) after AMI. The thallium images were divided into 15 segments in 3 projections and assessed qualitatively and quantitatively. Fixed perfusion defects were present in at least 1 segment in 23 patients (92%) in group 1 and in 8 patients (50%) in group 2 (Fig. 2-3). All but 1 patient in group 1 (4%) and 3 patients in group 2 (19%) had perfusion defects (fixed or reversible). The number of segments with perfusion defects was 5.6 ± 2.6 in group 1 and 2.9 ± 2.3 in group 2 (p = 0.02); the peak creatine kinase was 1,280 ± 880 U/L in group 1 and 360 ± 340 in group 2; the LVEF was 38 ± 14% in group 1 -vs- 43 ± 15% in group 2. Thus, fixed perfusion defects are present in 92% of patients with Q waves and in 50% of patients with no Q waves; reversible perfusion defects tended to be more frequent in non-Q-wave AMI.

Plotnick and associates[29] from Baltimore, Maryland, performed exercise RNA in 65 normal subjects (group I), in 31 patients with exercise-induced transient thallium defects after AMI (group II), and in 16 patients without exercise-induced transient thallium defects, angina pectoris, or ECG changes after AMI (group III). Absolute LV volumes were measured using a correction for attenuation in each patient. Similar peak heart rate-BP products were achieved in groups II and III. Absolute LV volumes were measured using a correction for attenuation in each patient. Similar peak heart rate-BP products were achieved in groups II and III. Although the mean LVEF re-

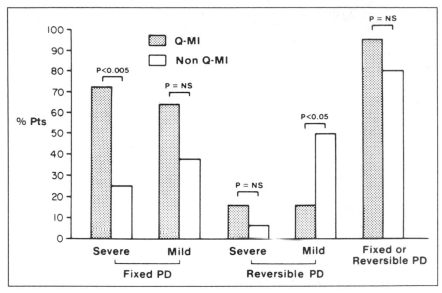

Fig. 2-3.   Distribution of perfusion defects (PD) in patients with Q-wave AMI and those with non-Q-wave AMI. Reproduced with permission from Wahl et al.[28]

sponse to exercise in group III (increase of 0.11 ± 0.10 units) closely resembled that of normal persons (increase of 0.14 ± 0.09 units) and was significantly different from that of group II (decrease of 0.04 ± 0.12), there was considerable individual variation. An abnormal EF response to exercise, defined as failure of EF to increase by at least 0.05 units, was found in 6 subjects (9%) in group I, 26 patients (84%) in group II, and 2 patients (13%) in group III. End-systolic volume failed to decrease in 10 subjects (15%) in group I, 25 patients (81%) in group II and 7 patients (44%) in group III. New regional wall motion abnormalities were found in no subject in group I, in 16 patients (52%) in group II, and in only 1 patient (6%) in group III. Thus, although group response of EF or end-systolic volume appeared to correlate with the presence or absence of ischemia, some patients with exercise-induced transient thallium defects after AMI responded normally and others abnormally to exercise RNA stress testing. The development of a new motion abnormality in the post-AMI patient was a relatively specific but insensitive indicator of myocardial ischemia.

Comparison of echo and radionuclide studies

Freeman and associates[30] from Sydney, Australia, assessed the diagnostic ability of RNA and 2-D echo to assess regional LV wall motion and compared the findings with contrast angiography in 52 patients with healed myocardial infarction. After 5 patients were excluded for inadequate 2-D echo studies, the LV images of 47 patients obtained by all 3 techniques were divided into 7 segments for analysis. Both 2-D echo and RNA showed close agreement with contrast angiography in assessing normal -vs- abnormal wall motion in the anterobasal (91%, 91%), anterolateral (87%, 79%), and posterolateral segments (77%, 79%). The sensitivity in detecting wall motion abnormalities was highest for 2-D echo and RNA in the anterolateral (83%, 77%) and apical (95%, 84%) segments and lowest for the inferior segment (48%, 48%). Specificity of 2-D echo and RNA was high, ranging from 94% in the anterolateral segment to 71% in the septal segment for 2-D echo, and from 91% in the inferior segment to 81% in the posterobasal and septal segments for RNA. Major discrepancies with contrast angiography occurred more often in the posterobasal, posterolateral, inferior, and septal LV segments. Thus, in comparison with contrast angiography, 2-D echo and RNA are reliable for detecting anterior and apical wall motion abnormalities, but relatively less sensitive for detecting wall motion abnormalities involving the inferior, posterobasal, and posterolateral LV segments.

Magnetic resonance imaging

The capability of magnetic resonance imaging (MRI) in the detection and characterization of alterations in signal intensity and T_2 relaxation time in acutely infarcted relative to normal myocardium was evaluated by McNamara and coworkers[31] from San Francisco, California, in 16 adult patients and normal volunteers by ECG-gated proton MRI. The 7 volunteers were asymptomatic and had no history of cardiovascular abnormality. Each of the 9 patients had had an AMI within 5–12 days before the MRI studies. The diagnosis in each patient was confirmed by ECG criteria and elevated levels of fractionated creatine kinase (CK) isoenzymes. ECG-gated MRI was performed with a superconducting system operating at 0.35 tesla. MRI demonstrated infarcted myocardium as a region of high signal intensity relative to that of adjacent normal myocardium; regions of high intensity corresponded anatomically to the site of AMI as defined by the ECG changes. The mean percent differences between normal and infarcted myocardium was substantially greater on 56 ms images compared with 28 ms images. Region of interest analysis revealed that infarcted myocardium had a significantly prolonged T_2 relaxation time relative to that in normal myocardium and relative to the mean T_2 of LV myocardium in the volunteers. Each patient with AMI had a high intraluminal flow signal on 56 msec images, but this also was observed in normal subjects and was therefore a nonspecific finding. Thus, MRI detects AMI as a region of high signal intensity relative to that of adjacent normal myocardium and identifies significant prolongation of infarct T_2 relaxation time in the damaged region. Quantification of T_2 relaxation times provides differential characterization of tissue in normal and infarcted myocardium.

Indications for coronary angiography after infarction

Veenbrink and associates[32] from Utrecht, The Netherlands, performed coronary angiography and exercise stress tests in 91 consecutive patients <60 years of age having either no or only mild angina pectoris, with or without medication, after a first AMI. Nine patients had angiographic high risk CAD defined as 3-artery CAD, significant LM stenosis, or significant proximal stenosis of the LAD coronary artery. Eighteen patients had a positive ECG exercise stress test, including 8 of the 9 patients with angiographic high risk CAD. The investigators concluded that coronary angiography to detect high risk CAD in this group can be restricted to patients with a positive exercise stress test. This policy would obviate the need for about 80% of coronary angiograms performed in this age group.

Relation to angina pectoris

Matsuda and associates[33] from Yamaguchi, Japan, interviewed 197 patients with AMI to evaluate the character of angina pectoris relative to physical activity before AMI and at the onset of AMI: 92 patients had no angina before AMI and 105 had angina. Among the 105 patients with angina, 58 had chronic stable angina that did not change before AMI, 22 noted worsening of symptoms within 2 weeks before AMI, and 25 had onset of angina within 2 weeks before AMI. In the 92 patients without angina before AMI, AMI occurred during heavy exertion in 10 (11%), mild exertion in 43 (47%), at rest in 28 (30%), and during sleep in 11 (12%). In the 58 patients with chronic stable angina, 47 had angina during exertion, 7 during rest, and 4 during both. Subsequent AMI occurred during heavy exertion in 9 (16%), during mild exertion in 16 (28%), at rest in 25 (43%), and during sleep in 8 (14%). In the patients without angina, or with chronic stable angina without worsening of symptoms, AMI occurred unpredictably or differently from the mode of physical activity precipitating angina before AMI.

Outcome

Connolly and Elveback[34] from Rochester, Minnesota, reviewed outcome in 1,221 residents of Rochester who were ≥30 years of age who had an AMI as a first manifestation of CAD during the period 1960–1979. Patients who had a prior diagnosis of CHF or valvular heart disease were excluded. Of the 1,221 patients, 784 were considered to have had a transmural AMI and 353 a subendocardial AMI and 84 patients had an AMI that could not be classified. (Most of the unclassified patients with AMI died suddenly outside the hospital.) The age- and sex-adjusted 30-day case fatality rate was 18% among those with transmural and 9% among those with subendocardial AMI. No significant difference was found in subsequent survivorship or in net survivorship free of reinfarction during the first 5 years of follow-up. Five-year net survivorship free of reinfarction, CABG, and cardiac death was not significantly different between the 2 groups, nor was net survivorship free of 5 established events (the 3 aforementioned events plus the development of CHF or angina) (Figs. 2-4–2-7). When these 5 events were considered indepen-

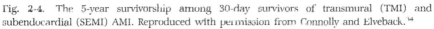

Fig. 2-4. The 5-year survivorship among 30-day survivors of transmural (TMI) and subendocardial (SEMI) AMI. Reproduced with permission from Connolly and Elveback.[34]

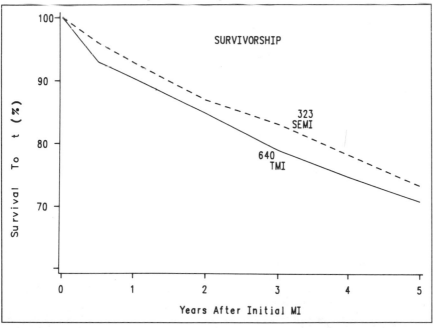

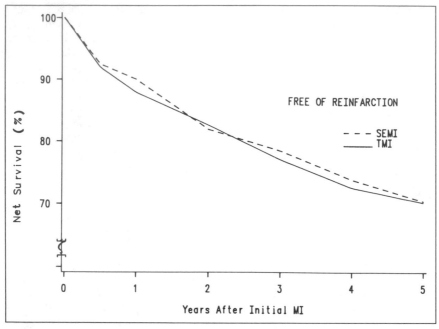

Fig. 2-5. The 5-year survivorship free of reinfarction among 30-day survivors of transmural (TMI) and subendocardial (SEMI) AMI. Reproduced with permission from Connolly and Elveback.[34]

dently in the 2 infarction cohorts, however, development of CHF was more common among patients with transmural AMI, whereas the development of angina was more common among patients with subendocardial AMI.

Frequency and outcome in a large employed population

Pell and Fayerweather[35] from Wilmington, Delaware, analyzed long-term trends in the incidence of a first AMI and in case-fatality rates among employees of the DuPont Company from 1957–1983. A steady decline in incidence was observed among male employees. The annual age-adjusted rate in the 1957–1959 period was 3.19/1,000, compared with 2.29/1,000 in the 1981–1983 period, a decline of 28%. The rate of decline was higher among salaried (white-collar) employees than among production workers receiving hourly wages. No trend was seen among female employees, but the number of cases may have been too small to detect a decline. Beginning in 1969, the 24-hour case-fatality rate showed a moderate decline, but after 1975, there was a sharp drop in the 30-day case-fatality rate among persons who survived 24 hours after the attack. These declines did not begin until several years after the decline in incidence had begun. This study and others suggest that improved medical care probably made some contribution to the decline in mortality associated with CAD, but the major source of the decline has been a reduction in the incidence of the disease.

This article was followed by an editorial by Stamler[36] entitled "Coronary Heart Disease, Doing the Right Things."

Several letters to the editor commented on the article by Pell and Fayerweather. Tyler[37] from Sacramento, California, suggested that the reason a decrease in AMI rates at the DuPont Company from 1957–1983 was not

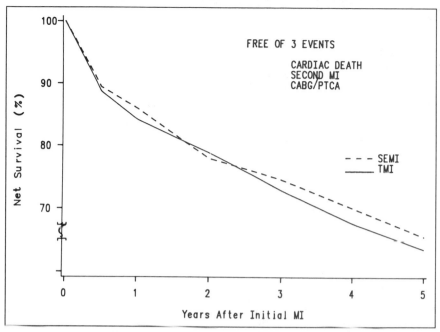

Fig. 2-6. The 5-year survivorship free of cardiac death, second AMI, and CABG or PTCA among patients with subendocardial (SEMI) and transmural (TMI) AMI. Reproduced with permission from Connolly and Elveback.[34]

observed in women was that the numbers of women were too small to see a trend. National figures for mortality from cardiovascular disease on an age-adjusted basis suggests that the rate for women dropped from 3.0/100,000 population in 1960 to 1.9 in 1980 (Table 2-1). If the decrease in AMI rates was the same or similar, then these figures might be useful for comparison with the rates for men at DuPont

---

COMPLICATIONS

Recurrence

Ulvenstam and associates[38] from Goteborg, Sweden, followed 1,306 men <68 years of age who survived a first AMI during 1968–1977. These patients were followed 2 and 12 years (mean, 6.5) after discharge from the hospital (Fig. 2-8). The patients were unselected and paid regular visits to a Post-AMI Clinic where treatment was standardized. The diagnosis of a nonfatal reinfarction was based on conventional clinical criteria, and the diagnosis of a fatal reinfarction, on autopsy findings of a recent myocardial injury or a fresh coronary thrombus, or both. The total cumulative rate of endpoint-free patients was 64% at 5 years and 50% at 10 years of follow-up. The total mortality rate was 19% at 5 years and 33% at 10 years. The total cumulative rate of a first reinfarction was 28% at 5 years and 37% at 10 years (80% nonfatal and 20% fatal) (Fig. 2-9). Sixty-three patients had >1 reinfarction. The mortality rate was strongly associated with age. In contrast, the rate of nonfatal reinfarction was independent of age.

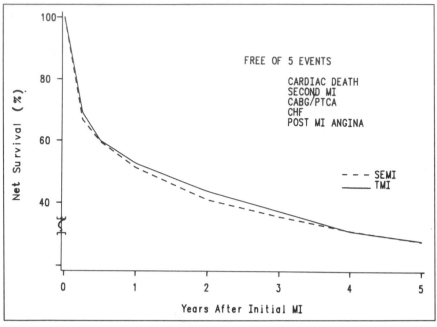

Fig. 2-7. The 5-year survivorship free of 5 events: cardiac death, second AMI, CABG or PTCA, CHF, and angina after AMI. SEMI = subendocardial AMI; TMI = transmural AMI. Reproduced with permission from Connolly and Elveback.[34]

TABLE 2-1. *Age-adjusted death rates for mortality from cardiovascular disease in the United States between 1900 and 1980.* *Reproduced with permission from Tyler.[37]*

	MEN		WOMEN	
YEAR	DEATH RATE	AGE-ADJUSTED DEATH RATE	DEATH RATE	AGE-ADJUSTED DEATH RATE
1980	457.7	343.0	416.2	187.9
1970	551.0	447.7	443.9	251.5
1960	584.2	493.6	448.0	303.7
1950	562.5	508.9	427.3	346.2
1940	452.9	462.8	360.1	350.7
1930	349.9	419.1	305.1	357.3
1920	280.3	370.0	284.8	361.1
1910	294.1	391.2	280.0	349.7
1900	269.3	339.9	259.2	311.3

*Rates are per 100,000 population and ha e been adjusted for age by the direct method, using the 1940 population as the standard. The rates for men and women were adjusted separately, using the same standard population. (Source: National Center for Health Statistics, U.S. Department of Health and Human Services.)

RV infarction and/or dysfunction

Kopelman and coworkers[39] from Nashville, Tennessee, evaluated the relation between RV hypertrophy and RV AMI in patients with chronic lung disease, including 28 with chronic lung disease, inferior AMI, and significant CAD (group I), and 20 patients with RV hypertrophy, chronic lung disease without inferior AMI or significant CAD (group II). Patients in group I were

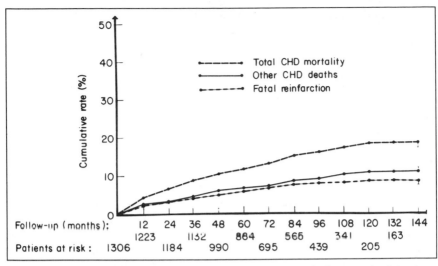

Fig. 2-8. Cumulative CHD mortality (total, fatal reinfarctions and other CAD deaths) among men with a first AMI. The numbers below the time axis denote patients at risk at the beginning of each interval. Reproduced with permission from Ulvenstam et al.[38]

classified into 2 subgroups: group Ia without RV hypertrophy and group Ib with RV hypertrophy. RV wall thickness was 3.3 mm ± 0.5 in group Ia, 6.0 mm ± 1.1 in group Ib, and 8.8 mm ± 2.4 in group II. Among group Ib patients, 11 (79%) had RV AMI compared with only 3 patients (22%) in group Ia. The 11 patients in group Ib had chronic lung disease with both RV hypertrophy and inferior AMI and those in group Ia had chronic lung disease without RV hypertrophy and with inferior AMI. RV AMI occurred in 4 patients (20%) in group II. There was no significant difference in the extent of CAD in patients in groups Ia and Ib. These data suggest that patients with RV

Fig. 2-9. Cumulative reinfarction rates (total, nonfatal, and fatal) among men with a first AMI. The numbers below the time axis denote patients at risk at the beginning of each interval. Reproduced with permission from Ulvenstam et al.[38]

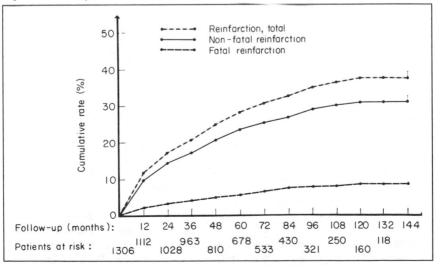

hypertrophy resulting from chronic lung disease are susceptible to RV AMI during inferior AMI. Isolated RV AMI may occur in patients with chronic lung disease, RV hypertrophy, and relatively less severe CAD. The data suggest a possible role for both an increased myocardial oxygen demand and decreased supply as factors in determining these relations.

Shah and associates[40] from Los Angeles, California, determined clinical and hemodynamic correlates and therapeutic and prognostic implications of RV dysfunction complicating AMI in 43 consecutive patients with scintigraphic evidence of RV dysfunction (wall motion abnormalities and a depressed RVEF <0.39) and a normal LVEF. Each of these 43 patients had inferior AMI, and they represented 40% of the patients with inferior AMI evaluated during the same time period. The clinical and scintigraphic findings in these patients were surprising. Only 8 (24%) had elevated jugular venous pressure on admission; 74% had a depressed cardiac index (<2.5 L/min/m²), but 30% of the patients did not have a RA pressure ≥10 mmHg. The LV end diastolic volume was reduced to 49 ± 11 ml/m² in 22 patients; this correlated significantly with the stroke volume index and cardiac index. During follow-up, RVEF determined in 33 patients increased ≥10% in 26 (79%) from a mean value of 0.30 ± 0.06–0.40 ± 0.09 without a significant change in the mean LVEF (0.56 ± 0.10–0.56 ± 0.11). Complications of the infarcts occurred frequently in patients with RV infarction, including bradycardia with hypotension in 25 (58%), hypotension or shock in 18 (42%), complete AV block in 6 (14%), VT or VF in 7 (16%), VSD and free wall rupture in 1 patient, and severe MR in 1 patient. Only 1 patient with a low output state improved hemodynamically with volume loading; the remainder required additional inotropic or vasodilator therapy or both, including intra-aortic balloon pumping in 2 patients and atrial pacing in 1 patient. Two patients with VSD died. These data indicate the following in patients with inferior AMI and evidence of predominant RV dysfunction: clinical and hemodynamic abnormalities occur variably; reduced LV end diastolic volume occurs frequently, resulting in reduced cardiac output; there is an important improvement in RVEF with time; and there is a good short-term prognosis in those patients who do not develop added mechanical complications. Patients with hypotension or shock often do not respond well to volume loading alone, and they may require additional inotropic support.

Haines and coworkers[41] from Charlottesville, Virginia, studied 74 consecutive patients with inferior AMI to determine the functional and prognostic significance of RV dysfunction in these patients. Gated equilibrium RNA at rest, submaximal exercise testing with thallium-201 scintigraphy at the time of hospital discharge, and coronary angiography before hospital discharge were obtained. Symptom-limited stress thallium-201 scintigraphy also was performed in 61 patients at 3 months, and all patients were followed clinically for 23 ± 15 months. Among these patients, 47 had normal RV function (group I); 12 patients (group II) had mild to moderate RV dysfunction; and 15 patients (group III) had severe RV dysfunction. There were no differences among these patients with respect to age, history of prior AMI, peak serum creatine kinase values, maximal Killip functional classification, number or type of in-hospital complications, LVEF, prevalence of multivessel CAD, or the distribution and severity of CAD affecting the infarct-related vessel. The data obtained indicate that exercise tolerance as assessed by treadmill time, BP-heart rate product, and peak work load were comparable among the 3 patient groups, both before hospital discharge and 3 months thereafter. There were no differences in the variables indicating exercise-induced ischemia among the 3 patient groups. Finally, cardiac mortality, reinfarction rate, and the incidence of medically refractory angina pectoris also were similar in patients in the 3 groups. Thus, RV dysfunction after inferior AMI does not appear to have important clinical or prognostic significance during short-term follow-up.

Atrial fibrillation

To elucidate the genesis and effect of AF, Sugiura and associates[42] from Osaka, Japan, studied 102 patients with AMI. Eighteen had AF during the first 72 hours in the coronary care unit. The hospital mortality rate was 23%. Discriminant analysis was used to determine the important variables contributing to the genesis of AF and hospital mortality based on the following variables: cardiac output, PA wedge pressure, RA pressure, systolic BP (at admission and before the onset of AF or most abnormal value), age, location of AMI, sex, and pericarditis. PA wedge pressure and age were important for hospital mortality. Therefore the hemodynamic change imposed on the left atrium and aging are the major factors related to the occurrence of AF and hospital mortality.

Pericardial effusion

Although a pericardial friction rub occurs in about 10% of patients after AMI, the frequency of pericardial effusion (PE) is not known. M-mode echo was done 1, 3, and 5 days after AMI in 43 consecutive patients admitted within 24 hours of AMI by Kaplan and associates[43] from Chicago, Illinois, and PE was detected in 16 (37%). The PE was small in 7 patients, moderate in 6, and large in 3. A pericardial friction rub developed in 8 (19%), of whom only 4 had PE. Pleuritic chest pain diminished by sitting up and was relieved by anti-inflammatory agents in 12 (28%), of whom only 5 had PE. The peak creatine kinase level was significantly higher in patients with PE (1,769 ± 1,003 U) than in those without (1,181 ± 838 U). More patients with PE were in Killip classification II, III, or IV (11 of 16 [69%] -vs- 9 of 27 [33%]). The presence of PE was not associated with age, site of AMI, development of Q waves, use of heparin, or previous AMI. In conclusion, PE as detected by M-mode echo is frequently present after AMI, and its presence is not closely associated with the occurrence of a pericardial friction rub or typical pericardial pain.

LV thrombi

Sharma and associates[44] from Springfield, Illinois, and Little Rock, Arkansas, studied prospectively 30 patients with AMI treated with intracoronary streptokinase (SK) ($7 \times 10^5 \pm 3 \times 10^5$ IU) followed by 10 days of intravenous heparin (800 to 1,500 IU/h) therapy by serial 2-D echo for LV thrombus. Within the first 24 hours, evidence of a thrombolytic state appeared as indicated by fibrin and fibrinogen degradation products (123 ± 45 mg/dl at 24 hours). Throughout the course of this study, partial thromboplastin times were maintained within therapeutic range (40–100 s). Apical LV thrombus developed in 8 of 30 patients (27%). Apical thrombus developed within 24 hours in 3 patients with anterior AMI and persisted through day 10. By day 10, apical thrombus developed in 3 additional patients with anterior AMI and 2 patients with inferior AMI. In these patients, anterior AMI and apical dysfunction were significant determinants of LV thrombus formation. Hence, the incidence of LV thrombus in patients treated with SK and heparin is similar to that reported earlier in comparable patients not receiving thrombolytic therapy.

LV aneurysm

Arvan and Badillo[45] from Pittsburgh, Pennsylvania, studied 25 patients with an anterior wall AMI by 2-D echo 3–5 days after the onset of chest pain, and serially over 3–24 months to determine if a particular pattern of contractility predisposed to LV aneurysm formation. No subject had a prior AMI. In 8 subjects LV aneurysm eventually developed (group I), usually within 2–4 weeks of AMI; in 17 patients LV aneurysm did not develop (group II). Percent fractional shortening of the basal and midventricular segments was significantly better in group I subjects than in group II subjects (29 ± 2 -vs- 20 ± 2%, respectively, for the basal segment, and 23 ± 1 -vs- 17 ± 2%, respectively, for the midventricular segment). Infarct size as determined by peak creatine kinase isoenzyme levels was large in both groups, and there was no statistically significant difference between their mean values (2,099 ± 620 IU -vs- 1,334 ± 249 IU for groups I and II, respectively). Severe asynergy of the infarcted myocardium was present in all group I subjects and in 9 of 27 group II subjects on the initial 2-D echo study. These results indicate that LV aneurysm formation depends on a critical imbalance of myocardial forces in which strong LV segments cause bulging of weakened ones.

Keenan and associates[46] from South Hampton, UK, analyzed results of cardiac operation for LV aneurysm in 100 patients operated on between February 1973 and January 1983. The principal indications for operation were LV failure in 58, angina in 23, both in 17, with arrhythmia and systemic emboli accounting for 1 case each. Eighty-five had had anterior AMI causing 82 anteroapical and 3 lateral aneurysms, and the remainder had had inferior infarcts resulting in 14 inferior aneurysms and 1 lateral aneurysm. Coronary angiography detected a single coronary narrowing in 46%. Three patients had aneurysmal plication and the remainder had aneurysmectomy. Eleven had MVR. Forty patients underwent CABG, with a mean number of grafts per patient of 1.4. The early mortality was 7% with no early deaths since 1978. The actuarial 5-year survival was 68%, and 82% of survivors are in New York Heart Association class I or II (mean follow-up, 3 years) (Fig. 2-10). LV

Fig. 2-10. Actuarial analysis of survival (a) showing influence of CABG according to preoperative symptoms (b), preoperative residual LV function (c), and the extent of CAD (d). Reproduced with permission from Keenan et al.[46]

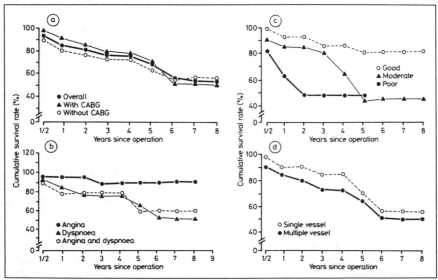

aneurysmectomy may be performed with a low operative mortality and good long-term results.

Mortality of surgical resection of a LV aneurysm is largely determined by size and function of nonaneurysmal or residual LV myocardium. Visser and associates[47] from Amsterdam, The Netherlands, determined a residual myocardial index using 2-D echo in 56 consecutive patients scheduled for LV aneurysmectomy, and these results were correlated with surgical outcome. The index was calculated using 3 apical cross-sections: the 2- and 4-chamber views and the long-axis view (Fig. 2-11). These views were recorded at mutual angles of 60°. In each view the end-diastolic length of normally moving endocardium of the 2 opposite walls was expressed as a fraction of the end-diastolic LV long axis. The index was assessed by averaging the 6 ratios obtained. In 41 survivors the index ranged from 40–71% (mean ± SD, 53 ± 8) and in 15 nonsurvivors from 29–67% (mean, 38 ± 9). With 1 exception, this echo index sharply separated survivors from nonsurvivors. The lower limit to survive aneurysmectomy was 40%.

Lapeyre and colleagues[48] from Rochester, Minnesota, and New York City evaluated 76 patients with chronic LV aneurysm to determine the incidence and prevention of systemic embolism. This retrospective study was performed during an 8-year interval (1971–1979). The median interval from AMI to ventriculography was 11 months and subsequent median follow-up was 5 years. Among these patients, 20 received anticoagulant therapy and 69 patients did not. Twenty-eight patients died during follow-up and the 3- and 5-year survival rates were 75 and 61%, respectively. Among these patients, only 1 not receiving anticoagulant therapy had an embolic event. The inci-

Fig. 2-11. Method of evaluating the residual myocardial index of the LV (RMI$_{LV}$). Arrows indicate the separation between the normally moving endocardium and the apical aneurysm. The end-diastolic length of the normally moving endocardium of each of the 6 walls was expressed as a fraction of the end-diastolic long axis of the left ventricle. 2C = 2-chamber view; 3C = apical long-axis or 3-chamber view; 4C = 4-chamber view.

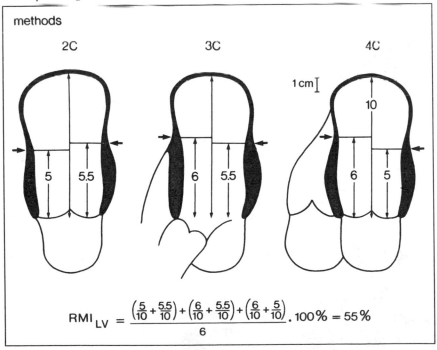

$$RMI_{LV} = \frac{\left(\frac{5}{10} + \frac{5.5}{10}\right) + \left(\frac{6}{10} + \frac{5.5}{10}\right) + \left(\frac{6}{10} + \frac{5}{10}\right)}{6} \cdot 100\% = 55\%$$

dence of systemic embolism was 0.35/100 patient-years. Thus, there is a low incidence of systemic emboli in patients with LV aneurysm documented at least 1 month after AMI. These data do not justify the use of long-term anticoagulant therapy in such patients.

Rupture of LV free wall or ventricular septum

Dellborg and associates[49] from Gothenberg, Sweden, studied the occurrence of LV free wall and/or ventricular septal rupture from AMI and they compared the patients who died of rupture with 2 control groups. Criteria for AMI were fulfilled in 1,746 patients. The diagnosis of rupture was made at either necropsy or at cardiac operation. Two control subjects were selected for each patient and matched for age and sex: 1 (control group A) with AMI having died in hospital but not of rupture (nonrupture cardiac death) and 1 (control group B) with AMI having survived the hospital stay. Necropsy was performed in 75% of all fatal cases with AMI. The total hospital mortality was 19%, the highest mortality being among women >70 years (29%). Rupture occurred in 56 patients or in 17% of the hospital deaths or 3% of all cases of AMI. Women aged <70 had the highest incidence of rupture, 42% of deaths being due to rupture. The mean age for patients with rupture and controls was 71 years. The median time after admission to death was approximately 50 hours for patients and control group A (Fig. 2-12). In 30% of patients, rupture occurred within 24 hours of the initial symptoms. Angina and previous AMI were more common among control group A. Patients with rupture and control group B were mostly relatively free of previous cardiovascular or other diseases (chronic angina pectoris and previous AMI). Sustained systemic hypertension during admission to the coronary care unit was more common in patients than in control group A. Hypotension and shock were more common among control group A. Most (79%) patients who subsequently had a rupture did not receive any corticosteroids during the hospital

Fig. 2-12.   Time from onset of symptoms to death for patients with myocardial rupture (●) and control group A (nonrupture cardiac death; ○). Reproduced with permission from Dellborg et al.[49]

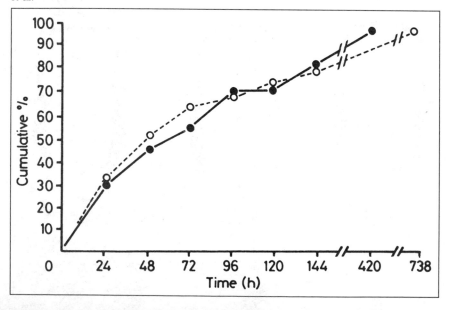

stay. Severe CHF and antiarrhythmic treatment were more uncommon among patients than among control group A. Patients with rupture received analgesics approximately 3 times a day throughout their stay. Control group B received analgesics mostly during the first 24 hours. Thus, female patients, patients with first infarcts, and patients with sustained chest pain should be investigated for the possibility of rupture. As many as one third (32%) of ruptures may be subacute, and therefore time is available for diagnosis and surgery.

Boden and Sadaniantz[50] from Providence, Rhode Island, encountered 4 patients who developed VSD during AMI in a 16-month period and 3 of the 4 patients were receiving ibuprofen therapy for concomitant pericarditis. Retrospective review of their patients with AMI between 1976 and 1984 yielded 5 more patients with pericarditis during AMI in whom a rupture of the ventricular septum developed; only 1 of the 5 was receiving concomitant treatment with an anti-inflammatory agent (salicylates). Whether ibuprofen per se resulted in the appreciably higher case occurrence rate of postinfarction VSD observed in the last 6-month period is unclear. Nevertheless, the incidence of postinfarction VSD increased 4-fold in their hospital since early 1983, during a period when ibuprofen therapy for pericarditis has been widely prescribed.

Rupture of papillary muscle

Come and associates[51] from Boston, Massachusetts, performed emergency echo and established the diagnosis of partial or complete papillary muscle rupture in 4 patients admitted to their hospital in 1983 and 1984. Echo played a pivotal role in diagnosis. In the first patient with complete papillary muscle rupture there was no audible precordial murmur and the initial PA wedge pressure tracing did not reveal large V waves. In the second patient, MR was audible but the patient improved markedly with vasodilator therapy. Emergency surgery was performed because of the echo diagnosis of partial papillary muscle rupture. Severe MR had not been suspected before echo in the third patient with partial rupture. In the fourth patient the presence of a mechanical defect in the setting of preserved septal and anterior wall motion prompted surgery. Complete papillary muscle rupture was characterized by 1 or more 2-D findings: abnormal cutoff of 1 papillary muscle; a mobile mass attached to chordae and to the mitral valve, which could simulate a valvular tumor, thrombus or vegetation; and a pattern of MVP or of a flail mitral leaflet. Partial papillary muscle rupture also had some abnormal features that were detectable by echo.

PROGNOSTIC INDEXES

Creatine kinase level

Fioretti and associates[52] from Rotterdam, The Netherlands, investigated in 266 patients who survived the first 48 hours from onset of AMI the extent to which patients with low peaks serum creatine kinase (CK) at their first AMI differ from patients with high CK levels in terms of risk for subsequent ischemic events. All patients were followed for 1 year. Four groups were formed, based on peak CK $\leq$200, 201–400, 401–800, and >800 IU/L^{-1}. During follow-up, the incidence of death was 15% (n = 39), nonfatal reinfarction 9% (n = 23), and angina 53% (n = 140). Hospital mortality was significantly higher in the highest CK group (16%), but the incidence of nonfatal reinfarction, angina pectoris, and late death was similar in the 4 groups. In-hospital survivors, ischemic ST changes during predischarge symptom-limited bicycle stress test and multiple vessel CAD were equally distributed in all 4 groups. The investigators concluded that while hospital mortality is directly related to peak CK, there is no relation between peak CK and late mortality, nonfatal reinfarction, or recurrent angina.

Grande and associates[53] from Durham, North Carolina, determined the strength of the relation between serum CK-MB isoenzyme estimated AMI size, other prognostic variables, and mortality after AMI. Serum CK-MB estimated AMI size and 11 other prognostic variables were obtained in 317 patients. By Cox regression analysis, the prognostic variables significantly related to mortality were identified: CHF, estimated AMI size, New York Heart Association class, number of previous AMIs, and age (Fig. 2-13). CHF and estimated AMI size were most strongly related to mortality. The relation between the prognostic variables and mortality was nonlinear, and the variables influenced each others' relation to mortality. A prognostic index based on all 5 prognostic variables provided the best means of estimating the probability of survival after AMI. Neither serum CK-MB estimated AMI size nor any of the other prognostic variables had a significant independent influence on mortality, and the probability of survival was high in the absence of any of the prognostic variables in combination.

White and associates[54] from Durham, North Carolina, studied CK-MB changes using agarose gel electrophoresis in 244 patients admitted to a coronary care unit for suspected AMI. A range of minimally elevated CK-MB levels, from 1–24 IU/L, was identified as representing uncertain AMI events. Positive AMI events were defined by elevations of ≥24 IU/L documented in patients with new Q waves or abnormalities in all enzyme and isoenzyme levels. Negative AMI events were defined by elevation of 0 IU/L, observed in all control subjects. The 1-year cardiac mortality rates in the "positive" AMI and "uncertain" AMI groups were identical (22%), and significantly higher than that in the "negative" AMI group (6%). However, when a larger uncertain AMI group of 115 patients was compiled by 2 collaborating centers, the 1-year cardiac mortality rate in the 39 patients with chest pain alone was 0 -vs- 33% in the 76 patients with accompanying severe medical problems,

Fig. 2-13. Probability of survival as a function of time for patients with different combinations of the prognostic variables. For the quantitative variables relevant constants were chosen: age 62 years (mean of the study population); estimated infarct size 200 U/L and 2000 U/L. The qualitative prognostic variables were: presence of previous infarct; New York Heart Association class >1; presence of heart failure. Reproduced with permission from Grande et al.[53]

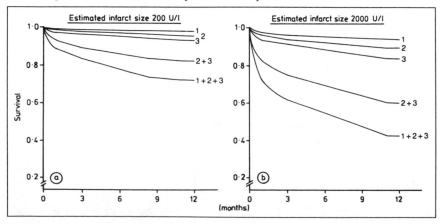

such as cardiac or respiratory failure. Whether minimal CK-MB elevations represent AMI of limited extent is not clear. These elevations occur most often in association with severe medical problems, and in patients without such problems, they may not indicate a poor prognosis.

Type A score

Shekelle and associates[55] from Houston, Texas, and Chicago, Illinois, administered the Jenkins Activity Survey (JAS), a questionnaire developed to assess the type A behavior pattern, to 2,314 participants in the Aspirin Myocardial Infarction Study. All had had an AMI before entering the study and all were followed for at least 3 years. The JAS type A score was not significantly related to risk of recurrent major coronary events (definite nonfatal AMI and coronary death) in the group of 244 women, the group of 2,070 men, or the subgroup of 671 men who were employed full-time in professional, technical, or managerial positions. These results indicate that the JAS type A score is not useful in assessing prognosis after AMI. By inference, traits measured by the JAS type A score, such as competitiveness, orientation toward achievement, and preference for a rapid pace of life, appear not to be associated with increased risk of recurrent major coronary events.

Initial ECG

Brush and associates[56] from New Haven, Connecticut, and Burlington, Vermont, evaluated the initial ECG as a predictor of complications in 469 patients with suspected AMI. An ECG was classified as positive if it showed ≥1 of the following: evidence of AMI, ischemia, or strain; LV hypertrophy; left BBB; or paced rhythm. Forty-two (14%) of 302 patients with a positive ECG had ≥1 life-threatening complication (VF, sustained VT, or heart block), compared with 1 (0.6%) of 167 patients with a negative ECG (Fig. 2-14). Life-threatening complications were therefore 23 times more likely if the initial ECG was positive. Other complications were 3–10 times more likely, and death was 17 times more likely in patients with a positive ECG (Fig. 2-15). The investigators concluded that patients with a negative initial ECG have a low likelihood of complications and could be admitted to an intermediate care unit instead of a coronary care unit. This would reduce admissions to the coronary care unit by 36% and thereby save considerable hospital cost without compromising patient care.

ECG ST segment depression

To study the mechanism and prognostic importance of precordial ST-segment depression during inferior wall AMI, Hlatky and associates[57] from Durham, North Carolina, studied 162 patients during a 3-year period. Patients with ST depression in leads V_1-V_3 had a significantly larger AMI as assessed by a QRS scoring system. Hospital mortality was 4% (3 of 75) among patients without ST depression, and 13% (11 of 87) in patients with ST depression. The relation between the amount of ST depression and hospital mortality was significant and remained significant after adjusting for other potentially prognostic factors. Among patients discharged from the hospital, the 5-year survival was 92% in those without precordial ST depression and 80% in those with precordial ST depression (Fig. 2-16). Precordial ST-segment depression on the admission ECG during an inferior AMI indicates a larger AMI, predicts a higher hospital mortality, and suggests a worse long-term prognosis after discharge.

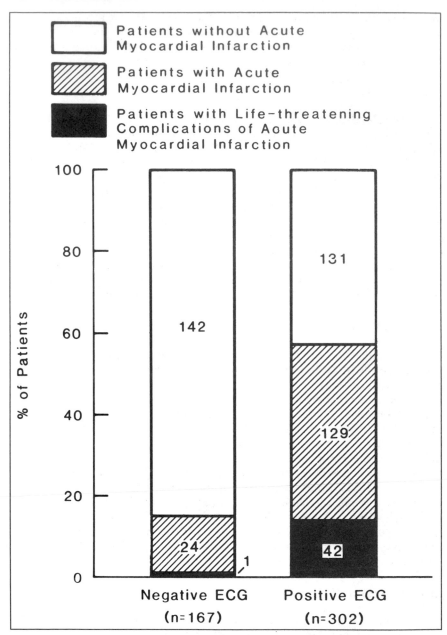

Fig. 2-14.   Percent of patients with AMI and immediate life-threatening complications (VF, sustained VT, or heart block), according to initial ECG. Numbers of patients shown within bars. The differences in the rates of AMI and in the rates of complications between the 2 ECG groups are statistically significant (p <0.001). Reproduced with permission from Brush et al.[56]

LV thrombi

Improved detection for 2-D echo recently has demonstrated that LV thrombi are common in patients with AMI. Spirito and coworkers[58] from Genoa, Italy, studied 58 patients with transmural AMI prospectively to determine the prognostic significance of LV thrombi during an AMI, the incidence of systemic embolization, and the possible occurrence of spontaneous regres-

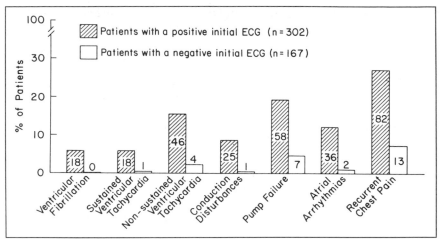

Fig. 2-15. Percent of patients with individual complications of AMI, according to initial ECG. Numbers of patients are shown within or above bars. The differences in complication rates between the 2 ECG groups are statistically significant (p <0.01). Reproduced with permission from Brush et al.[56]

sion of LV thrombi. The patients were not treated with anticoagulants or platelet inhibitors. Two-D echo was obtained within 24 hours of AMI, every 24 hours until day 5, every 48 hours until day 15, and every month for 11 months in the surviving patients. Of 774 echoes, LV thrombi were identified

Fig. 2-16. Cumulative survival of patients discharged from the hospital, according to the presence or absence of precordial ST-segment depression on the admission ECG.

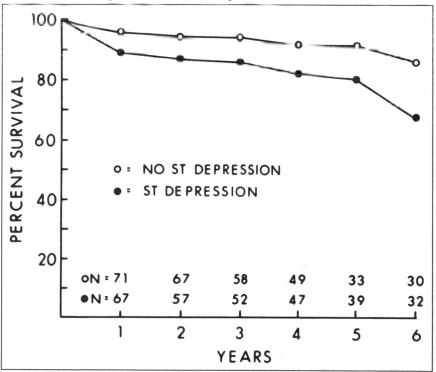

in 24 (41%) of the 58 study patients, and developed within 48 hours of AMI in 11 patients (Fig. 2-17). Ten of the 11 patients with thrombus died early during hospitalization or during follow-up, whereas only 2 of 13 who developed thrombus after 48 hours of AMI died. Killip class III or IV, total lactic dehydrogenase values, and extent of wall motion abnormalities were significantly higher in patients with thrombus within 48 hours of AMI than in patients without thrombus. In patients developing a thrombus after 48 hours of AMI, these parameters were not different from those in patients not developing a thrombus. Spontaneous regression of thrombi was documented in 3 of the 15 patients who survived the acute phase of AMI. One of the 24 patients with LV thrombi had transient ischemic attacks, and no embolic events were detected in patients without thrombus. These investigators concluded that development of LV thrombi within 2 days of AMI occurs in patients with the most extensive infarcts and is predictive of high mortality. These data also demonstrate that spontaneous regression of thrombi occurs.

Fig. 2-17.   Patients who developed LV thrombus (LVT) within 48 hours of AMI, those who developed LVT after 48 hours, and those without LVT are compared with regard to incidence of Killip class III or IV. Reproduced with permission from Spirito et al.[58]

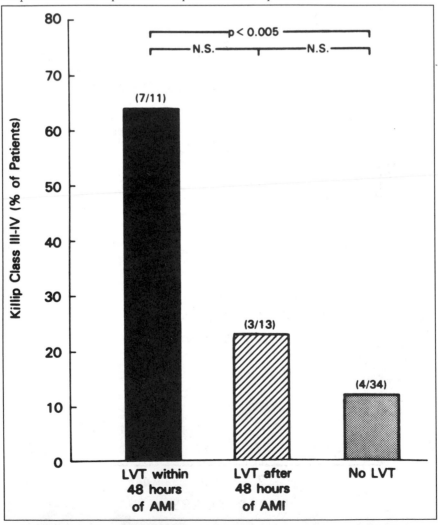

Takamoto and associates[59] from Stanford, California, assessed in 47 patients, 11 of whom underwent resection of a LV aneurysm and 36 of whom underwent cardiac transplantation, the diagnostic accuracy of cross-sectional echo and cineangiography in detecting LV mural thrombi and the effect of anticoagulation treatment on the incidence of such thrombi. Cross-sectional echo in 37 patients and cineangiography in 26 (16 patients were examined by both methods) were analyzed independently by 2 observers experienced in the respective methods. Mural thrombus was confirmed anatomically in 14 of 47 (30%) cases; 11 of these 14 patients had intra-aneurysmal thrombi. The negative predictive value was quite good for both methods, but cross-sectional echo had a superior positive predictive value. Mural thrombi were present in 3 of 20 patients with preceding anticoagulation and in 10 of 29 patients without anticoagulation. The results emphasize that cross-sectional echo is more reliable than cineangiography in recognizing thrombi.

Location of infarction

Maisel and associates[60] from San Diego, California, and Vancouver, Canada, studied prognostic differences between patients with anterior or inferior AMI in 997 hospital survivors of Q-wave AMI (anterior in 449, inferior in 548) who were matched closely with regard to age, sex, prior AMI, and CHF. There were no differences in peak serum creatine kinase values between patients in the 2 groups. In patients with anterior AMI dying during the first year of follow-up, 56% died in the first 2 months after hospital discharge compared with 18% of those with inferior AMI. Thereafter, survival curves became nearly identical and remained so for 1 year when the total mortality rate was 10% for patients with anterior AMI and 7% for those with inferior AMI. Those patients with anterior AMI had more clinical evidence of CHF; rales above the scapulae and ventricular gallop sounds were the strongest predictors of 1-year mortality by both univariate and multivariate analysis. Age and peripheral edema also were strong predictors of mortality in patients with anterior AMI, and prior AMI was predictive of mortality risks in patients with both types of infarctions (Table 2-2). Thus, these data indicate that in matched patients with anterior or inferior AMI who survive hospitalization, there is a higher mortality up to 60 days in those with anterior infarcts. Moreover, signs of CHF in the hospital, especially in patients with prior AMI, identify those patients at highest risk of death during follow-up.

LV ejection fraction

Kelly and associates[61] from Nedlands, Australia, determined by radionuclide first-pass portable probe method within a mean of 24 hours after the onset of major symptoms in 171 patients after AMI. The results were related prospectively to the subsequent incidence of EF in hospital and to hospital and postdischarge deaths in a mean follow-up of 15 months (range, 9–21). All 8 episodes of primary VF, all 12 deaths due to pump failure in hospital, and 12 of 13 postdischarge deaths occurred in that minority of 81 patients whose initial postinfarction LVEF was ≤0.35. Multivariate correlation with clinical, enzymatic, and ECG indicators of AMI showed that the prognostic significance of these indicators could largely be explained by their association with low LVEF. LVEF measured within the initial 24 hours after AMI predicts prognosis throughout the subsequent year.

TABLE Table 2-2. *Univariate predictors of 1-year mortality after hospital discharge. Reproduced with permission from Maisel et al.[60]*

RANK VARIABLE*	SURVIVORS	NONSURVIVORS	P VALUE
Anterior Infarction[+]			
1. Mean age (yr)	61 ± 12	70 ± 10	0.0001
2. Peripheral edema (%)	6	22	0.0001
3. Diuretic on discharge (%)	31	53	0.0001
4. Digitalis on discharge (%)	42	64	0.0004
5. Cardiothoracic ratio	0.485 ± 0.05	0.514 ± 0.06	0.0007
6. Blood urea nitrogen (mg/dl)	21	28	0.0058
7. EF (%)	41 ± 11	32 ± 11	0.02
8. Final heart rate (per min)	73	77	0.023
9. Maximal heart rate (per min)	98 ± 20	106 ± 22	0.02
10. Pulmonary congestion (%)	19	35	0.04
Inferior Infarction[+]			
1. Rales above scapulae (%)	6	27	0.0001
2. Ventricular gallop (%) (final examination)	3	21	0.0001
3. Previous infarction (%)	19	48	0.0001
4. Sinus tachycardia (%)	16	41	0.0002
5. Maximal heart rate (per min)	89	105	0.0008
6. Cardiothoracic ratio	0.48 ± 0.05	0.53 ± 0.05	0.0018
7. Systolic murmur (%)	2	14	0.003
8. EF (%)	52 ± 11	43 ± 11	0.003
9. Pulmonary congestion	2	15	0.0035
10. Diuretic on discharge (%)	19	39	0.026

*Total variables = 65; rank based on p values; mean values are ± 1 SD.
[+]There were 400 survivors and 49 nonsurvivors.
[+]There were 510 survivors and 38 nonsurvivors.

Infarct extension

Maisel and coworkers[62] from San Diego, California, examined whether or not subsets of patients with extension of AMI were at high risk for early and late mortality. They hypothesized that infarct extension in patients with non-Q-wave infarcts might be associated with a poorer prognosis than for patients with extension of Q-wave AMI. A total of 1,253 patients with AMI were included and followed prospectively. The patients were classified according to ECG results into the following groups: those with non-Q-wave infarcts (n = 277) and those with Q-wave anterior infarcts (n = 462) and Q-wave inferior infarcts (n = 497). Extension was diagnosed by 2 of the following criteria: 1) recurrent chest pain ≥24 hours after admission to the hospital, 2) new persistent ECG changes, and 3) elevation or reappearance of elevated creatine kinase levels. By these criteria 85 (6%) had extension (8% of non-Q-wave infarcts, 6% of Q-wave anterior infarcts, and 6% of Q-wave inferior infarcts). Hospital mortality with extension was 15% in those with Q-wave infarcts and 43% in those with non-Q-wave infarcts. Of the 1,253 patients 952 were followed for 1 year. In 24% of those who did not survive 1 year, there was extension of infarct: only 6% of survivors had extension. The 1-year cumulative survival rates for patients with Q wave -vs- non-Q-wave infarcts with no extension were nearly identical: 82 and 84% (Fig. 2-18). For patients

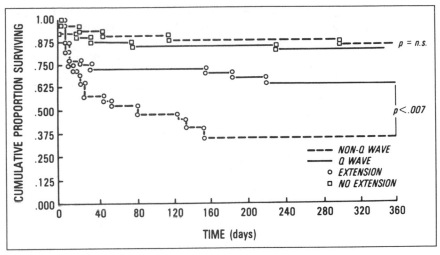

Fig. 2-18. Cumulative survival in Q-wave (solid line) and non-Q-wave (dashed line) infarctions with (○) and without (□) extension. Each point on the survival curve represents at least 1 new death. In patients with no extension the survival curves were similar for the 2 groups. The 1-year survival for those with non-Q-wave infarcts with extension was 35 -vs- 66% for those with Q-wave infarction with extension (p <0.01) and 84% for those with non-Q-wave infarct without extension (p <0.001). Among hospital survivors of non-Q-wave infarcts, the time to death was shorter in the group with extension compared with those without extension (70 ± 18 -vs- 168 ± 28 days, p <0.01). Reproduced with permission from Maisel et al.[62]

with extension, 1-year survival rates for those with Q-wave -vs- non-Q-wave AMI were 66 and 35%. In hospital survivors of non-Q-wave AMI, death occurred twice as early with extension as without. Of 60 variables examined for prognostic significance, extension was not a predictor in patients with Q-wave AMI but was the strongest univariate predictor of 1-year mortality in those with non-Q-wave infarcts. These investigators concluded that patients with non-Q-wave AMI with extension represent a subset of patients at high risk for early and late mortality.

Exercise testing

Handler[63] from London, UK, evaluated the prognostic value of abnormalities resulting from predischarge submaximal treadmill exercise testing in 222 patients after AMI. The presence of the following variables—ST-segment depression and elevation, an abnormal BP response, limited exercise duration, angina pectoris, ventricular arrhythmias—were predictive of subsequent cardiac events among the 154 patients with ≥1 of these abnormalities. When the presence or absence of specific variables was assessed, only an abnormal BP response, limited exercise duration, and ST segment elevation and shift were significantly associated with cardiac death. Exercise-induced angina was predictive only of the development of subsequent angina, and ST depression was associated only with future CABG. Ventricular arrhythmias had no independent prognostic value. Markers of LV dysfunction elicited by submaximal exercise testing are therefore valuable in identifying patients at high risk of death after AMI. Hallmarks of residual reversible myocardial ischemia are of limited prognostic importance. The test result may be useful in selecting patients for coronary angiography.

Of 866 patients enrolled by Krone and the Multicenter Postinfarction Research Group[64] from St. Louis, Missouri, 667 performed a low-level exercise test early after AMI. Excluding the 7 patients who died before the test could be considered, there was a 14% 1-year mortality in 192 patients who did not take the test compared with 5% in those who did. Of those who took the test, 12% subsequently underwent CABG compared with 14% of those who did not. Decreased mortality in the year after the AMI in those taking the test was associated with an increase in BP to 110 mmHg or higher, ability to complete the 9-minute test, and the absence of couplets or any VPC before, during, or after exercise. Achievement of a BP of 110 mmHg or higher during exercise in patients with no evidence of pulmonary congestion on the chest radiograph identified a group of 454 patients (70% of those taking the test) with a 1-year cardiac mortality of 1% compared with 13% in the remaining patients. Logistic models showed that the exercise test contributed independent prognostic information for cardiac death, new AMI, and CABG. Thus, the results of low-level exercise testing before hospital discharge combined with clinical features of the AMI can effectively identify patients at low risk for subsequent cardiac mortality.

Madsen and associates[65] from San Diego, California, and Vancouver, Canada, evaluated whether an ischemic exercise test response or functional capacity could be predicted from data available during hospitalization in patients discharged after AMI. The value of exercise test variables for predicting death and new AMI within 1 year also was examined. Among 1,469 patients, 466 (32%) underwent treadmill exercise testing around the time of discharge. An ischemic exercise test response (ST-segment depression or angina) could not be predicted. Good functional capacity (>4 METs) could be predicted from age and ST-segment changes at rest. Among the 60% of patients who were predicted to have functional capacity of >4 METs, only 15% had poor functional capacity at the time of testing. Multivariate analysis for predicting death and new AMI selected only functional capacity (continuous variable in METs), which classified 72% of the patients into a low risk group with a <2% rate of death and new AMI in the first year. The high risk group (29% of the patients) had an 18% rate of death or new AMI. It was concluded that functional capacity is the most important exercise test variable and that patients likely to have good functional capacity can be identified on the basis of age and ST-segment changes at rest. Further, the level of functional capacity on exercise testing can identify groups of patients with very low and relatively high risk of death or new AMI within 1 year.

Teo and associates[66] from Edmonton, Canada, studied the heart rate and BP responses to standardized exercise tests in 37 patients with ECG evidence of inferior wall AMI. The tests were done on a bicycle ergometer at 8–10 days and 10–12 weeks after AMI. At 8–10 days after AMI, those with ST AMI (n = 12) had a significantly reduced heart rate response to exercise compared with patients with Q-wave AMI (n = 25). This difference was not evident at 10–12 weeks. The systolic BP response in patients with ST AMI was lower than that of Q-wave AMI patients during the first exercise test, although the difference did not attain statistical significance but was significantly lower than the responses of both groups at the second test. The patients with ST AMI had smaller amounts of myocardial damage than those with Q-wave AMI as indicated by plasma creatine kinase values.

Fioretti and associates[67] from Rotterdam, The Netherlands, studied the predictive value of a predischarge symptom-limited stress test in 405 consecutive survivors of AMI: 300 patients performed bicycle ergometry; 105 could not perform it. Among these latter 105 patients, the stress test was contraindicated in 43 because of angina or CHF and in 62 because of noncardiac limitations. One-year survival was 44% in the cardiac-limited group (19 of 43) and 92% in the noncardiac-limited group (57 of 62). One-year survival among the patients who performed an exercise test at discharge was 93% (280 of 300). The best stress test predictor of mortality by univariate analysis was the extent of BP increases: 42 ± 24 mmHg in 280 survivors -vs- 21 ± 14 mmHg in 20 nonsurvivors. Among the 212 patients in whom BP increased ≥30 mmHg, mortality was 3%, whereas it was 16% among the 88 patients in whom BP increased <30 mmHg. Angina, ST changes, and arrhythmias were not as predictive. Stepwise discriminant function analysis showed inadequate BP increase to be an independent predictor of mortality. A high risk group can be identified at discharge on clinical grounds in patients unable to perform a stress test, whereas intermediate and low risk groups can be identified by the extent of BP increase during exercise.

To determine the prognostic value of submaximal exercise testing in patients after AMI, Waters and associates[68] from Montreal, Canada, studied 225 survivors of AMI by a limited exercise test 1 day before hospital discharge. These patients were followed for 5 years. Mortality rate was 11% during the first year, but averaged 3%/year from the second to fifth years. The 5 variables that predicted mortality by multivariate analysis were QRS score, an exercise-induced ST-segment shift, previous AMI, failure to achieve target heart rate or workload, and ventricular arrhythmias during the exercise test. The factors that were predictive of mortality during the first year were an exercise-induced ST shift, a failure to increase systolic BP by ≥10 mmHg during exercise, and angina in the hospital ≥48 hours after admission. These data indicate that exercise test variables are useful predictors of mortality after AMI during the first year. Thereafter, mortality risk correlates more strongly with evidence of LV dysfunction.

Echocardiography

Bhatnagar and colleagues[69] from Kuwait, Arabian Gulf, performed 2-D echo in 47 consecutive survivors (mean age, 47 years) of a first AMI to assess its value in predicting major cardiac complications (MCC) during the post-hospital phase. Two-D echo was done 1 day before hospital discharge (mean, 15 days). A wall motion score was derived by analyzing endocardial motion in 11 LV segments. During a mean 17-month follow-up, 17 patients had MCC: 8 (47%) had significant angina; 2 (12%) had a reinfarction, and 7 (41%) died. Wall motion scores of patients with MCC (9 ± 1) (±SEM) were significantly higher compared with those without MCC (4 ± 0.5). A wall motion score ≥8 was present in 82% (14 of 17) of patients with MCC compared with 7% (2 of 30) who remained asymptomatic. Patients who died had significantly higher wall motion scores compared with those who survived (11 ± 1 -vs- 5 ± 1). Stepwise logistic regression and discriminant analysis, by means of age, infarct site, maximal Killip class, cardiac enzymes, and wall motion score, identified wall motion score and Killip class as the most significant predictors of MCC. Thus, predischarge 2-D echo is capable of identifying high risk patients prone to developing MCC after a first AMI.

Radionuclide angiography

Morris and associates[70] from Durham, North Carolina, studied the value of rest and exercise RNA for predicting specific events, including death, recurrent AMI, coronary care unit readmission for unstable chest pain, and medically refractory angina after AMI in 106 consecutive survivors of AMI. Analysis of the RNA variables using the Cox proportional hazards regression model yielded significant associations of the time to death with EF at rest and during exercise ($X^2 = 11$ and 14, respectively). Both variables added significant prognostic information to the clinical assessment ($X^2 = 4$ and 6, respectively). The change in EF from rest to exercise predicted the time to CABG for medically refractory angina before ($X^2 = 21$) and after ($X^2 = 13$) adjustment for the clinical descriptors, but did not predict death or other nonfatal events. Significant correlations were found between RNA variables and a variety of clinical descriptors previously reported to have prognostic significance. Clinical and RNA variables that are measures of LV function were predictive of subsequent mortality, whereas those that reflect residual potentially ischemic myocardium were predictive of subsequent nonfatal ischemic events. Rest and exercise RNA after AMI provides significant prognostic information regarding specific events during follow-up independent of that provided by clinical assessment.

Ventricular arrhythmias

Maisel and coworkers[71] from San Diego, California, examined whether or not subsets of patients with complex ventricular arrhythmias after AMI are at high risk with respect to 1-year mortality after hospital discharge. Based on previous studies showing increased risk for patients with non-Q-wave infarcts, these investigators hypothesized that complex VPC in this group might be associated with a poorer prognosis than complex VPC in patients with Q-wave infarcts; 777 patients with AMI were followed prospectively for 1 year after undergoing a predischarge 24-hour ambulatory ECG. Patients were classified by ECG criteria into the following groups: Non-Q wave (n = 191), Q-wave anterior (n = 261), and Q-wave inferior aMI (n = 325). The following arrhythmias were classified as complex: multiform VPC, couplets, and VT; 62% of patients with non-Q-wave infarcts who did not survive 1 year had complex VPC compared with 32% of survivors (Fig. 2-19). No differences were seen in the Q-wave subgroups. The survival for patients with Q-wave and non-Q-wave AMI without complex VPC was nearly identical at 1 year (93 and 90%), whereas in patients with complex VPC survival for those with Q-wave and non-Q-wave AMI was 92 and 76%, respectively. Of those with non-Q-wave AMI, only 4% of nonsurvivors were free of any VPC compared with 28% of nonsurvivors in the Q-wave group. Stepwise linear discrimination analysis revealed that complex VPC were independent of EF in those with non-Q-wave AMI, but were closely associated with EF in those with Q-wave AMI. Thus, the presence of complex VPC at the time of hospital discharge is an important predictor of 1-year mortality in the presence of non-Q-wave, but not Q-wave AMI.

Schwartz and associates[72] from Milan, Italy, performed a case-controlled study in 250 post-AMI patients to examine whether an episode of VF during the in-hospital period modified the long-term prognosis for patients with either an anterior or an inferior wall AMI. After identification of 70 patients with an anterior AMI and 55 patients with an inferior AMI, all complicated by VF and discharged alive, they selected 125 additional patients who had an AMI not complicated by VF (control subjects). To minimize the potential sources of differences in outcome, cases and controls were matched for the following variables: sex (all men), age (same ± 2 years), coronary care unit (same), epoch of AMI (same ± 3 months), and site of AMI (same). LV dysfunction and prior AMI were present in only a few patients. Patients receiving β-adrenergic blocking agents were not included. The average follow-up was 59 months (range, 12–120). The cumulative mortality during the first 5 years for the patients with inferior AMI without VF (6, 11, 13, 13 and 13%) was modest and not significantly different from that of inferior AMI complicated by VF (6, 11, 20, 20, and 26%) (Fig. 2-20). In contrast, a striking

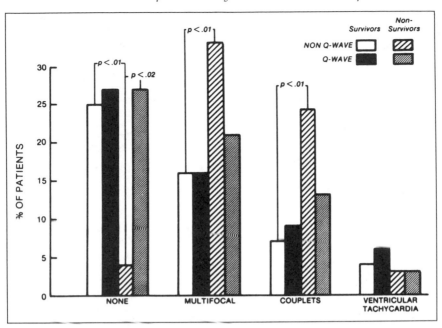

Fig. 2-19. Arrhythmias present at duscharge (Holter) as related to 1-year survival in Q-wave and non-Q-wave infarction groups. Multifocal VPCs and couplets were present with greater frequency in nonsurvivors with non Q-wave infarction than in survivors (33 and 24% -vs- 16 and 7%, respectively, p <0.01), but did not differ in survivors and nonsurvivors of Q-wave infarctions. Only 4% of nonsurvivors of non Q-wave infarction were free of any ventricular arrhythmias compared with 25% of survivors (p <0.01). Reproduced with permission from Maisel et al.[71]

difference appeared when the cumulative mortality of patients with anterior AMI without VF (9, 13, 17, 27, and 29%) was compared with that of patients with anterior AMI complicated by VT (32, 40, 46, 49, and 54%). This group also had a high incidence of sudden death (71%), particularly in the first year after AMI. This finding is in contrast with the current view that VF does not modify the long-term post-AMI prognosis. In conclusion, patients who are discharged alive after an anterior AMI complicated by VF represent a subgroup at very high risk of sudden cardiac death. For patients with an inferior AMI, the occurrence of VF in the acute phase does not modify the long-term prognosis.

Luria and associates[73] from Cleveland, Ohio, followed 248 patients for at least 12 years, all of whom survived an AMI. The cumulative survival at 1 year was 89%, at 5 years 68%, at 10 years 53%, and at 12 years, 43%. When patients were assessed with 5 routinely obtained clinical factors, significant prognostic stratification of high and low risk survival groups extended throughout the follow-up period. Sudden coronary death was found to be twice as frequent as nonsudden coronary death, but a significant relation between sudden death and complex ventricular and complex VPC could not be defined. The extent of complex features of VPC, such as pairs, multiform, repetitive, and R-on-T, was inversely related to survival (Fig. 2-21). During the first year after AMI, frequency of VPC also was inversely related to survival. A long-term effect of frequency on survival, however, could not be demonstrated.

DiMarco and coworkers[74] from Charlottesville, Virginia, studied 53 patients surviving an initial episode of sustained VT or VF between 3 and 60

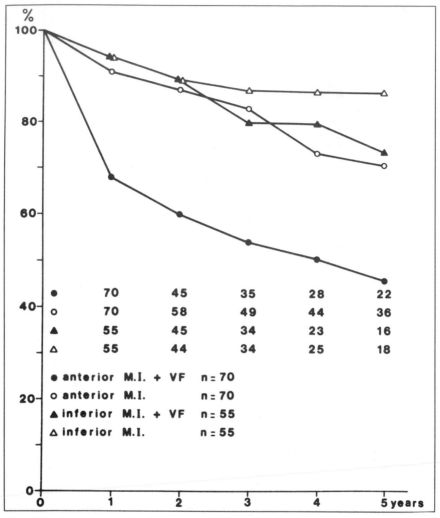

Fig. 2-20. Survival curves for the 4 groups of patients (total 250) after hospital discharge. The numbers represent the number of patients studied at each interval.

days after AMI. Most patients had a large complicated AMI. Forty-two (79%) had repetitive sustained ventricular arrhythmias and 19 patients could not be stabilized with drug therapy. Twenty-eight patients had either infarctectomy of aneurysmectomy because of coexistent CHF or angina and sustained ventricular arrhythmias. In 16 of the patients, the procedure was done on an emergency basis. Intraoperative mapping was attempted in all patients but was successful in only 13 (52%). Operative mortality was 16%, with deaths occurring in patients who were in shock before the procedure. Five of 21 surgically treated survivors required long-term antiarrhythmic therapy. Twenty-one of 24 patients treated medically were alive and well 15 ± 10 months into their follow-up and 19 of 21 medically treated patients were alive and well after 18 ± 11 months. These data indicate a poor medical prognosis for patients with sustained ventricular tachyarrhythmias in the initial weeks after AMI, but demonstrate that an acceptable rate of survival can be achieved with a combined medical and surgical therapeutic approach.

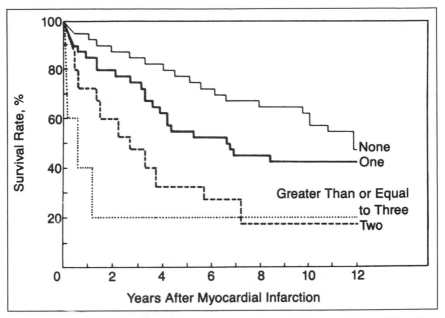

Fig. 2-21.   Long-term Kaplan-Meier cumulative survival rate after recovery from AMI based on number of features of complex VPC (pairs, VT, multiform, R-on-T). Reproduced with permission from Luria et al.[73]

Programmed ventricular stimulation

Since survivors of AMI represent a large and easily identifiable population of patients at risk for sudden cardiac death, considerable efforts have been made to identify those survivors at highest risk with subsequent fatal arrhythmic events. The prognostic significance of programmed ventricular stimulation and its usefulness in relation to other forms of invasive and noninvasive testing was evaluated by Roy and coworkers[75] from Montreal, Canada, on 150 survivors of AMI. Ventricular arrhythmias of ≥6 beats were induced in 35 (23%) patients. No significant differences existed between patients with inducible ventricular tachyarrhythmias and those without inducible VT with respect to occurrence of spontaneous ventricular arrhythmias in the acute and early recovery phase of AMI or predischarge exercise-induced ischemia or arrhythmias, severity of CAD, or degree of LV dysfunction. A higher incidence of inferior AMI was observed in patients with inducible VT compared with those without inducible VT (66 -vs- 41%). During a mean follow-up of 10 ± 5 months, there were 2 sudden deaths, 3 nonsudden deaths, and additional patients developed sustained ventricular tachyarrhythmias. There was no significant difference between patients with and without inducible ventricular tachyarrhythmias with respect to the occurrence of these events. In this study population, a lower mean EF, the presence of LV aneurysm, and exercise-induced VPC were predictors of sudden death and spontaneous VT. Thus, these findings do not support the hypothesis that the induction of VT in patients recovering from AMI identifies a group at high risk for sudden cardiac death.

Bhandari and associates[76] from Los Angeles, California, Everett, Washington, and Taipai, Taiwan, performed electrophysiologic study, 24-hour ambulatory ECG monitoring, treadmill exercise test, and angiographic evaluation in 45 patients 14 ± 3 days after AMI. Electrophysiologic study protocol included burst ventricular pacing and 1–3 ventricular extrastimuli at 2-cycle

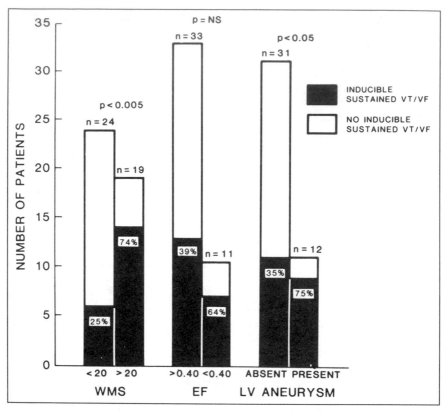

Fig. 2-22. LV angiographic data in patients with and without inducible sustained VT or VF.
WM = wall motion score.

lengths from RV apex, RV outflow, and left ventricle. Sustained monomorphic VT (13 patients) or VF (7 patients) was induced in 20 patients (44%)
(group I). In these 20 patients, VT/VF was inducible with 2 extrastimuli in 10
patients, 3 extrastimuli in 9 patients, and burst pacing in 1 patient. In the
remaining 25 patients (56%), induction of ≥ 7 VPC were noted (group II).
Severe LV wall motion abnormalities occurred in 70% of group I patients and
22% of group II patients. There was no difference in the site of AMI, frequency and grade of VPC on ambulatory ECG monitoring, double product on
submaximal exercise, LVEF, and number of obstructed coronary arteries
($\geq 70\%$ in diameter) between group I and group II patients (Fig. 2-22). During a mean follow-up of 10 ± 3 months, 1 patients in each group died suddenly, and in 1 group 1 patient spontaneous-sustained VT developed, which
was identical in morphologic configuration to that induced during electrophysiologic study. In conclusion, electrical induction of sustained VT or VF
during electrophysiologic study is common in patients 2 weeks after AMI.
These patients have an increased incidence of LV wall motion abnormalities.
The prognostic significance of this finding requires further follow-up study
but appears to be of limited value.

Denniss and associates[77] from Sydney, Australia, investigated the ability
of programmed ventricular stimulation in exercise testing to predict 1-year
mortality after AMI in 228 clinically well survivors of AMI. Patients with
inducible VT or VF had a higher mortality rate than those without inducible
arrhythmias (26 -vs- 6%) (Table 2-3). Exercise-induced ST-segment change
of ≥ 2 mm was associated with a higher mortality rate than ST change of

TABLE 2-3. *One-year mortality in study group*

GROUP	#	DEATHS	MORTALITY (%)	P
All patients	228	22	10	
Underwent PS	175	18	10	
VT/VF	38	10	26	< 0.001
No VT/VF	137	8	6	
Underwent ET	191	12	6	
≥2 mm ST change	61	7	11	< 0.01
<2 mm ST change	130	5	4	
Underwent PS + ET	138	8	6	
VT/VF and/or ≥2 mm ST change	53	7	13	< 0.001
No VT/VF and <2 mm ST change	85	1	1	

ET = exercise testing; PS = programmed stimulation.

<2 mm (11 -vs- 4%). Of patients who had both tests, 62% had no inducible VT or VF and ST change of <2 mm, and only 1% died during the first year. Thus, in clinically well survivors of AMI, programmed stimulation is a powerful predictor of first year mortality; programmed stimulation and exercise testing together predict virtually all deaths within the first year, and they can identify a large group of patients with a very low mortality rate.

Santarelli and associates[78] from Chicago, Illinois, studied the prevalence, characteristics, and clinical significance of ventricular electrical instability with programmed ventricular stimulation in 50 hemodynamically stable patients 17–40 days after AMI using double extrastimuli at 2 and 10 mA intensity and from 2 RV sites. Ventricular electrical instability was defined as induction of ≥10 consecutive intraventricular reentrant beats. Of 50 patients, 23 (46%) had ventricular electrical instability (10 of these had sustained VT induced). No significant differences were observed between patients with and without ventricular electrical instability with respect to age, site of AMI, coronary prognostic index, maximal level of creatine kinase, number of narrowed coronary arteries, and presence of severe wall motion abnormalities. During a mean follow-up of 11 months, no patient died suddenly. During repeated Holter recordings, patients with ventricular electrical instability had a higher incidence of nonsustained VT than did patients without ventricular electrical instability.

Waspe and coworkers[79] from New York City evaluated the prognostic significance of ventricular arrhythmias induced by programmed electrical stimulation in 50 survivors of AMI complicated by major new conduction disturbance (38 patients), CHF (33 patients), or sustained ventricular tachyarrhythmias (22 patients), alone or in combination. Programmed stimulation was performed in patients in stable condition 7–36 days (mean, 16) after AMI using 1–3 extrastimuli. Two groups of patients were identified by their response to programmed stimulation: 17 patients developed sustained (>15 s) or nonsustained (>7 beats but <15 s) VT (group I), and 33 patients had 0–7 intraventricular reentrant complexes with maximal stimulation (group II). The group I patients had a higher incidence of anterior AMI (71 -vs- 42%, respectively), lower LVEF (mean, 0.35 -vs- 0.48, respectively), and were more often treated with antiarrhythmic drugs (47% -vs- 18%). There were no differences among the patients in the 2 groups in the frequency of CHF, new conduction abnormalities or sustained ventricular arrhythmias with AMI, or in the numbers of patients treated with β-receptor blocking agents, CABG, or a pacemaker. The mean follow-up was 23 months for the 2 groups of patients. The responses to programmed stimulation identified a subset of group I patients with high risk of late sudden death or spontaneous VT. These patients could be identified by their developing sustained or non-sustained VT with electrical stimulation (sensitivity, 100%). However, triple extrastimuli were required to induce prognostically significant arrhythmias in 5 of these 7 patients, thus the specificity of this protocol was only 57%. Response to programmed electrical stimulation had a stronger association with the risk of late sudden death than it did with any other variable examined. Thus, programmed ventricular stimulation using a maximum of 3 extrastimuli is a sensitive but relatively nonspecific method for identifying survivors of complicated AMI at high risk of late sudden death or spontaneous ventricular arrhythmias.

TREATMENT

Morphine

Despite a lack of clinical data, conventional wisdom holds that morphine sulfate induces vagally mediated conduction defects, especially in patients with inferior wall AMI. To assess the accuracy of this thesis, Semenkovich and Jaffe[80] from St. Louis, Missouri, reviewed the records of 244 patients admitted to Barnes Hospital Cardiac Care Unit with suspected AMI to determine the frequency of deleterious cardiovascular effects related to the administration of morphine sulfate. Of 184 patients (156 subsequently documented to have AMI) who received morphine sulfate, 4 patients had symptomatic systemic hypertension temporally associated with morphine sulfate administration. These 4 patients represented a frequency of 2.2% of all patients treated with morphine sulfate and a frequency of 2.6% in those with proved AMI. In each instance, the heart rate response was inappropriate, decreased or less markedly accelerated than might be expected given the reduced BP, suggesting a vagal mechanism for the adverse effects. Only 1 of the 4 patients had inferior AMI, and in 3 of 4 instances, the adverse effect occurred after the first dose. All patients subsequently received morphine sulfate without evidence of toxicity. No case of narcotic-induced conduction abnormality was identified. This series, which is the most extensive evaluation of the topic, documents that adverse cardiovascular effects due to morphine sulfate are rare and do not conform to preconceived clinical doctrine. They consist of inappropriate heart rate responses to hypotension rather than conduction defects and are not particularly associated with inferior AMI.

Lidocaine

Dunn and associates[81] from Belfast, North Ireland, studied 402 patients with suspected AMI seen within 6 hours of the onset of symptoms, in a double-blind randomized trial of lidocaine -vs- placebo. During the 1 hour after administration of the drug, the incidence of VF or sustained VT among the 204 patients with AMI was 1.5%. Lidocaine, given in a 300 mg dose intramuscularly followed by 100 mg intravenously, did not prevent sustained VT, although there was a significant reduction in the number of patients with warning arrhythmias between 15 and 45 minutes after the administration of lidocaine. The average plasma lidocaine level 10 minutes after administration for patients without an AMI was significantly higher than that for patients with an AMI. The mean plasma lidocaine level of patients on β-

blocking agents was no different from that in patients not on β-blocking agents. During the 1-hour study period, the incidence of central nervous system side effects was significantly greater in the lidocaine group; hypotension occurred in 11 patients, 9 of whom had received lidocaine, and 4 patients died from asystole, 3 of whom had had lidocaine. Thus, these investigators are adverse to the administration of lidocaine prophylactically in the early hours of suspected AMI.

In a randomized control study examining the value of an intramuscular injection of lidocaine in the prehospital phase of suspected AMI, Koster and Dunning[82] from Amsterdam, The Netherlands, reported a study in which paramedics used an automatic injector to administer 400 mg of the drug into the patient's deltoid muscle before transport to the hospital. In a 33-month period, 7,026 patients with chest pain were seen. Of the 6,024 patients randomized (2,987 to the lidocaine group and 3,037 to the control group), 1,935 (32%) proved to have an AMI. In the 60-minute period of observation by continuous ECG, primary VF was observed in 8 treated and in 17 control patients. However, from 15 minutes after randomization onward, when plasma lidocaine levels were in the therapeutic range, only 2 cases of VF occurred in the treated group, compared with 12 in the control group. VT terminated a mean of 10 minutes after injection in 6 of 9 lidocaine-treated patients with AMI but in none of 5 control patients with AMI. Mean plasma lidocaine levels were 3 μg/ml 11–20 minutes after injection in 369 consecutive patients. In 65 patients, levels were <2μg/ml and in 15 patients, levels were >6μg/ml. Side effects were rare and did not contribute to mortality. Koster and Dunning concluded that intramuscular lidocaine may be useful if given by a paramedic, another person, or the patient himself when AMI is suspected outside the hospital.

This article was followed by an editorial by Lown entitled, "Lidocaine to Prevent Ventricular Fibrillation, Easy Does It."[83]

Wong and Hurwitz[84] from Kansas City, Kansas, modified the lidocaine infusion rate on the basis of the 4-hour serum lidocaine level. In a group of 32 patients, after dosage adjustment, the mean lidocaine level did not increase and all levels remained within the 2–4 mg/L therapeutic range for 24 hours. Thus, a simple formula can be used to adjust prophylactic lidocaine infusion rates to attain levels that remain therapeutic, yet nontoxic.

Digitalis

The use of digitalis soon after AMI has come under intense scrutiny as evidence accrues to suggest its deleterious effects. Digitalis could aggravate myocardial ischemia, increasing myocardial oxygen demand because of its direct inotropic action or by increasing systemic vascular resistance. Intravenous digitalis can decrease oxygen supply by causing coronary vasoconstriction. In addition, digitalis can cause arrhythmic toxicity to which the ischemic myocardium may be particularly sensitive. Finally, digitalis produces a relatively small improvement in LV failure in AMI. To determine whether treatment with digitalis is associated with decreased survival after AMI, Bigger and associates[85] from New York City analyzed data from 502 patients who were enrolled in the post-AMI natural history study. At the time of discharge, 229 patients (46%) were taking digitalis. After 3 years of follow-up, the cumulative survival rate for patients discharged on digitalis was 66% compared with 87% of those not treated. Univariate analysis showed that statistically significant differences existed between the 2 groups with respect to age, previous AMI, LV failure in the coronary care unit, AF in the coronary care unit, peak creatine kinase levels, enlarged heart and pulmonary vascular

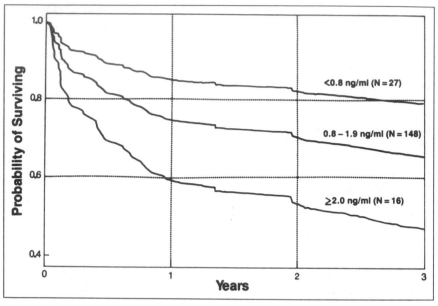

Fig. 2-23. Survival curves for patients treated with digitalis classified by serum digoxin concentration: <0.8, 0.8–1.9, and ≥2.0 ng/ml. The survival curves were fitted by Cox's method and were not adjusted for covariates. In the group with the lowest serum digoxin concentration, there were 27 patients at the start of follow-up and 3 were known to be alive at 3 years; the respective numbers of patients for the intermediate level were 148 and 22 and for the highest level were 16 and 2.

congestion on the discharge chest radiograph, ventricular arrhythmias, and treatment with diuretic, antiarrhythmic, and β-blocking drugs. Survival analysis using Cox's regression model showed that the association between digitalis and decreased survival was of borderline significance after adjustment for AF and LV failure. Serum digoxin concentration was measured in 83% of the patients who took digitalis. Survival was inversely and significantly related to serum digoxin—the higher the serum digoxin concentration, the lower the long-term survival rate (Fig. 2-23). After adjusting for AF and LV failure, serum digoxin was not significantly related to survival. Taken together with the results of 3 other large, nonrandomized studies of digitalis treatment after AMI, this study suggests that digitalis treatment may have adverse effects on survival during follow-up. Until this question is definitively answered by controlled, randomized clinical studies, clinicians should ask themselves, in each case, whether treatment is really needed for LV dysfunction after AMI and, if so, which treatment has the best risk to benefit ratio.

Byington and colleagues[86] from Houston, Texas, and Detroit, Michigan, evaluated the influence of digitalis therapy on survivors of AMI in the placebo-treated patients from the Beta-Blocker Heart Attack Trial (BHAT). Among the 1,921 placebo-treated patients, 250 (13%) were receiving digitalis at the time of randomization. The patients receiving digitalis differed in several clinical characteristics, including age, prior history of CHF, prior AMI, and angina pectoris. In addition, they also had a higher proportion of in-hospital complications, including pulmonary edema, persistent hypotension, AF, and CHF and a greater frequency of complex VPC. In digitalis-treated patients during a mean 25 month follow-up, the total mortality rate was 20% compared with 8% in patients not receiving digitalis. However, when the patients receiving and not receiving digitalis were compared by a multiple logistic regression analysis adjusting for 17 independent variables predictive of mortality, digitalis usage was not independently predictive of total mortality. Therefore these data indicate that patients receiving digitalis after AMI generally have more extensive cardiovascular disease and greater morbidity than those not receiving digitalis, but their subsequent higher mortality rate appears to be more likely related to the extent of cardiovascular disease than to the use of digitalis per se.

Anticoagulants

Nordrehaug and associates[87] from Bergen, Norway, randomized 53 patients with a suspected first anterior wall AMI to intervention with intravenous heparin followed by oral warfarin (26 patients) or matching placebo (27 patients). The regimen was started within 12 hours after the onset of AMI. Anticoagulation was maintained at a therapeutic level (for heparin, activated partial thromboplastin time 70–140 seconds; for warfarin, thrombotest 5–10%) for 10 days, and no bleeding episodes occurred. The baseline characteristics of the 2 study groups were well matched. In 7 patients in the placebo group and in none in the anticoagulant group, LV thrombus developed during the study, as detected by serial 2-D echo. Early intervention with high-dose anticoagulant drugs may prevent the development of LV thrombus in anterior wall AMI.

Dobutamine or nitroprusside

RV AMI may present with a spectrum of hemodynamic characteristics and when decreased cardiac index and systolic arterial BP are associated, volume loading has been advocated. To assess the value of volume loading and to determine the relative efficacy of dobutamine compared with nitroprusside therapy in RV AMI, Dell'Italia and coinvestigators[88] from San Antonio, Texas, evaluated 13 patients with clinical, hemodynamic, and RNA evidence of RV AMI. In 10 patients who had an initial PA wedge pressure of 18 mmHg, volume loading did not improve cardiac index, despite significant increases in mean RA pressure (11 to 15 mmHg) and PA pressure (10 to 15 mmHg). Nine patients received dobutamine or nitroprusside in random order while hemodynamic measurements and RNA were obtained simultaneously. Compared with nitroprusside, dobutamine produced a statistically significant increase in cardiac index (2.0–2.7 -vs- 2.1 -2.3 L/min/m^2), stroke index (29–36 -vs- 29–30 ml/m^2), and RVEF (30–42 -vs- 34–37%) by 2-way analysis of variance. The investigators concluded that volume loading does not improve cardiac index in patients with acute RV AMI despite an increase in cardiac filling pressures and that infusion of dobutamine, after appropriate volume loading, produces a significant improvement in cardiac index and RVEF over those after infusion of nitroprusside.

Beta blockers

Brown and associates[89] from Auckland, New Zealand, assessed LV function and exercise capacity in 79 patients randomized to receive intravenous and oral propranolol (n = 44) or conventional therapy (n = 35) within 4 hours of onset of their first AMI. Cineangiocardiography and exercise testing were performed 4 weeks after AMI to allow for maximum recovery of myocardial function. Left ventriculography showed no improvement in EF or preservation of regional contractile function in patients treated with propranolol compared with controls. A trend toward smaller end-diastolic volumes was seen in the propranolol group (mean, 151 ± 42 ml) compared with controls (167 ± 42 ml). Exercise duration and frequency of angina were not significantly different in the 2 groups. It is concluded that limitation of infarct size by propranolol does not lead to a significant improvement in ventricular systolic function, although LV dilation may be reduced. These findings are consistent with the known effect of early intravenous β-blockade that limits infarct size by preservation of subepicardial myocardium.

Low serum potassium concentrations have been associated with increased frequency of cardiac arrhythmias in AMI and an inverse relation has been shown between serum potassium concentrations of <5.2 mM/L and the occurrence of VF. Serum potassium concentrations correlate inversely with catecholamine concentration, which is increased in AMI and certain β-blocking drugs impair the potassium response to infused catecholamines. A small increase in serum potassium concentration has been reported in hypertensive patients treated with β-blockers. Nordrehaug and associates[90] from Danderyd, Sweden, and Sandvika, Norway, examined the effects of intravenous timolol on serum potassium concentration and determined the incidence of hypokalemia during the first 24 hours after hospital admission in patients with AMI: 106 patients with AMI hospitalized within 4 hours after the onset of symptoms were randomized to treatment with intravenous timolol (54 patients) or placebo (52 patients). Serum potassium concentrations were estimated at frequent intervals during the first 24 hours of admission. Patients in both treatment groups, who did not receive subsequent diuretic treatment, had a transient increase in serum potassium concentration, which was maximal after 4 hours (Fig. 2-24). This increase was abolished by diuretic treatment in the placebo group but not in the timolol group, in which there was a pronounced and prolonged increase in serum potassium concentration. The change in serum potassium concentration in the first 4 hours after admission correlated with cumulative creatine kinase release in the placebo group, but not in the timolol group. Hypokalemia (serum potassium concentration <3.5 mM/L) occurred in 15 (29%) patients in the placebo group and in 7 (13%) in the timolol group and was independent of infarct size. The frequency of hyperkalemia was not increased in the timolol group. By increasing the serum potassium concentration and preventing hypokalemia, the use of intravenous timolol early in AMI may have important clinical effects in addition to reducing infarct size.

Ronnevik and associates[91] from Stavanger, Norway, analyzed the effect of smoking habits before and after AMI and their relation to mortality and reinfarction rate after treatment of timolol in 1,884 patients included in the Norwegian multicenter group study. The follow-up period ranged from 12–33 months (mean, 17). No relation was found between initial smoking habits and risk category after AMI or between initial smoking habits and later outcome. At the time of their first infarct, smokers were 7 years younger than nonsmokers. One month after AMI nearly 60% of the smokers had stopped smoking completely. A significantly lower incidence of early cardiac death and lower total mortality was found in patients treated with timolol in both those who continued smoking and in the combined nonsmoking groups and a significantly lower reinfarction rate among nonsmokers (Fig. 2-25). Cessation of smoking alone was associated with a reduced reinfarction rate by 45% but a nonsignificant reduction in mortality by 26%. The investigators concluded that treatment with timolol and cessation of smoking have an additive effect in reducing mortality and reinfarction rate after AMI.

Salathia and associates[92] from Belfast, North Ireland, carried out a double-blind randomized study of 800 patients to determine if very early intervention with metoprolol (15 mg intravenously followed by oral adminis-

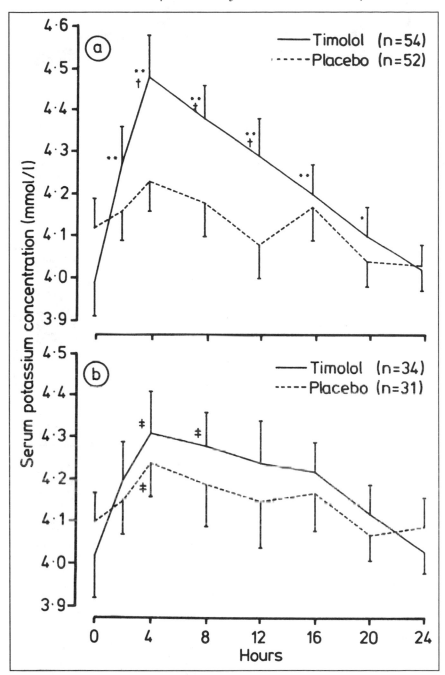

Fig. 2-24. Mean (SEM) serum potassium concentration during 0–24 hours of drug administration in all patients (a) and patients not treated with diuretics either on admission or during the first 24 hours (b). *p <0.05; **p <0.01 compared with baseline; †p <0.05 comparison of timolol and placebo; ‡p <0.05 each time interval compared with baseline. Reproduced with permission from Nordrehaug et al.[90]

tration) in suspected AMI affected overall mortality in selected subgroups (age, site of infarct, delay to intervention). Sudden death occurred less frequently in patients allocated to metoprolol, but there was no significant difference in total mortality on discharge, at 3 months, and at 12 months. VF

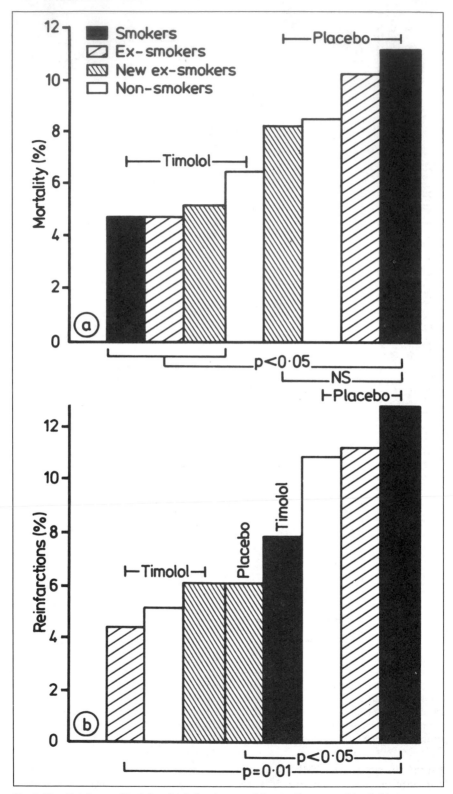

Fig. 2-25. Total mortality (a) and reinfarction rate (b) according to smoking habit in patients treated with timolol or placebo. Reproduced with permission from Ronnevik et al.[91]

after intervention was not significantly reduced. Adverse reactions did not occur significantly more frequently in patients assigned to metoprolol.

The MIAMI Trial Research Group chaired by Hjalmarson[93] from Goteborg, Sweden, compared the effect of metoprolol on mortality and morbidity after 15 days with that of placebo in a double-blind randomized international trial in patients with definite or suspected AMI. Treatment with intravenous metoprolol (15 mg) or placebo was started shortly after the patient's arrival at the hospital within 24 hours of the onset of symptoms, and then oral treatment (200 mg daily) was continued for the study period (15 days). Of the 5,778 patients, 2,901 were allocated to placebo and 2,877 to metoprolol. Definite AMI was confirmed in 4,127 patients. There were 142 deaths in the placebo group (4.9%) and 123 deaths in the metoprolol group (4.3%), a difference at 13% and 95% confidence limits of −8 and +33%, not statistically significant. Previously recorded risk indicators of mortality were analyzed in retrospect. These indicated that there was a category that showed higher risk, which contained approximately 30% of all randomized patients. In these, the mortality rate in the metoprolol-treated group was 29% less than in the placebo group. In the remaining lower risk categories there was no difference between the treatment groups. This subset analysis must be interpreted with caution in view of the findings from other similar studies. Positive effects were observed on the incidence of definite AMI and on serum enzyme activity in patients treated early (<7 hours). There was no significant effect on VF, but the number of episodes tended to be lower in the metoprolol-treated patients during the later phase (6–15 days; 24 -vs- 54 episodes). The incidence of SVT, the use of cardiac glycosides and other antiarrhythmics, and the need for pain-relieving treatment were significantly diminished by metoprolol among all randomized patients. Adverse events associated with metoprolol were infrequent, expected, and relatively mild.

In a prospective study carried out by Nordrehaug and colleagues[94] from Bergen, Norway, 20 patients with a first AMI and no current treatment with diuretics or cardioactive drugs were randomized to treatment with intravenous timolol (10 patients) or placebo (10 patients). Plasma epinephrine, norepinephrine, and serum potassium were estimated at baseline (3.6 ± 0.8 hours after the onset of AMI) and 4 hours after the start of treatment. The patient selection criteria embraced a low risk study population. Before treatment, the serum potassium concentrations correlated inversely with plasma epinephrine, but not with plasma norepinephrine concentrations. An increase of serum potassium from 4.1 ± 0.3–4.4 ± 0.4 mM/L in the placebo group and from 4.0 ± 0.4–4.5 ± 0.5 in the timolol group was in multivariate analysis associated in the placebo group with infarct size, estimated as cumulative creatine kinase release, and in the timolol group with the mean individual plasma epinephrine concentrations. By reversing the effect of epinephrine from a decrease to an increase in the serum potassium concentrations, timolol changed the relations between circulating epinephrine, potassium, and infarct size.

The original Norwegian Multicenter Study on Timolol after Myocardial Infarction was a double-blind, randomized study comparing the effect of timolol with that of placebo for up to 33 months after AMI. The initial results showed that the cumulated mortality was 39% lower among 943 patients randomly assigned to timolol treatment than among 939 patients randomly assigned to placebo. After the end of the double-blind period, most participating patients in the timolol group continued to receive β-adrenergic blockade, whereas most placebo-treated patients continued without such blockade. During an extended follow-up of participating patients up to 72 months after randomization, Pedersen,[95] representing the Norwegian Multicenter

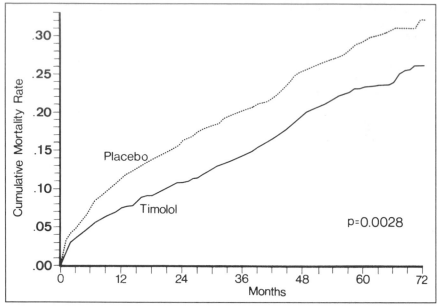

Fig. 2-26.   Life-Table cumulative rates from all causes among all patients randomly assigned to treatment with either placebo or timolol. Reproduced with permission from Pedersen et al.[95]

Study Group, found that the mortality curves of the 2 groups continued to increase in parallel (Fig. 2-26). Continued mortality rates were 32% in the placebo group and 26% in the timolol group. It was concluded that the previously observed early beneficial effect of β-adrenergic therapy is maintained for at least 6 years after AMI.

Bethge and coworkers[96] from Gotingen, West Germany, for the European Infarction Study Group, studied 736 patients after AMI to determine the efficacy of slow release oxprenolol or placebo on ventricular tachyarrhythmias. Twenty-four ECG recordings were obtained 14–36 days after AMI and before the start of this randomized study. Follow-up 24-hour ECG recordings were obtained 5–12 days (mean, 10) and at 3, 6, and 12 months after the administration of the study medication. In patients treated with oxprenolol, there were slower daytime heart rates compared with the placebo group, but no difference was found at night. During the 1-year follow-up, the prevalence of ventricular arrhythmias did not change significantly in either treatment group. There was a trend toward a reduction in the daytime frequency of ventricular couplets in patients treated with oxprenolol, but only multiform VPC were significantly less frequent in the patients treated with oxprenolol (47 and 43% -vs- 60 and 58%, respectively). Twelve months after the infarct, multiform VPC frequency was the same in both groups of patients. These data indicate that oxprenolol has a weak suppressant effect on ventricular tachyarrhythmias in survivors of AMI.

Calcium channel blockers

Crea and associates[97] from London, UK, performed in 17 patients admitted to the coronary care unit with transmural AMI a single-blind placebo-controlled trial the effects of verapamil on angina and reinfarction after initial AMI. The study was terminated because results obtained in the initial 17 patients indicated that verapamil is not effective in treating angina after

AMI, as it is in angina before AMI, and does not prevent reinfarction. Continuous ECG monitoring during the first 3 days after AMI showed the presence of transient episodes of ST-segment elevation in 4 patients taking verapamil and 4 patients taking placebo. The total number and duration of transient ischemic episodes were similar in the 2 groups (46 -vs- 41 and 23 ± 22 -vs- 17 ± 15 minutes, respectively). Transient ischemic episodes accompanied by chest pain was 10% in both groups. The ischemic episodes were never preceded by important increases of heart rate. Four patients taking verapamil and 4 taking placebo had reinfarction within the first 10 days after the incident AMI. These findings suggest that the prevailing mechanisms of myocardial ischemia in the immediate post-AMI period could be different from those operating in angina before AMI.

To assess the contribution of coronary vasospasm to chest pain in patients with nontransmural AMI, Eisenberg and associates[98] from St. Louis, Missouri, performed a controlled trial of prophylactic antivasospastic therapy. As soon as AMI was diagnosed, 50 patients with nontransmural AMI received either nifedipine or placebo in a double-blind randomized trial and were evaluated during subsequent hospitalization. Chest pain occurred in 52% of treated patients (38 episodes on 35 days) compared with 48% of control patients (42 episodes on 33 days). Concurrent therapy was comparable in the 2 groups. Recurrent AMI occurred in 12% and was comparable between groups. EF was similar and was unchanged throughout the study in both groups. Logistic regression failed to identify predictors for recurrent chest discomfort. These data indicate that potent antivasospastic therapy does not reduce the incidence of recurrent chest pain or AMI. Thus, remediable coronary vasospasm is not likely to be a major cause of early postinfarction ischemia in patients with nontransmural AMI.

Tiapamil is a new verapamil congener; but in a direct comparison with verapamil, tiapamil did not depress myocardial contractility in dogs over a wide range. Eichler and coinvestigators[99] from Cape Town, South Africa, studied the hemodynamic effects of this drug (1 mg/kg followed by 25 µg/kg/min over 36 hours) in 30 patients randomly assigned in a double-blind manner to a tiapamil or control group within 12 hours of the onset of AMI as diagnosed by Swan-Ganz catheterization and gated blood pool scans. Tiapamil reduced heart rate from 83 before to 74 beats/minute after the drug, arterial pressure from 128–118 mmHg, rate-BP product from 10,695 to 8,880 U, and systemic vascular resistance from 1,732–1,400 dynes · sec · cm^{-5}. Tiapamil also increased stroke volume index from 35–42 ml/m^2, LVEF from 50–56% (at 24 hours), LV end-diastolic volume index from 71–81 ml/m^2, and peak diastolic filling rate from 2.1–2.6 end-diastolic volumes/second. Cardiac index, PA wedge pressure, LV end-systolic volume, and PR interval remained unchanged. Without precipitating LV failure, tiapamil reduced afterload and heart rate and maintained cardiac index while apparently improving diastolic compliance. Thus, like β-blocking drugs tiapamil reduces heart rate and arterial BP, but in contrast to β-blockers it maintains cardiac output and improves diastolic compliance. Therefore, tiapamil might become a potential and a useful alternative to β-blockers for early intervention after AMI.

Intracoronary thrombolysis

Raizner and associates[100] from Houston, Texas, designed a prospective, randomized trial to assess the efficacy of intracoronary thrombolytic therapy with streptokinase (SK) in AMI. Sixty-four patients with AMI were randomized within 6 hours of onset of symptoms to 1 of 3 groups. Sixteen patients were treated by conventional means (control group). Nineteen patients underwent coronary arteriography and received corticosteroids and intracoronary (IC) and intravenous nitroglycerin (NTG group). Twenty-nine patients received management identical to that of the NTG group, with the addition of IC SK therapy (SK group). Recanalization was demonstrated in 21 patients (72%) in the SK group. Global and regional EF was determined by radionuclide ventriculography before any intervention and 7–10 days later. No significant improvement in global EF was achieved in the control and NTG groups. In SK patients as a group, global EF did not increase significantly; however, in patients recanalized with SK, EF improved from 42 ± 17–49 ± 16%. All groups had wide variability of response. Improvement in global EF of >5% occurred in 44% of patients recanalized with SK. When subgrouped on the basis of initial global EF of ≤45% or >45%, only patients recanalized with SK with an initial EF of ≤45% had an improved global EF (from 30 ± 10–42 ± 10%). Regional EF of all involved infarct regions was improved only in the SK group (from 34 ± 19–42 ± 23%) and SK-recanalized subgroup (from 33 ± 18–45 ± 24%). When only the most involved infarct regions were analyzed, control, NTG, and SK groups improved, with patients recanalized with SK having the greatest degree of improvement. Thus, this trial demonstrates a beneficial effect of thrombolytic therapy in global and, more strikingly, in regional function in patients in whom recanalization with SK is successful, with predominant benefit in those with initially depressed LV function.

Kennedy and associates[101] from Seattle, Washington, randomly assigned 134 patients who had had an AMI to treatment with IC SK, 4,000 U/minute, begun approximately 4.5 hours after the onset of symptoms, for a total of 286,000 ± 78,000 U over 72 ± 24 minutes, after cardiac catheterization and coronary angiography; 116 control patients received standard care after they returned to the coronary care unit immediately after angiography. Preliminary results of this trial had been published in the *New England Journal of Medicine* (1983; 309: 1477–81). During the first 30 days, 5 deaths occurred in the SK group and 13 occurred in the control group (3.7 -vs- 11.2%); during the first year, the corresponding figures were 11 and 17 deaths (8.2 -vs- 14.7%) (Fig. 2-27). However, when a minor imbalance in the EF and infarct location between the 2 groups was adjusted by logistic regression, the difference in 1-year mortality became significant. In the SK group, 2 of the 80 patients in whom perfusion was reestablished (2.5%) had died by 1 year, whereas 3 of the 13 with partial reperfusion (23.1%) and 6 of the 41 with no reperfusion (14.6%) had died. Mortality among patients with partial reperfusion was not significantly different from that among those without reperfusion. No baseline clinical, angiographic, or hemodynamic variable was predictive of successful reperfusion, according to univariate and multivariate analyses. The investigators concluded that IC SK reduced 1-year mortality among patients with AMI, but this improvement occurred only among those in whom thrombolysis resulted in coronary artery reperfusion.

The Society for Cardiac Angiography maintains a registry of IC SK therapy in patients with AMI. Between July 1981 and August 1984, 1,029 patients were entered into the registry. The baseline and clinical characteristics of patients were determined, the early results of therapy were evaluated, and baseline characteristics of those in whom reperfusion was achieved was compared with those in whom it was not. The present report was prepared by Kennedy and associates[102] from Seattle, Washington. Multivariate discriminant analysis was used to identify the predictors of reperfusion and hospital mortality. The overall rate of reperfusion was 71.2%. Reperfusion was positively associated with hypotension, absence of cardiogenic shock, and early treatment. The hospital mortality rate for all patients was 8.2%

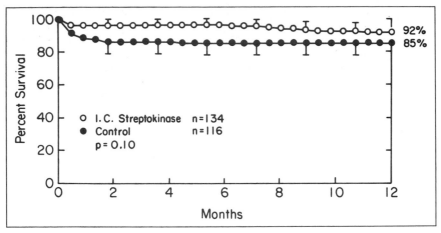

Fig. 2-27. One-year survival curves for the streptokinase and control groups. Reproduced with permission from Kennedy et al.[101]

and was higher for women and the elderly. The hospital mortality was significantly lower among patients in whom reperfusion was achieved compared with those in whom it was not (5.5 -vs- 14.7%) and for several high risk subgroups. Thus, coronary artery reperfusion induced by IC SK significantly reduced hospital mortality in high risk patients with AMI. High risk patients in whom reperfusion failed with IC SK therapy should be considered for early PTCA or CABG.

In a randomized trial of IC SK therapy in AMI, Decoster and associates[103] from Brussels, Belgium, performed sequential thallium-201 planar imaging before angiography and after 4 hours, 4 days, and 6 weeks in 44 patients (21 controls and 23 patients treated with SK). Patients were classified according to the presence or absence of angiographic reperfusion of the infarct-related artery. The semiquantitative score of myocardial thallium uptake was expressed as percent of maximal defect score. Both in control and in SK-treated groups, thallium defect scores decreased over time, but this decrease was smaller in the control group (before angiography, 33 ± 4%; redistribution, 29 ± 4%; 4 days, 25 ± 4%; 6 weeks, 22 ± 4%) than in the SK group (44 ± 4%, 38 ± 4%, 26 ± 4%, 21 ± 3%, respectively). In patients in whom reperfusion was achieved (20 SK-treated, 6 control subjects), a marked decrease in thallium score was observed (before angiography, 40 ± 4%; redistribution, 32 ± 4%; 4 days, 20 ± 5%; 6 weeks, 14 ± 22%) compared with patients in whom reperfusion was not achieved (37 ± 4%, 36 ± 5%, 33 ± 5%, 33 ± 4%, respectively). These results indicate that serial thallium imaging is an accurate method of assessing changes in myocardial perfusion after AMI. Restoration of thallium uptake was observed after reperfusion of the infarct-related artery whether this recanalization was seen spontaneously or after successful thrombolysis.

In an evaluation of the role of coronary collaterals in the early period of AMI, Saito and associates[104] from Hamamatsu City, Japan, treated 30 patients with acute total coronary occlusion with intracoronary thrombolysis 2–8 hours after the onset of symptoms. Thirteen patients with well-developed collaterals in the early period of AMI and successful thrombolysis showed improvement of global and regional EF from the acute phase to the chronic phase (global EF from 50–71%); regional EF from 25–49%. In patients with no less well-developed collaterals and successful thrombolysis, global and regional EF were similar to those in patients in whom thrombosis was unsuccessful. Among the 19 patients with successful thrombolysis, there was no significant correlation between the duration of ischemia and the improvement of regional EF. These data suggest that the extent of coronary collateral vessels in the early period of AMI is an important determinant of restoration of LV function after intracoronary thrombolysis.

The restoration of antegrade coronary flow long after coronary thrombosis may be of benefit to patients with continuing ischemia. To determine whether old intracoronary thrombi are susceptible to lysis with thrombolytic agents, Shapiro and associates[105] from Baltimore, Maryland, treated 18 patients with angina at rest during evolving AMI and total occlusion of the infarct artery with IC SK 3–13 days after onset of AMI. In 12 of the 18 patients, successful recanalization of the artery was achieved 6.9 ± 2.7 days after AMI. To evaluate the efficacy of this approach in reducing post-AMI ischemia, the number of episodes of angina at rest was compared in patients with successful and unsuccessful attempts at recanalization. The mean number of daily episodes of angina decreased from 1.02 ± 0.6–0.09 ± 0.2 in patients in whom reperfusion was achieved, and from 1.07 ± 0.8–0.88 ± 0.8 in those in whom it was not. Thus, in patients with early post-AMI angina, IC SK can restore flow in the occluded artery and may decrease the frequency of angina.

Verani and colleagues[106] from Houston, Texas, evaluated the effects of coronary artery recanalization by IC SK on RV function during AMI. Fifty-four patients who participated in a prospective, controlled, randomized trial of recanalization therapy during AMI were studied. Nineteen of 30 patients with inferior wall AMI had RV dysfunction on admission. Patients with successful recanalization (n = 6) had improved RVEF from admission to day 10 (26 ± 7–39 ± 14%). However, control patients (n = 6) and patients who did not have recanalization (n = 7) also had improvement in RVEF during the same time periods (20 ± 7–29 ± 11%, and 30 ± 8–40 ± 6%, respectively). Thus, in patients with RV dysfunction associated with inferior wall AMI, the RVEF tends to improve with time irrespective of early recanalization of the infarct-related vessel.

Stratton and coworkers[107] from Seattle, Washington, determined whether intracoronary SK improves late regional wall motion or reduces LV aneurysm or thrombus formation in patients with AMI using 2-D echo performed at 8 ± 3 weeks after AMI in 83 patients randomized to SK (n = 45) or standard therapy (n = 38) in the Western Washington Intracoronary Streptokinase Trial. The average time to treatment with SK was 4.7 ± 2.5 hours after the onset of chest pain and 67% of patients had successful reperfusion. Echo evaluations of regional wall motion were made in 9 LV segments using a qualitative grading scheme. LV thrombus formation was interpreted as positive, equivocal, or negative from the echo findings. All patients received anticoagulant therapy in the hospital and 52 received such therapy after hospital discharge. The data obtained in this study failed to demonstrate an improvement in global or regional wall motion scores in the SK-treated patients compared with those in the control group. The prevalence of LV aneurysm was 16% in both groups. LV thrombus was identified in only 5 patients and each was in the SK-treated group. These data suggest that the relatively late administration of IC SK does not improve global or regional wall motion or reduce the frequency of LV thrombus or LV aneurysm formation.

Sheehan and colleagues[108] from Seattle, Washington, and Hamburg, West Germany, quantitatively analyzed the coronary and ventricular angiograms of 47 patients with AMI in whom reperfusion was achieved by IC SK to determine the factors that affect recovery of regional LV function after reperfusion. Hypokinesis in the infarct region was measured by the center line method and expressed in terms of SD from normal. Severity of CAD was measured quantitatively. Hypokinesis showed more significant improvement after thrombolysis in patients with minimum stenosis diameter of >0.4 mm than in those with severe residual stenosis, that is, stenosis producing a minimum diameter of ≤0.4 mm. Improvement in hypokinesis was greater in patients who received thrombolytic therapy within 2 hours than in those treated later. These results indicate that angiographic reperfusion alone may not be sufficient: reperfusion must provide adequate flow and be achieved early to salvage myocardial function.

Von Essen and associates[109] from Aachen, West Germany, summated the ST-segment depression and elevation in ECG limb leads I, II, and III for each of 56 patients with AMI before and immediately after IC SK infusion and the results were compared with angiographic findings. Forty-three patients had angiographically confirmed reperfusion of an initially occluded vessel and had a significant decrease in summated ST shift. The ST-segment changes in the limb leads virtually returned to normal in all 43 patients, and, in most, inverted T waves developed. Thrombolysis was unsuccessful in 10 patients, and the infarct-related coronary artery was already patent in 3. When these 2 groups were combined, all 13 patients without reperfusion had no significant change in summated ST-segment shift. During PTCA inflation of the balloon in the artery that was previously occluded, simulated reocclusion was followed by new ST elevation if the artery supplied viable myocardium. In another consecutive study of 54 patients with anterior AMI, the precordial R waves and Q waves were studied over the 4–6 months after AMI using a standardized 48 electrode mapping system. All patients underwent a repeat angiogram after 4–6 months. In 36 patients with unsuccessful thrombolysis or reocclusion there was a further reduction in mean summated R-wave amplitude and an increased number of precordial leads not showing R waves. Precordial R-wave mapping seems to be a valuable noninvasive method of assessing the salvage of myocardium after reperfusion and the damage caused by reocclusion. Loss of R waves in the acute phase of AMI does not necessarily mean an irreversibly damaged myocardium.

Wei and associates[110] from Boston, Massachusetts, analyzed the time course of serum creatine kinase (CK), the CK-MB isozyme, lactate dehydrogenase (LDH), and SGOT activity and calculated rates of increase and decline for CK in 24 consecutive patients with AMI who received IC SK or urokinase. In 19 patients with successfully reperfused infarcts, peak CK activity occurred at 14 ± 1 hours after onset of symptoms, the maximal rate of CK increase was 595 ± 102 IU/L/hour, and the fractional disappearance rate (K_d) was $(86 \pm 6) \times 10^{-5}$/minute. The peak CK-MB activity occurred at 13 ± 1 hours and the MB K_d was $(223 \pm 39) \times 10^{-5}$/minute. In 5 patients in the nonreperfused group the peak CK (25 ± 5 hours) and CK-MB (23 ± 3 hours) activity occurred later, the maximal rate of CK increase (281 ± 37 IU/L/hour) was less, and the CK K_d [$(68 \pm 5) \times 10^{-5}$/min] and MB K_d [$(116 \pm 28) \times 10^{-5}$/min] were lower. The peak CK, CK-MB, cumulative CK release, and area under the curve were not different. Except for a shortened time to peak SGOT in the reperfused (17 ± 1 hours) compared with the nonreperfused (29 ± 6 hours) groups, the time course of LDH and SGOT were not different. Thus, the initial serum CK kinetics and time to peak SGOT may be useful in assessing the reperfusion status in patients with AMI receiving thrombolytic therapy without coronary angiography or in those who may have spontaneous recanalization.

Blanke and associates[111] from New York City and Goettingen, West Germany, described the effects on patients treated with IC SK during AMI and long-term follow-up. The mortality and the incidence of cardiac events were assessed during a follow-up period of 35 ± 5 months. CABG was done in 37% of the patients. Hospital mortality was 11% (n = 8); none of these deaths was due to LV rupture. The postdischarge mortality was 10%; 3 patients died suddenly. Serial assessment of LV function in 35 patients showed an increase of angiographic EF before intervention from 50 ± 4%–58 ± 12% 36 ± 53 days later. Gated blood pool imaging after 16 ± 7 months (n = 35) and 32 ± 9 months (n = 31) revealed no change in EF. Angina pectoris recurred in 4 of the 35 patients. Also studied was a historical comparison group that consisted of 66 patients who were treated at the same institution before the advent of IC intervention techniques; this group was followed for 48 ± 9 months. Baseline clinical and angiographic parameters were comparable in the 2 groups. CABG was performed in 18 of these patients. Mortality during hospitalization and postdischarge was not significantly different in the 2 groups. EF decreased significantly in the comparison group from the first to the second evaluation and remained unchanged during the follow-up period. It was concluded that no major adverse effects were associated with IC SK infusion over a long follow-up period. This may be related to the high frequency of CABG after reperfusion.

Melin and associates[112] from Brussels, Belgium, tested the hypothesis that IC SK increases coronary patency rates after AMI and thus may lead to a greater exercise-induced myocardial ischemia. They studied 39 patients enrolled in an angiographically randomized trial of IC SK (19 treated with SK and 20 control subjects); all patients underwent thallium-201 scintigraphy at rest before acute angiography and at rest and during stress 5 and 6 weeks after AMI. The patients were classified into 2 groups based on the presence or absence of complete obstruction of the infarct-related coronary artery at the end of the acute angiography. Semiquantitative score of myocardial thallium uptake was expressed as percent of maximal defect score. Thallium defect score at rest between admission and 5–6 weeks' study decreased from 10 ± 16% U in the control group and from 23 ± 14% U in the SK group. This decrease was related to opening of the infarct-related artery (opening 23 ± 16% -vs- occlusion 5 ± 10%). The change in exercise-induced defect score was significantly larger in patients in the SK group (11 ± 6% U) than in those in the control group (5 ± 7% U). The perfusion defect during exercise was larger in patients with incomplete obstruction or reperfusion (10 ± 6% U) than in patients with complete obstruction (3 ± 7%). This difference was independent of the number of narrowed coronary arteries. Radionuclide ventriculography during submaximal exercise was performed within 2–3 weeks after AMI in 21 of the 39 patients studied. The exercise-induced increase in EF was significantly smaller in patients with opened arteries (4 ± 7%) than in those with closed arteries (13 ± 9%). Thus, in this group of patients who were studied 5–6 weeks after AMI, patients treated with SK had scintigraphic improvement at rest compared with results at admission, but had more exercise-induced ischemia; this was related to incomplete coronary obstruction or reperfusion.

Kambara and associates[113] from Kyoto, Japan, evaluated the efficacy of IC urokinase in 514 patients with AMI (anterior, 296 patients; inferior, 195; lateral or posterior, 18; and anterior and inferior, 5). The time between onset of chest pain and coronary arteriography was 0.5–81 hours with an average of 5 hours. Initial administration of nitrates resulted in recanalization of the coronaries in 9.3%. Subsequently, urokinase was infused into the coronary arteries, and coronary thrombolysis was successfully achieved in 67%. The success rate was low in a group with average infusion speed of >30,000 U/ minute or with a total dose of urokinase of ≤480,000 U. Complications, mainly arrhythmias, were present in 111 patients (33%) of the 334 who had successful thrombolysis and in 18 patients (11%) of the 166 with unsuccessful thrombolysis, but serious hemorrhage was rare and no fatal case was reported. Patients who had successful thrombolysis had less in-hospital mortality than those who did not (6.3 -vs- 13.3%). Thus, coronary thrombolysis can be achieved effectively and relatively safely with a sufficient amount of IC urokinase administration in AMI.

To test the hypothesis that AMI size rather than location determines the LV response to reperfusion, Timmis and associates[114] from Royal Oak, Michigan, studied 69 patients receiving IC SK within 5 hours of chest pain onset, all of whom had sustained reperfusion at 8.4 ± 3.4 days. Twenty reperfusion failures served as controls. There were 31 patients with anterior AMI, 18 of which were estimated to be large, based on an EF at reperfusion of <50%; 14 of 38 patients with inferior AMI also had a large AMI. The EF increased at follow-up by 6 ± 3% in patients with large anterior AMI and by 8 ± 2% in those with large inferior AMI; in contrast, it increased by only 2 ± 3% in patients with small anterior AMI and significantly decreased by 6 ± 2% in patients with small inferior AMI. Six controls with a large AMI (4 anterior) had no change in EF; in 14 with small AMI (10 inferior), it decreased slightly. There were no significant group differences in the number of diseased arteries, residual stenosis, or collaterals. It was concluded that AMI size, not site, largely determines the ventricular functional response to early reperfusion; thus, patients with inferior AMI cannot be disqualified on this basis alone for thrombolytic therapy.

Verheught and associates[115] from Amsterdam, The Netherlands, determined the risk of bleeding associated with IC infusion of SK in AMI in a randomized controlled trial containing 302 patients <70 years of age. IC SK infusion was given to 152 patients and 150 patients were treated conventionally. Bleeding was seen in 24 (16%) patients in the SK group and in 2 of the conventionally treated patients. Bleeding was most common (28%) in patients >60 years of age. The groin was the site of bleeding in all patients except 1. In the first 48 hours after admission, the hematocrit in SK-treated patients with manifest bleeding decreased by 0.07 ± 0.04, by 0.05 ± 0.04 in the SK-treated patients without manifest bleeding, and by 0.03 ± 0.04 in the conventionally treated patients. Sixty-six units of packed cells were transfused in the SK group (50 U to those who bled); the control group required only 17 units. There were no deaths due to bleeding. The occurrence of bleeding and the decrease in hematocrit in the SK group correlated with the occurrence of systemic fibrinolysis but not with the dose of SK given. Thus, in about 15% of patients treatment with IC SK resulted in significant nonfatal bleeding from the femoral puncture site that required substantial transfusion support. Furthermore, there was a significant decrease in hematocrit in patients without manifest bleeding. These results emphasize the need for more specific fibrinolytic agents.

Intravenous thrombolysis

Schroder and associates[116] from Berlin, West Germany, determined short- and long-term changes in residual coronary stenosis of the AMI-related coronary arteries in patients with successful reperfusion by intravenous streptokinase (SK). In 15 patients the residual diameter stenosis decreased significantly from 62 ± 9% after 24 hours to 55 ± 13% in the fourth week. Quantitative angiographic analyses in 61 patients with patent infarct-related coronary arteries in the fourth week revealed a mean diameter stenosis of 61 ± 13%. The patients were followed up 34 ± 10 months. Sixteen had elective CABG or PTCA. Eighteen without CABG or PTCA had undergone repeat angiography after 26 ± 9 months. Twenty-five (41%) have had a residual diameter stenosis >65% in the fourth week. A stenosis >65% was found in: 4 of 5 patients with late reinfarction; 3 of 7 with 1-vessel CAD and persistent angina, in none of 11 with stenosis <65%; 6 of 7, whose silent reocclusion had been found at long-term follow-up and in 1 of 9 with a residual stenosis <65%. In 8 patients with persistent patency of the infarct artery, the stenosis had decreased significantly from 55 ± 6–36 ± 12%. Correspondingly, there was a significant improvement in the infarct-related LV wall motion disorders. These data indicate that in patients with less severe residual stenosis in the fourth week after successful intravenous SK the long-term course is relatively uneventful, whereas reocclusion or reinfarction in the same myocardial territory is frequent in patients with a stenosis >65%. PTCA may be advisable in these latter patients.

Wheelan and coworkers[117] from Dallas, Texas, studied 14 patients with transmural "Q-wave" AMI who were treated with intravenous SK 4 ± 1 hours after chest pain and underwent technetium-99m stannous pyrophosphate (^{99m}Tc-PPi) scintigraphy 7 ± 2 hours after the onset of chest pain. The hypothesis tested in these studies was that an abnormal ^{99m}Tc-PPi scintigram immediately after thrombolytic therapy would be indicative of successful reperfusion and lysis of a coronary thrombus. Eleven of 14 patients had early peaking (within 16 hours) serum creatine kinase (CK) isoenzyme levels at a mean of 11 ± 3 hours. Ten of 14 patients had 3+ or 4+ acute ^{99m}Tc-PPi images. Eight of 11 patients had patent infarct-related vessels at cardiac catheterization 15 days later. One patient who had both an early positive ^{99m}Tc-PPi image and CK-B peak level had an occluded infarct-related artery at catheterization. The LVEF obtained acutely with RNA was compared with the LVEF on day 15 and improved from 0.37 ± 0.13 to 0.50 ± 0.16 in the 10 patients with strongly positive acute ^{99m}Tc-PPi images. LVEF also improved from 0.37 ± 0.12–0.49 ± 0.15 in 11 patients with early peaking serum CK-B values. In 3 patients without evidence of reperfusion, the LVEF failed to improve from the initial value to that obtained at hospital discharge. Six control patients had acute ^{99m}Tc-PPi images 10 ± 2 hours after chest pain; none had strongly positive images and the mean time to CK-B peak was 19 ± 5 hours. Thus, these data suggest that strongly positive early ^{99m}Tc-PPi images may be reliable markers of successful reperfusion in patients receiving intravenous SK therapy after AMI.

Hillis and colleagues[118] from Dallas, Texas, and Bethesda, Maryland, determined the efficacy of intravenous SK in causing thrombolysis in 40 patients with AMI receiving 1,500,000 U of SK intravenously in 1 hour. In these patients, SK was given 270 ± 86 (mean $\pm$ SD) minutes after the onset of chest pain suggestive of AMI. Repeat coronary arteriography was performed to assess the efficacy of the SK. Among these 40 patients, 34 had total or near total coronary occlusion before SK administration. In 14 (41%) patients, some reperfusion occurred during the 90 minutes after the administration of SK, but in only 11 of 14 was reperfusion present at 90 minutes. All patients received heparin for 8–10 days after the administration of SK. Subsequently, they were given aspirin and dipyridamole. Clinical evidence of rethrombosis during the first 24 hours of heparin therapy occurred in only 1 patient. These data indicate that when SK is administered intravenously, an average of 4.5 hours after the onset of symptoms suggestive of AMI, reperfusion is achieved in only about 40% of patients acutely and sustained reperfusion occurs in only approximately 30% of such individuals.

Koren and associates[119] from Jerusalem, Israel, evaluated the effectiveness of early intravenous administration of 750,000 U of SK in 53 patients with acute myocardial ischemia treated by a mobile care unit at home (9 patients) or in the hospital (44 patients). Treatment was begun an average ($\pm$SD) of 1.7 $\pm$ 0.8 hours from the onset of pain. Non-Q-wave AMI developed subsequently in 8 patients, whereas all others had typical Q-wave infarct patterns. In 81% of the patients the infarct-related artery was patent at angiography performed 4–9 days after admission. Artery patency was independent of the time of treatment, but residual LV function was time dependent. Patients treated <1.5 hours after the onset of pain had a significantly higher EF (56 $\pm$ 15 -vs- 47 $\pm$ 14%) and infarct-related regional EF (51 $\pm$ 19 -vs- 9 $\pm$ 6) than patients receiving treatment between 1.5 and 4 hours after the onset of pain. Patients treated earlier by the mobile care unit also had better preserved LV function than patients treated in the hospital. It was concluded that thrombolytic therapy with SK is most effective if given within the first 1.5 hours after the onset of symptoms of AMI.

Lew and coworkers[120] from Los Angeles, California, studied the influence of the following variables on the time interval from initiation of an intravenous infusion of 750,000 U of SK until reperfusion (reperfusion time) in 140 consecutive patients with an evolving AMI: the rate of infusion of SK, the duration of chest pain before initiation of treatment, patient age, sex, location of AMI, history of previous AMI, and pretreatment pathologic Q waves. The time of reperfusion was recognized by clinical criteria that were completely concordant with the anatomic findings in all 119 patients in whom patency or occlusion of the artery of AMI was established at delayed angiography or at necropsy. The mean reperfusion time for the 129 patients for whom data were available was 49 $\pm$ 36 minutes. The reperfusion time was inversely related to the rate of infusion of SK, but this effect of infusion rate appeared to plateau at rates of <500 U/kg/min. In the 64 patients receiving infusions at rates of $\leq$500 U/kg/min, the mean reperfusion time was 60 $\pm$ 40 minutes, whereas in the 58 patients receiving the drug at rates >500 U/kg/minute it was 35 $\pm$ 22 minutes. The duration of chest pain before treatment was the only other studied variable found to influence the reperfusion time, but only at infusion rates of <250 U/kg/min. These investigators indicated that in patients with AMI who received high dose intravenous SK, the time interval to reperfusion can be minimized by increasing the infusion rate up to at least 500 U/kg/min and by shortening the delay from onset of symptoms to treatment.

Lew and coworkers[121] from Los Angeles, California, studied the hypotensive effect of a rapid intravenous infusion of high-dose SK in 98 patients with an AMI. The systolic BP decreased from 132–97 mmHg at an average of 15 minutes after the commencement of the SK infusion, accompanied by a decrease in diastolic BP from 80–61 mmHg. The decrease in BP was associated with an increase in heart rate from 73–78 beats/minute, preceded the appearance of clinical signs of reperfusion by 37 minutes and was similar in magnitude and timing in patients with anterior and inferior AMI. There were direct relations between the rate of infusion of SK and both the magnitude and the rate of decrease of systolic BP and both the magnitude and rate of decrease of diastolic BP. In most patients, the decrease in BP was transient, ranging from 2–30 minutes, and easily managed by slowing or stopping the infusion, placing the patient in the Trendelenburg position, or by administering an infusion of low dose norepinephrine or dopamine. In 4 patients with severe LV dysfunction, severe hypotension persisted for >60 minutes. These data indicate that in patients with either anterior or inferior AMI, a rapid infusion of high dose SK may frequently cause transient and sometimes severe hypotension, the magnitude of which is directly related to the rate of infusion of SK.

Mathey and associates[122] from Hamburg, West Germany, and Seattle,

Washington, administered an intravenous bolus of 2,000,000 U of urokinase (UK) in 50 patients with transmural AMI 1.8 ± 2.5 hours after the onset of symptoms. Coronary angiography performed 1.1 ± 0.6 hours after UK therapy revealed patent coronary arteries in 30 patients (60%), with no significant difference between those with anterior and those with inferior AMI. Reocclusion occurred in only 1 of 24 patients restudied. Failure to achieve reperfusion was not related to the degree of systemic fibrinolytic activity, which was equally high in patients who did and did not achieve reperfusion, as was evident from serially obtained fibrinogen measurements (77 ± 52 -vs- 84 ± 24 mg/dl, difference not significant). Plasmin activity, measured serially from 15 minutes to 24 hours after UK in 7 patients, was maximal at 15 minutes and undetectable after 3 hours. Wall motion at the infarct site measured from contrast ventriculograms was significantly better at follow-up only in patients in whom reperfusion was achieved and who received UK within 2 hours after the onset of symptoms compared with patients in whom reperfusion was not achieved (−1.2 ± 1.4 -vs- −2.4 ± 0.9 SD from normal). Peak serum CK level was significantly lower in patients in whom reperfusion was achieved than in those in whom it was not or those who had rethrombosis (802 ± 763 -vs- 1,973 ± 1,071 U/L). No complications related to UK therapy were observed. Thus, thrombolysis with an intravenous bolus injection of 2,000,000 U of UK is effective and safe and can be used to achieve reperfusion rapidly in the short term, when salvage of myocardium is more likely to occur.

Kremer and coworkers[123] from Hamburg, West Germany, administered UK for systemic thrombolysis in 16 patients with recent AMI (3–12 weeks old) and large LV thrombi. The LV thrombi were diagnosed by 2-D echo and in all patients the mural thrombi were located in the area of the recent AMI. Each of 3 patients had an embolic episode before the initiation of thrombolytic therapy and a stroke resulted in 1 individual. UK was infused intravenously at a rate of 60,000 U/hour for 2–8 days in combination with intravenous heparin. LV thrombi were successfully lysed in 10–16 patients, as determined by 2-D echo. In 4 of the 6 remaining patients only partial thrombolysis was achieved and in 2 thrombolytic treatment failed. There was no evidence of embolic events during thrombolysis in any of the 16 patients. The success of thrombolysis seemed to depend on the age of the thrombus: the thrombus was dissolved in 8 of 9 patients undergoing thrombolysis within 4 weeks of AMI -vs- 2 of 7 patients receiving treatment later. The presence of a LV aneurysm or depressed LV function also appeared to reduce the likelihood of successful thrombolysis. All patients were discharged on oral anticoagulants. At 6 months follow-up, no recurrence of LV thrombus was found. The results of this study show that LV thrombi can be safely lysed by intravenous UK, but the investigators cautioned that further investigation is necessary for definition of the risk and benefit of this new therapy.

Tiefenbrunn and coworkers[124] from St. Louis, Missouri, studied selected pharmacologic properties and effects on the fibrinolytic system of tissue-type plasminogen activator (t-PA) synthesized by recombinant DNA technology in 12 patients treated for coronary thrombosis. t-PA was infused parenterally for 30–60 minutes in the drug-induced coronary thrombolysis in 10 of the 12 patients treated (83%), including 6 of the 8 given t-PA intravenously. No bleeding complications were encountered. Peak plasma values were generally proportional to the dose of t-PA and approximately 90% of peak level was reached in 30 minutes, with a plateau at peak reached within 40 minutes. Changes in concentration of fibrinogen were transient and modest. Plasminogen and α_2-antiplasmin levels declined moderately to 51 and 32% of pretreatment values at the end of infusion of t-PA. Prothrombin time, prota-mine-corrected thrombin time, and assay of fibrinogen degradation products corroborated the lack of a lytic state. Thus, these investigators concluded that desirable levels of t-PA can be achieved consistently with short-term infu-sions of appropriately selected doses without induction of a systemic lytic state predisposing to bleeding.

The National Heart, Lung, and Blood Institute (NHLBI) established the Thrombolysis in Myocardial Infarction (TIMI) study group in 1983 to assess the efficacy of intravenous SK and other thrombolytic agents in the treatment of AMI. The study group includes 13 clinical sites, a data coordinating center, a drug distribution center, and core laboratories for radiographic, radionuclear, electrocardiographic, coagulation, and pathologic studies. TIMI includes a number of consecutive efforts, in open-label phase, and phases I and II. Phase I is designed to assess the relative thrombolytic activity and side effects of intravenous t-PA and intravenous SK in patients with AMI and angiographic documentation of an infarct-related total occlusion of a coronary artery. The primary endpoint is recanalization of the totally oc-cluded infarct-related coronary artery 90 minutes after the start of drug infu-sion. Phase II, a placebo-controlled trial, is being planned at present. On February 5, 1985, the NHLBI stopped Phase I on the recommendation of the TIMI Policy Advisory and Data Monitoring Board, because of substantial, statistically significant differences in recanalization rates between the pa-tients given t-PA and those given SK. The findings were summarized in an article developed by the TIMI study group.[125] Patients with ≥30 minutes of ischemic chest pain and ST-segment elevation (>0.1 mm) in ≥2 ECG leads were eligible for study. Eligible consenting patients were given intravenous heparin (5,000 U) after placement of an arterial sheath. Left ventriculogra-phy was performed followed by coronary arteriography with the infarct-related arteries studied last. Repeated opacification of the infarct-related ar-tery was obtained after administration of intracoronary nitroglycerin (200 µg). Patients with <50% reduction in the diameter of the infarct-related artery after intracoronary nitroglycerin were not given thrombolytic therapy. Repeat injections were performed 10, 20, 30, 45, 60, 75, and 90 minutes after the start of intravenous administration of the assigned thrombolytic agent. Intravenous heprin was begun at a dose of 1,000 U/hour and started 3 hours after the initial bolus dose. Each patient was randomly assigned to receive simultaneously either a 1-hour infusion of 1,500,000 U of SK and a 3-hour infusion of t-PA placebo or a 3-hour infusion of t-PA (40 mg, 20 mg, and 20 mg in the first, second, and third hours) and a 1-hour infusion of SK placebo. The primary endpoint, grade 2 or 3 patency at 90 minutes in pa-tients who had grade 0 initially, was therefore measured 30 minutes after infusion of 1,500,000 U of SK or after infusion of 50 mg of the total dose of 80 mg of t-PA. Data regarding the course during hospitalization are available for the initial 226 randomized patients, 112 treated with t-PA and 114 treated with SK. Thus, data presented in the article include recanalization rates for all treated patients with grade 0 or with grade 0 or 1 baseline occlusion; complications reported during hospitalization are referable to the first 226 treated patients regardless of arteriographic findings at baseline. From August 20, 1984, to February 5, 1985, 316 patients were randomly assigned to t-PA or to SK. Twenty-six patients were not treated; 8 had <50% diameter reduction, 9 became sufficiently unstable to require termination of the study before administration of the assigned thrombolytic agent, and 6 technical difficulties precluded completion of the protocol, and there were 3 protocol violations involving randomization of ineligible patients. Of the 290 treated patients, 76 did not have total coronary occlusion before drug infusion. Among these were 19 in the t-PA group and 7 in the SK group who had TIMI grade 1 perfusion at baseline and were excluded from primary endpoint consideration by the grade 0 requirement. The remaining 50 patients had baseline grade 2 or 3 perfusion, that is, complete opacification of the distal artery with either normal or sluggish flow. Thus, there were 214 patients who had an absolute (grade 0) total occlusion of the infarct-related artery at baseline; 99 were assigned to t-PA and 115 to SK. Baseline clinical and arteriographic findings were similar in the 2 treatment groups. The mean time from the onset of pain to the start of drug infusion was 287 minutes in the t-PA group and 286 minutes in the SK group. Of the patients with total occlusion at baseline, 59 (60%) of those assigned to t-PA had 90-minute reperfusion (grade 2 or 3) compared with only 40 (35%) of those assigned to SK. This was the preliminary phase I endpoint comparison. The median time from the start of drug infusion to the highest grade of reperfusion was 60 minutes in the successfully treated patients in both groups. If the 26 patients with grade 1 perfusion are added to those with grade 0, there were 240 treated patients with a less rigorously defined baseline coronary occlusion—118 given t-PA and 122 given SK. The diagnosis of AMI was confirmed by ECG evolution or CK enzyme elevation in all patients treated with t-PA and 97% of those treated with SK. At 90 minutes, 78 patients given t-PA and 44 given SK had recanalization. Comparison of local and central assessment of patency in the initial 181 patients revealed very close agreement; a discrepancy of >1 reperfusion grade occurred in 2% at time 0 and 1% at 90 minutes. Nineteen of the treated patients died during hospitalization: 7 of 143 (5%) assigned to t-PA and 12 of 147 (8%) assigned to SK. Of the 226 patients for whom complete hospital data are available, 112 were treated with t-PA, and 114 with SK. There were no clear-cut instances of fatal or central nervous system hemorrhages in either group. Extension of the AMI or reinfarction occurred in 12 (11%) of the patients given t-PA and 16 (14%) of those given SK. Hematoma at the catheterization site occurred in 43% of the t-PA group and 47% of the SK group. Gastrointestinal tract bleeding occurred in 6% and 10%, respectively.

An editorial by Relman, entitled "Intravenous Thrombolysis in Acute Myocardial Infarction," followed this report.[126] Relman concluded that the phase I TIMI trial clearly established that t-PA holds more promise as an intravenous thrombolytic agent in AMI than does SK and clearly deserves further study.

Verstraete and associates[127] from 7 European medical centers in a single-blind randomized trial in patients with AMI of <6 hours duration also found the patency to be higher after intravenous administration of t-PA than after intravenous SK. Sixty-four patients were allocated to t-PA, 0.75 mg/kg over 90 minutes and the infarct-related coronary artery was patent in 70% of 61 assessable coronary angiograms taken 75–90 minutes after the start of infusion; 65 patients were allocated to 1,500,000 IU SK over 60 minutes, and the infarct-related artery was patent in 55% of 62 assessable angiograms. The 95% confidence interval of the difference ranges from ±30--2%. Bleeding episodes and other complications were less common in the t-PA patients than in the SK group. Hospital mortality was identical in the 2 treatment groups. At the end of the t-PA infusion, the circulating fibrinogen level was 61 ± 35% of the starting value, as measured by a coagulation-rate assay, and 69 ± 25% as measured by sodium sulfite precipitation. After SK infusion, corresponding fibrinogen levels were 12 ± 18% and 20 ± 11%. In the t-PA group only 4.5% of the fibrinogen was measured as incoagulable fibrinogen degradation products compared with 30% in the SK group. Activation of the systemic fibrinolytic system was far less pronounced with t-PA than with SK.

When human recombinant t-PA became available for clinical investigation in Europe, 2 randomized multicenter trials were launched simultaneously. One involved 7 centers[127] and Verstraete and coworkers[128] summarize the findings in a 6-center study, which was a double-blind randomized trial of 129 patients with their first AMI of <6 hours duration when they were allocated to treatment with t-PA given intravenously over 90 minutes or to placebo infusion. Coronary angiography at the end of this infusion showed that the infarct-related artery was patent in 61% of 62 accessible coronary angiograms in the t-PA-treated group compared with 21% in the control group. Treatment with t-PA was not accompanied by any major complications. In the t-PA group the circulating fibrinogen level at the end of the catheterization was $52 \pm 29\%$ of the starting value.

Topol and coworkers[129] from Baltimore, Maryland, evaluated functional recovery in 20 consecutive patients with AMI receiving t-PA using serial 2-D echo performed before and after t-PA administration and at 1 and 10 days after AMI. t-PA was administered intravenously to 17 patients or by intracoronary infusion (3 patients) after angiographic confirmation of total coronary occlusion. Reperfusion documented by angiography occurred in 13 of the 20 patients at a mean time from onset of chest pain of 5 ± 1 hours. There was no immediate or 24-hour improvement in segmental wall motion. At day 10 compared with pretreatment, 28 of 33 reperfused infarct zone segments -vs- 6 of 20 nonreperfused infarct segments had improved segmental wall motion. Among reperfused infarct zone segments in the distribution of coronary artery balloon dilation, 19 of 23 segments had improvement -vs- 7 of 17 that were reperfused without angioplasty and 6 of 20 nonreperfused without angioplasty. Infarct zone segments reperfused at the time of ongoing chest pain also demonstrated functional recovery compared with segments reperfused in the absence of chest pain (18 of 23 compared with 10 of 20, respectively). These data suggest there is improvement in segmental function of reperfused infarct segments 10 days after coronary thrombolysis with t-PA and that this recovery occurs predominantly in patients who also have PTCA, ongoing chest pain, or both at the time of coronary thrombolysis.

Certain risk factors for AMI have been linked with disturbances in fibrinolytic activity. Hamsten and associates[130] from Stokholm, Sweden, recently developed a new sensitive and specific method for determining tissue plasminogen activator (t-PA) activity and antigen and discovered a new rapid inhibitor of this enzyme that enabled them to study fibrinolytic function in detail in a representative population of postinfarction patients. Seventy-one patients (62 men and 9 women) who had survived an AMI before the age of 45 years were compared with 50 healthy subjects of similar age, 3 years after AMI. Low t-PA activity after venous occlusion, mostly explained by high plasma levels of the t-PA inhibitor and to some extent by impaired release of t-PA from the vessel wall, was a frequent finding in the patients. The level of t-PA inhibitor was positively and significantly correlated with levels of serum triglycerides. The data suggest that reduced fibrinolytic capacity due to increased plasma levels of a rapid inhibitor of t-PA may have pathogenetic importance in AMI, particularly in patients with hypertriglyceridemia.

Sherry[131] from Philadelphia, Pennsylvania, in an editorial, issued a word of caution on the various plasminogen activators more specific for fibrin than SK. Sherry suggested that t-PA is being considered to be an ideal thrombolytic agent a bit too prematurely. t-PA, at least theoretically, is more specific for effecting clot dissolution and without significant hazard compared with the plasminogen activators, SK and UK, which are effective in dissolving thrombi and emboli, but not specific for fibrin. SK and UK activated plasminogen in the circulation and also that bound to fibrin, whereas the latter action was responsible for clot dissolution, the former action increased the proteolytic activity of blood and resulted in the degradation of fibrinogen and blood-clotting Factors V and VIII. The latter lead to marked hemostatic abnormality and increase the risk of bleeding complications. Sherry pointed out that in the 2 trials thus far reported comparing recombinant t-PA to SK in patients with AMI success in lysing coronary thrombi after a short-term intravenous infusion was reported as favoring t-PA (the TIMI trial: t-PA, 66% -vs- SK, 36%; European Cooperative Study: t-PA, 70% -vs- SK, 55%). Sherry raised the questions, is t-PA really a more effective thrombolytic agent than SK and is t-PA really a safer agent than is SK? Sherry emphasized that although t-PA is more selective for fibrin than is SK or UK, nevertheless t-PA will produce a serious hemostatic defect when given in the amounts used in the 2 recent trials in AMI. Sherry concluded that many questions, including how much it will cost, must also be answered before an accurate appraisal can be made of t-PA as a thrombolytic agent.

Intracoronary -vs- intravenous thrombolysis

Valentine and associates[132] from Indianapolis, Indiana, studied 164 consecutive patients with AMI in a prospective trial of coronary thrombolysis with streptokinase (SK): the first 98 patients received intracoronary (IC) SK after coronary angiography and the next 66 received high dose rapid infusion of SK (900,000 IU) intravenously (IV) before angiography. First-pass radionuclide EF was performed early (within 24 hours of admission) and late (10–14 days after admission) to evaluate LF function. In the IV group, 42 of 66 (64%) of infarct-related arteries were patent at the initial angiogram and 6 (9%) opened with subsequent IC SK. In the IC group, 13 of 98 (13%) of infarct-related arteries were patent at the initial angiogram and 50 of 85 (59%) opened with the IC SK. The IV and IC groups did not differ in time from onset of chest pain to presentation, type of infarct, or underlying severity of CAD. In the IV group, SK was begun 67 minutes earlier than in the IC group. In 62 patients in whom reperfusion was successful, mean EF increased from 39 ± 11% early to 48 ± 13% late. In 30 in whom it was not, the mean EF increased from 36 ± 10–40 ± 12%. The increase in EF was significantly greater in patients in the reperfused group. In 18 patients who underwent reperfusion by IV SK, the mean EF increased 11 ± 12%, whereas in 44 patients who had reperfusion by IC SK, the mean EF increased 9 ± 10% (difference not significant). Complications of the lysis procedure were similar in both groups. Thus, IV and IV SK are of comparable efficacy and safety in establishing reperfusion of the infarct-related artery in patients with AMI.

Simoons and associates[133] from 3 medical centers in The Netherlands compared 2 strategies for treatment of AMI in a randomized trial of 533 patients admitted within 4 hours of the onset of symptoms of myocardial ischemia: 264 patients were allocated to conventional treatment and 269 patients to a strategy aimed at rapid recanalization of the occluded coronary artery. At first IC SK (≤250,000 U) was given immediately after PTCA. In the last 117 patients IC administration was preceded by IV SK (500,000 U). No angiography was done in 35 patients allocated to thrombolytic therapy.

Among the 234 patients who underwent angiography, the infarct-related coronary artery was patent on admission or recanalized in 198 (85%). The median time between onset of symptoms and angiographic confirmation of a patent infarct-related artery was 200 minutes. Mortality was lower in patients randomized to thrombolysis than in controls at 28 days (16 -vs- 31 patients) and at 8 months (23 -vs- 42); 1-year survival was higher after thrombolysis (91%) than conventional treatment (84%). The clinical course in the hospital was more favorable in patients allocated to thrombolysis, with a lower incidence of VF (38 -vs- 61), pericarditis (19 -vs- 46), and cardiogenic shock (13 -vs- 24), although they had a higher frequency of bleeding episodes (53 -vs- 7). Nonfatal reinfarction was more common after thrombolysis than after conventional therapy (36 -vs- 16 patients).

Yusuf and associates[134] from Oxford, UK, Bethesda, Maryland, and Boston, Massachusetts, reviewed findings in 24 randomized trials of IV fibrinolytic treatment during the past 25 years involving some 6,000 patients with AMI. Most tested IV SK, but a few tested IV urokinase (UK). In the past 2 or 3 years numerous small randomized trials of IC SK have been started, 9 of which, involving a total of about 1,000 patients, have been reported. Because all of these IV and IC trials were small (the largest including only 747 patients), their separate results appear contradictory and unreliable. An overview of the data from these trials indicates that IV treatment produces a highly significant (22% ± 5%) reduction in the odds of death, an even larger reduction in the odds of reinfarction, and an absolute frequency of serious adverse effects. The apparent size of the mortality reduction in the IV trials was similar whether anticoagulants were compulsory or optional, whether treatment was in a coronary care unit or an ordinary ward, and, surprisingly, whether treatment began early (<6 hours from onset of symptoms) or late (generally 12–24 hours). In addition, there was no evidence that UK was more effective than the less expensive SK, or that, despite their technical complexity, the new IC regimens were more effective than the IV regimens. Even the IV schedules that have been studied in randomized trials were, however, quite complex, and the IC schedules were far more so. Perhaps partly because of this, none of them is widely used. If so, then some much simpler, and hence more widely practicable, IV SK regimens should be developed and tested. For example, a simple 1-hour high dose intravenous SK infusion, without anticoagulation, will successfully convert virtually all of the available plasminogen into plasmin. But, it may be several years before the net effects on mortality of any more widely practicable IV SK regimens can be agreed on unless many of the hospitals that do not wish routinely to use IC regimens or the complex previous IV regimens will collaborate in multicenter randomized trials that can, if necessary, continue rapid intake until some tens of thousands of patients have been randomized, and some thousands of deaths have been observed among the control and treated patients.

PTCA with or without thrombolysis

Holmes and associates[135] from Rochester, Minnesota, analyzed the treatment strategy of 66 consecutive patients who underwent invasive therapy for AMI with specific attention focused on the role of PTCA. The following 4 treatment regimens were used: PTCA alone (11 patients), PTCA followed immediately by administration of streptokinase (SK) (15 patients), SK therapy alone (11 patients), and SK therapy followed by PTCA (29 patients). Reperfusion was achieved in 91%, 80%, 82%, and 72% of these subgroups, respectively. PTCA was particularly helpful in patients with severe residual stenoses after intracoronary administration of SK and in patients in whom SK therapy failed to reopen the occluded artery. PTCA further reduced the residual stenosis in 11 of 15 patients with successful thrombolysis, and it restored blood flow in 10 of 14 patients in whom thrombolysis had failed to do so. The incidence of reinfarction after therapy was similar in all 4 treatment groups. Patients in whom PTCA was used either alone or in combination with SK therapy had a significantly decreased incidence of subsequent revascularization (<30% compared with 82%).

Although thrombolytic therapy can result in lysis of a coronary artery thrombus, salvage of myocardium as measured by enzymatic, ECG, and wall motion evaluation has not been clearly documented. Many patients after successful reperfusion continue to have recurrent chest pain. The presence of recurrent chest pain suggests salvaged myocardium. Controlled reocclusion of the infarct vessel with the use of coronary angioplasty may support evidence for myocardial salvage. Statler and associates[136] from Washington, D.C., reviewed experiences in 50 patients who underwent PTCA. Of the 50 patients, 16 had ECG or clinical evidence of ischemia at the time of balloon inflation. Prospectively, all patients who underwent PTCA after they had received SK were evaluated, and 5 of 5 patients had chest pain and ST-segment elevation during balloon inflation. The development of ischemic changes during balloon catheter inflation suggests the presence of persistently viable, salvaged myocardium after successful thrombolysis.

Coronary artery bypass grafting

Singh and colleagues[137] from Providence, Rhode Island, studied 108 consecutive patients undergoing urgent CABG procedures for postinfarction angina within 30 days of AMI. There were 84 men and 24 women, and mean age was 60 ± 10 years. Patients were divided as follows: Group I (15 patients) had CABG within 48 hours of the AMI; group II (47 patients) had CABG between 3 and 7 days; and group III (46 patients) had CABG within 30 days of their AMI. Among these patients, 59 (55%) had Q-wave infarcts. LVEF was <40% in 21 patients and LV end-diastolic pressure was ≥20 mmHg in 42 patients. Single, 2-vessel, and 3-vessel significant stenoses and ≥70% LM coronary stenosis were found in 4, 20, 59, and 17%, respectively. There were 2 deaths (1.8%) within 30 days of CABG. The requirement for intra-aortic balloon pumping was higher in group I patients, but there were no differences in the need for inotropic agents or the frequency of arrhythmias or postoperative AMI among patients in the 3 groups. Four patients had late AMI and 8 died. Actuarial survival was 87% at 5 years and 73% of 108 patients were free of angina. Thus, these data indicate that CABG may be accomplished with an acceptable morbidity and mortality in patients having such a procedure within the first 30 days after AMI.

At home -vs- group rehabilitation

DeBusk and associates[138] from Stanford, Redwood City, and Santa Clara, California, compared medically directed at-home rehabilitation with group rehabilitation that began 3 weeks after clinically uncomplicated AMI in 127 men (mean age, 53 ± 7 years). Between 3 and 26 weeks after AMI, adherence to individually prescribed exercise was equally high (≥71%), the increase in functional capacity equally large (1.8 ± 1.0 METs) and nonfatal reinfarction and dropout rates equally low (both ≤3%) in the 66 men randomized to home training and the 61 randomized to group training. No training-related complications occurred in either group. The low rate of reinfarction and death (5% and 1%, respectively) in the study as a whole, which included 34 patients with no training and 37 control patients, reflected a stepwise process of clinical evaluation, exercise testing at 3 weeks, and frequent telephone surveillance of patients who underwent exercise training. Medically directed at-home rehabilitation has the potential to increase the availability and to decrease the cost of rehabilitating low risk survivors of AMI.

Exercise

To evaluate potential benefits that elderly cardiac patients might gain from early exercise programs, Williams and associates[139] from Omaha, Nebraska, studied early exercise programs in 361 such patients: Group 1 had 60 patients aged ≤44 years; group 2 had 114 patients aged 45–54 years; group 3 had 111 patients aged 55–64 years; and group 4 had 76 patients aged ≥65 years. All patients participated in a 12-week exercise program within 6 weeks of AMI or CABG. All patients performed symptom-limited exercise tests before and after completion of the exercise program. Between tests, elderly patients manifested significant differences in body weight (77–75 kg), percent body fat (22–21 kg), heart rate at rest (77–68 beats/min), maximal heart rate (126–138 beats/min), maximal METs (5–8), submaximal average double product (17,305–14,071), and submaximal average rating of perceived exertion (12–10). Magnitudes of change were similar among groups, although the elderly patient group had a significantly lower absolute physical work capacity at testing after training than the other 3 groups. In the 25 elderly patients who received β-blocking drugs, METs increased from 5.1–7.8. In the remaining 51 elderly patients not receiving β-blocking drugs, METs increased from 5–8. The magnitude of increase in patients who received β-blocking drugs was not significantly different from that in patients not receiving β blocking drugs. Results suggest that benefits of early exercise programs seen in young cardiac patients may also be expected in elderly cardiac patients.

Taylor and associates[140] from Stanford, California, compared the effects of wives' involvement in their husbands' performance of treadmill exercise testing 3 weeks after clinically uncomplicated AMI; 10 wives did not observe the test, 10 observed the test, and 10 observed and participated in the test. In a counseling session after the treadmill test, couples were fully informed about the patient's capacity to perform various physical activities. Wives' final ratings of confidence (perceived efficacy) in their husbands' physical and cardiac capability were significantly higher in those who also performed the test than in the other 2 groups. Only wives who walked on the treadmill increased their ratings of their husbands' physical and cardiac efficacy to a level equivalent to those of their husbands. Spouses' and patients' perceptions of patients' cardiac capability after treadmill testing and counseling at 3 weeks were significantly correlated with peak treadmill heart rate and workload at 11 and 26 weeks. Efficacy ratings at 3 weeks were slightly better than peak 3-week treadmill heart rate and workload as predictors of treadmill performance at 11 and 26 weeks. Participation in treadmill testing early after AMI is an effective means for reassuring spouses about the capacity of their partners to resume their customary physical activities with safety.

References

1. THOMPSON DR, BLANDFORD RL, SUTTON TW, MARCHANT PR: Time of onset of chest pain in acute myocardial infarction. Int J Cardiol 1985 (Feb); 7:139–146.

2. MULLER JE, STONE PH, TURI ZG, RUTHERFORD JD, CZEISLER CA, PARKER C, POOLE WK, PASSAMANI E, ROBERTS R, ROBERTSON T, SOBEL BE, WILLERSON JT, BRAUNWALD E, MILIS STUDY GROUP: Circadian variation in the frequency of onset of acute myocardial infarction. N Engl J Med 1985 (Nov 21); 313:1315–1322.

3. INGWALL JS, KRAMER MF, FIFER MA, LORELL BH, SHEMIN R, GROSSMAN W, ALLEN PD: The creatine kinase system in normal and diseased human myocardium. N Engl J Med 1985 (Oct 24); 313:1050–1054.

4. TURI ZG, RUTHERFORD JD, ROBERTS R, MULLER JE, JAFFE AS, RUDE RE, PARKER C, RAABE DS, STONE PH, HARTWELL TD, LEWIS SE, PARKEY RW, GOLD HK, ROBERTSON TL, SOBEL BE, WILLERSON JT, BRAUNWALD E, COOPERATING INVESTIGATORS FROM THE MILIS STUDY GROUP: Electrocardiographic, enzymatic and scintigraphic criteria of acute myocardial infarction as determined from study of 726 patients (a MILIS study). Am J Cardiol 1985 (June 1); 55:1463–1468.

5. ROSENBERG L, KAUFMAN DW, HELMRICH SP, MILLER DR, STOLLEY PD, SHAPIRO S: Myocardial infarction and cigarette smoking in women younger than 50 years of age. JAMA 1985 (May 24); 253:2965–2969.

6. ARONOW WS, STARLING L, ETIENNE F, D'ALBA P, EDWARDS M, LEE NH, PARUNGAO RF: Unrecognized Q-wave myocardial infarction in patients older than 64 years in a long-term health-care facility. Am J Cardiol 1985 (Sept 1); 56:483.

7. KANNEL WB, DANNENBERG AL, ABBOTT RD: Unrecognized myocardial infarction and hypertension: the Framingham Study. Am Heart J 1985 (Mar); 109:581–585.

8. CREAN PA, WATERS DD, BOSCH X, PELLETIER GB, ROY D, THEROUX P: Angiographic findings after myocardial infarction in patients with previous bypass surgery: explanations for smaller infarcts in this group compared with control patients. Circulation 1985 (Apr); 71:693–698.

9. JANSEN DE, CORBETT JR, WOLFE CL, LEWIS SE, GABLIANI G, FILIPCHUK N, REDISH G, PARKEY RW, BUJA LM, JAFFE AS, RUDE RE, SOBEL BE, WILLERSON JT: Quantification of myocardial infarction: a comparison of single photon-emission computed tomography with pyrophosphate to serial plasma MB-creatine kinase measurements. Circulation 1985 (Aug); 72:327–333.

10. RENNERT G, SALTZ-RENNERT H, WANDERMAN K, WEITZMAN S: Size of acute myocardial infarcts in patients with diabetes mellitus. Am J Cardiol 1985 (June 1); 55:1629–1630.

11. FREEDMAN SB, DUNN RF, BERNSTEIN L, MORRIS J, KELLY DT: Influence of coronary collateral blood flow on the development of exertional ischemia and Q wave infarction in patients with severe single-vessel disease. Circulation 1985 (Apr); 71:681–686.

12. SELZER A, ROKEACH S: Clinical, electrocardiographic, and ventriculographic consequences of isolated occlusion of the right coronary artery. Am J Med 1985 (May); 78:749–753.

13. NITZBERG WD, NATH HP, ROGERS WJ, HOOD WP, WHITLOW PL, REEVES R, BAXLEY WA: Collateral flow in patients with acute myocardial infarction. Am J Cardiol 1985 (Nov 1); 56:729–736.

14. CORTINA A, AMBROSE JA, PRIETO-GRANADA J, MORIS C, SIMARRO E, HOLT J, FUSTER V: Left ventricular function after myocardial infarction: clinical and angiographic correlations. J Am Coll Cardiol 1985 (Mar); 5:619–624.

15. SCHWARTZ H, LEIBOFF RL, KATZ RJ, WASSERMAN AG, BREN GB, VARGHESE PJ, ROSS AM: Arteriographic predictors of spontaneous improvement in left ventricular function after myocardial infarction. Circulation 1985 (Mar); 71:466–472.

16. STADIUS ML, MAYNARD C, FRITZ JK, DAVIS K, RITCHIE JL, SHEEHAN F, KENNEDY JW: Coronary anatomy and left ventricular function in the first 12 hours of acute myocardial infarction: the western Washington randomized intracoronary streptokinase trial. Circulation 1985 (Aug); 72:292–301.

17. CASE RB, HELLER SS, CASE NB, MOSS AJ, MULTI-CENTER POST-INFARCTION RESEARCH GROUP: Type A behavior and survival after acute myocardial infarction. N Engl J Med 1985 (Mar 21); 312:737–741.

18. FRIEDRICH T, LICHEY J, NIGAM S, PRIESNITZ M, WEGSCHEIDER K: Follow-up of prostaglandin

plasma levels after acute myocardial infarction. Am Heart J 1985 (Feb); 109:218–222.

19. MUELLER HS, RAO PS, GREENBERG MA, BUTTRICK PM, SUSSMAN II, LEVITE HA, GROSE RM, PEREZ-DAVILA V, STRAIN JE, SPAET TH: Systemic and transcardiac platelet activity in acute myocardial infarction in man: resistance to prostacyclin. Circulation 1985 (Dec); 72:1336–1345.

20. EISENBERG PR, SHERMAN LA, SCHECTMAN K, PEREZ J, SOBEL BE, JAFFE AS: Fibrinopeptide A: a marker of acute coronary thrombosis. Circulation 1985 (May); 71:912–918.

21. HOFFMAN JR, IGARASHI E: Influence of electrocardiographic findings on admission decisions in patients with acute chest pain. Am J Med 1985 (Dec); 79:699–707.

22. LEW AS, MADDAHI J, SHAH PK, WEISS AT, PETER T, BERMAN DS, GANZ W: Factors that determine the direction and magnitude of precordial ST-segment deviations during inferior wall acute myocardial infarction. Am J Cardiol 1985 (Apr 1); 55:883–888.

23. TZIVONI D, CHENZBRAUN A, KEREN A, BENHORIN J, GOTTLIEB S, LONN E, STERN S: Reciprocal electrocardiographic changes in acute myocardial infarction. Am J Cardiol 1985 (July 1); 56:23–26.

24. LEVINE HD: Subendocardial infarction in retrospect: pathologic, cardiographic, and ancillary features. Circulation 1985 (Oct); 72:790–800.

25. GASH AK, WARNER HF, ZADROZNY JH, CARABELLO BA, SPANN JF: Electrocardiographic ST-T wave patterns, extent of coronary artery disease, and left ventricular performance following non-Q-wave myocardial infarction. Cathet Cardiovasc Diagn 1985 11:223–233.

26. ARVAN S, VARAT MA: Two-dimensional echocardiography versus surface electrocardiography for the diagnosis of acute non-Q wave myocardial infarction. Am Heart J 1985 (July); 110:44–49.

27. CHANDRARATNA PAN, ULENE R, NIMALASURIYA A, REID CL, KAWANISHI D, RAHIMTOOLA SH: Differentiation between acute and healed myocardial infarction by signal averaging and color encoding two-dimensional echocardiography. Am J Cardiol 1985 (Sept 1); 56:381–384.

28. WAHL JM, HAKKI A-H, ISKANDRIAN AS, YACONE L: Scintigraphic characterization of Q wave and non-Q-wave acute myocardial infarction. Am Heart J 1985 (Apr); 109:769–775.

29. PLOTNICK GD, BECKER LC, FISHER ML: Value and limitations of exercise radionuclide angiography for detecting myocardial ischemia in healed myocardial infarction. Am J Cardiol 1985 (July 1); 56:1–7.

30. FREEMAN AP, GILES RW, WALSH WF, FISHER R, MURRAY IPC, WILCKEN DEL: Regional left ventricular wall motion assessment: comparison of two-dimensional echocardiography and radionuclide angiography with contrast angiography in healed myocardial infarction. Am J Cardiol 1985 (July 1); 56:8–12.

31. MCNAMARA MT, HIGGINS CB, SCHECHTMANN N, BOTVINICK E, LIPTON MJ, CHATTERJEE K, AMPARO EG: Detection and characterization of acute myocardial infarction in man with use of gated magnetic resonance. Circulation 1985 (Apr); 71:717–724.

32. VEENBRINK TWG, VAN DER WERF T, WESTERHOF PW, ROBLES DE, MEDINA EO, MEIJLER FL: Is there an indication for coronary angiography in patients under 60 years of age with no or minimal angina pectoris after a first myocardial infarction? Br Heart J 1985 (Jan); 53:30–35.

33. MATSUDA M, MATSUDA Y, OGAWA H, MORITANI K, KUSUKAWA R: Angina pectoris before and during acute myocardial infarction: Relation to degree of physical activity. Am J Cardiol 1985 (May 1); 55:1255–1258.

34. CONNOLLY DC, ELVEBACK LR: Coronary heart disease in residents of Rochester, Minnesota. VI. Hospital and posthospital course of patients with transmural and subendocardial myocardial infarction. Mayo Clin Proc 1985 (June); 60:375–381.

35. PELL S, FAYERWEATHER WE: Trends in the incidence of myocardial infarction and in associated mortality and morbidity in a large employed population, 1957–1983. N Engl J Med 1985 (Apr 18); 312:1005–1011.

36. STEMLER J: Coronary heart disease: Doing the "right things". N Engl J Med 1985 (Apr 18); 312:1053–1055.

37. TYLER B: Letter to the Editor. N Engl J Med 1985 (Oct 10); 313:957.

38. ULVENSTAM G, ABERG A, BERGSTRAND R, JOHANSSON S, PENNERT K, VEDIN A, WEDEL H, WILHELMSEN L, WILHELMSSON C: Recurrent myocardial infarction. 1. Natural history of fatal and nonfatal events. Eur Heart J 1985 (Apr); 6:294–302.

39. KOPELMAN HA, FORMAN MB, WILSON BH, KOLODGIE FD, SMITH RF, FRIESINGER GC, VIRMANI R: Right ventricular myocardial infarction in patients with chronic lung disease: possible role of right ventricular hypertrophy. J Am Coll Cardiol 1985 (June); 5:1302–1307.

40. Shah PK, Maddahi J, Berman DS, Pichler M, Swan HJC: Scintigraphically detected predominant right ventricular dysfunction in acute myocardial infarction: clinical and hemodynamic correlates and implications for therapy and prognosis. J Am Coll Cardiol 1985 (Dec); 6:1264–1272.

41. Haines DE, Beller GA, Watson DD, Nygaard TW, Craddock GB, Cooper AA, Gibson RS: A prospective clinical, scintigraphic, angiographic and functional evaluation of patients after inferior myocardial infarction with and without right ventricular dysfunction. J Am Coll Cardiol 1985 (Nov); 6:995–1003.

42. Sugiura T, Iwasaka T, Ogawa A, Shiroyama Y, Tsuji H, Onoyama H, Inada M: Atrial fibrillation in acute myocardial infarction. Am J Cardiol 1985 (July 1); 56:27–29.

43. Kaplan K, Davison R, Parker M, Przybylek J, Light A, Bresnahan D, Ribner H, Talano JV: Frequency of pericardial effusion as determined by M-mode echocardiography in acute myocardial infarction. Am J Cardiol 1985 (Feb 1); 55:335–337.

44. Sharma B, Carvalho A, Wyeth R, Franciosa JA: Left ventricular thrombi diagnosed by echocardiography in patients with acute myocardial infarction treated with intracoronary streptokinase followed by intravenous heparin. Am J Cardiol 1985 (Sept 1); 56:422–425.

45. Arvan S, Badillo P: Contractile properties of the left ventricle with aneurysm. Am J Cardiol 1985 (Feb 1); 55:338–341.

46. Keenan DJM, Monro JL, Ross JK, Manners JM, Conway N, Johnson AM: Left ventricular aneurysm: the Wessex experience. Br Heart J 1985 (Sept); 54:269–272.

47. Visser CA, Kan G, Meltzer RS, Moulijn AC, David GK, Dunning AJ, Van Corler M, De Koning H: Assessment of left ventricular aneurysm resectability by two-dimensional echocardiography. Am J Cardiol 1985 (Nov 15); 56:857–860.

48. Lapeyre AC III, Steele PM, Kazmier FJ, Chesebro JH, Vlietstra RE, Fuster V: Systemic embolism in chronic left ventricular aneurysm: incidence and the role of anticoagulation. J Am Coll Cardiol 1985 (Sept); 6:534–538.

49. Dellborg M, Held P, Swedberg K, Vedin A: Rupture of the myocardium: occurrence and risk factors. Br Heart J 1985 (July); 54:11–16.

50. Boden WE, Sadaniantz A: Ventricular septal rupture during ibuprofen therapy for pericarditis after acute myocardial infarction. Am J Cardiol 1985 (June 1); 55:1631–1632.

51. Come PC, Riley MF, Weintraub R, Morgan JP, Nakao S: Echocardiographic detection of complete and partial papillary muscle rupture during acute myocardial infarction. Am J Cardiol 1985 (Nov 1); 56:787–789.

52. Fioretti P, Sclavo M, Brower RW, Simoons ML, Hugenholtz PG: Prognosis of patients with different peak serum creatine kinase levels after first myocardial infarction. Eur Heart J 1985 (June); 6:473–478.

53. Grande P, Nielsen A, Wagner GS, Christiansen C: Quantitative influence of serum creatine kinase isoenzyme MB estimated infarct size and other prognostic variables on one year mortality after acute myocardial infarction. Br Heart J 1985 (Jan); 53:9–15.

54. White RD, Grande P, Califf L, Palmeri ST, Califf RM, Wagner GS: Diagnostic and prognostic significance of minimally elevated creatine kinase-MB in suspected acute myocardial infarction. Am J Cardiol 1985 (June 1); 55:1478–1484.

55. Shekelle RB, Gale M, Norusis M: Type A score (Jenkins Activity Survey) and risk of recurrent coronary heart disease in the Aspirin Myocardial Infarction Study. Am J Cardiol 1985 (Aug 1); 56:221–225.

56. Brush JE, Brand DA, Acampora D, Chalmer B, Wackers FJ: Use of the initial electrocardiogram to predict in-hospital complications of acute myocardial infarction. N Engl J Med 1985 (May 2); 312:1137–1141.

57. Hlatky MA, Califf RM, Lee KL, Pryor DB, Wagner GS, Rosati RA: Prognostic significance of precordial ST-segment depression during inferior acute myocardial infarction. Am J Cardiol 1985 (Feb 1); 55:325–329.

58. Spirito P, Bellotti P, Chairella F, Domenicucci S, Sementa A, Vecchio C: Prognostic significance and natural history of left ventricular thrombi in patients with acute anterior myocardial infarction: a two-dimensional echocardiographic study. Circulation 1985 (Oct); 72:774–780.

59. Takamoto T, Kim D, Urie PM, Guthaner DF, Gordon HJ, Keren A, Popp RL: Comparative recognition of left ventricular thrombi by echocardiography and cineangiography. Br Heart J 1985 (Jan); 53:36–42.

60. Maisel AS, Gilpin E, Hoit B, LeWinter M, Ahnve S, Henning H, Collins D, Ross Jr. J: Survival after hospital discharge in matched populations with inferior or anterior myocardial infarction. J Am Coll Cardiol 1985 (Oct); 6:731–736.

61. KELLY MJ, THOMPSON PL, QUINLAN MF: Prognostic significance of left ventricular ejection fraction after acute myocardial infarction: A bedside radionuclide study. Br Heart J 1985 (Jan); 53:16–24.

62. MAISEL AS, AHNVE S, GILPIN E, HENNING H, GOLDBERGER AL, COLLINS D, LEWINTER M, ROSS J: Prognosis after extension of myocardial infarct: the role of Q wave or non-Q wave infarction. Circulation 1985 (Feb); 71:211–217.

63. HANDLER CE: Submaximal predischarge exercise testing after myocardial infarction: prognostic value and limitations. Eur Heart J 1985 (June); 6:510–517.

64. KRONE RJ, GILLESPIE JA, WELD FM, MILLER JP, MOSS AJ: Low-level exercise testing after myocardial infarction: usefulness in enhancing clinical risk stratification. Circulation 1985 (Jan); 71:80–89.

65. MADSEN EB, GILPIN E, AHNVE S, HENNING H, ROSS J: Prediction of functional capacity and use of exercise testing for predicting risk after acute myocardial infarction. Am J Cardiol 1985 (Nov 1); 56:839–845.

66. TEO KK, HSU L, RAMANADEN I, ROSSALL RE, KAPPAGODA T: Cardiovascular responses to early exercise in inferior wall ST acute myocardial infarction. Am J Cardiol 1985 (May 1); 55:1277–1281.

67. FIORETTI P, BROWER RW, SIMOONS ML, BOS RJ, BAARDMAN T, BEELEN A, HUGENHOLTZ PG: Prediction of mortality during the first year after acute myocardial infarction from clinical variables and stress test at hospital discharge. Am J Cardiol 1985 (May 1); 55:1313–1318.

68. WATERS DD, BOSCH X, BOUCHARD A, MOISE A, ROY D, PELLETIER G, THÉROUX P: Comparison of clinical variables and variables derived from a limited predischarge exercise test as predictors of early and late mortality after myocardial infarction. J Am Coll Cardiol 1985 (Jan); 5:1–8.

69. BHATNAGAR SK, MOUSSA MAA, AL-YUSUF AR: The role of prehospital discharge two-dimensional echocardiography in determining the prognosis of survivors of first myocardial infarction. Am Heart J 1985 (March); 109:472–477.

70. MORRIS KG, PALMERI ST, CALIFF R, MCKINNIS RA, HIGGINBOTHAM MB, COLEMAN E, COBB FR: Value of radionuclide angiography for predicting specific cardiac events after acute myocardial infarction. Am J Cardiol 1985 (Feb 1); 55:318–324.

71. MAISEL AS, SCOTT N, GILPIN E, AHNVE S, LE WINTER M, HENNING H, COLLINS D, ROSS J JR: Complex ventricular arrhythmias in patients with Q wave versus non-Q wave myocardial infarction. Circulation 1985 (Nov); 72:963–970.

72. SCHWARTZ PJ, ZAZA A, GRAZI S, LOMBARDO M, LOTTO A, SBRESSA C, ZAPPA P: Effect of ventricular fibrillation complicating acute myocardial infarction on long-term prognosis: importance of the site of infarction. Am J Cardiol 1985 (Sept 1); 56:384–389.

73. LURIA MH, DEBANNE SM, OSMAN MI: Long-term follow-up after recovery from acute myocardial infarction: observations on survival, ventricular arrhythmias, and sudden death. Arch Intern Med 1985 (Sept); 145:1592–1595.

74. DIMARCO JP, LERMAN BB, KRON IL, SELLERS TD: Sustained ventricular tachyarrhythmias within 2 months of acute myocardial infarction: results of medical and surgical therapy in patients resuscitated from the initial episode. J Am Coll Cardiol 1985 (Oct); 6:759–768.

75. ROY D, MARCHAND E, THEROUX P, WATERS D, BOURASSA MG: Programmed ventricular stimulation in survivors of an acute myocardial infarction. Circulation 1985 (Sept); 72:487–494.

76. BHANDARI AK, ROSE JS, KOTLEWSKI A, RAHIMTOOLA SH, WU D: Frequency and significance of induced sustained ventricular tachycardia or fibrillation two weeks after acute myocardial infarction. Am J Cardiol 1985 (Nov 1); 56:737–742.

77. DENNISS AR, BAAIJENS H, CODY DV, RICHARDS DA, RUSSELL PA, YOUNG AA, ROSS DL, UTHER JB: Value of programmed stimulation and exercise testing in predicting one-year mortality after acute myocardial infarction. Am J Cardiol 1985 (Aug 1); 56:213–220.

78. SANTARELLI P, BELLOCCI F, LPERFIDO F, MAZZARI M, MONGIARDO R, MONTENERO AS, MANZOLI U, DENES P: Ventricular arrhythmia induced by programmed ventricular stimulation after acute myocardial infarction. Am J Cardiol 1985 (Feb 1); 55:391–394.

79. WASPE LE, SEINFELD D, FERRICK A, KIM SG, MATOS JA, FISHER JD: Prediction of sudden death and spontaneous ventricular tachycardia in survivors of complicated myocardial infarction: value of the response to programmed stimulation using a maximum of three ventricular extrastimuli. J Am Coll Cardiol 1985 (June); 5:1292–1301.

80. SEMENKOVICH CF, JAFFE AS: Adverse effects due to morphine sulfate: challenge to previous clinical doctrine. Am J Med 1985 (Sept); 79:325–337.

81. DUNN HM, MCCOMB JM, KINNEY CD, CAMPBELL NPS, SHANKS RG, MACKENZIE G, ADGEY AAJ: Prophylactic lidocaine in the early phase of suspected myocardial infarction. Am Heart J

1985 (Aug); 110:353–362.

82. KOSTER RW, DUNNING AJ: Intramuscular lidocaine for prevention of lethal arrhythmias in the prehospitalization phase of acute myocardial infarction. N Engl J Med 1985 (Oct 31); 313:1105–1110.

83. LOWN D: Lidocaine to prevent ventricular fibrillation, easy does it (letter). N Engl J Med 1985 (Oct 31); 313:1154–1155.

84. WONG BYS, HURWITZ A: Simple method for maintaining serum lidocaine levels in the therapeutic range. Arch Intern Med 1985 (Sept); 145:1588–1591.

85. BIGGER JT, FLEISS JL, ROLNITZKY LM, MERAB JP, FERRICK KJ: Effect of digitalis treatment on survival after acute myocardial infarction. Am J Cardiol 1985 (Mar 1); 55:623–630.

86. BYINGTON R, GOLDSTEIN S, BHAT RESEARCH GROUP: Association of digitalis therapy with mortality in survivors of acute myocardial infarction: observations in the beta-blocker heart attack trial. J Am Coll Cardiol 1985 (Nov); 6:976–982.

87. NORDREHAUG JE, JOHANNESSEN KA, VON DER LIPPE G: Usefulness of high-dose anticoagulants in preventing left ventricular thrombus in acute myocardial infarction. Am J Cardiol 1985 (June 1); 55:1491–1493.

88. DELL'ITALIA LJ, STARLING MR, BLUMHARDT R, LASHER JC, O'ROURKE RA: Comparative effects of volume loading, dobutamine, and nitroprusside in patients with predominant right ventricular infarction. Circulation 1985 (Dec); 72:1327–1335.

89. BROWN MA, NORRIS RM, BARNABY PF, GEARY GG, BRANDT PW: Effect of early treatment with propranolol on left ventricular function four weeks after myocardial infarction. Br Heart J 1985 (Oct); 54:351–356.

90. NORDREHAUG JE, JOHANNESSEN KA, VON DER LIPPE G, SEDERHOLM M, GROTTUM P, KJEKSHUS J: Effect of timolol on changes in serum potassium concentration during acute myocardial infarction. Br Heart J 1985 (Apr); 53:388–393.

91. RONNEVIK PK, GUNDERSEN T, ABRAHAMSEN AM: Effect of smoking habits and timolol treatment on mortality and reinfarction in patients surviving acute myocardial infarction. Br Heart J 1985 (Aug); 54:134–139.

92. SALATHIA KS, BARBER JM, McILMOYLE EL, NICHOLAS J, EVANS AE, ELWOOD JH, CRAN G, SHANKS RG, BOYLE DMCC: Very early intervention with metoprolol in suspected acute myocardial infarction. Eur Heart J 1985 (Mar); 6:190–198.

93. THE MIAMI TRIAL RESEARCH GROUP: Metoprolol in acute myocardial infarction (MIAMI). A randomized placebo-controlled international trial. Eur Heart J 1985 (Mar); 6:199–226.

94. NORDREHAUG JE, JOHANNESSEN K-A, VON DER LIPPE G, MYKING OL: Circulating catecholamine and potassium concentrations early in acute myocardial infarction: effect of intervention with timolol. Am Heart J 1985 (Nov); 110:944–948.

95. PEDERSEN TR: Six-year follow-up of the Norwegian Multicenter Study on timolol after acute myocardial infarction. N Engl J Med 1985 (Oct 24); 313:1055–1058.

96. BETHGE K-P, ANDRESEN D, BOISSEL J-P, VON LEITNER E-R, PEYRIEUX J-C, SCHRÖDER R, TIETZE U: Effect of oxprenolol on ventricular arrhythmias: the European infarction study experience. J Am Coll Cardiol 1985 (Nov); 6:963–972.

97. CREA F, DEANFIELD J, CREAN P, SHAROM M, DAVIES G, MASERI A: Effects of verapamil in preventing early postinfarction angina and reinfarction. Am J Cardiol 1985 (Apr 1); 55:900–904.

98. EISENBERG PR, LEE RG, BIELLO DR, GELTMAN EM, JAFFE AS: Chest pain after nontransmural infarction: the absence of remediable coronary vasospasm. Am Heart J 1985 (Sept); 110:515–521.

99. EICHLER HG, MABIN TA, COMMERFORD PJ, LLOYD EA, BECK W, OPIE LH: Tiapamil, a new calcium antagonist: hemodynamic effects in patients with acute myocardial infarction. Circulation 1985 (Apr); 71:779–786.

100. RAIZNER AE, TORTOLEDO FA, VERANI MS, VANREET RE, YOUNG JB, RICKMAN FD, CASHION WR, SAMUELS DA, PRATT CM, ATTAR M, RUBIN HS, LEWIS JM, KLEIN MS, ROBERTS R: Intracoronary thrombolytic therapy in acute myocardial infarction: a prospective, randomized, controlled trial. Am J Cardiol 1985 (Feb 1); 55:301–308.

101. KENNEDY JW, RITCHIE JL, DAVIS KB, STADIUS ML, MAYNARD C, FRITZ JK: The western Washington randomized trial of intracoronary streptokinase in acute myocardial infarction. N Engl J Med 1985 (Apr 25); 312:1073–1078.

102. KENNEDY JW, GENSINI GG, TIMMIS GC, MAYNARD C: Acute myocardial infarction treated with intracoronary streptokinase: A report of the society for cardiac angiography. Am J Cardiol 1985 (Apr 1); 55:871–877.

103. DECOSTER PM, MELIN JA, DETRY JMR, BRASSEUR LA, BECKERS C, COL J: Coronary artery reperfu-

sion in acute myocardial infarction: assessment by pre- and postintervention thallium-201 myocardial perfusion imaging. Am J Cardiol 1985 (Apr 1); 55:889–895.

104. SAITO Y, YASUNO M, ISHIDA M, SUZUKI K, MATOBA Y, EMURA M, TAKAHASHI M: Importance of coronary collaterals for restoration of left ventricular function after intracoronary thrombolysis. Am J Cardiol 1985 (May 1); 55:1259–1263.

105. SHAPIRO EP, BRINKER JA, GOTTLIEB SO, GUZMAN PA, BULKLEY BH: Intracoronary thrombolysis 3 to 13 days after acute myocardial infarction for postinfarction angina pectoris. Am J Cardiol 1985 (May 1); 55:1453–1458.

106. VERANI MS, TORTOLEDO FE, BATTY JW, RAIZNER AE: Effect of coronary artery recanalization on right ventricular function in patients with acute myocardial infarction. J Am Coll Cardiol 1985 (May); 5:1029–1035.

107. STRATTON JR, SPECK SM, CALDWELL JH, STADIUS ML, MAYNARD C, DAVIS KB, RITCHIE JL, KENNEDY JW: Late effects of intracoronary streptokinase on regional wall motion, ventricular aneurysm and left ventricular thrombus in myocardial infarction: results from the Western Washington randomized trial. J Am Coll Cardiol 1985 (May); 5:1023–1028.

108. SHEEHAN FH, MATHEY DG, SCHOFER J, DODGE HT, BOLSON EL: Factors that determine recovery of left ventricular function after thrombolysis in patients with acute myocardial infarction. Circulation 1985 (June); 71:1121–1128.

109. VON ESSEN R, SCHMIDT W, UEBIS R, EDELMANN B, EFFERT S, SILNY J, RAU G: Myocardial infarction and thrombolysis: Electrocardiographic short term and long term results using precordial mapping. Br Heart J 1985 (July); 54:6–10.

110. WEI JY, MARKIS JE, MALAGOLD M, GROSSMAN W: Time course of serum cardiac enzymes after intracoronary thrombolytic therapy: creatine kinase, creatine kinase MB isozyme, lactate dehydrogenase, and serum glutamic-oxaloacetic transaminase. Arch Intern Med 1985 (Sept); 145:1596–1600.

111. BLANKE H, SCHICHA H, COHEN M, KAISER H, KARSCH KR, NEUMANN P, RENTROP KP: Long-term follow-up after intracoronary streptokinase therapy for acute myocardial infarction. Am Heart J 1985 (Oct); 110:736–742.

112. MELIN JA, DECOSTER PM, RENKIN J, DETRY JMR, BECKERS C, COL J: Effect of intracoronary thrombolytic therapy on exercise-induced ischemia after acute myocardial infarction. Am J Cardiol 1985 (Nov 1); 56:705–711.

113. KAMBARA H, KAWAI C, KAMMATSUSE K, SATO H, NOBUYOSHI M, CHINO M, MIWA H, UCHIDA Y, KODAMA K, MITSUDO K, HAYASHI T, KAJIWARA N, SEKIGUCHI M, YASUE H: Coronary thrombolysis with urokinase infusion in acute myocardial infarction: multicenter study in Japan. Cathet Cardiovasc Diagn 1985, 11:349–360.

114. TIMMIS GC, WESTVEER DC, HAUSER AW, STEWART JR, GANGADHARAN V, RAMOS RG, GORDON S: The influence of infarction site and size on the ventricular response to coronary thrombolysis. Arch Intern Med 1985 (Dec); 145:2188–2193.

115. VERHEUGT FWA, VAN EENIGE MJ, RES JCJ, SIMOONS ML, SERRUYS PW, VERMEER F, VAN HOOGEN-HUYZE DCA, REMME PJ, DE ZWAAN C, BAER F: Bleeding complications of intracoronary fibrinolytic therapy in acute myocardial infarction: assessment of risk in a randomized trial. Br Heart J 1985 (Nov); 54:455–459.

116. SCHRODER R, VOHRINGER H, LINDERER T, BIAMINO G, BRUGGEMANN T, LEITNER E: Follow-up after coronary arterial reperfusion with intravenous streptokinase in relation to residual myocardial infarct artery narrowings. Am J Cardiol 1985 (Feb 1); 55:313–317.

117. WHEELAN K, WOLFE C, CORBETT J, RUDE RE, WINNIFORD M, PARKEY RW, BUJA LM, WILLERSON JT: Early positive technetium-99m stannous pyrophosphate images as a marker of reperfusion after thrombolytic therapy for acute myocardial infarction. Am J Cardiol 1985 (Aug 1); 56:252–256.

118. HILLIS LD, BORER J, BRAUNWALD E, CHESEBRO JH, COHEN LS, DALEN J, DODGE HT, FRANCIS CK, KNATTERUD G, LUDBROOK P, MARKIS JE, MUELLER H, DESVIGNE-NICKENS P, PASSAMANI ER, POWERS ER, RAO AK, ROBERTS R, ROBERTS WC, ROSS A, RYAN TJ, SOBEL BE, WILLIAMS DO, ZARET BL, Co-investigators: High dose intravenous streptokinase for acute myocardial infarction: preliminary results of a multicenter trial. J Am Coll Cardiol 1985 (Nov); 6:957–962.

119. KOREN G, WEISS AT, HASIN Y, APPELBAUM D, WELBER S, ROZENMAN Y, LOTAN C, MOSSERI M, SAPOZNIKOV D, LURIA MY, GOTSMAN MS: Prevention of myocardial damage in acute myocardial ischemia by early treatment with intravenous streptokinase. N Engl J Med 1985 (Nov 28); 313:1384–1389.

120. LEW AS, LARAMEE P, CERCEK B, RODRIGUEZ L, SHAH PK, GANZ W: The effect of the rate of intravenous infusion of streptokinase and the duration of symptoms on the time interval

to reperfusion in patients with acute myocardial infarction. Circulation 1985 (Nov); 72:1053–1058.

121. Lew AS, Laramee P, Cercek B, Shah PK, Ganz W: The hypotensive effect of intravenous streptokinase in patients with acute myocardial infarction. Circulation 1985 (Dec); 72:1321–1326.

122. Mathey DG, Schofer J, Sheehan FH, Becher H, Tilsner V, Didge HT: Intravenous urokinase in acute myocardial infarction. Am J Cardiol 1985 (Apr 1); 55:878–882.

123. Kremer P, Fiebig R, Tilsner V, Bleifeld W, Mathey DG: Lysis of left ventricular thrombi with urokinase. Circulation 1985 (July); 72:112–118.

124. Tiefenbrunn AJ, Robison AK, Kurnik PB, Ludbrook PA, Sobel BE: Clinical pharmacology in patients with evolving myocardial infarction of tissue-type plasminogen activator produced by recombinant DNA technology. Circulation 1985 (Jan); 71:110–116.

125. The TIMI Study Group: The Thrombolysis in Myocardial Infarction (TIMI) trial: Phase I findings. N Engl J Med 1985 (Apr 4); 312:932–936.

126. Relman AS: Intravenous thrombolysis in acute myocardial infarction: a progress report. N Engl J Med 1985 (Apr 4); 312:915–916.

127. Verstraete M, Bory M, Collen D, Erbel R, Lennane RJ, Mathey D, Michels HR, Schartl M, Uebis R, Bernard R, Brower RW, DeBono DP, Huhmann W, Lubsen J, Meyer J, Rutsch W, Schmidt W, Von Essen R: Randomised trial of intravenous recombinant tissue-type plasminogen activator versus intravenous streptokinase in acute myocardial infarction. Lancet 1985 (Apr 13); 1:842–847.

128. Verstraete M, Brower RW, Collen D, Dunning AJ, Lubsen J, Michel PL, Schofer J, Vanhaecke J, Van De Werf F, Bleifeld W, Charbonnier B, De Bono DP, Lennane RJ, Mathey DG, Raynaud P, Vahanian A, Van De Kley GA, Von Essen R: Double-blind randomized trial of intravenous tissue-type plasminogen activator versus placebo in acute myocardial infarction. Lancet 1985 (Nov 2); 2:965–969.

129. Topol EJ, Weiss JL, Brinker JA, Brin KP, Gottlieb SO, Becker LC, Bulkley BH, Chandra N, Flaherty JT, Gerstenblith G, Gottlieb SH, Guerci AD, Ouyang P, Llewellyn MP, Weisfeldt ML, Shapiro EP: Regional wall motion improvement after coronary thrombolysis with recombinant tissue plasminogen activator: importance of coronary angioplasty. J Am Coll Cardiol 1985 (Aug); 6:426–433.

130. Hamsten A, Wiman B, Defaie U, Blomback M: Increased plasma levels of a rapid inhibitor of tissue plasminogen activator in young survivors of myocardial infarction. N Engl J Med 1985 (Dec 19); 313:1557–1563.

131. Sherry S: Tissue plasminogen activator (t-PA): Will it fulfill its promise? (Editorial.) N Engl J Med 1985 (Oct 17); 313:1014–1017.

132. Valentine RP, Pitts DE, Brooks-Brunn JA, Williams JC, Van Hove E, Schmidt PE: Intravenous versus intracoronary streptokinase in acute myocardial infarction. Am J Cardiol 1985 (Feb 1); 55:309–312.

133. Simoons ML, Brand M, De Zwaan C, Verheugt FWA, Remme WJ, Serruys PW, Bar F, Res J, Krauss XH, Vermeer F, Lubsen J: Improved survival after early thrombolysis in acute myocardial infarction: a randomized trial by the Interuniversity Cardiology Institute in The Netherlands. Lancet 1985 (Sept 14); 2:578–581.

134. Yusuf S, Collins R, Peto R, Furberg C, Stampfer MJ, Goldhaber SZ, Hennekens CH: Intravenous and intracoronary fibrinolytic therapy in acute myocardial infarction: overview of results on mortality, reinfarction and side-effects from 33 randomized controlled trials. Eur Heart J 1985 (July); 6:556–585.

135. Holmes DR, Smith HC, Vlietstra RE, Nishimura RA, Reeder GS, Bove AA, Bresnahan JF, Chesebro JH, Piehler JM: Percutaneous transluminal coronary angioplasty, alone or in combination with streptokinase therapy for acute myocardial infarction. Mayo Clin Proc 1985 (July); 60:449–456.

136. Satler LF, Rackley CE, Green CE, Pallas RS, Pearle DL, Del Negro AA, Kent KM: Ischemia during angioplasty after streptokinase: a marker of myocardial salvage. Am J Cardiol 1985 (Nov 1); 56:749–752.

137. Singh AK, Rivera R, Cooper Jr. GN, Karlson KE: Early myocardial revascularization for postinfarction angina: results and long-term follow-up. J Am Coll Cardiol 1985 (Nov); 6:1121–1125.

138. DeBusk RF, Haskell WL, Miller NH, Berra K, Taylor CB, Berger WE, Lew H: Medically directed at-home rehabilitation soon after clinically uncomplicated acute myocardial infarction: a new model for patient care. Am J Cardiol 1985 (Feb 1); 55:251–257.

139. WILLIAMS MA, MARESH CM, ESTERBROOKS DJ, HARBRECHT JJ, SKETCH MH: Early exercise training in patients older than age 65 years compared with that in younger patients after acute myocardial infarction or coronary artery bypass grafting. Am J Cardiol 1985 (Feb 1); 55:263–266.

140. TAYLOR CB, BANDURA A, EWART CK, MILLER NH, DEBUSK RF: Exercise testing to enhance wives' confidence in their husbands' cardiac capability soon after clinically uncomplicated acute myocardial infarction. Am J Cardiol 1985 (Mar 1); 55:635–638.

3

Arrhythmias, Conduction Disturbances, and Cardiac Arrest

ARRHYTHMIAS IN HEALTHY INDIVIDUALS

Kennedy and associates[1] from St. Louis, Missouri, followed 73 asymptomatic healthy subjects who were discovered to have frequent and complex ventricular ectopic activity. Ventricular ectopic activity in these subjects was measured by 24-hour ambulatory ECG, which showed a mean frequency of 566 VPC per hour (range, 78–1,994), with multifocal VPC in 63%, ventricular couplets in 60%, and VT in 26% (Fig. 3-1). Asymptomatic healthy status was confirmed by extensive noninvasive cardiologic examination, although cardiac catheterization of a subsample of subjects disclosed serious CAD in 19%. Follow-up for 3.0–9.5 years (mean, 6.5) was accomplished in 70 subjects (96%) and documented 1 sudden death and 1 death from cancer. Calculation of a standardized mortality ratio for 448 person-years of follow-up indicated that 7.4 deaths were expected, whereas 2 occurred (standardized mortality ratio, 27). A comparison of survival of the study cohort with that of persons without CAD or with mild CAD, patients with moderate CAD, and men with unrecognized AMI showed a favorable prognosis for the study cohort over 10 years (Fig. 3-2). The investigators concluded that the long-term prognosis in asymptomatic healthy subjects with frequent and complex ventricular ectopic activity is similar to that of the healthy United States population and suggests no increased risk of death. This article was followed by an editorial by Ruskin.[2]

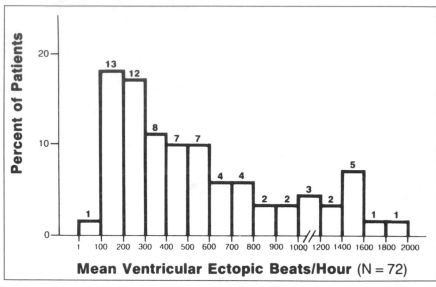

Fig. 3-1. Distribution of frequencies of mean VPC in 72 subjects. Reproduced with permission from Kennedy et al.[1]

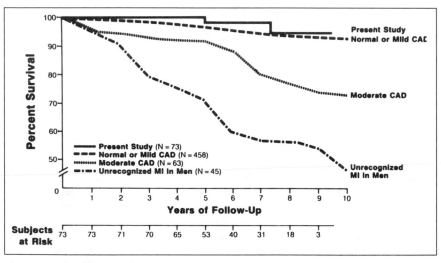

Fig. 3-2. Life-table survival experience of the study cohort compared with that of patients with normal coronary arteries or mild CAD, moderate CAD, and unrecognized AMI. The data in the present study were analyzed by the Kaplan-Meier method because of the small sample size, and the results are independent of the follow-up time. Reproduced with permission from Kennedy et al.[1]

ATRIAL FIBRILLATION/FLUTTER

In infants and children

Dunnigan and associates[3] from Minneapolis, Minnesota, studied clinical features and treatment of atrial flutter in 8 infants <2 months of age; 4 had associated structural or functional heart disease. In 6 infants flutter waves were not obvious on standard ECG, but transesophageal electrograms demonstrated the presence of flutter with second degree AV block. The atrial cycle length during flutter ranged from 135–180 ms (mean atrial rate, 403 beats/min) with a 2:1 ventricular response. Successful termination of flutter was accomplished using DC cardioversion in 1, transvenous atrial pacing in 1, and transesophageal pacing in 5. One infant converted to sinus rhythm 24 hours after digoxin administration and 1 infant had multiple recurrences and required chronic procainamide therapy. Seven had no recurrences in 6 months to 3.5 years of follow-up.

Campbell and associates[4] from Ann Arbor, Michigan, studied 23 pediatric patients with 27 episodes of sustained atrial flutter. Ten of 16 episodes were converted using intracardiac techniques and 8 of 11 were converted using transesophageal techniques. Hemodynamic, electrophysiologic, and radiographic characteristics were not predictive of conversion by either technique.

Garson and associates[5] from Houston, Texas, reported on a collaborative study of 380 patients, aged 1–25 years (mean age at onset, 10 years) with atrial flutter. Flutter continued to occur for a mean of 2.5 years after onset. Repaired congenital heart disease was present in 60%, palliated congenital heart disease in 13%, unoperated congenital heart disease in 8%, a normal heart in 8%, cardiomyopathy in 6%, and rheumatic heart disease in 4%. Drugs were effective in eliminating flutter in 58% of patients with digoxin alone, digoxin and amiodarone plus quinidine and amiodarone alone the most useful. Atrial flutter was easier to control or resolved in 52% of 66 patients who had corrective surgery. In a mean follow-up of 6.5 years, 83% of patients were alive and 49% no longer had flutter. Death occurred in 17%: 10% was sudden, 6% was nonsudden cardiac cause, and 1% was noncardiac cause. Cardiac death occurred in 20% of those for whom an effective drug could not be found compared with 5% of those who had effective drug therapy. These investigators show that the goal of medical therapy should be to eliminate flutter, since the incidence of death is four times higher in patients who continue to have episodes of flutter -vs- those who resolve. The chance of obliteration of atrial flutter by corrective surgery outweighs the risk of worsening flutter after surgery by a factor of 10.

Lone

Brand and associates[6] from Framingham and Boston, Massachusetts, and Bethesda, Maryland, found AF in 193 men and in 183 women among 5,209 participants in the Framingham Study followed for 30 years. Among this group, lone AF occurred in 32 men and in 11 women free of CAD, CHF, rheumatic valve disease, and hypertensive cardiovascular disease (Table 3-1). To determine the characteristics and prognosis of lone AF, each case was matched to a control in the remaining Framingham sample. Comparisons indicated that levels of several risk factors associated with CAD were similar between the 2 groups. AF cases, however, had significantly higher rates of preexisting nonspecific T- or ST-wave abnormalities and intraventricular block as determined by ECG. Follow-up for new cardiovascular events indicated similar rates of CAD and CHF, but the rate of strokes was significantly greater in the lone AF group. Findings suggest that subjects with lone AF, despite similar cardiovascular risk profiles to controls, have a distinct preponderance of preexisting ECG abnormalities. Furthermore, contrary to general belief, lone AF is not a benign condition; it has a serious prognosis.

TABLE 3-1. *Age distribution of lone AF among all AF cases. Reproduced with permission from Brand et al.[6]*

	MEN			WOMEN			BOTH SEXES		
AGE, YR*	AF CASES	LONE AF	%	AF CASES	LONE AF	%	AF CASES	LONE AF	%
<50	10	1	10.0	7	1	14.3	17	2	11.8
50–59	27	2	7.4	21	1	4.8	48	3	6.3
60–69	65	11	16.9	51	3	5.9	116	14	12.1
70–79	64	13	20.3	62	5	8.1	126	18	14.3
>79	27	5	18.5	42	1	2.4	69	6	8.7
Total	193	32	16.6	183	11	6.0	376	43	11.4

*Age at diagnosis.

Alcohol related

Heavy alcohol use has been suspected to cause acute AF, but an association between the 2 common problems has never been demonstrated. Rich and associates[7] from St. Paul, Minnesota, retrospectively reviewed 64 cases of idiopathic acute AF and 64 age- and sex-matched controls, randomly selected from among general medical admissions: 62% of cases and 33% of controls had documentation as heavy users of alcohol. Furthermore, patients with alcohol-related AF were significantly more likely to manifest alcohol withdrawal syndrome than were other inpatients with heavy alcohol use. Patients with alcohol-related acute AF were not different from other patients with acute AF with respect to clinical evidence of CHF, ECG abnormalities, cardiomegaly, electrolyte disturbance, or response to therapy. Heavy alcohol use is an important potential cause for acute AF; alcohol withdrawal may represent a particular risk for such alcohol-related AF.

Diltiazem treatment

Theisen and associates[8] from Munich, West Germany, studied the effect of oral diltiazem on the mean ventricular rate in 10 patients with stable AF. The profile of mean ventricular rate was analyzed by means of 24-hour ECG recordings. Both single-dose (120 mg) and maintenance therapy (80 mg 3 times daily) reduced the mean ventricular rate significantly. After the single dose, the effect set in after 120 ± 40 minutes (mean $\pm$ SD) and persisted for 347 ± 84 minutes. Histograms of RR intervals were plotted and their changes after diltiazem therapy also were analyzed. The shortest and longest AV conduction times were defined as 5 and 95% values of the cumulative frequency curve, respectively. There were 2 distinct types of the RR-interval histographic changes: In 50% of the patients, the longest and shortest RR intervals were prolonged proportionately; in the other 50%, the longest intervals increased disproportionately. Results indicate that oral diltiazem treatment can significantly decrease the mean ventricular rate in patients with AF by influencing the concealed conduction in the AV node. The changes of the RR-interval histograms suggest that in 50% both increased AF rate and prolonged refractory period in the AV node contributed to the increase of concealed conduction.

Amiodarone treatment

Horowitz and coworkers[9] from Philadelphia, Pennsylvania, assessed the effects of amiodarone in 38 patients with AF resistant to quinidine: 29 had organic heart disease and 9 did not. Eleven patients had persistent and 27 had paroxysmal AF. Amiodarone therapy resulted in no recurrent symptomatic AF in 15 (56%) of 27 patients with paroxysmal and 5 (45%) of 11 patients with persistent AF. Amiodarone failed to have an important effect in 5 (19%) of 27 patients with paroxysmal and 6 of 11 patients with persistent AF. Amiodarone had a modest effect in 7 (26%) of the 27 patients with paroxysmal AF. The efficacy of amiodarone appeared related to ECG measurements of LA dimension and LVEF in all patients, and the duration of the arrhythmia in patients with persistent AF. Thus, amiodarone provides an alternative therapeutic intervention for patients with quinidine-resistant AF.

SUPRAVENTRICULAR TACHYCARDIA WITH OR WITHOUT SHORT P-R INTERVAL SYNDROMES

Natural history

Deal and associates[10] from Houston, Texas, reviewed the records of 90 patients with WPW presenting with SVT in the first 4 months of life. Structural heart disease was present in 20%, most commonly Ebstein's anomaly. All patients presented with a regular narrow QRS tachycardia. Only 1 had atrial flutter and none had AF. Type A WPW was most common with heart disease occurring in only 5% of these patients, whereas heart disease was identified in 45% of those with type B WPW. Initially, sinus rhythm was achieved in 88% of 66 infants treated with digoxin, with no deaths. Sinus rhythm resumed after DC cardioversion in 87% of 15 infants so treated. The WPW pattern disappeared in 36% of patients. Four infants died of cardiac causes during the follow-up period of 6.5 years: 2 of the 4 had congenital heart disease and the third with a normal heart initially developed VF and died from cardiomyopathy considered related to resuscitation; the remaining infant with a normal heart died suddenly. All were receiving digoxin. A wide QRS tachycardia later appeared in 3 patients (all with heart disease and 1 of these patients died). After age 1 year, 33% of infants had recurrent SVT; recurrences were more frequent in patients with type B WPW and in those requiring >1 drug to maintain sinus rhythm during hospitalization. These investigators document quite well the well-known effectiveness of digoxin therapy on achieving sinus rhythm initially in infants with SVT. In addition they document the disappearance of the WPW pattern in a little more than one third of patients. Of particular interest is the fact that 4 infants died during the follow-up under conditions that were suggestive of an acute rhythm abnormality. There continues to be controversy as to whether infants and young children are susceptible to the well-known but rare problem of AF in association with rapid antegrade conduction over the accessory pathway leading to VF in adults with WPW who are on digitalis therapy. For this reason, many clinicians hesitate to use digitalis in the adult with WPW unless it is proved that they do not have a short antegrade accessory pathway refractory period either before or after digitalis therapy.

Caused by theophylline

Multifocal atrial tachycardia is defined as an atrial rate >100 beats/minute with >50% of the atrial complexes being ectopic and at least 3 different P-wave morphologies with varying PR and PP intervals. Multifocal atrial tachycardia commonly develops in elderly persons during periods of acute exacerbation of underlying pulmonary disease. Since improvement in the respiratory disease is generally associated with a resolution of multifocal atrial tachycardia, aggressive respiratory therapy, including the use of intravenous theophylline, remains the standard treatment for multifocal atrial tachycardia. Levine and associates[11] from Baltimore, Maryland, identified 16 patients with multifocal atrial tachycardia who were taking theophylline during a 6-month period. After theophylline was discontinued, the atrial rate decreased and multifocal atrial tachycardia resolved in all 16 patients. Five patients were challenged with intravenous aminophylline to investigate the role of theophylline in the genesis of multifocal atrial tachycardia. Multifocal atrial tachycardia with a rapid ventricular response occurred in all 5, even though metabolic and respiratory variables did not change. Multifocal atrial tachycardia returned on challenge in 3 patients in whom serum theophylline levels were within the generally accepted therapeutic range (10–20 mg/L). In individual patients, theophylline had a dose-related effect on the atrial rate and the amount of ectopic atrial activity. Thus, theophylline may commonly precipitate multifocal atrial tachycardia and treatment with the drug should be carefully considered in patients with respiratory insufficiency and multifocal atrial tachycardia.

Arrhythmias produced by antitachycardia pacing

Pacing is being used frequently for the treatment of drug resistant paroxysmal SVT. SVT can usually be terminated by pacing, but arrhythmias may be induced that interfere with the safety of antitachycardia pacing. To quantify these pacing-induced arrhythmias, Waldecker and associates[12] from Maastricht, The Netherlands, analyzed 453 attempts to terminate SVT in 111 patients. The patients were 6–73 years old (mean, 41); 62 were male. Seventy-six patients had SVT using an accessory AV bypass, and 35 patients had intranodal SVT. Single and then, if required, multiple ventricular and atrial premature beats and overdrive pacing were delivered from the atrium and ventricle. A pacing-induced arrhythmia occurred in 9% of all attempts (34% of patients). Atrial flutter or AF was the most frequent arrhythmia (in 8% of all attempts and sustained in 75%). Atrial -vs- ventricular pacing resulted in a 12 -vs- 2% incidence of AF. AF was unrelated to age, sex, atrial size, and SVT type, and was predominantly induced by multiple VPC. In 6 patients a different SVT and in 2 patients a nonsustained VT was induced. In 6 patients SVT could only be terminated by initiating another arrhythmia. Thus, AF is frequently induced during attempted pacing termination of SVT. In 6% of patients, SVT can only be terminated by inducing another arrhythmia. Therefore careful investigation of the properties of the clinical SVT by programmed electrical stimulation of the heart is mandatory before considering pacing as therapy for these patients.

Transesophageal atrial pacing

Benson and associates[13] from Minneapolis, Minnesota, used transesophageal atrial pacing to initiate and terminate SVT in 24 infants aged 1–34 days. Six infants received no chronic treatment and chronic oral digoxin prophylaxis was administered to 18. In these 18 infants the initiation of SVT by transesophageal pacing was compared with its ability to prevent spontaneous recurrences of SVT. Tachycardia could be reinitiated in 15 (83%) of the infants while on digoxin therapy, at which time the serum digoxin concentration was 1.9 ng/ml. In these infants the cycle length of the SVT and the AV interval were the same before and during digoxin treatment. Three infants in whom SVT could not be initiated during digoxin therapy had no spontaneous recurrence during 6 months of follow-up, whereas 10 of 15 (67%) infants in whom SVT could be reinitiated had clinically significant recurrence. Thus, digoxin was effective in preventing significant spontaneous recurrences of SVT in only 8 of 18 (44%) of infants treated.

This interesting study indicates that the ability to initiate SVT with transesophageal pacing may be useful in determining which digoxin-treated infants are at risk for recurrence. There was a marked variability in terms of both number of episodes and severity of recurrences in infants who initially present with SVT. They provided important documentation that chronic therapy is not necessary in a number of infants with SVT and that digoxin may not be the drug of choice.

Adenosine

DiMarco and colleagues[14] from Charlottesville, Virginia, and Danville, Pennsylvania, evaluated the influence of adenosine to alter sinus node automaticity and AV nodal conduction. Increasing doses of intravenous adenosine were given to 46 patients with SVT. Adenosine predictably terminated episodes of SVT in all 16 patients with AV reciprocating tachycardia, in 13 of 13 patients with AV nodal reentrant tachycardia, and 1 of 2 patients with junctional tachycardia with long RP intervals. Adenosine resulted in transient high grade AV block without any effect on atrial activity in 6 patients with intra-atrial reentrant tachycardia, 4 patients with atrial flutter, 3 patients with AF, and in 1 patient with either sinus node reentry or automatic atrial tachycardia. The dose of adenosine required to abolish episodes of SVT ranged from 2–23 mg and side effects were minor and of short duration. These data indicate that adenosine may be useful in the acute therapy of SVT whenever reentry through the AV node is involved.

Amiodarone

Brugada and Wellens[15] from Maastricht, The Netherlands, studied the refractory periods during cardiac pacing in 13 patients with the WPW syndrome. The RA and RV refractory periods and refractory period of the accessory pathway (antegradely and retrogradely) was studied at 2 pacing cycle lengths before and after therapy with oral amiodarone (8,400–11,200 mg given in 4–6 weeks). The RA and RV effective refractory period shortened significantly when the pacing rate was increased during the control study, and also after oral amiodarone administration. The antegrade and retrograde effective refractory period of the accessory pathway also shortened significantly at control study, but not during treatment with oral amiodarone. This indicated that amiodarone blunted the rate-dependent shortening in the refractory period of the accessory pathway. The rate-dependent increase in refractoriness of the accessory pathway could not be predicted or determined in all patients. In 5 patients a rate-dependent increase in the effective refractory period of the accessory pathway was observed in the antegrade direction and in 3 patients in the retrograde direction while they were receiving oral amiodarone therapy. When these data were correlated with the mode of induction and termination of tachycardia, however, a possible effect was found in only 1 patient. Further investigation of new antiarrhythmic drugs should include the development of components resulting in a reliable and predictable increase in refractoriness when the heart rate increases. This would result in prompt termination of reentrant tachycardia by creating block for the circulating impulse.

Propafenone

Manz and associates[16] from Munich, West Germany, evaluated the electrophysiologic effects of intravenous and oral propafenone in 14 patients with the WPW syndrome and in 10 patients with AV nodal reentrant tachycardia. The effective refractory periods of the right atrium and the AV node increased after both preparations. In patients with WPW syndrome, intravenous propafenone blocked antegrade accessory pathway conduction in 2 patients and retrograde conduction in 1; during oral therapy, accessory pathway conduction block occurred in 2 additional patients. The mean cycle length of the SVT increased from 338 ± 60–387 ± 56 ms after intravenous application, and from 336 ± 65–367 ± 65 ms during oral propafenone. The shortest pacing interval maintaining a 1:1 AV conduction increased from 325 ± 65–368 ± 81 ms after intravenous infusion, and from 333 ± 57–369 ± 75 ms during oral therapy. There was no difference in the electrophysiologic effects between intravenous and oral propafenone. The induction of SVT was prevented by intravenous propafenone in 10 of 20 patients and in 4 additional patients with oral propafenone. During follow-up, 6 of 7 patients, whose SVT could not be initiated by electrophysiologic drug testing, remained free from recurrences, whereas 5 of 7 patients with inducible tachycardia had recurrences of SVT. Thus, in patients with SVT, propafenone prolonged accessory pathway and AV nodal conduction and had a beneficial effect on circus movement tachycardia. Electrophysiologic drug testing with propafenone predicts its efficacy during chronic therapy in most patients.

Verapamil

Multifocal atrial tachycardia is a distinct ECG entity characterized by an atrial rate of >100 beats/minute, the presence of at least 3 different P-wave forms, and variation in the PR and PP intervals. The condition usually occurs episodically in the setting of an acute clinical decompensation in seriously ill patients and it usually resolves with management of the underlying illness. The rapid ventricular response, however, may lead to myocardial eschemia or CHF and thus the need to treat multifocal atrial tachycardia may arise. Conventional therapy with digoxin and quinidine is ineffective and β-blockers are often contraindicated because of underlying airway disease. Although the mechanism underlying multifocal atrial tachycardia is unknown, its behavior suggests that it is caused by autosomal atrial automaticity. Levine and associates[17] from Baltimore, Maryland, studied the effects of verapamil in 8 consecutive episodes of multifocal atrial tachycardia in 6 patients aged 54–84 years. Predisposing factors to the multifocal atrial tachycardia included severe chronic pulmonary disease, hypokalemia, recent surgery, and theophylline. Five of 8 episodes occurred in conjunction with respiratory embarrassment. The atrial rate, ventricular rate, and number of nonconducted P-waves before and after verapamil were recorded. Although multifocal atrial tachycardia is an irregular rhythm, the atrial and ventricular rates varied little throughout the 20 minutes before verapamil therapy. In 6 of the 8 episodes, nonconductive P-waves were present before verapamil therapy.

These blocked atrial beats were more prevalent in patients with faster atrial rates, presumably because of the physiologic refractor in this of the AV node and the His-Purkinje system. Before verapamil therapy the number of different P-wave forms varied between 6 and 14/minute. In all episodes verapamil slowed the atrial and ventricular rates; it decreased the mean atrial rate from 138–108 beats/minute and the ventricular rate from 130–109 beats/minute. The number of nonconducted P-waves was unchanged by verapamil, but the drug did decrease the number of different P-wave forms per minute in 7 of 8 episodes, from a mean of 11 to 1 of 7. The changes caused by verapamil were noted within 5 minutes of its administration and persisted throughout the short-term study. In 3 separate patients, verapamil therapy converted multifocal atrial tachycardia to normal sinus rhythm with occasional atrial premature beats. Conversion to sinus rhythm occurred gradually over the space of several minutes. The decrease in ventricular rate was due to a decrease in the atrial rate rather than to an increase in the number of blocked P-waves. Verapamil did not significantly effect the serum digoxin or arterial blood gas levels. No complications occurred with verapamil therapy. Thus, verapamil may be helpful as an adjunct in caring for patients while the underlying disordered physiologic conditions are corrected. Verapamil consistently reduces the atrial and ventricular rates and occasionally converts multifocal atrial tachycardia to normal sinus rhythm. The mechanism for this appears to be a decrease in atrial ectopic activity. The response to verapamil suggests that multifocal atrial tachycardia may be a triggered arrhythmia.

This article was followed by an editorial by Graboys.[18]

Esmolol -vs- propranolol

The Esmolol Multicenter Study Research Group (Laddu and associates[19] from Chicago, Illinois) studied the efficacy of intravenous esmolol infusion and compared it to that of intravenous propranolol injection in patients with SVT during a double-blind parallel study: 127 patients were randomized to either the esmolol (n = 64) or propranolol (n = 63) group. Therapeutic response was achieved in 72% of esmolol and 69% of propranolol patients. The average dose of esmolol in responders was 115 ± 11 μg/kg/min. Therapeutic response was sustained in the 4-hour maintenance period in 67% of esmolol and 58% of propranolol patients. Rate of conversion to normal sinus rhythm was similar in the 2 treatment groups. After discontinuation, rapid recovery from β-blockade (decrease in heart rate reduction) was observed in esmolol patients (within 10 minutes) compared with propranolol patients (no change in heart rate up to 4.3 hours). The principal adverse effect was hypotension, reported in 23 esmolol (asymptomatic in 19) and 4 propranolol (asymptomatic in 3) patients. In most esmolol patients, hypotension resolved quickly (within 30 minutes) after esmolol was discontinued. It was concluded that esmolol was comparable in efficacy and safety to propranolol in the treatment of patients with SVT. Unlike propranolol, because of the short half-life of esmolol, rapid control of β-blockade is possible with esmolol in clinical conditions when required.

Surgical ablation

Ott and associates[20] from Houston, Texas, reported 67 children who underwent surgical therapy for refractive SVT using intraoperative mapping followed by surgical excision or cryoablation of an abnormal conduction pathway or atrial ectopic focus. Patients ranged in age from 4 months to 18 years (mean, 11 years); 55 patients had an abnormal conduction pathway crossing the AV junction with 36 of these 55 having classic WPW with delta wave on the ECG; 19 had only retrograde conduction across the Kent bundle and had a normal ECG. Kent bundles were isolated to the right anterior lateral aspect in 19 (35%), left posterior lateral in 22 (40%), posterior septal in 10 (18%), anteroseptal in 2 (4%), and both right and left in 2 (4%). Follow-up evaluation to 8 years (mean, 35 months) has showed 7 immediate failures and 1 late recurrence of arrhythmia. There were only 2 failures (8%) in the last 25 attempts. Twelve patients had surgery for atrial ectopic focus by cryoablation in 7, excision in 1, and excision and cryoablation in 4. At a mean follow-up of 17 months, there was 1 late recurrence.

Holmes and associates[21] from Rochester, Minnesota, performed ablation of the accessory AV pathway in 27 patients aged ≤21 years (mean, 15) with asymptomatic tachycardia. Six patients had associated Ebstein's malformation. SVT had been present for a mean of 5 years. At electrophysiologic study, 4 patients had 2 accessory pathways. LV free wall pathways were found in 14 patients, RV free wall pathways in 10, and septal pathways in 6. Successful initial ablation of all the pathways was achieved in 26 of the 27 patients. No patient died perioperatively and none had persistent complete heart block. During a mean follow-up of 11 months, no patients had recurrence of an arrhythmia related to the accessory pathway. Thus, the surgical treatment of children and young adults with accessory AV pathways and symptomatic SVT is safe and effective.

Kramer and associates[22] from St. Louis, Missouri, performed simultaneous intraoperative computer mapping from multiple sites before surgical division of the accessory pathways in 16 patients with the WPW syndrome. A 16-bipolar electrode band was positioned around the AV groove. Ventricular epicardial electrograms from single beats were recorded simultaneously during atrial pacing, resulting in maximal preexcitation, and atrial electrograms were recorded during orthodromic SVT. Electrograms were processed separately using a guarded signal conditioner that isolates, amplifies, filters, and analog-to-digitally converts synchronously at 2 kHz with 12-bit accuracy. Digital data were transmitted by fiber optics to a high density digital recorder and processed with a computer having rapid interactive graphics. Results in the 16 patients revealed 20 distinct Kent bundles. Two patients had only nonsustained SVT induced intraoperatively, and 1 patient manifested intermittent antegrade ventricular preexcitation. Multiple pathways were identified in 4 patients. This simultaneous multiple electrode mapping procedure facilitates intraoperative mapping by requiring only a single beat for analysis of antegrade and retrograde activation times, decreases cardiac manipulation during mapping, obviates the need for cardiopulmonary bypass, and permits analysis of transmural activation patterns. This approach decreases markedly the time required for mapping and permits accurate study of nonsustained arrhythmias and rapid identification of multiple accessory pathways.

Cox and colleagues[23] from St. Louis, Missouri, reported results of operation for WPW in 118 patients. There were 72 male and 46 females aged 9 months to 70 years (mean, 28 ± 6 years). The major indications for operation were medical refractoriness or drug intolerance (60%) and previous cardiac arrest (14%). Ebstein's anomaly was present in 12%. Other arrhythmias were noted in 34%; 22% had congenital heart disease other than Ebstein's anomaly. Twenty percent of patients had multiple (2–4) accessory pathways. Distribution of the accessory pathways was as follows: 58% left free wall, 24% posterior septal, 13% right free wall, and 5% anterior septal. Of the 149 accessory pathways present, 148 were successfully divided in the

118 patients. The surgical results document an increase in the success rate for division of accessory pathways from 86–99%, a decrease in the reoperation rate from approximately 15% to zero, and a decrease in the incidence of permanent complete heart block from 11–1%. The mortality was 5%, but only 1 death occurred after elective operation in the absence of associated cardiac abnormalities.

VENTRICULAR ARRHYTHMIAS

Diagnosis

Chronic recurrent VT is a life-threatening disorder and its recognition is therefore important. Diagnosis is complicated by the fact that characteristic broad QRS complexes of VT may be simulated by SVT with aberrant intraventricular conduction. Confusion of the 2 conditions remains common. Dancy and associates[24] from London, UK, studied 24 patients with recurrent VT who were repeatedly misdiagnosed as having SVT. SVT was recorded as the diagnosis 163 times in these patients. The researchers reviewed 72 12-lead ECGs together with the notes made at the time of the ECG to discover the reasons for misdiagnosis. Retrospective application of established criteria used to distinguish VT from SVT with aberrancy enabled the diagnosis of VT to be made in 22 of 24 patients (92%). In all but 2 of 72 episodes the only differentiating criterion noted by the attending physicians was disassociated atrial activity, and there seemed to be considerable bias in favor of the diagnosis of SVT. Of the 24 patients, 20 were given inappropriate treatment, which had dangerous consequences in 5.

Morady and associates[25] from Ann Arbor, Michigan, asked 75 internal medicine house officers, 73 internists or general practitioners, and 48 cardiologists whether or not they were influenced by a patient's BP and clinical status when attempting to distinguish between VT and SVT with BBB. Of the 196 physicians who completed the questionnaire, 59% indicated that they were influenced by patient's BP and clinical status. Thus, a sizable proportion of physicians are unaware that VT need not be associated with shock. The differentiation of VT from SVT should be based on ECG findings and not on the patient's BP or clinical status.

Dongas and associates[26] from Milwaukee, Wisconsin, examined in 18 patients who had preexisting left or right BBB the relation between the morphologic configuration of QRS complexes during wide QRS tachycardia induced during physiologic studies and sinus rhythm. Representative QRS complexes during sinus rhythm and during tachycardia were isolated from each patient and juxtaposed for comparison. The QRS complexes that constituted each pair were judged by 4 observers as being identical, different, or, if the decision was equivocal, similar. Nine patients had SVT. In 8 of the 9 patients, all 4 observers found the QRS complexes during sinus rhythm and SVT identical in morphologic configuration. In the other patient, 2 observers found the QRS complexes identical and 2 found them similar. In 12 patients VT was induced. In 11 of these 12, all 4 observers found the QRS complexes during VT different from their respective sinus beats. In the other patient, 3 observers found the QRS complexes different, whereas the fourth found them similar. During SVT, the QRS duration was unchanged from the corresponding value during sinus rhythm, whereas in patients with VT, QRS width increased by a mean of 56 ± 20 ms. These results suggest that the ECG differentiation of wide QRS tachycardia in patients with preexisting BBB can be accomplished easily and accurately by comparing the QRS complexes during tachycardia with those during sinus rhythm: if the complexes are identical, the tachycardia is supraventricular, but if they are different, the arrhythmia is ventricular in origin.

Wren and associates[27] from New Castle upon Tyne, UK, examined 16 consecutive patients with spontaneous sustained broad QRS complex tachycardia with heart rates of 120–225 beats/minute. Echo evidence of 1:1 conduction was seen in 3 cases and 2:1 AV conduction in 1 (all 4 had SVT, confirmed by intracardiac ECG in 3). Evidence of retrograde block was seen in 12 (all had VT, with electrophysiologic confirmation in 10). Satisfactory views of the mitral valve were obtained in all patients. Patients with VT had a variable mitral valve opening time (range, 42–110%) compared with those who had SVT (9–15%). Aortic root and LA views gave direct evidence of atrial contraction in 3 cases, and subcostal RA wall views were diagnostic in 4 of 5 cases. Seven patients with VT had been wrongly diagnosed elsewhere as having SVT. This study confirms that echo is a simple and rapid aid to accurate diagnosis in patients with broad QRS complex tachycardia.

Relation to psychologic factors

Because there is little systemic information available on the psychologic profile of patients with various cardiac arrhythmias, Katz and associates[28] from New Hyde Park, Stoney Brook, and Brooklyn, New York, administered a battery of 12 standardized personality inventories to 102 patients aged 19–69 years, 38 of whom had VPC without a history of AMI, 34 were medical/surgical control patients with no history of VPC or AMI, and 30 had VPC with healed AMI. The 38 patients with frequent VPC (>30/hour) without AMI were significantly more psychologically symptomatic than were the 34 age- and sex-matched general medical/surgical patients. The variables found to be significant portray the patient with frequent VPC without AMI as follows: high scores for hysteria, less moral orientation, more anxiety, depression and social alienation, and an inhibited and low respectful style. This combination of psychologic variables produced a discriminant function that accounted for 53% of the variance between the arrhythmia/no AMI group and the medical/surgical control group and could correctly predict group membership in 83% of cases. These results may have further implications in nonpharmacologic and psychotropic adjuncts to antiarrhythmic therapy.

Overdose of tricyclic antidepressant drug

There is a need for a rapid predictor of potential clinical severity to guide therapy in patients with an acute overdose of tricyclic antidepressant drugs. Boehnert and Lovejoy[29] from Boston, Massachusetts, performed a prospective study of 49 such patients to observe the associations among serum drug levels and maximum limb-lead QRS duration and the incidence of seizures and ventricular arrhythmias. Patients were divided into 2 groups on the basis of maximal limb-lead QRS duration. Group A (13 patients) had a duration of <0.10 second, and group B (36 patients) had a QRS duration of ≥0.10 second. No seizures or ventricular arrhythmias occurred in group A. In group B there was a 34% incidence of seizures and a 14% incidence of ventricular arrhythmias. All patients survived. Serum drug levels failed to predict the risk of seizures or ventricular arrhythmias accurately. Seizures occurred at any QRS duration ≥0.01 second, but ventricular arrhythmias were seen only with a QRS duration of ≥0.16 second. It was concluded that determination of the maximal limb-lead QRS duration predicts the risk of seizures and ventricular arrhythmias in acute overdose with tricyclic antidepressants. Serum drug levels are not of predictive value. This article was followed by an editorial by Salzman entitled "Clinical Use of Antidepressant Blood Levels and the Electrocardiogram."[30]

Thousands of people in the United States poison themselves with tricyclic antidepressants each year. These patients often require cardiac monitoring for potential arrhythmias, but clinical practice is highly variable in regard to the hours of monitoring required. Clarification of this issue is important because of the impact on resources. Goldberg and associates[31] from Providence, Rhode Island, retrospectively reviewed the monitoring practices and cardiac complications following tricyclic antidepressant overdose in 75 adults. The patients received an average of 62 hours of monitoring. Most ECG changes, including 3 cardiac arrests, appeared within the first 24 hours. No patient who had a normal level of consciousness and a normal ECG for 24 hours went on to develop any significant arrhythmia. On the basis of these data and a review of previous publications, the investigators proposed that current guidelines for cardiac monitoring following tricyclic antidepressant overdose be reconsidered.

Spontaneous variability

Pratt and associates[32] from Houston, Texas, reported results of analysis of the variability of complex ventricular arrhythmias in a cohort of 110 patients selected for the presence of VT. All patients were enrolled in investigational antiarrhythmic drug trials and had an average of 4 consecutive days of placebo ambulatory ECG recording to serve as the database for this study. Using a statistical approach incorporating analysis of variance, the minimum percent reductions of VPC, couplets, and VT were calculated to establish "drug effect" rather than variability at a significance level of 0.05. The relative variability of ventricular arrhythmias in prognostically important groups also was analyzed: 1) CAD -vs- no CAD; 2) patients with a LVEF of ≤40% -vs- those with an EF >40%; and 3) patients with frequent runs of VT (≥10 runs/day) -vs- infrequent VT. Multiple regression analysis revealed that patients with CAD had significantly greater VPC variability than patients without CAD (Fig. 3-3). Also, patients with frequent VT runs had greater VT variability than that previously reported in smaller studies, thus requiring greater VT reductions to establish drug effect. Whether the variability of ventricular arrhythmia is itself an independent risk factor for sudden cardiac death is unknown.

Initial baseline ECGs are used to assess the efficacy of treatment of ventricular arrhythmias. This approach assumes that in the absence of treatment the frequency of arrhythmia would remain constant. To test the validity of this assumption, Pratt and associates[33] from Houston, Texas, studied 26 clinically stable patients with symptomatic but not life-threatening ventricular arrhythmias during 2 periods of placebo treatment separated by a mean of 17 months. Compared with the initial placebo period, there were significant reductions in VPC (50%), pairs (65%), and VT (83%) during the second period of placebo administration. More than a third of the patients gave the appearance of receiving successful therapy during the second placebo period even when the reported spontaneous variability of ventricular arrhythmia was taken into consideration. If unrecognized, these long-term spontaneous changes in the frequency of arrhythmia could result in continuation of unnecessary and potentially toxic therapy and lead to incorrect conclusions regarding the efficacy of antiarrhythmic drugs in clinical trials. The investigators therefore recommended that the frequency of arrhythmia be

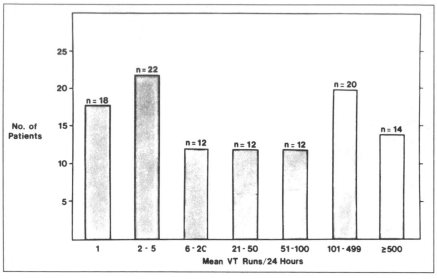

Fig. 3-3. Distribution of frequency of VT runs in 110 patients referred for investigational antiarrhythmic therapy—results of 4 consecutive days of ambulatory ECG monitoring.

reassessed annually in the absence of treatment in patients similar to those in their study. These recommendations should not be applied to patients with life-threatening ventricular arrhythmias.

Reproducibility of responses to programmed electrical stimulation

Brugada and Wellens[34] from Maastricht, The Netherlands, prospectively studied in 24 consecutive patients with documented VT (22 patients) or VF (2 patients) the results of 2 programmed ventricular stimulation protocols to initiate VT/VF. Seventeen patients had VT/VF after a healed AMI and 7 patients had idiopathic VT. In both protocols (designated 1 and 2), the RV apex was paced at 100 beats/minute, using a maximum of 2 VPC given at twice diastolic threshold. This protocol had a sensitivity of 25%. In protocol 1, the pacing site was changed to the RV outflow tract and the previous steps were repeated; in protocol 2, the pacing rate was increased to 120 and 140 beats/minute at the RV apex, also using a maximum of 2 VPC. The next step in protocol 1 consisted of an increase of current strength to 20 mA and repeating previous steps at the RV apex and RV outflow tract, with a maximum of 2 VPC; in the next step in protocol 2, 3 VPC were used during sinus rhythm and pacing was performed at rates of 100, 120, and 140 beats/minute. In protocol 1 only stimulation site and current strength were changed, whereas in protocol 2 only pacing rate and number of VPC were modified. Protocol 1 had a sensitivity of 54% and protocol 2 a sensitivity of 83%. The sensitivity of protocol 2 was statistically higher than that of protocol 1. In the group of patients with VT after AMI, the sensitivity was 66% for protocol 1 and 93% for protocol 2. Protocol 2 combined with administration of isoproterenol had a sensitivity of 95% (100% in the patients with VT after AMI). These observations have important implications for the design of the most successful order of programmed ventricular stimulation in patients with documented VT/VF. Stimulation at the RV apex using a single pacing rate and 2 VPC is a much more effective means of initiating VT than changing the stimulation site to RV outflow tract or increasing the current strength to 20 mA.

McPherson and associates[35] from New Haven and West Haven, Connecticut, studied the day-to-day reproducibility of responses to RV programmed electrical stimulation in 77 patients in the baseline state twice within 72 hours. Of 66 in whom VT was inducible at the first study (C1), VT was reproduced in 53 (80%) at the second control study (C2). Among 41 patients in whom VT was inducible using 1 or 2 programmed electrical stimuli at C1, VT remained inducible in 39 (95%) at C2, whereas only 14 of 25 patients (56%) who required 3 or more programmed electrical stimuli for VT induction at C1 had VT reproduced at C2. The difference in the reproducibility of VT induction in these 2 patient groups was highly significant. Although VT was inducible in 50% of patients using the identical stimulation mode at each study, 35% required a more intense mode for VT induction at C2; this included 11 of 35 patients (31%) in whom VT was initially inducible with 1 or 2 programmed electrical stimuli who required ≥3 for induction of VT at C2. Thus, patients in whom VT is initially inducible with 1 or 2 programmed electrical stimuli demonstrate reproducible day-to-day responses to programmed electrical stimulation and appear to be excellent candidates for electrophysiologically guided antiarrhythmic drug therapy. Because VT induction was significantly less reproducible in patients who required ≥3 programmed electrical stimuli at C1, day-to-day reproducibility of VT induction should be confirmed in such patients if electropharmacologic therapy is attempted. Because a more intense stimulation mode is often required to reproduce VT induction at C2, such a change cannot serve as a reliable index of drug efficacy when multiple antiarrhythmic agents are serially tested.

Morady and associates[36] from Ann Arbor, Michigan, performed programmed stimulation at 2 RV sites with 1–3 extrastimuli at current strengths of twice diastolic threshold (1.0 ± 0.2 mA, mean $\pm$ SD) and 10 mA in 41 patients undergoing an electrophysiologic study because of sustained VT (11 patients), nonsustained VT (19 patients), or unexplained syncope (11 patients). In 26 patients, VT was not induced by programmed stimulation at twice diastolic threshold. Programmed stimulation at 10 mA induced VT or VF in 16 of these 26 patients (62%). In 4 of 16 patients, the coupling intervals of the extrastimuli that induced VT/VF at 10 mA were all equal to or longer than the shortest coupling intervals resulting in ventricular capture at twice diastolic threshold. Fifteen patients had inducible VT at twice diastolic threshold. Programmed stimulation at 10 mA induced a similar VT in 12 patients, but resulted in no VT induction in 3 of 15 patients, despite ventricular capture at the same coupling intervals that had induced VT at twice diastolic threshold. This study shows that programmed stimulation at a high current strength may either facilitate or prevent induction of VT. Facilitation of VT induction usually is attributable to a shortening of ventricular refractoriness and the ability of extrastimuli at 10 mA to capture the ventricle at shorter coupling intervals than possible at twice diastolic threshold. However, in 25% of cases, the facilitation of VT induction by 10 mA stimuli is not explained by a shortening of ventricular refractoriness. In these cases, and in the patients in whom 10 mA stimuli prevent the induction of VT that was inducible at twice diastolic threshold, the effects of high current strength appear to be mediated through some other mechanism.

Significance of induction of ventricular arrhythmias by programmed electrical stimulation

Gradman and coworkers[37] from New Haven, Connecticut, evaluated the relation between spontaneous and induced ventricular arrhythmias, ambulatory ECG monitoring, and programmed electrical stimulation in 48 adult patients with suspected life-threatening ventricular arrhythmias. Nine patients had no inducible arrhythmia, 11 had 1–2 beats of intraventricular reentry, 19 had nonsustained VT, and 9 had sustained VT during electrophysiologic studies. Patients without arrhythmia inducibility had a higher incidence of multiform VPC (66%) and bigeminy (44%), but they also had a reduced incidence of VPC couplets (11%) on continuous ECG monitoring. With increasing degrees of ventricular inducibility, a corresponding increase in the complexity of VPC was found. Specifically, in patients with induced sustained VT, multiform VPC were present in 100%, bigeminal VPC and couplets in 89%, and spontaneous VT in 78%. In addition, the frequency of VPC, couplet frequency, and the ratio of couplets to VPC also were directly correlated to the likelihood of being able to induce VPC. Three arrhythmia variables predicted the ability to induce VT among these patients. Specifically, a mean VPC frequency of ≥100/1,000 normal beats; a mean VPC couplet frequency of ≥1/1,000 beats; and a mean ratio of VPC couplets to VPC of ≥15/1,000 VPC suggested a high likelihood of the patient having inducible VT. These data demonstrate that spontaneous and induced VPC have certain predictable relations. Sustained ECG monitoring can be used to identify patients who may have VT induced by programmed electrical stimulation.

Spielman and colleagues[38] from Philadelphia, Pennsylvania, evaluated the vulnerability of patients with nonsustained VT to symptomatic and potentially life-threatening arrhythmias. Electrophysiologic studies were performed in 58 patients with clinically documented nonsustained VT (≥3 complexes, but <15 seconds of self-terminating VT by 24 hours ambulatory ECG or telemetry monitoring) and abnormal LV function EF <50% by RNA. The stimulation protocol included the introduction of single, double, and triple ventricular extrastimuli at 3 cycle lengths and 2 RV sites. Sustained VT was produced in 23 patients (40%) and a nonsustained VT in 14 patients (24%). The induction of sustained VT correlated with the presence of LV akinesis or aneurysm, or both, but not with the LVEF or the presence or absence of CHD. These data indicate that patients with nonsustained VT and chronic LV dysfunction have a high incidence of inducible sustained VT or VF, and electrophysiologic testing may allow subsetting of patients at risk for sudden cardiac death.

VT induced at electrophysiologic studies is believed to be clinically significant if the morphology of the induced arrhythmia and the spontaneous arrhythmia are similar. Yet many times an adequate 12-lead ECG does not exist to permit determination of the VT morphology. Since the significance of differences in induced and spontaneous arrhythmias has not been clearly established, Torres and colleagues[39] from New York City reviewed the records of 153 patients and correlated induced VT morphology with the incidence of sudden death. Polymorphic VT was induced in 88 patients (58%) and monomorphic VT, in 65 patients (43%). The total mortality and sudden death rates were similar in the 2 groups despite antiarrhythmic therapy, 12 and 7% (polymorphic) -vs- 10 and 5% (monomorphic). All sudden deaths occurred in patients who presented with cardiac arrest and hemodynamically symptomatic VT and none in the asymptomatic VT group, regardless of VT morphology. The induced VT morphology cannot be used to predict the potential efficacy of antiarrhythmic drugs, since patients with either morphology are as likely to respond to conventional or experimental agents. Thus, induced polymorphic VT can be a useful index of electrical instability in high risk patients (cardiac arrest and hemodynamically symptomatic VT) and may be of utility in guiding antiarrhythmic therapy.

Schoenfeld and coworkers[40] from Boston, Massachusetts, evaluated those factors predictive of the ability to both initiate and suppress ventricular tachyarrhythmias during electrophysiologic study. Programmed electrical cardiac stimulation results were evaluated in 261 patients: 66 of these presented with nonsustained VT, 91 with sustained VT, and 104 with VF. Multivariate logistic regression analysis demonstrated that the presenting arrhythmia was a potent and independent predictor of the ability to provoke ventricular arrhythmias at electrophysiologic study. A history of prior AMI and male sex were also significant independent predictors. Among patients presenting with sustained VT, 89% had inducible ventricular arrhythmias compared with 61 and 66% of patients with nonsustained VT and VF, respectively. Complete suppression of ventricular arrhythmias was achieved in only 52% of the patients; these included 34 of 66 patients with sustained VT and 73 patients presenting with nonsustained VT and VF, respectively. Multivariate analysis demonstrated that the major independent determinants of the ability to induce VT were the number of drug trials performed before the electrophysiologic study (inversely correlated) and the nature of the induced arrhythmias. Thus, these data indicate that the presenting clinical arrhythmia is a highly significant and independent predictor of the ability to induce ventricular arrhythmias during electrophysiologic testing, and an important determinant of the ability to suppress induced arrhythmias in patients with spontaneous VT.

Veltri and associates[41] from Baltimore, Maryland, studied 33 patients with VT ($\geq$3 beats, <30 seconds in duration, rate >100 beats/minute) on 24-hour Holter monitoring and no history of clinical arrhythmia (presyncope, syncope, or sudden death) using programmed electrical stimulation. VT was induced in 14 patients (42%), sustained VT, in 7 (21%), and nonsustained VT, in 7 (21%). Inducible VT was associated with underlying heart disease in 9 of 19 patients with CAD, 3 of 6 patients with idiopathic dilated cardiomyopathy, and 2 of 4 patients with MVP. Patients without structural heart disease did not have inducible VT. EF was not significantly different in patients with or without inducible VT. Twenty-three patients were discharged with drug therapy and 10 patients without therapy. At 23 ± 16 months (mean ± SD) follow up, 28 patients (85%) were alive, 4 (12%) had died from a cardiac cause (EF 40 ± 17 vs 28 + 20%). Another patient died from stroke. Twenty-six patients (79%) were free of clinical arrhythmia and 7 patients (21%) had arrhythmic events (EF 49 ± 18 -vs- 31 ± 17%). Two of 8 patients with noninducible VT who were discharged without drug treatment had clinical arrhythmic events and neither of 2 patients with inducible VT discharged off drugs had such events. Thus, in asymptomatic, nonsustained VT, underlying heart disease makes inducible VT more likely, an incidence of progression to clinical arrhythmic events is apparent, and EF appears predictive of subsequent cardiac death and clinical arrhythmic events, but not the ability to induce VT.

Controversy persists among groups carrying out programmed ventricular stimulation as to which criteria should be used to define a positive test. To examine this question, Platia and Reid[42] from Baltimore, Maryland, carried out in 50 patients with documented sustained VT or VF the results of programmed ventricular stimulation analyzed retrospectively. All patients underwent serial programmed ventricular stimulation using single and double extrastimuli and ventricular burst pacing in the right ventricle and, when necessary, the left ventricle, with sustained VT elicited during the control study in each patient. Antiarrhythmic drugs were then administered, with therapy tailored to both programmed ventricular stimulation result and ambulatory Holter monitoring, when possible. All patients were maintained and followed on the same drugs and dosages as at the time of predischarge programmed ventricular stimulation. After a mean of 20 months follow-up,

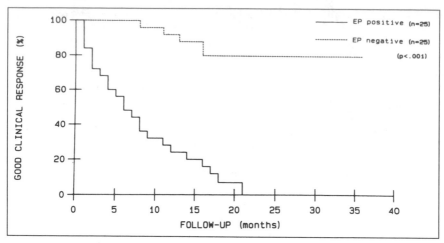

Fig. 3-4. Kaplan-Meier life-table analysis of 50 patients who underwent programmed ventricular stimulation. A positive test is defined as the induction of VT 5 or more beats in duration. Good clinical response is defined as the absence of sudden death or recurrent symptomatic VT during follow-up. EP = electrophysiologic.

8 patients died suddenly and 20 had documented sustained VT (Fig. 3-4). The ability to induce nonsustained or sustained VT on predischarge programmed ventricular stimulation was associated with a significantly higher likelihood of subsequent sudden death or VT recurrence than if VT could not be induced. In addition, using the criterion of ≥5 beats of induced VT to define a positive study maximized the predictive value of programmed ventricular stimulation and provided a significantly higher predictive accuracy than if only sustained VT were used to define a positive study (Fig. 3-5). Thus, in patients with a history of serious ventricular arrhythmias, the persistent ability to induce either nonsustained or sustained VT despite drug therapy predicts a high likelihood of subsequent VT or sudden death, and using the induction of VT of ≥5 beats duration as a criterion for a positive study on drug therapy maximizes the overall predictive accuracy of programmed ventricular stimulation.

Fig. 3-5. Predictive accuracy of programmed ventricular stimulation as a function of the number of induced ventricular responses defining a positive test in a population of 50 patients. Error bars indicate 95% confidence limits.

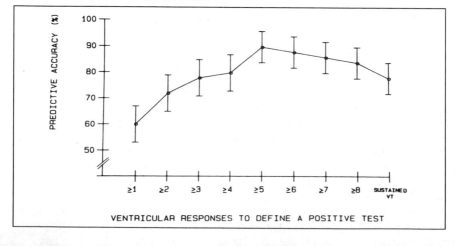

Comparison of Holter monitoring to electrophysiologic study

Swerdlow and Peterson[43] from Stanford, California, compared baseline 24-hour Holter monitoring and electrophysiologic study in 43 consecutive patients with CAD who had sustained ventricular tachyarrhythmias to determine the fraction of patients in whom each could be performed and the fraction in whom each could be used to guide therapy. Patients were excluded from Holter monitoring if sustained VT requiring termination occurred and from electrophysiologic study if CHF was sufficiently severe to cause excessive risk. More patients completed electrophysiologic study than Holter monitoring (90 -vs- 71%), but this difference was not statistically significant. Overall, Holter detected arrhythmias suitable for antiarrhythmic drug assessment in 50% of patients: ≥30 VPC/hour in 50%, ≥10 VPC pairs in 44%, ≥5 runs in 19%, and ≥10 pairs and runs in 44%. Sustained monomorphic VT suitable for electropharmacologic testing was induced in 82%. Drug efficacy could be assessed in 70% of patients evaluated by Holter monitoring, compared with 96% evaluated by electrophysiologic study. Thus, in consecutive coronary patients with sustained ventricular tachyarrhythmias, electrophysiologic study could be used to guide therapy more frequently than Holter monitoring.

Antiarrhythmic drug efficacy—general

Rae and associates[44] from Philadelphia, Pennsylvania, evaluated the efficacy and proarrhythmic potential of antiarrhythmic agents. Programmed ventricular stimulation was performed in 160 consecutive patients with CAD during a baseline study and 432 subsequent drug studies. The tachyarrhythmias induced during baseline studies were sustained VT (121 patients), VF (16 patients), and symptomatic nonsustained VT (23 patients). Regimens were completely successful if <6 repetitive ventricular responses were inducible during therapy and partially successful if ≤15 repetitive ventricular responses were inducible (Fig. 3-6). Procainamide and quinidine were the most successful single agents, with overall success rates of 24 and 35%, respectively. Either procainamide or quinidine combined with mexiletine was the most successful combination (overall success of 23%). Each antiarrhythmic regimen had a proarrhythmic potential. The incidence of proarrhythmic effects ranged from 4–13%, with no significant difference between regimens. In 13% of patients at least 1 regimen produced a proarrhythmic effect. Patients treated with an antiarrhythmic regimen that prevented induction of arrhythmia had significantly fewer arrhythmia recurrences than patients treated with a regimen that failed to prevent it. In conclusion, identification of an effective drug regimen is possible in 38% of patients with lethal ventricular arrhythmias, proarrhythmic effects occur in a significant number of patients during electrophysiologic testing of antiarrhythmic regimens, and the clinical outcome in patients in whom ventricular arrhythmias are not inducible with ventricular stimulation have a better prognosis than those in whom arrhythmias continue to be inducible on therapy.

Arrhythmogenicity of antiarrhythmic agents

Torres and associates[45] from New York City studied 181 patients who were referred for programmed electrical stimulation because of ventricular arrhythmias. Forty-three patients (24%) had worsening of the induced arrhythmia by at least 1 of the 10 drugs tested. There were no differences in the

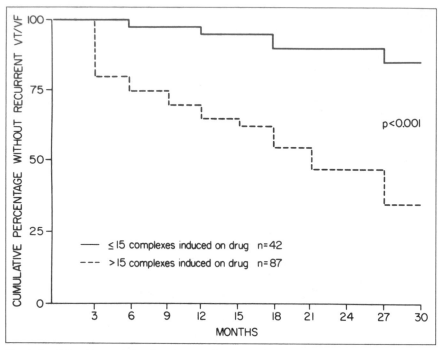

Fig. 3-6. Life-table analysis of patients with sustained ventricular tachyarrhythmias. Time from the electrophysiologic study is denoted on the abscissa and the cumulative percentage of patients without recurrent VT/VF is shown on the ordinate. Patients followed on regimens that prevented induction of more than 15 complexes (solid line) had a significantly better outcome than patients in whom more than 15 complexes (broken line) were induced on antiarrhythmic therapy.

clinical characteristics of the patients who had an arrhythmogenic response and the rest of the study population. The incidence of arrhythmia facilitation was 13% (63 of the 478 drug tests). An arrhythmogenic response was spontaneous VT during drug infusion (which occurred in 1% of drug tests), decrease in the number of stimuli needed to induce VT (7.5%), nonsustained VT converting to sustained VT (1.8%), VF developing for the first time (2.3%), and new inducible VT after drug administration (0.6%). The incidence of arrhythmia aggravation was similar to that reported using ambulatory monitoring techniques. Programmed electrical stimulation studies can be useful in rapidly identifying drugs that might facilitate arrhythmias in a particular patient and in determining the extent of arrhythmogenicity of antiarrhythmic drugs.

Poser and associates[46] from Boston, Massachusetts, performed electrophysiologic tests in 63 patients who had a history of malignant, sustained ventricular tachyarrhythmias. Monitoring and exercise tests showed low frequency or nonreproducible ventricular arrhythmia. Criteria for definite drug-induced aggravation of arrhythmia included conversion of nonsustained VT to a sustained ventricular arrhythmia and provocation of the endpoint with 1 extrastimulus when 3 were required during control. Aggravation was deemed possible when, compared with a control group, the endpoint resulted with the use of 1 less extrastimulus and sustained tachycardia with a more rapid rate was provoked. A total of 216 single drug studies were performed (3.4/patient). In general, definite or possible aggravation occurred in 35 tests (16%). In 28 cases (13%) aggravation was categorized as definite, while in 7 cases (3%) the induced arrhythmia was deemed as possibly related to the use of the antiarrhythmic drugs. Drug tests with multiple agents caused aggravation of arrhythmia in 19 patients (30%). Therefore, exacerbation of arrhythmia by antiarrhythmic drugs also occurs during electrophysiologic study. The incidence approximates that reported when monitoring and exercise tests are used for evaluating drug efficacy.

Amiodarone

To determine whether combined intravenous and oral loading with amiodarone can shorten its onset of action, Kerin and associates[47] from Detroit, Michigan, conducted a comparative study in 20 patients with refractory ventricular arrhythmias who were treated with amiodarone. All patients had frequent and complex VPC on a 24-hour baseline Holter recording. Ten patients (group A) received oral loading alone: 800 mg/day for 7 days, 600 mg/day for 3 days, then a maintenance dose 200–400 mg/day. Ten patients (group B) received intravenous and oral loading: 5 mg/kg intravenous, and then the same regimen as for group A. Follow-up 24-hour Holter recordings were obtained daily for 7 days, weekly for 1 month, and then monthly. Arrhythmia control was defined as ≥70% reduction in VPC, a ≥90% reduction in couplets, and abolition of VT. The time to optimal ventricular arrhythmia control was shorter for group B (20 ± 18 -vs- 105 ± 83 days) and the cumulative amiodarone dose at the time of control was smaller for group B (10 ± 8 -vs- 48 ± 39 g). No complications were encountered with intravenous amiodarone. Thus, initial loading with intravenous amiodarone can shorten the time to optimal ventricular arrhythmia control and lower the cumulative dose required.

Horowitz and associates[48] from Philadelphia, Pennsylvania, prospectively studied in 100 consecutive patients the prognostic importance of electrophysiologic studies in 100 patients with sustained ventricular tachyarrhythmias treated with amiodarone. Sustained VT/VF was inducible in all patients before amiodarone therapy. After amiodarone administration, 2 groups of patients were identified. In group 1 patients the ventricular tachyarrhythmia was no longer inducible and in group 2 patients the arrhythmia remained inducible. In group 1, no recurrent arrhythmia occurred during a follow-up of 18 ± 10 months. In group 2, 38 of 80 patients (48%) had arrhythmia recurrence during a follow-up of 12 ± 9 months. The difference between group 1 and 2 could not be explained by clinical variables, amiodarone doses, plasma concentrations, or ECG variables. In 12 patients in whom cardiovascular collapse or other severe symptoms where noted during electrophysiologic study after amiodarone treatment, recurrences caused sudden death. In 26 patients in whom the induced arrhythmia produced moderate symptoms, the recurrent arrhythmia was nonfatal VT. Electrophysiologic testing provides clinical guidance and predicts prognosis in patients treated with amiodarone as it does for the evaluation of other antiarrhythmic agents.

DiCarlo and associates[49] from San Francisco, California, performed multivariate analysis of 11 clinical variables in 104 patients with sustained symptomatic VT or VF treated with amiodarone to determine variables predictive of subsequent fatal or nonfatal cardiac arrest. Twenty-five patients (24%) had fatal or nonfatal cardiac arrest after 7.3 ± 6.2 months (mean ± SD) of therapy. Multivariate analysis identified an EF ≤0.40, syncope or cardiac arrest before amiodarone therapy, and VT (≥3 consecutive VPC) during predischarge ambulatory ECG monitoring as variables associated with a high risk of subsequent fatal or nonfatal cardiac arrest. Patients who had these 3 clinical variables had a much higher predicted incidence of cardiac arrest at

6 months (62%) and 12 months (76%) than did patients with an EF >0.40 without syncope or cardiac arrest before amiodarone therapy and without VT during predischarge ambulatory ECG monitoring (2 and 5%, respectively). Risk stratification using clinical variables can predict which patterns indicate a high risk of recurrent cardiac arrest or sudden death during amiodarone therapy.

Veltri and associates[50] from Baltimore, Maryland, performed electrophysiologic testing in 13 patients with refractory, recurrent, life-threatening VT before and after long-term amiodarone therapy. Nine patients (69%) had CAD, 3 (23%) had nonischemic cardiomyopathy, and 1 (8%) had MVP. At control electrophysiologic study, programmed electrical stimulation induced VT in all patients: sustained VT in 11, and nonsustained VT in 2 (9 and 31 beats). After oral loading with amiodarone, 1,200 mg/day for 14 days, followed by maintenance therapy with 408 ± 20 mg/day (mean ± SEM), repeat programmed electrical stimulation at 6 ± 2 months revealed inducible VT in 12 of 13 patients: sustained VT in 11 and nonsustained VT (32 beats) in 1. Inducible VT was suppressed in only 1 patient. Amiodarone significantly increased sinus cycle length, P-R interval, QRS duration, and RV effective refractory period. Insignificant increases in A-H, H-V, and Q-Tc intervals were noted. At 24 ± 2 months, 8 patients (62%), all with inducible VT at late programmed electrical stimulation, were free of clinical arrhythmic events (syncope or sudden death), compared with 5 patients (38%; 4 with inducible VT at late programmed electrical stimulation) with events. There were no significant differences in the induced VT cycle length, VT cycle length change, ease of inducibility, or hemodynamic response to induced VT of late programmed electrical stimulation in patients with and without arrhythmic events. Thus, in patients who receive long-term amiodarone treatment, late programmed electrical stimulation does not predict clinical efficacy, and the frequency of conversion from inducible VT to noninducible VT is low. Despite ventricular electrical instability, as judged by late programmed electrical stimulation testing, amiodarone is clinically effective in patients at high risk.

Marchlinski and associates[51] from Philadelphia, Pennsylvania, did Holter monitoring in 74 patients with sustained ventricular tachyarrhythmias before and after 11 ± 6 days of amiodarone therapy. On controlled Holter recordings, 55 patients (group I) had frequent (>10/hour VPC) and/or complex (at least couplets) ventricular ectopic activity (VEA); and 19 patients (group II) had infrequent and simple VEA. A positive Holter monitor response to amiodarone was defined as a decrease in VEA by >85% and abolition of all complex VEA. In group I, 34 patients (62%) had a positive Holter monitor response. In group II, 16 patients (84%) had persistent, infrequent, and simple VEA and 3 had frequent and/or complex VEA. During a mean follow-up of 13 ± 12 months, 22 patients (30%) had VT or sudden death. In group I, VT or sudden death occurred in 6 of 34 (18%) patients with a positive Holter monitor response and 11 of 21 (52%) with a negative Holter monitor response, and in group II, VT or sudden death occurred in 5 of 16 patients (31%) with persistent, infrequent and simple VEA. All episodes of VT or sudden death occurred after ≥2 weeks of amiodarone therapy (mean, 5 ± 6 months). The predictive accuracy of a positive Holter monitor response as an indicator for subsequent prevention of sustained ventricular tachyarrhythmias and sudden cardiac death was 82%, and for a negative Holter monitor response as an indicator of tachyarrhythmia or sudden death recurrence on therapy, it was 52%. Thus, in patients with sustained ventricular tachyarrhythmias, 1) VEA on the Holter recording too infrequent to index a response to amiodarone will be present in 25% of patients; 2) amiodarone is usually effective in suppressing frequent and complex VEA; 3) abolition of complex and frequent ectopic activity during amiodarone therapy predicts control of sustained ventricular arrhythmias; and 4) failure to control VEA does not preclude control of sustained ventricular arrhythmias with amiodarone therapy in 50% of patients.

Veltri and colleagues[52] from Baltimore, Maryland, studied 42 patients with refractory, recurrent, life-threatening VT and spontaneous VT treated with amiodarone to determine the value of Holter recordings in predicting future prognosis. After 1 week of amiodarone therapy and during the follow-up period of 22 ± 11 months, these patients had serial 24-hour recordings. VT was suppressed on all follow-up serial Holter recordings in 17 patients (40%). During follow-up, 24 (57%) patients were free of important ventricular arrhythmias. These data were utilized to determine the sensitivity, specificity, and positive and negative predictive values and accuracy of identifying VT on 24-, 48- and 72-hour Holter recordings during the second week of amiodarone therapy for predicting subsequent arrhythmic events. Positive and negative predictive values were 100 and 71% for 24-hour Holter recordings, 88 and 71% for 48-hour recordings, and 89 and 75% for 72-hour recordings. Overall predictive accuracy was 76, 76, and 79%, respectively. Specificity decreased slightly from 100% on 24-hour Holter recordings to 94% on 48- or 72-hour recordings, and sensitivity increased from 44% on 24-hour recordings to 62% on 72-hour recordings. Thus, Holter monitoring during the second week of amiodarone therapy can be used to identify patients at relatively low or high risk for future important arrhythmic events.

Optimal loading and maintenance regimens for amiodarone are undefined. Kennedy and associates[53] from New Haven, Connecticut, used serial electrophysiologic testing in 25 patients with VT to assess the adequacy of a 1-week oral loading regimen at 1,200 mg/day to modify maintenance dosing at the conclusion of loading and to evaluate the appropriateness of maintenance dosing after 2 months of therapy. During the loading period, highly significant increases occurred in the A-H interval (88 ± 22 -vs- 120 ± 31 ms), H-V interval (49 ± 10 -vs- 61 ± 11 ms), AV nodal Wenckebach cycle length (390 ± 92 -vs- 537 ± 147 ms), ventricular refractory period (247 ± 17 -vs- 276 ± 23 ms), mean VT cycle length (254 ± 38 -vs- 298 ± 52 ms), and return cycle length (294 ± 55 -vs- 360 ± 87 ms). VT inducibility decreased in a few cases, and when observed in association with a >10% increase in ventricular refractory period, resulted in a lower maintenance dose. After 2 months of maintenance therapy, no additional change occurred in any of these parameters except for an increase in VT cycle length (298 ± 52 -vs- 330 ± 65 ms). VT inducibility again showed no consistent response. It is concluded that patients can be discharged after 1 week of therapy with oral amiodarone loading at 1,200 mg/day and that maintenance dosing modified by electrophysiologic assessment results in steady perpetuation of the cardiac amiodarone effect, as indicated by the time course of change in electrophysiologic variables consistently affected.

Adams and coworkers[54] from London, UK, measured tissue concentrations of the amiodarone and its major metabolite, desethylamiodarone, in human tissues. These were obtained from 18 patients at autopsy (9), surgery (7), or biopsy (2) after treatment with amiodarone for varying periods of time. High concentrations of amiodarone were found in fat, but amiodarone and desethylamiodarone concentrations also were high in liver, lung, adrenal gland, testis, and lymph node. High concentrations of both were found in abnormally pigmented (blue) skin from patients with amiodarone-induced skin pigmentation. These values were 10-fold higher than those in unpigmented skin from the same patients. These high concentrations were associated with lysosomal inclusion bodies in dermal macrophages in the pigmented skin. The inclusion bodies were intrinsically electron dense and contained iodine by energy dispersive x-ray microanalysis. Lysosomal inclusion bodies shown by electron microscopy to be multilamellar were seen in other tissues, including terminal nerve fibers in pigmented skin, pulmonary macrophages, blood neutrophils, and hepatocytes and Kupffer cells. These characteristic ultrastructural findings occurred in both genetic lipidoses and lipidoses induced by other drugs, such as perhexiline. The investigators concluded that during therapy with amiodarone, widespread deposition of amiodarone and desethylamiodarone occurs. This leads to ultrastructural changes typical of a lipidosis. These changes are seen clearly in tissues associated with the unwanted effects of amiodarone, such as skin, liver, and lung.

To assess the effects of amiodarone on cardiac function, Ellenbogen and colleagues[55] from Durham, North Carolina, studied 41 consecutive patients with first-pass or equilibrium RNA before and 3 months after drug therapy was initiated. The mean heart rate, systolic BP, and diastolic BP were not significantly altered by treatment. The mean EF was 36% at the time of drug initiation and 36% 3 months later. Nineteen patients had an EF >30% and 16 had an EF <30%. The mean change in EF for these 2 subgroups showed no significant difference. No correlation between amiodarone dose and change in EF was noted. There was no correlation between baseline EF and change in EF over this 3-month period. In summary, amiodarone does not depress LV function and as a result can be used safely in patients with mild to moderate impairment of LV function.

To assess the incidence of adverse effects associated with long-term amiodarone therapy, Raeder and associates[56] from Boston, Massachusetts, evaluated the records of 217 consecutive patients who were treated for refractory arrhythmia. After an average of 12 months of therapy, ≥1 side effects occurred in 113 patients (52%). These were considered clinically significant in 42 patients (19%), mandating discontinuation of amiodarone in 18 (8%). The untoward reactions requiring discontinuation of amiodarone included thyroid dysfunction, visual disturbances, pulmonary infiltrates, ataxia, cardiac conduction abnormalities, and drug interactions. The mild side effects included corneal microdeposits, skin rashes, and gastrointestinal symptoms. There was weak correlation between blood levels of amiodarone, the daily dose, and the cumulative dose. Drug levels were higher in symptomatic patients, although they received lower doses of amiodarone. Amiodarone is associated with frequent side effects, but they are generally mild and do not necessitate drug discontinuation. Careful monitoring of therapy is essential to detect the potentially serious adverse reactions that are encountered in nearly 20% of patients.

Bepridil

Somberg and associates[57] from New York City studied bepridil, a new calcium blocker that prolongs the Q-T interval, to determine the antiarrhythmic and possible arrhythmogenic properties of this agent. Programmed electrical stimulation was employed to evaluate bepridil in 15 patients with symptomatic VT. Bepridil prevented VT induction in 7 of 15 patients. Bepridil prolonged the Q-T and refractoriness and a linear correlation was demonstrated between the percent change in Q-Tc and refractory period prolongation for the bepridil-protected group. Bepridil thus possesses antiarrhythmic properties with a minimal proarrhythmic effect.

Encainide

To establish long-term efficacy and safety of encainide, 48 patients with chronic VPC underwent 6 months of therapy with encainide in a multicenter French study carried out by Dumoulin and associates[58] from Paris, France. A 24-hour ambulatory ECG was obtained at baseline for each daily dosage of 75, 150, and 225 mg of encainide during the in-hospital titration period and at the end of the first and sixth months during the follow-up period. There was a significant reduction in the median hourly total VPC rates from 481 at baseline to 2 at the end of the titration period with the highest dosage and to 22 at the last visit of the chronic dosing period. Nearly total suppression of VPC was observed in 56% of the patients at the end of the titration period and in 30% at the end of the 6-month follow-up period. The most common side effects were vertigo, vision disturbance, and headache. P-R, QRS, and Q-Tc intervals consistently significantly increased from baseline during the various encainide trial periods. Encainide may have worsened ventricular arrhythmia in 4 patients who received >200 mg of encainide daily. Plasma concentrations of encainide and encainide metabolites varied widely, and no relation was found between antiarrhythmic efficacy and plasma levels of encainide, O-demethyl-encainide, or 3-methoxy-O-demethyl-encainide.

Duff and associates[59] from Nashville, Tennessee, studied 37 patients with drug resistant ventricular arrhythmias. Eleven patients in group I had sustained VT and 26 in group II had nonsustained ventricular arrhythmias. In group I, 8 patients had remote AMI, CHF, and sustained VT requiring repeated cardioversion (group Ia). No patient responded to encainide treatment, but 6 did have an antiarrhythmic response (complete in 3 and only partial in 3) to other investigational antiarrhythmic agents. Three patients in group I, all without CAD (group Ib), had an excellent antiarrhythmic response to encainide, as did 21 of 26 patients in group II. In 4 of 5 patients in group II who did not respond, the dosage was limited due to the development of sinus pauses, AV block, or BBB, and in 3 of these 4 patients preexisting conduction disease was evident (P-R >0.2 second or QRS >0.12 second). Diplopia occurred while taking the maximal oral dosage in the fifth patient. At 22 months follow-up, 14 of the original 24 patients who responded to encainide continued to receive it; 3 had died (all due to natural progression of LV dysfunction) and encainide was discontinued in 7: in 2 because of syncope, in 2 because of new-onset AF, in 1 because of exercise-induced polymorphic VT, in 1 because of diplopia, and in 1 because of skin exanthem. Paradoxical worsening of ventricular arrhythmias occurred more frequently in patients in group Ia (4 of 8 patients) than in those in group Ib and II (3 of 29 patients). Although no significant relation could be established, paradoxical responses tended to be associated with higher encainide concentrations and greater prolongation of the QRS interval.

Flecainide

Flowers and associates[60] from New York City prescribed flecainide initially at a dose of 200 mg twice daily in 21 patients with sustained VP and in 19 with nonsustained VT provoked during controlled electrophysiologic study. After early toxicity in the VT patients, the dosage was reduced to 100 mg twice daily. The effects of flecainide were studied in the 40 patients, all of whom underwent programmed electrical stimulation at the reduced dose. Sustained VT was induced in 21 patients and nonsustained in 19. Flecainide prevented VT induction in 26 patients (65%). At a mean dose of 1.5 ± 0.1 mg/kg, prolongation occurred in the effective refractory period of the first (280 ± 5 -vs- 249 ± 5 ms) and second (254 ± 6 -vs- 209 ± 9 ms) extrastimuli. In the patients protected by flecainide, the effective refractory periods increased by 17 ± 2 and 21 ± 3%, in contrast to only a 7 ± 3 and 6 ± 4% increase in the nonprotected group, despite a higher mean dose (1.9 ± 0.1 -vs- 1.35 ± 0.1 mg/kg). Twenty-one patients were discharged on flecainide therapy, 100 mg twice daily, and were followed for a mean of 11 months. Sixteen patients were alive and well, 1 died suddenly, 1 died from a noncardiac cause, and 1 had a "break-through" arrhythmia. Thus, flecainide therapy guided by programmed electrical stimulation is effective at a reduced dose.

Josephson and colleagues[61] from Los Angeles, California, administered flecainide to 22 patients with CAD. Intravenous infusions of 1 and 2 mg/kg resulted in respective increases in RA pressure (12 and 15%), mean PA pressure (27 and 28%), and PA wedge pressure (44 and 33%). Cardiac index decreased 8% after 1 mg/kg flecainide and 12% after the 2 mg/kg dose. The mean LVEF decreased by 15 and 16%, respectively, 10 minutes after 1 and 2 mg/kg of flecainide. Minimal increases in the heart rate (<5%) and no significant change in arterial pressure occurred 5–10 minutes after flecainide and were associated with borderline and variable increases in pulmonary and systemic vascular resistances. Flecainide diluent did not induce changes in PA wedge pressure or LVEF. Thus, flecainide exerts a moderate but significant negative inotropic effect that may be clinically significant in patients with severely compromised ventricular function.

Platia and associates[62] from Baltimore, Maryland, performed intracardiac electrophysiologic studies and when possible ambulatory monitoring before and after therapy with flecainide (mean dose, 418 ± 87 mg) in 22 patients with CAD and spontaneous VT or VF. An average of 4 antiarrhythmic agents were used and were unsuccessful before therapy with flecainide was begun. During 64 ± 16 hours of control Holter monitoring in 16 patients, all had ≥1 salvos of VT and VPC. Programmed stimulation during the control period induced VT in 17 of 22 patients. After flecainide therapy, Holter monitoring showed elimination of all forms of VT in all but 1 patient and significant reduction of paired VPC by 95% and single VPC by 70%. Electrophysiologic study during flecainide therapy showed significant increases in A-H, H-V, P-R, QRS, and Q-Tc intervals, and the ventricular effective refractory period. Programmed stimulation in 17 patients taking flecainide, with a mean plasma level of 1,075 ± 521 ng/ml, showed ablation of inducible VT in only 2 patients, a worsening in 5, and continued VT inducibility in 10. Adverse effects that required drug withdrawal were infrequent and encountered in patients who received higher drug levels: 1 patient with CHF and 1 with severe sinus bradycardia. Thus, although flecainide suppresses complex ventricular arrhythmias on Holter recordings, it rarely alters the response to programmed stimulation. Caution is recommended in its use for recurrent sustained VT or VF and in the interpretation of electrophysiologic studies until the predictive value of programmed stimulation with flecainide therapy is established.

Lal and coworkers[63] from St. Louis, Missouri, Milwaukee, Wisconsin, and Houston, Texas, evaluated 38 patients with organic heart disease and a history of sudden cardiac arrest or recurrent sustained VT treated with flecainide. Flecainide is thought to be a sodium channel blocking agent with substantially more potency than procainamide, quinidine, and lidocaine. Twenty-eight patients had electrophysiologic testing before and during flecainide treatment. Sustained VT became noninducible in 5 patients, nonsustained in 5 patients, and slowed in 13 patients. Thirteen of 14 patients with cardiac arrest and 15 of the 24 patients with recurrent sustained VT remained on long-term flecainide therapy. The mean LVEF in 16 of these 18 patients was 37%. The administration of flecainide caused nonserious side effects in 7 patients (18%) and proarrhythmic effects in 4 patients (11%). After 11 ± 3 months, 15 patients (39%) had no recurrence of their serious ventricular arrhythmias. In the 18 patients receiving long-term therapy, 3 late deaths occurred, and 1 was caused by a cardiac arrhythmia. These data indicate that flecainide is effective in approximately 40% of patients with otherwise severe and refractory ventricular arrhythmias.

Dubner and associates[64] from Buenos Aires, Argentina, studied the effects on ventricular arrhythmias of flecainide and compared them with those of amiodarone in 10 patients with frequent, chronic, and stable VPC. The study consisted of an initial 1-week, placebo-controlled, baseline period followed by 2 12-day, randomized, crossover, double-blind treatment periods with incremental dosage and 1 month of placebo between drug periods. Frequent VPC, which were present in all 10 patients during both placebo control periods (≥30 VPC/hour every hour, during 24-hour Holter monitoring), were markedly suppressed (reduction >80%) in 9 patients with both drugs. There was almost total abolition of the VPC in 6 patients with flecainide, and the satisfactory results with a minimal dose in 3 demonstrated its fast onset of action. Side effects from either agent were infrequent and no discontinuation was necessary. It was concluded that flecainide is a highly effective antiarrhythmic agent.

Mexiletine

Rutledge and coworkers[65] from Davis and Sacramento, California, evaluated the efficacy of oral mexiletine on ventricular arrhythmias in 58 patients in whom conventional drugs were unsuccessful. The mean daily dose of mexiletine was 652 mg (range, 250–1,500) and mean duration of therapy was 14 months. Mexiletine therapy was associated with a decrease of 52% in total VPC during 24 hours compared with control and 19 patients had a >83% decrease in ventricular ectopic rhythm frequency. Five patients (26%) had side effects after a mean period of 30 weeks and 1 died suddenly. Thus, mexiletine appeared to suppress ventricular ectopic rhythms without serious side effects in 13 of 52 patients during long-term therapy. There was no correlation between drug dose and therapeutic effectiveness. The administration of mexiletine also was associated with a 48% decrease in the frequency of VT and 5 of 10 patients with a history of cardiac arrest remain without symptomatic VT for 15 months. Important side effects requiring discontinuation of mexiletine occurred in 12 patients (21%) and were primarily related to central nervous system and gastrointestinal tract alterations. Thus, mexiletine was effective in a subset of patients with serious ventricular arrhythmias in whom conventional antiarrhythmic therapy had failed. However, substantial side effects occur in patients treated with this agent.

Nademanee and associates[66] from Sepulveda and Los Angeles, California, studied the antiarrhythmic effects of mexiletine (n = 14) and compared them to procainamide (n = 16) by a double-blind parallel protocol in 30 patients (group I) with frequent VPC (>20/hour), and to amiodarone by an open-label sequential approach in 25 patients (mean LVEF 33 ± 13%) with life-threatening ventricular arrhythmias (group II) resistant to ≥2 conventional agents. The predetermined endpoint of therapy in group I patients was met in 6 of 14 given mexiletine, with 7 requiring drug discontinuation for severe gastrointestinal or central nervous system side effects and only 3 of 16 patients (19%) given procainamide, with 5 (31%) developing limiting side effects. Increases in dose led to a higher efficacy rate for VPC suppression with a corresponding increase in side effects with mexiletine; with procainamide, the higher dose was not associated with greater VPC suppression. In group II patients, mexiletine was effective in 4 (16%), with 1 patient discontinuing the drug during long-term therapy; mexiletine was ineffective in 16 (64%) and early side effects developed in 5 (20%). Patients not responding to or not tolerating mexiletine were given amiodarone; 20 of 21 (95%) responded with arrhythmia control after the loading dose. During a mean follow-up period of 2 years, sudden death occurred in 2 patients, death from CHF in 2, and death from subarachnoid hemorrhage in 1 patient; 15 (75%) patients were alive and free of arrhythmia. It was concluded that in patients with refractory life-threatening arrhythmias mexiletine is significantly less potent than amiodarone; its potency for VPC suppression is similar to that of procainamide, but its use is associated with a high incidence of limiting side effects.

Greenspan and associates[67] from Philadelphia, Pennsylvania, studied the efficacy of combination therapy using a type 1A agent (quinidine or procainamide) and a type 1B agent (mexiletine) in suppressing inducible sustained ventricular tachyarrhythmias in 23 patients undergoing serial drug testing with programmed stimulation. All patients had CAD with previous AMI and abnormal LV function (mean EF, 35%); 55% presented with syncope or cardiac arrest. In 19 patients therapy had failed during empiric trials of 1–3 antiarrhythmic agents. All 23 patients had inducible sustained VT (18 had uniform morphology sustained VT and 5 had VF during control electrophyiologic study), and therapy had failed with a type 1A agent and mexiletine and the type 1A agent prevented induction of VT in 8 of 23 patients. In 15 patients, the combination significantly prolonged the tachycardia cycle length and reduced the symptoms associated with the induced arrhythmia. Patients more likely to respond to the combination had shorter cycle lengths and polymorphic configuration of the control-induced arrhythmia. The increased efficacy of the combination therapy could not be attributed to higher plasma drug levels for the combination, since there was no significant difference in plasma levels for each drug when given alone or in combination. Thus, the increased efficacy most likely reflects a synergistic electropharmacologic effect of the 2 agents. These findings suggest that combination therapy with type 1A and 1B agents may be an important addition to pharmacologic therapy of life-threatening ventricular arrhythmias.

Lorcainide and norlorcainide

Echt and colleagues[68] from Stanford, California, studied 50 patients with drug-refractory (failed 7 ± 2 other drug trials) sustained VT or VF and treated them with oral lorcainide. Twenty-three patients underwent programmed stimulation both before and after oral lorcainide, and all 23 remained inducible, although VT cycle length was prolonged and mean arterial pressure was higher. Lorcainide was discontinued in 23 patients before hospital discharge because of death in 4 patients, side effects in 5 patients, spontaneous clinical arrhythmia recurrence in 6 patients, and ventricular tachyarrhythmias induced at electrophysiologic study in 8 patients. Twenty-seven patients were discharged on an average dosage of 169 ± 56 mg twice a day, including 15 in whom VT remained inducible. During long-term follow-up, the drug was discontinued in 15 patients; 3 because of side effects, 3 because of clinical nonfatal arrhythmia recurrence, 2 who selected other alternative therapy, and 7 patients who died suddenly due to ventricular tachyarrhythmias. Twelve patients remained on long-term lorcainide. The actuarial 1-year chance of being arrhythmia free was 39%, and 1-year cardio-vascular and arrhythmia survival rates were 57 and 60%, respectively. Based on these data, it was concluded that: 1) in this extremely drug-resistant patient population the clinical efficacy of lorcainide is low; 2) lorcainide should not be used empirically in such highly drug-resistant patients; 3) persistent ventricular tachyarrhythmia inducibility at electrophysiologic study implies a poor prognosis in patients treated with oral lorcainide; 4) the incidence of becoming noninducible during oral lorcainide therapy in highly drug-resistant patients appears low; and 5) for patients in whom the drug seems partially beneficial, it could be used in conjunction with a backup automatic implantable cardioverter/defibrillator.

Somberg and associates[69] from New York City carried out in 100 patients inducible at electrophysiologic studies serial drug testing with procainamide, lidocaine, and lorcainide to determine comparative efficacy. Acute intravenous administration was followed by repeat programmed electrical stimulation studies on separate days for each antiarrhythmic drug. Lorcainide prevented VT induction in 69% of the 100 patients, procainamide was effective in 50% of 75 patients studied, and lidocaine prevented VT induction in 30% of 53 patients. After programmed electrical stimulation and serial drug testing, 46 patients were started on lorcainide, 9 patients on procainamide, and 45 patients were started on other antiarrhythmic drug regimens. Seventy percent of the patients have remained on lorcainide therapy, and 47% have continued on other drug therapies started over a 21 ± 3-month mean follow-up period. Despite sleep-wake disturbances and a need for sedation at night, lorcainide therapy was tolerated well and remained an effective antiarrhythmic agent on prolonged administration.

Anastasiou-Nana and colleagues[70] from Salt Lake City, Utah, gave lorcainide long-term orally to 24 patients controlled initially with intravenous therapy—19 with frequent (>1/min) complex VPC on a baseline 24-hour Holter monitor and 5 with ongoing sustained VT or frequent paroxysmal sustained VT, for a mean of 13 months (range, 0.03–39). Long-term lorcainide was given in divided doses of 200–800 mg/day (median, 260; mean, 269 ± 90 mg/day). Response to long-term lorcainide therapy was assessed at a mean of both 26 days and 12 months. Median frequency of VPC decreased by 94 and 97% at the first and second lorcainide efficacy assessments, respectively. Couplets decreased by a median of 99 and 100% at the first and second assessments, respectively. VPC runs were suppressed by a median of 100% at both evaluations. Only 3 (16%) patients with complex VPC failed to respond to therapy. No recurrence during lorcainide occurred in the 5 patients with ongoing sustained VT or recurrent episodes of VT. Three continued on therapy, 1 was discontinued after corrective cardiac surgery, and 1 was discontinued because of side effects. P-R and QRS intervals increased mildly but significantly during therapy. Adverse effects were frequent and led to drug discontinuation in 6 (25%) because of severe insomnia in 2, dizziness and metallic taste, impotence, arrhythmia exacerbation, and CHF in 1 each. Thus, lorcainide is an effective antiarrhythmic long-term agent in patients initially responding to intravenous therapy, but is associated with a relatively high incidence of adverse effects.

Mead and associates[71] from Stanford, California, evaluated the long-term efficacy of lorcainide in suppressing chronic symptomatic VPC and examined the relation of arrhythmia suppression to plasma concentrations of lorcainide and norlorcainide. Fourteen patients were treated with lorcainide, 200–400 mg/day, 12 of whom achieved nearly complete suppression of arrhythmias after treatment for 1 year. Chronic lorcainide treatment was well tolerated; no patient discontinued treatment because of adverse effects.

Lorcainide and norlorcainide plasma concentrations remained stable after the first week of therapy. Antiarrhythmic activity persisted throughout the year. On drug withdrawal, the mean lorcainide washout half-life was 14 ± 4 hours and the mean norlorcainide washout half-life was 32 ± 9 hours. The return of arrhythmias occurred well after the lorcainide plasma concentration had decreased to subtherapeutic levels, suggesting an antiarrhythmic effect of norlorcainide. Thus, long-term lorcainide therapy is effective in treating chronic symptomatic VPC and is well tolerated by most patients. The metabolite norlorcainide appears to have antiarrhythmic activity independent of lorcainide.

Procainamide

Benson and colleagues[72] from Minneapolis, Minnesota, evaluated the efficacy of a single oral dose of procainamide to terminate paroxysmal tachycardia when procainamide was taken shortly after onset of tachycardia, a regimen termed "periodic procainamide." In 12 patients with nonlife-threatening tachycardia (orthodromic reciprocating tachycardia, 8 of 12; VT, 3 of 12: atrial flutter, 1 of 12) in whom intravenously administered procainamide terminated tachycardia, efficacy of a single oral dose of procainamide (25 mg/kg) was tested during electrophysiologic study. After oral administration of procainamide, tachycardia was terminated and could not be reinitiated in 11 of 12 patients. Time of tachycardia termination approximately coincided with the time peak serum concentration of procainamide after the single oral dose. Delayed response or failure of procainamide to terminate tachycardia was associated with delayed and diminished peak serum procainamide concentration. After evaluation, 10 responders were instructed to take a single dose of procainamide when tachycardia occurred. During a mean follow-up of 9 months (range, 2–17) 7 of 10 patients had an opportunity to use periodic procainamide on 1–>100 occasions; 4 of 10 patients did not have recurrence of tachycardia. Tachycardia was successfully terminated in 6 of 7 patients using the periodic regimen and could not be terminated on the first out-of-hospital use in 1 of 7 patients. The success of periodic procainamide was predicted during evaluation by rapid termination of tachycardia after oral administration.

Rae and coworkers[73] from Philadelphia, Pennsylvania, determined whether failure of procainamide to prevent initiation of ventricular tachyarrhythmias during electrophysiologic testing predicted failure of other antiarrhythmic regimens. Eighty-one consecutive patients with CAD whose VT remained inducible during procainamide administration were evaluated. Twenty-six (12%) of 216 subsequent drug studies were successful and at least 1 effective drug regimen was identified in 22 (27%) of the 81 patients. Drug success was related to the arrhythmia induced at baseline study: 7% of drug studies were successful in patients with sustained VT, 24% in patients with VF, and 29% in patients with nonsustained VT. An effective drug regimen was found in 11 (19%) of 59 patients with sustained VT, in 4 of 8 patients with VF, and in 7 of 14 patients with nonsustained VT. Failure of procainamide to suppress the arrhythmia correlated with failure of other agents used singly, but not in combination. Therefore when procainamide fails to prevent initiation of the arrhythmia in patients with inducible sustained VT, it is unlikely that other individual standard agents will be effective. However, combination regimens may suppress the arrhythmia and should be evaluated.

Oseran and associates[74] from Los Angeles, California, prospectively evaluated 20 patients with inducible sustained VT to determine whether the response to intravenous procainamide administration, as assessed by programmed ventricular stimulation, predicted the response to oral procainamide and oral quinidine treatment. Six patients (30%) responded to intravenous procainamide (<10 beats of inducible VT). Ten of 20 patients responded to oral quinidine and 5 responded to oral procainamide. Mean drug serum levels were 11 ± 2 $\mu g/ml$ for intravenous procainamide, 5.4 ± 0.8 $\mu g/ml$ for oral quinidine, and 12 ± 3 $\mu g/ml$ for oral procainamide. There was no significant difference in serum levels between those who responded and those who did not. Fifteen patients (75%) had a concordant drug response for intravenous and oral procainamide. Ten patients had a concordant response for intravenous procainamide and oral quinidine. Fifteen patients (75%) had a concordant drug response for oral procainamide and oral quinidine. Thus, in patients with sustained VT, the response to intravenous procainamide does not reliably predict the response to oral quinidine or oral procainamide, and serial day drug testing with these agents is necessary. Furthermore, high dose quinidine therapy may be more effective in controlling VT in these patients than procainamide.

N-acetylprocainamide

N-acetylprocainamide (NAPA), the N-acetylated metabolite of procainamide, has been shown to have antiarrhythmic properties in humans. Wynn and associates[75] from New York City studied in 12 patients with CAD who presented with cardiac arrest or documented sustained VT the antiarrhythmic properties of NAPA by programmed electrical stimulation. The 12 patients were aged 15–80 years (mean, 63) and they had a LVEF of 16–69% (mean, 33). All patients tested had inducible VT provoked by programmed electrical stimulation without antiarrhythmic therapy. Patients were then tested with procainamide, 1,000 mg administered intravenously. VT could be provoked after procainamide treatment in 8 of 10 patients. Twenty-four to 36 hours later NAPA was administered, 18 mg/kg body weight intravenously, and programmed electrical stimulation was performed after 20 minutes. NAPA did not significantly change heart rate, mean arterial BP, ECG intervals and AH or HV conduction times. The Q-T interval lengthened, but not significantly. The mean serum NAPA levels were 16 ± 4 $\mu g/ml$ in the group protected and not protected by NAPA. Five patients were discharged with NAPA therapy, 1.5 g orally every 8 hours. Two patients have been maintained with chronic NAPA therapy (10 ± 3 months), and 2 patients had breakthrough VT on follow-up Holter monitoring and alternative therapy was given. One patient died while taking oral therapy. NAPA demonstrates antiarrhythmic efficacy in preventing induction of VT by programmed electrical stimulation in a high-risk group of patients. During chronic oral therapy in some patients, NAPA appears to be well tolerated, with antiarrhythmic efficacy that may be enhanced with further upward dose titration.

Propafenone

Dinh and associates[76] from Little Rock, Arkansas, evaluated the efficacy of oral propafenone and oral quinidine in suppressing VPC in a double-blind, randomized study involving 25 men who were studied for 3 weeks. Twelve were randomized to the quinidine group and 13 to the propafenone group. Small doses of the drugs were administered for 1 week (200 mg of quinidine every 6 hours or 300 mg of propafenone every 12 hours) and large doses were administered for another week (400 mg of quinidine every 6 hours or 300 mg of propafenone every 8 hours). Strict criteria were used to define responders to antiarrhythmic therapy. For >85% reduction in total VPC/hour, during the low dose week, 36% in the quinidine group and 50% in the propafenone group were responders, and during the high dose week, 33% and 64% were responders. For >95% reduction of ventricular couplets/hour, during the low dose week, 45% in each group were responders, and during the high dose week, 56% and 60% were responders. For 100% abolition of VT beats/24 hours, during the low dose week, 60% in the quinidine group and 56% in the propafenone group were responders, and during the high dose week, 80% and 67% were responders. There was no significant difference in the 2 groups in incidence of side effects. This study shows comparable efficacy and tolerance of propafenone and quinidine for the control of ventricular arrhythmias in ambulatory patients with diverse forms of heart diseases.

Brodsky and colleagues[77] from Irvine, California, administered propafenone to 12 patients (10 with CAD) with ventricular tachyarrhythmias and LVEF <40%. Propafenone significantly reduced isolated VPC, couplets, and VT on ambulatory monitoring. Propafenone eliminated all exercise provocable VT and additionally abolished VT inducible by programmed stimulation in 5 of 6 patients. In 8 patients studied before and during therapy, there was no significant change in LVEF determined by RNA. Propafenone was discontinued in 3 patients due to side effects. All patients remain alive and without recurrence of clinically significant arrhythmia over a mean follow-up period of 14 months. Propafenone is an effective drug for the management of ventricular tachyarrhythmias and may be used in patients with impaired LV function.

In a double-blind, placebo-controlled study Naccarella and associates[78] from Bologna, Italy, compared the efficacy of propafenone to that of disopyramide. Sixteen patients with frequent and complex VPC were studied by serial 24-hour ambulatory monitoring, while they were receiving both propafenone, 300 mg, and disopyramide, 200 mg, every 8 hours. A reduction in the mean frequency of VPC/hour, in comparison to the placebo period, $574 \pm 535–100 \pm 130$, was observed after propafenone and $629 \pm 455–231 \pm 280$ after disopyramide. A >70% reduction in VPC in comparison to placebo was observed in 11 of 14 after propafenone and 9 of 15 after disopyramide. A ≥90% reduction in VPC was observed in 9 of 16 with propafenone and in 4 of 15 with disopyramide. The suppression of complex VPC (repetitive, polymorphic, or >5/minute with bigeminy) was observed in 11 of 14 after propafenone and in 9 of 14 after disopyramide. The abolition of nonsustained VT was observed in 6 of 6 and 3 of 5, respectively, after propafenone and disopyramide. A lower incidence of side effects, 4 of 16 -vs- 8 of 16, was observed during propafenone than during disopyramide treatment. It was concluded that propafenone, in a dose of 900 mg daily, is more effective than disopyramide, in a dose of 600 mg daily, in the treatment of frequent and complex VPC and nonsustained VT. Propafenone also showed a lower incidence of side effects.

Quinidine

Duff and associates[79] from Calgary, Canada, used a computer simulation to devise quinidine sulfate infusions to produce pseudo-steady state concentrations in the low and high (14 μM/L) therapeutic ranges, avoiding high peak concentrations. Using this infusion, efficacy and electrophysiologic actions of quinidine sulfate were assessed in 21 patients with sustained inducible VT when concentrations were 12.6 ± 11 μM/L (mean, $\pm$SD) and 18 ± 9 μM/L. Although mean concentrations approximated target levels, there was substantial individual variation. A reciprocal linear relation was noted between resultant serum concentrations and drug-free EF. Transient hypotension occurred early in 3 patients, 2 of whom had a normal LVEF. No hemodynamic compromise was seen in patients with LVEF <30%. Induced VT was suppressed in 5 patients at low concentrations and in an additional 4 at high concentrations (total, 9 of 21, 43%). Concentration-dependent changes in the ventricular effective refractory period of the beat induced by S_3 paralleled antiarrhythmic efficacy. Independent of response or lack of response to intravenous quinidine, 17 patients received gradually increasing oral quinidine dosages adjusted to reproduce plasma levels that had been effective during intravenous administration, or to maximal well-tolerated dosage (if side effects occurred). VT was still inducible during oral treatment in 4 of 5 patients in whom VT had been suppressed during the intravenous infusion. Side effects frequently limited oral dosage to less than that required to reproduce effective concentrations. In contrast, 11 of 12 patients who did not respond to intravenous quinidine also did not respond to its oral preparation. Response to intravenous quinidine also accurately predicted whether response would ultimately occur to any oral antiarrhythmic agent. In conclusion, acute drug testing with quinidine is safe and efficacious.

Morganroth and Hunter[80] from Philadelphia, Pennsylvania, performed a comparative, fixed-dose, parallel, randomized, blinded trial to define the efficacy and safety of a new once-a-day quinidine preparation, Quiniday, at 1,200 mg/day, and compared it to quinidine sulfate (as Quinora, 300 mg 4 times daily, and Quinidex Extentabs, 600 mg twice daily) and to quinidine gluconate (as Quinaglute Dura-Tabs, 648 mg twice daily). After placebo washout from all prior antiarrhythmic agents, 76 patients with at least 30 VPC/hour on 48-hour ambulatory monitoring were randomized to 3 weeks of treatment with 1 of the 4 study drugs. There was no difference in the etiologic, demographic, New York Heart Association therapeutic classification, or ventricular arrhythmia frequency at baseline between the patients randomized to the 4 groups. There was no statistically significant difference between the percent efficacy for VPC reduction on any drug compared with baseline or in the percent efficacy of reduction in beats of VT. There was no difference between the 4 agents in terms of types of side effects noted nor in their overall prevalence or need for premature discontinuation of therapy. This study demonstrated that a variety of quinidine preparations exists that do not differ in terms of their efficacy or safety, but that a long-acting, once-a-day preparation (Quiniday) was as effective and safe as other forms of quinidine despite its dosing schedule.

To determine the prevalence and importance of proarrhythmic events secondary to the initiation of quinidine therapy in outpatients with benign or potentially lethal ventricular arrhythmias, Morganroth and Horowitz[81] from Philadelphia, Pennsylvania, retrospectively reviewed data from 360 patients treated with quinidine as part of 3 outpatient drug trials. These patients had ≥30 VPC/hour during placebo treatment and had no evidence of unstable clinical states, hypokalemia, digitalis toxicity, AF, or a prolonged Q-T interval (>0.50 second). The quinidine dose varied from 200–400 mg 4 times a day for 2–4 weeks. Proarrhythmic effect was defined on Holter monitoring as a 400% increase in frequency of VPC, the presence of new VT not previously identified, or a 10-fold increase in the number of beats of VT. There was no difference in the demography, response to quinidine therapy or side effects on quinidine among the 3 trials. Six of 360 patients (2%) had a proarrhythmic response and no patient had hemodynamic symptoms, required hospitalization, or died from the proarrhythmic event. Thus, quinidine can be safely initiated to outpatients who meet the inclusion criteria cited herein.

Kim and associates[82] from New York City studied the efficacy and tolerance of quinidine and procainamide individually and in combination in 19 patients with frequent VPC. During single-drug treatment, the maximum tolerated dose of quinidine without extracardiac dose-related side effects was 1.6 ± 0.21 g/day and that of procainamide was 4.1 ± 1.05 g/day. During combination therapy with smaller doses of quinidine (1.2 ± 0.3 g/day) and procainamide (2.8 ± 1.0 g/day), no patient had side effects. Before treatment, all patients had frequent (>60/hour) VPC and 17 had VT on Holter monitoring. The frequency of VPC was reduced to 22 ± 19% with quinidine, 47 ± 40% with procainamide, and 9 ± 11% with combination therapy (combination -vs- procainamide or quinidine alone). Individually, an effective regimen (>83% reduction of VPC and abolition of VT) was found in 5 patients (26%) receiving quinidine alone at maximal tolerated dose, in 4 (21%) receiving procainamide alone at maximal tolerated dose, and in 14 (74%) receiving combination therapy. Thus, the antiarrhythmic effects of quinidine and procainamide are additive. When quinidine or procainamide is ineffective because dose-related extracardiac side effects limit the maximal tolerated dose, combination therapy in smaller and tolerable doses avoids side effects and is more effective than either drug alone at the maximal tolerated dose.

Sotalol

Sotalol is a unique β-blocker that lengthens cardiac repolarization and effective refractory period (ERP). Its efficacy after intravenous (1.5 mg/kg) and oral (160–480 mg twice daily) administration was evaluated by Nademanee and colleagues[83] from Los Angeles, California, in 37 patients with refractory recurrent VT/VF. Thirty-five patients, 33 with inducible VT/VF, underwent electrophysiologic testing. Intravenous sotalol lengthened the ERP in the atrium by 25%, AV node by 25%, the ventricle by 15%. It also significantly lengthened the sinus node recovery time, corrected Q-T interval, and the A-H interval, but not the H-V interval. Sotalol prevented reinduction of VT/VF in 15 patients (46%). Twenty-five of the 33 patients (15 with positive results of electrophysiologic tests; 10 with negative results) were given oral sotalol. The drug was ineffective in 7 (28%) and aggravated arrhythmia in 1. In 4 patients sotalol was withdrawn because of side effects; arrhythmias recurred late in 2 (8%). Eleven patients have continued on oral sotalol over a mean follow-up period of 9 months. Sotalol reduced total VPC count on the Holter ECG by 73%, paired VPC by 89%, and VT by 95%. In 11 (52%) total reduction in VPC was at least 85%, and incidence of paired and tachycardia beats was reduced ≥90% (group A). In the remaining 10 patients VPC suppression was not significant (group B). Group A included 9 patients with nonreinducible VT/VF and 2 in whom it was reinduced; in group B, 8 of 10 patients had reinducible VT/VF. The prevention of reinducible VT/VF by intravenous sotalol and suppression of spontaneously occurring arrhythmias by the oral drug were both predictive of long-term drug efficacy. Sotalol is a significance advance in the short- and long-term management of life-threatening ventricular arrhythmias.

In a multicenter open, randomized, crossover study Lidell and colleagues[84] from Uppsala and Danderyd, Sweden, Seinäjoki, Finland, and Stavanager, Norway, examined the efficacy of sotalol compared with procainamide in 33 patients with frequent chronic VPC. A 75% reduction in VPC/24 hours (2 24-hour recordings) was arbitrarily considered to constitute an adequate therapeutic effect. Sotalol was started at a dose of 160 mg once daily for 1 week, followed by a 24-hour recording. In the absence of any therapeutic effect, the same procedure was repeated with 320, 480, and 640 mg daily. Procainamide, 1 g 3-times daily, was given or, if plasma concentrations were insufficient, 1.5 g 3 times/day for 1 week. VPC control was obtained in 22 (67%) patients on sotalol, including all 12 with CAD. Procainamide was successful in 13 (39%) patients. Effects on the number of attacks of VT were achieved by both drugs in those patients in whom VPC were reduced by ≥75%. Sotalol caused side effects in 5 patients, who could not accept planned increases in dosage. Side effects were noted by 12 patients with procainamide. Nine patients responded to both drugs, 7 to neither. Thirteen responded to sotalol only and 4 to procainamide only. It was concluded that sotalol is a useful alternative to procainamide in controlling chronic VPC, especially in patients with CAD.

Tocainide

Morganroth and associates[85] from Philadelphia, Pennsylvania, Rochester, New York, and Denver, Colorado, compared the antiarrhythmic efficacy and safety of oral tocainide hydrochloride and quinidine sulfate in a double-blind, 3-center, parallel trial involving 133 patients with benign and potentially lethal ventricular arrhythmias. Baseline demographic, etiologic, functional, and ventricular arrhythmia data were not significantly different between the 2 groups. Two weeks of an initial placebo period were followed by 8 weeks of active drug treatment, concluding with 4 weeks of washout. Frequent 24-hour ambulatory ECG monitoring was used to judge efficacy. Ten of 27 patients (37%) receiving tocainide and 12 of 24 patients receiving quinidine had a 75% reduction with drug treatment compared with the initial placebo period. Total abolition of VT occurred in 6 of 16 patients (37%) receiving tocainide and 6 of 13 patients (43%) receiving quinidine. Conditions that required discontinuation of therapy occurred in 18 of 67 patients (27%) receiving quinidine. More patients had dizziness during tocainide treatment and diarrhea during quinidine treatment. Quinidine caused a prolongation in the Q-T interval (0.03 s), tocainide caused a slight reduction (0.01 s). No important changes in vital signs or laboratory measurements were observed in LVEF when measured. Thus, tocainide, the new oral analog of lidocaine, appears to be as safe as quinidine but is slightly less effective in suppressing ventricular arrhythmias.

Verapamil

Woelfel and associates[86] from Chapel Hill, North Carolina, determined the antiarrhythmic efficacy of verapamil by serial treadmill testing in 16 patients with reproducible exercise-induced VT. Twelve patients responded to verapamil, 0.2 mg/kg intravenously; in 8 of the 12 responders, an oral verapamil regimen of 160–320 mg given every 8 hours also prevented exercise-induced VT. Plasma verapamil concentration was significantly higher in the responders than in the nonresponders to intravenous verapamil, but levels were similar in responders and nonresponders to oral therapy. The 8 responders to the oral drug were followed while receiving verapamil therapy for 6–22 months (mean, 15), and exercise-induced VT did not recur in any patient. Five of the 8 responders also had concomitant spontaneous VT unrelated to exercise, which verapamil suppressed initially as well: 4 remained free of spontaneous VT and 1 patient had recurrence of spontaneous VT.

Danger of cardioversion with therapeutic serum digoxin levels

Mann and coworkers[87] from San Diego, California, determined the risk of cardioversion-induced ventricular arrhythmias in patients with therapeutic serum levels of digoxin. Nineteen patients (average age, 61 ± 12 years; mean ± SD) undergoing elective direct cardioversion for AF were evaluated. Each patient had a therapeutic serum digoxin level (range, 0.5–1.9 ng/ml; mean, 1.1 ± 0.5) at the time of cardioversion. Patients with acute myocardial ischemia, important electrolyte abnormalities, or those requiring class I antiarrhythmic agents for control of ventricular or supraventricular arrhythmias were excluded. In these studies, an ambulatory ECG was recorded 24 hours before and 6 hours after cardioversion. No patient developed serious ventricular arrhythmias in the immediate 3-hour period after cardioversion. There were no differences in the frequency of VPC or couplets before and after cardioversion. In addition, there was no significant relation between the strength of the applied shock and the development of postcardioversion arrhythmias. Thus, patients with therapeutic serum levels of digoxin may safely undergo cardioversion.

Antitachycardia pacemaker

Echt and colleagues[88] from Stanford, California, reviewed their clinical experience, complications, and survival in the first 70 patients with automatic implantable cardioverter/defibrillator. Seventy patients received the automatic implantable defibrillator, 5 original devices and 72 modified second-generation devices using only bipolar rate sensing and delivering an R-wave synchronous cardioverting/defibrillating shock, for either VT or VF. The primary clinical arrhythmia was sustained VT in 32 patients, VF in 20 patients, and both VT and VF in 18 patients. Before implantation of the device, the patients had survived 3.1 arrhythmic episodes, including 1.9 cardiac arrests, and had received 4 antiarrhythmic drugs without improvement. Sixty-eight patients ultimately received devices. After a follow-up period of 8.9 months (range, 1–33), 37 patients received 463 discharges. Inability to determine the precise reason for most discharges and the unpleasant nature of the discharges were the major clinical problems encountered. Complications included postoperative death (1 patient), lead problems (6 patients), inadequate energy requiring explanation (2 patients), and pocket infection (1 patient). Life-table analysis revealed 6- and 12-month cardiovascular survival of 95 and 90% and sudden death survival of 98 and 98%. In the investigators' experience, survival with the automatic implantable cardioverter/defibrillator exceeds that with other forms of therapy.

Herre and coworkers[89] from Houston, Texas, used permanent pacemakers capable of triggered ventricular stimulation in 28 patients with a history of sustained VT or VF. Noninvasive programmed ventricular stimulation was performed on 125 occasions during follow-up periods ranging from 1–25 months and was used to determine the efficacy of the antiarrhythmic drug therapy, dose or dosage changes, and LV endocardial resection. Drug or dosage changes based on noninvasive programmed ventricular stimulation were made in 19 of the 28 patients; 126 episodes of spontaneous sustained VT were terminated noninvasively in 9 patients. Thus, a permanent pacemaker capable of triggered ventricular stimulation is useful in the treatment of patients with VT or VF that is otherwise difficult to control.

Since there has been no controlled prospective study of the comparative efficacy of transvenous cardioversion and rapid ventricular pacing in terminating sustained VT in the same patient population, Saksena and coworkers[90] from Newark, New Jersey, performed a prospective randomized crossover study to evaluate the efficacy of transvenous cardioversion and rapid ventricular pacing for termination of induced VT in patients with spontaneous VT and organic heart disease: 62 episodes of VT were induced in 15 patients during electrophysiologic studies. All patients underwent a preselected electrical therapy protocol in a randomized crossover sequence. Transvenous cardioversion was performed by an incremental protocol of 3 sequential shocks and 6 asynchronous sequential bursts of rapid ventricular pacing were used. The mean cycle length of VT for the study population was 391 msec. The morphology of the tachycardia was left BBB in 27, right BBB in 32, and indeterminate in 3. Characteristics of VT terminated by the 2 techniques were comparable. Rate of success for termination of tachycardia with the 2 methods also was comparable (transvenous cardioversion, 83%; rapid ventricular pacing, 80%). The incidence of acceleration of VT per episode with these preselected protocols also was comparable. Transient SVT was more frequent after transvenous cardioversion than after rapid ventricular pacing (23 -vs- 3%). Significant patient discomfort occurred only after transvenous cardioversion (57%). These investigators concluded that transvenous cardioversion and rapid ventricular pacing have comparable and usually concordant efficacy for termination of VT. Transvenous cardioversion results in a higher incidence of postcardioversion arrhythmias and poorer patient tolerance than does rapid ventricular pacing.

LV endocardial resection

Holt and associates[91] from Birmingham, UK, produced an ECG atlas of VT by pacing 27 epicardial sections of the heart and the mitral papillary muscles to simulate focal ventricular arrhythmias and simultaneously recorded their 12-lead ECG appearances (Fig. 3-7). In 5% of 129 patients undergoing cardiac surgery, all 27 epicardial sites were paced at operation and in 124, individual sections were paced postoperatively with temporary epicardial wires and the ECGs analyzed in terms of frontal and horizontal plan QRS axis, maximum limb lead QRS amplitude, and QRS duration. Each ventricular region paced produced a distinctive 12-lead QRS amplitude, and QRS duration.

Miller and associates[92] from Philadelphia, Pennsylvania, performed mapping-guided subendocardial resection for control of arrhythmias from 3 weeks to 10 years after AMI in 119 patients with drug refractory VT. Patients were separated into 2 groups: those treated early (within 4 months, group I) and those treated later (>1 year, group II) after AMI. There were 32 patients in group I and 72 in group II. Both groups had similar clinical, angiographic, and hemodynamic characteristics. Patients in group I had VT with a shorter mean cycle length than patients in group II (322 ± 71 -vs- 349 ± 88 ms). The groups did not differ with respect to operative mortality (12 -vs- 7%), late mortality (31 -vs- 33%; mean follow-up, 23 months), or frequency with which subendocardial resection without any adjunctive therapy prevented postoperative spontaneous or inducible VT (21 -vs- 34%). Group I was further divided into patients who underwent subendocardial resection within 1 month of AMI (n = 7) and those who underwent subendocardial resection >2 months of AMI (n = 14). Although patients in group I were characterized by having more spontaneous morphologically distinct tachycardias, their operative mortality, total mortality, and surgical success rates were comparable to those in group II. The results of the study suggest that in a patient population with drug-refractory VT after AMI: 1) there are no clini-

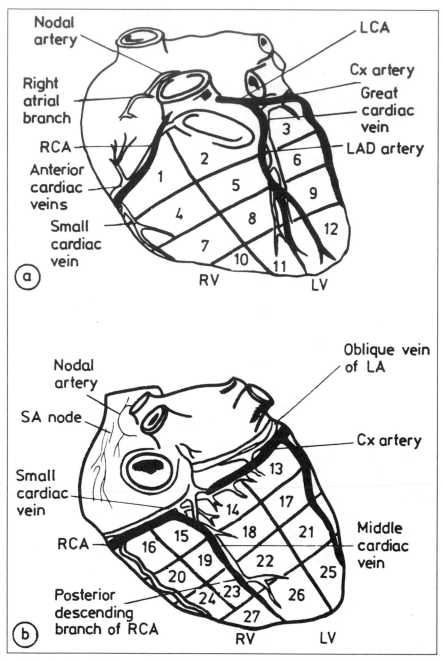

Fig. 3-7. Diagram of the anterior and posterior ventricular epicardium divided in 27 sections, 12 anteriorly and 15 posteriorly in (a) the sternocostal aspect and (b) the diaphragmatic aspect. RCA, right coronary artery; LCA, left coronary artery; Cx, circumflex; SA, sinoatrial; LA, left atrium; RV, right ventricle; LV, left ventricle. Reproduced with permission from Holt et al.[91]

cal, angiographic, or hemodynamic variables that distinguish patients in whom VT develops early (≤4 months) from those in whom it develops late (>1 year) after AMI; 2) VT early after AMI tends to have faster rates and increased number of distinct morphologies; and 3) subendocardial resection early (≤4 months, but even within 1 or 2 months) after AMI is associated with acceptable operative mortality and control of VT.

Miller and colleagues[93] from Philadelphia, Pennsylvania, evaluated 55 patients with sustained VT caused by prior AMI to determine patterns of ventricular activation in these patients. Mapping data obtained during intra-operative endocardial activation mapping were utilized to determine the pattern of endocardial activation during VT. Of 122 tachycardias, 101 had endocardial activation as follows: a) in 90 (89%), endocardial activation spread centrifugally from the site of origin and b) 11 (11%) had a continuous loop of electrical activity around an aneurysm. There were no significant differences in the preoperative clinical characteristics, operative survivals, or the frequency of cure of the tachycardia between patients having VT of the continuous loop pattern -vs- those with centrifugal spread of activation. These data indicate that most sustained VT is characterized by centrifugal spread of endocardial activation from a site of origin that is small. They also suggest that guided ablative surgery may abolish the tachycardia circuit in these patients and in patients with continuous loop tachycardias; in the latter group, presumably a critical portion of the circuit is removed by ablative surgery.

CARDIAC ARREST

In persons ≤21 years of age

Neuspiel and Kuller[94] from Pittsburgh, Pennsylvania, studied the descriptive epidemiology of sudden nontraumatic death from persons aged 1–21 years in a defined population. In 9 years, the 207 deaths in this group (4.6/100,000 population/per year) comprised 22% of nontraumatic mortality. Age-specific rates were highest between 1 and 4 years (mainly infections and undetermined causes) and 14 and 21 years (mainly cardiovascular, epilepsy, intracranial hemorrhage, and asthma). Nonwhite rates were higher than whites, and white males had higher rates than white females. Referral for medicolegal evaluation was inconsistent. Only 18% died at university hospitals. Infections included lower respiratory tract and septic shock. The main cardiac diagnosis was myocarditis. Most epilepsy deaths were unwitnessed and had absent or low anticonvulsant levels. Eighty-five cases had a known associated chronic illness and 111 reported prodromal symptoms. Prevention of these events requires improved identification and management of antecedent conditions. Fifty-one individuals died with cardiac lesions including 14 (27%) with myocarditis, 7 (14%) with cardiomyopathy, 6 (12%) with previously diagnosed arrhythmias, 5 (10%) with "myocardial fibrosis," 3 (6%) with coronary artery abnormalities, 3 (6%) with aortic aneurysm, 2 (4%) with Ebstein's anomaly, and 1 each of 11 other congenital and acquired defects. The arrhythmias were 2 prolonged QT syndrome, 1 WPW syndrome type B, 1 congenital AV block, and 2 nonspecific. Of the 51 patients with fatal cardiovascular conditions, 21 had the cardiovascular abnormality diagnosed clinically before death.

Nonfatal cardiac arrest out of hospital

Ritchie and associates[95] from Seattle, Washington, studied 154 survivors of out-of-hospital VF with CAD by RNA an average of 4.2 months after VF. All patients were studied at rest, and 91 of them also were studied using supine bicycle exercise. Clinical histories and a 24-hour ambulatory ECG also were assessed, and patients were followed for an average of 3.1 years after ventriculography. The mean LVEF at rest was $40 \pm 16\%$; in 34% of patients, it was ≤30%; in 37%, 31–50%; and in 29%, >50%. Regional LV wall motion was normal in 18%. The most severe segmental abnormality was hypokinesia in 22%, akinesia in 45%, and dyskinesia in 14%. Wall motion abnormalities were usually located at the apex. During exercise, only 3% of patients (3 of 91) had a normal increase in EF of >5%, and the main EF decreased from 42–38%. New exercise-induced wall motion abnormalities occurred in 30%. During the follow-up period, 54 patients died (35%): 48 from cardiac causes and 42 from unexpected and sudden causes. Predictors of death included EF at rest, presence of akinesia or dyskinesia on the ventriculogram at rest, the number of abnormal LV segments, history of CHF, history of AMI, absence of AMI at the time of VF and the presence of ventricular arrhythmia. In a stepwise regression analysis, EF at rest, arrhythmia frequency, history of CHF, and absence of AMI at the time of VF were selected as independently predictive for death, with EF selected first. When all clinical variables were forced into the model, only EF added significant predictive information; other radionuclide measurements and ambulatory ECG arrhythmia frequencies were of no or borderline significance. In conclusion, the radionuclide LVEF at rest is the best predictor of death in patients resuscitated from out-of-hospital VF. The diversity of rest and exercise levels of LV function suggest multifactorial pathophysiologic mechanisms in this syndrome.

Goldstein and colleagues[96] from Ann Arbor, Michigan, added ambulatory ECG observations obtained within the first 3 months of cardiac arrest to the previous clinical predictors of death. Among 227 such patients in their study, 20% died at 1 year, and 50% were dead in slightly >3 years. Predictors of death were related to use of digitalis, elevated blood urea nitrogen, cerebral vascular accident, previous AMI, and age. In a subset of 103 patients in whom ambulatory ECG recordings were available within 3 months of the arrest event, the presence of complexity and high-frequency VPC (>25/hour) were added to the mortality predictors of digitalis and diuretic therapy and elevated blood urea nitrogen (Fig. 3-8). An almost equal number of patients died suddenly and nonsuddenly. Predictors of sudden death were treatment with quinidine and paired VPC. Occurrence of arrhythmias was an important addition to the previous mortality predictors related to LV dysfunction.

To determine whether LV function, coronary anatomy, or electrophysiologic characteristics could differentiate patients with sudden death from those with VT without sudden death, Stevenson and coworkers[97] from Maastricht, The Netherlands, compared results of cardiac angiography and programmed electrical stimulation in 42 patients referred for evaluation of sustained VT or surviving "aborted" sudden death for >9 days after AMI. By univariate analysis, there were no differences between patients with sudden death and those with VT in age, time from AMI to VT or sudden death, EF (0.31 -vs- 0.29), or the number of patients with a major area of contracting myocardium supplied by an artery with a ≥50% or a ≥70% diameter stenosis. Thirty-six percent of patients with sudden death but no patient with VT had 2 separate areas of AMI. During programmed electrical stimulation, a sustained ventricular arrhythmia was initiated in 100% of patients with VT and 73% of patients with nonfatal cardiac arrest and rapidly produced syncope in 67% of patients with "sudden death" but in only 5% of those with VT. The difference was due to the more frequent initiation of rapid polymorphic VT of VF and to the shorter VT cycle length when monomorphic VT was induced in the group with sudden death. No difference was found in the number of extrastimuli required for initiation of sustained ventricular arrhythmia.

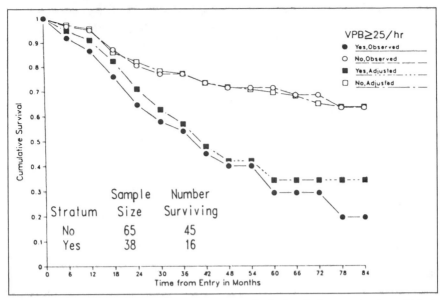

Fig. 3-8. Survival experience among 103 patients who had ambulatory ECG data within 3 months after cardiac arrest and who survived the first 3 months of follow-up. Patients were grouped by frequency of VPC (<25/hr and ≥25/hr). Reproduced with permission from Goldstein et al.[96]

Ambulatory ECG recordings at time of fatal cardiac arrest

The relation between arrhythmias at cardiac arrest and the outcome of arrest is poorly understood. Milner and associates[98] from Baltimore, Maryland, reviewed Holter monitor tracings of 13 patients after they sustained an in-hospital cardiac arrest during ambulatory ECG monitoring. All had a prior cardiac arrest or cardiac-induced syncope. Twelve patients had VT as the initial arrest arrhythmia and 1 patient had bradycardia followed by VF. VT degenerated to VF in 10 of 12 patients after a mean interval of 96 ± 31 seconds. The number of VT runs increased significantly during the hour immediately preceding arrest. Despite prompt resuscitation efforts in 12 patients, only 6 survived. The 6 survivors and 6 nonsurvivors were not different with regard to age, EF, extent of coronary narrowing, and time to first defibrillation. However, degeneration to VF within 30 seconds of arrest (5 of 6 nonsurvivors and 1 of 6 survivors) and a slower rate of VT at the onset of arrest (166 beats/minute in nonsurvivors and 227 beats/minute in survivors) were associated with unsuccessful resuscitation.

Usefulness of prehospital cardiopulmonary resuscitation

Cummins and Eisenberg[99] from Seattle, Washington, summarized evidence that early, bystander-initiated cardiopulmonary resuscitation (CPR) saves lives. From review of quasi-experimental studies in which a control group could be recognized, the balance of evidence leans heavily in favor of the concept that early, bystander-initiated CPR leads to better survival rates than delayed, emergency medical system (either paramedics or physicians) initiated CPR. No control study was located that suggested early CPR does harm.

During anesthesia

Keenan and Boyan[100] from Richmond, Virginia, studied patients who had cardiac arrest due solely to anesthesia in a large university hospital over a 15-year period. There were 27 cardiac arrests among 163,240 anesthetics given, for a 15-year incidence of 1.7/10,000 anesthetics: 14 patients (0.9/ 10,000) subsequently died. Detailed examination of the data from these 27 patients revealed that the pediatric age group had a 3-fold higher risk than adults and that the risk for emergency patients was 6 times that for elective patients. Failure to provide adequate ventilation caused almost half of the anesthetic cardiac arrests, and one-third resulted from absolute overdose of an inhalation agent. Hemodynamic instability in very ill patients was an association in 22%. Specific errors in anesthetic management could be identified in 75%. Progressive bradycardia preceding the arrest was observed in all but 1 patient.

This article was followed by an editorial entitled, "Cardiac Arrest: Signal of Anesthetic Mishap," by Vandam.[101]

SYNCOPE

Beder and associates[102] from Cleveland, Ohio, evaluated 6 children for syncope of unknown etiology. All had undergone previous neurologic evaluation, which was normal. Cardiac examination, chest roentgenograms, and 2-D echo also were normal in all patients. Abnormal noninvasive findings in 5 patients included Mobitz type II AV block (1 patient), sinus bradycardia (3 patients), and SVT (1 patient). Four patients had ≥1 abnormal findings at invasive electrophysiologic study, including evidence of sinus node dysfunction (3 patients), AV node dysfunction (3 patients), and distal His-Purkinje system disease (2 patients). All children had normal right-sided heart hemodynamics. It was concluded that arrhythmias are an important cause of syncope in some children with an otherwise normal heart when neurologic causes have been excluded.

Hysing and Grendahl[103] from Oslo, Norway, performed ambulatory 24-hour ECG and a follow-up by questionnaire after 2 years in 174 patients referred to a general hospital for unexplained syncope. The ambulatory ECG showed sinus rhythm in 113 patients, AF in 15, AV block in 10, sinoatrial block in 14, tachycardia or frequent VPC in 21, and no recording in 1. Ten patients received a permanent pacemaker and 7 were given antiarrhythmic drug therapy. Of the 174 patients, 121 responded to the questionnaire: 37 were dead and 16 were lost to follow-up. Of the 121 responders, 36 reported multiple episodes of syncope in the follow-up period and another 17, 1 episode of syncope. Eleven additional patients received a permanent pacemaker during the follow-up period.

Olshansky and coworkers[104] from Iowa City, Iowa, studied 105 patients to determine the frequency of inducible tachycardia in patients presenting with syncope whose noninvasive evaluation failed to reveal a cause; 97 patients were followed for a mean period of 26 months. Sixty-eight patients (65%) did not have inducible tachycardia, and 60 of the 68 patients were followed long-term and 12 (20%) had recurrent syncope. In contrast, VT or

SVT was inducible in 37 patients (35%). Three patients with inducible VT died suddenly or were resuscitated from cardiac arrest, and an additional 7 had recurrent syncope. Thus, among these patients, the recurrence rate for syncope was 27%. Of 23 patients undergoing effective therapy as predicted by electrophysiologic testing, 3 (14%) had a recurrent event. Ineffective therapy as judged by electrophysiologic testing was associated with more frequent recurrence of syncope or cardiac arrest (7 of 13 patients). Thus, these data indicate that tachycardia may be induced in patients with syncope of unknown origin whether or not organic heart disease is present. Effective treatment of inducible tachycardia often prevents the recurrence of syncope.

Doherty and associates[105] from Philadelphia, Pennsylvania, completed electrophysiologic studies in 119 patients with unexplained syncope (82%) or presyncope (18%). Symptoms were recurrent in 72% of the patients; 52% had structural heart disease. Forty-one patients had normal electrophysiologic study results and 78 had electrophysiologic abnormalities (VT in 31, induced AF in 17, vasovagal syncope in 8, hypersensitive carotid sinus syndrome in 7, SVT in 6, heart block in 5, and sick sinus syndrome in 4). The presence of structural heart disease and previous AMI were the only clinical or ECG predictors of a positive electrophysiologic study response. Therapy was guided by electrophysiologic study and patients were followed for 27 ± 20 months (mean ± SD). In the patients with negative electrophysiologic study results, 76 ± 11% were symptom-free at follow-up, compared with 68 ± 10% in the group with positive electrophysiologic study responses. No clinical variables helped to predict remission in the absence of therapy. One patient in the negative electrophysiologic study response group and 2 patients in the electrophysiologic study positive group died suddenly (cumulative survival 94 ± 4%). Total cardiovascular mortality was 13% in the positive electrophysiologic study response group. Thus, certain clinical characteristics are helpful in selecting patients for study. Electrophysiologically guided therapy is associated with a recurrence and sudden death rate similar to an untreated control group. Electrophysiologic study can identify a subgroup of patients at low risk of recurrence of symptoms and sudden death in the absence of therapy.

Teichman and colleagues[106] from New York City examined the diagnostic yield and therapeutic efficacy of electrophysiologic studies in 150 patients with syncope of undetermined origin (SUO). SUO was defined as those syncopal or near-syncopal events remaining unexplained after a standardized, noninvasive evaluation that included a history, physical examination, routine laboratory screening, electroencephalogram, nuclear brain scan or computed tomography scan, 12-lead ECG, chest radiograph, orthostatic vital signs, bedside carotid sinus massage, and ≥24 hours of continuous ECG monitoring. The 150 SUO patients included 95 men and 55 women (mean age, 62 years); 35 had recurrent SUO, 75 had organic heart disease, and 129 (86%) had an abnormal ECG. There were 162 abnormal electrophysiologic findings that could explain the SUO uncovered in 112 patients, a diagnostic yield of 75%: 1 finding in 71 patients, 2 findings in 32, and 3 in 9. These findings were: His-Purkinje disease in 49 patients (30%), inducible ventricular arrhythmias in 36 (22%), AV nodal disease in 20 (12%), sinus node disease in 19 (12%), inducible supraventricular arrhythmias in 18 (11%), carotid sinus hypersensitivity in 15 (9%), and hypervagotonia in 5 (3%). When electrophysiologic study findings were classified as clearly abnormal or borderline, 54 patients had ≥1 clearly abnormal finding, a diagnostic yield of 36%. Subgroups of patients presenting with only 1 SUO event, no evidence of organic heart disease, or normal baseline ECG all had substantial diagnostic yields during electrophysiologic studies. Follow-up data in 137 patients

(91%) (mean, 31 months) showed recurrences in 16 of 34 patients (47%) without and 15 of 103 (15%) with electrophysiologic findings despite therapy directed by electrophysiologic testing. This study and a review of the literature indicate that electrophysiologic testing is useful in elucidating the causes of SUO and directing therapy. A significant number of patients benefit from electrophysiologic studies, even when only clearly abnormal findings are considered diagnostic, when only a single syncopal event has occurred, or whether or not organic heart disease or an abnormal ECG is present.

To assess whether findings on ambulatory monitoring not obtained during syncope can be used to indicate the results that are found on electrophysiologic testing in patients with recurrent syncope, Reiffel and colleagues[107] from New York City reported on the ambulatory monitoring records of 59 such patients referred for electrophysiologic testing. Although 29 patients had abnormalities on electrophysiologic testing, 13 of which were severe, in only 6 were the findings suggested by the abnormalities recorded during ambulatory monitoring. Twenty-one patients had concordance between electrophysiologic testing and ambulatory monitoring results, but in 15 of the 21, results of both tests were normal. Severe abnormalities were more frequently detected in the patients by electrophysiologic testing than by ambulatory monitoring, especially if patients had organic heart disease.

TABLE 3-2.   *Causes of syncope—Yale patients*

	#
Vasovagal/psychogenic	80
Vasovagal episode	64
Gastrointestinal bleeding	6
Duodenal ulcer	3
Gastric ulcer	1
Gastritis	1
Diverticulosis	1
Postural hypotension	5
Diarrhea	3
Intravenous pyelographic dye reaction	1
Familial	1
Hyperventilation	2
Tussive syncope	2
Micturition syncope	1
Cardiac	15
VT	6
Complete heart block	3
Severe bradycardia	2
AMI	2
Aortic stenosis	1
Rapid AF	1
Metabolic/drug	7
Hypoglycemia	3
Ethanol intoxication	3
Nitrate syncope	1
Central nervous system	5
Seizure	2
Vertebrobasilar insufficiency	3
Unknown	69
Total	176

To evaluate 2 published sets of prognostic classifications for patients with syncope, Eagle and associates[108] from New Haven, Connecticut, and Boston, Massachusetts, studied 176 consecutive patients who presented to an emergency room with syncope (Table 3-2). The 2 previously published studies to which this report compares were by Day et al (*American Journal of Medicine*, 1982; 73:15–23) and Kapoor and associates (*New England Journal of Medicine*, 1983; 309:197–204). Although relatively few of the 176 patients had cardiac syncope, these data confirm their high 1-year mortality. At the other extreme, it also was confirmed that patients who were >30 years or <70 years of age and had vasovagal/psychogenic syncope or SUO had a benign prognosis, with only 2 deaths in 225 patients in pooled data. However, these data did not confirm the previously reported prognoses for "medium-risk patients" or for patients with diagnosable noncardiovascular causes of syncope, largely because of differences in criteria for patient eligibility. It was concluded that available data allow more than 70% of patients with syncope to be placed into either very high or very low risk groups.

LONG Q-T INTERVAL SYNDROME

During the past 4 years 196 patients with the idiopathic long Q-T syndrome were enrolled in a prospective international study by Moss and coworkers[109] from Rochester, New York. The patients qualified for enrollment if the Q-T interval in either lead II or V_1 was >0.44 seconds or ≥0.40 seconds; if the patient had unexplained syncope, or was a member of a family in which ≥1 blood relative had a QTc of >0.44 seconds. The mean patient age was 24 years, 64% were female and 88% had family members with Q-T prolongation. During an average follow-up of 26 months per patient, 4 patients died suddenly (1.3%/year) and 27 patients had ≥1 syncopal episodes (8.6%/year). Multivariate analysis identified congenital deafness, history of syncope, female gender, and a documented episode of torsades de pointes or VF as independent risk factors for postenrollment syncope or sudden death. Two types of treatment (left stellate ganglionectomy and β-blocker therapy) were associated with a significant reduction in the occurrence of cardiac events during follow-up.

Bhandari and coworkers[110] in Stanford, California, performed electrophysiologic studies in 15 patients with syncope and/or cardiac arrest who had the long Q-T syndrome and 11 control subjects who had normal Q-T intervals. The syndrome was familial in 5 patients and idiopathic in 10. All patients had a prolonged Q-T (546 ms) and corrected Q-T (550 ms). Incremental atrial pacing at cycle lengths of 600–400 ms resulted in shortening of the Q-T interval, but there was no significant difference in the magnitude or percent of the shortening of the Q-T interval between patients with the long Q-T syndrome and control subjects. Intravenous propranolol did not influence the Q-T interval measured at fixed atrial paced cycle lengths in patients with either the familial or idiopathic form of the syndrome. Programmed RV and LV stimulation with up to 3 extrastimuli before and during isoproterenol infusion did not induce sustained VT or VF in any patient. However, rapid polymorphic nonsustained VT was induced in 6 of the 15 patients (40%). Neither the inducibility of nonsustained VT nor the results of electropharmacologic testing with β-blockers proved to be of prognostic value during the mean follow-up period of 28 months. These investigators concluded that electrophysiologic studies are of limited value in the diagnosis and treatment of patients with the long Q-T syndrome.

Bharati and coworkers[111] from Browns Mills, New Jersey, Hershey and Philadelphia, Pennsylvania, studied the cardiac conduction system in 5 patients with Romano-Ward syndrome and in 1 patient with the Jervell and Lange-Nielsen syndrome to determine morphologic changes occurring in association with a prolonged Q-T interval. These patients were 9 and 15 months and 2, 5, and 19 years of age. A sixth girl was 16 years old and she died suddenly; several members of her family had a prolonged Q-T interval. The morphologic observations made in this study demonstrated marked fatty infiltration at the entrance to the AV node in all patients. In 4 patients, the AV bundle was lobulated with loop formation in 1. In 4 patients, the AV bundle and bundle branches were fibrotic. In all cases, the ventricular myocardium contained chronic inflammatory cells. Thus, each patient with a prolonged Q-T interval had morphologic abnormalities in their AV node or more distally. The relation of these morphologic abnormalities to sudden death and prolongation of the Q-T interval is unclear.

BUNDLE BRANCH BLOCK

To determine whether any associated ECG findings in persons with newly acquired complete left BBB correlate with the prevalence of associated clinically apparent cardiovascular abnormalities, Schneider and associates[112] from Cincinnati, Ohio, and Boston and Framingham, Massachusetts, reviewed ECGs from all 55 members of the Framingham study cohort in whom left BBB developed during 18 years of routine prospective biennial examinations. A QRS axis left of or equal to $0°$, LA conduction delay and an inverted T wave in lead V_6 on the first ECG with left BBB and an abnormal ECG in the Framingham examination preceding the appearance of left BBB each correlated with the prevalence of systemic hypertension, cardiomegaly, CAD, and CHF (Table 3-3). However, neither the P-R interval nor the duration of the QRS complex on the first ECG with left BBB correlated with the prevalence of any of the associated cardiovascular abnormalities. The 8 patients with neither LA conduction delay nor a QRS axis left of or equal to $0°$ on the first Framingham ECG with left BBB nor an abnormal ECG on the examination preceding the appearance of left BBB were 6 times more likely to remain free of all of the clinical cardiovascular abnormalities than the 47 patients with ≥ 1 of these 3 ECG findings.

Vasey and associates[113] from Indianapolis, Indiana, reviewed the records of 2,584 consecutive patients who underwent both treadmill exercise testing

TABLE 3-3. *ECG interpretation on the Framingham examination that preceded onset of left BBB.*

INTERPRETATION	%
Normal	44
LV hypertrophy*	24
AMI*	12
Nonspecific ST and/or T abnormalities	12
Isolated left-axis deviation	5
Incomplete left BBB	5

*Of the 55 patients, 2 with inferior infarction also had LV hypertrophy; thus, total is greater than 100%.

and coronary angiography to determine the relation between exercise-induced, acceleration-dependent left BBB and the presence of CAD. Rate-dependent left BBB during exercise was identified in 28 patients (1.1%), who were categorized according to their presenting symptoms: classic angina pectoris, atypical chest pain, symptomatic cardiac arrhythmia, and asymptomatic. Asymptomatic patients underwent a screening exercise test. CAD was present in 7 of 10 patients who presented with classic angina pectoris, but 12 of 13 patients presenting with atypical chest pain had normal coronary arteries. All 10 patients in whom left BBB developed at a heart rate of ≥125 beats/minute were free of CAD, whereas 9 of 18 patients in whom left BBB developed at a heart rate of <125 beats/minute had CAD. Normal coronary arteries were present in 3 patients who presented with angina and in whom both chest pain and left BBB developed during exercise. It was concluded that patients who present with atypical chest pain in whom rate-dependent left BBB develops on the treadmill are significantly less likely to have CAD than patients who present with classic angina; the onset of left BBB at a heart rate of ≥125 beats/minute is highly correlated with the presence of normal coronary arteries, regardless of patient presentation; and patients with angina in whom both chest pain and left BBB develop during exercise may have normal coronary arteries.

The presence of left BBB is believed by most electrocardiographers to invalidate the usual criteria for LV hypertrophy. Several autopsy studies, however, indicate that the commonly used criteria, as in normal conduction, remain specific but insensitive. Kafka and associates[114] from Kingston, Canada, tested ECG diagnosis of LV hypertrophy in the presence of left BBB by determining LV mass by echo in 125 patients. M-mode echo was technically adequate in 80% of patients. LV mass was calculated using previously validated M-mode formulas and then indexed to body surface area. The known shifts in the QRS voltage and axis with the onset of left BBB led to the selection of 4 ECG parameters for the diagnosis of LV hypertrophy: R in aVL > 11; QRS axis < 40° (or SII > RII); $SV_1 + RV_5$ to $RV_6 > 40$; $SV_2 > 30$ and $SV_3 > 25$; these parameters were used in cumulative fashion. This cumulative approach was superior to using single conventional criterion such as the $SV_1 + RV_5$ or RV_6. When LV hypertrophy was defined as an M-mode index of ≥115 g/m², the sensitivity was 75% and specificity 90%. Using an M-mode mass of ≥215 g as the standard, the sensitivity was 73% and the specificity 66%. LV hypertrophy can be diagnosed by ECG criteria in the presence of left BBB at least as reliably as in normal conduction.

ATRIOVENTRICULAR BLOCK

Shaw and associates[115] from Exeter, UK, followed 214 patients with chronic second degree AV block. The patients had been seen with block initially between 1968 and 1982. The patients were divided into 3 groups according to the type of block. In group 1 there were 77 patients with Mobitz type I block (mean age, 69 years), in group 2, 86 patients with Mobitz type II block (mean age, 74 years), and in group 3, 51 patients with 2:1 or 3:1 block (mean age, 75 years). The 5-year survival was similar in all groups, being 57, 61, and 53% in groups 1, 2, and 3, respectively (Fig. 3-9). The presence or absence of BBB did not appear to influence prognosis. In particular, patients in group 1 without BBB did not fare any better than those in group 2 both with and without BBB. One hundred and three of the patients were fitted with pacemakers, the proportion being greatest in group 2. In each group a

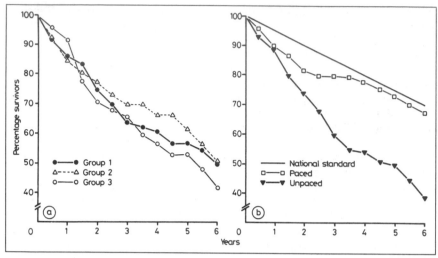

Fig. 3-9. (a) Overall survival of patients in the 3 different groups in relation to time in years since admission to the study. The curves are taken to 6 years to show that there are no sudden changes in the trends after the initial 5 years. (b) Survival of paced patients compared with that of unpaced patients. In both cases the time in years was estimated from the data of entry to the study. An additional line is plotted which represents the expected survival for the general population (National Standard) of similar age and sex. Reproduced with permission from Shaw et al.[115]

significantly larger number of paced patients survived than unpaced. The 5-year survival for all the paced patients in the study was 78% compared with 41% for the unpaced. Since the paced patients were slightly younger than the unpaced, 2 age-matched groups of 74 patients each were selected from the paced and unpaced patients, but the 5-year survival of those paced was still significantly better. It was concluded that in the patients in the present study chronic Mobitz type I block has a similar prognosis to that of Mobitz type II block. Unpaced patients with both types did badly, whereas those fitted with pacemakers had a 5-year survival similar to that expected for the normal population. These results refute the benign reputation of chronic Mobitz type I block and imply that patients with this condition should be considered for pacemaker implantation on similar criteria to those for patients with higher degrees of block.

PACEMAKERS AND CARDIOVERTERS

Guidelines for their use

The Council on Scientific Affairs of the American Medical Association[116] published current indications for the use of permanent pacemakers and the issue of overutilization of pacemakers, pacemaker follow-up, requirements for pacemaker facilities, and the physician-manufacture interphase. Similar guidelines have been published previously by a joint task force of the American Heart Association and the American College of Cardiology, by the North American Society for Pacing and Electrophysiology, and to some extent by the InterSociety for Heart Disease Resources on Optimal Resources for Implantable Cardiac Pacemakers. I (WCR) found this guideline piece published in the *Journal of the American Medical Association* to be the best of the guidelines published thus far for insertion of permanent pacemakers. This Committee recommended the following: Pacemakers should be permanently implanted only when they can correct or prevent symptoms that are proved to be related to an arrhythmia, usually a bradyarrhythmia. Such symptoms include confusion, dizziness, syncope, or seizures. Generalized weakness is a less specific symptom and some patients may have symptoms of CHF that are aggravated, or at least contributed to, by the bradyarrhythmia. Before permanent pacing is initiated, it is essential to ensure that the arrhythmia is not due to a drug, an electrolyte imbalance, or an acute inflammatory or ischemic process that may be reversible. (Drugs used for treatment of systemic hypertension [such as β-blockers, verapamil, diltiazem], CHF [for example, digitalis], arrhythmias [such as quinidine, procainamide], and various psychiatric conditions [such as amitriptyline] can effect sinoatrial nodal impulse formation, AV nodal conduction, and carotid sinus sensitivity. Also, some drugs may produce bradycardia by altering the pharmacokinetics of other drugs [such as cimetidine, quinidine, verapamil].) Rarely, the bradycardia must be treated even when it is induced by a drug, because the agent is essential in the patient's medical management. When a bradyarrhythmia that is responsible for intermittent or permanent symptoms is not reversible, implantation of a permanent cardiac pacemaker is indicated. The etiology in these symptomatic patients will usually be attributed to one of the following:

Atrioventricular block
- A. Complete (third degree)
- B. Incomplete (second degree)
    1. Mobitz type I (Wenckebach's disease: a rare indication)
    2. Mobitz type II
- C. Incomplete with 2-1 or 3-1 AV response

Sinus node dysfunction (symptomatic)
- A. Sinus bradycardia
- B. Sinoatrial block, sinus arrest
- C. Bradycardia-tachycardia syndrome

The following clinical entities are still controversial but have been proposed by ≥1 investigator as an indication in selected patients for pacemaker implantation: Bifascicular intraventricular block with syncope; alternating bilateral BBB (asymptomatic); second-degree AV block Mobitz type II (asymptomatic); transient complete or type II AV block with BBB in selected situations (such as AMI); congenital complete AV block (asymptomatic); and hypersensitive carotid syndrome.

Sinus node dysfunction in persons ≤ 40 years of age

To examine the clinical course of sinus node dysfunction that necessitates permanent pacing in young persons, Albin and associates[117] from Rochester, Minnesota, studied the records of 39 patients aged ≤40 years (mean age, 23) who underwent implantation of a permanent pacemaker for treatment at the Mayo Clinic between 1960 and 1983. The tachycardia-bradycardia syndrome was the most common rhythm disturbance, and syncope was the most frequent initial symptom. All symptomatic patients noted resolution of symptoms after pacemaker implantation. Twenty-five of the 39 patients (64%) had associated cardiovascular disease, most commonly TGA. In each of the 11 patients with this anomaly, sinus node dysfunction developed after a surgical procedure for correction of the defect. Of the total patient population, 20 patients (51%) had previously undergone a cardiac operation. The mean interval between pacemaker implantation and the previous operation was 105 months. After a mean follow-up of 51 months, the patients with no obvious underlying heart disease had done well. Each of the 8 patients who have died had underlying cardiovascular disease. None of the deaths was believed to be pacemaker related. Sinus node dysfunction should be considered in the differential diagnosis of young patients with syncope or dizziness, especially if they have undergone a reparative cardiac surgical procedure. If symptomatic sinus node dysfunction is confirmed, permanent pacing is an effective therapeutic modality. In the absence of associated heart disease, the prognosis seems to be excellent.

External noninvasive temporary cardiac pacing

Zoll and coworkers[118] from Boston, Massachusetts, introduced an external cardiac pacemaker-monitor in 1981 that provided safe, effective noninvasive ventricular stimulation well tolerated in conscious patients and allowed clear recognition of ECG response. The noninvasive temporary pacemaker (NTP) now has been applied in 134 patients in 5 hospitals. Stimulation was tolerated well in 73 of 82 conscious patients, and 9 found it intolerable. The NTP was effective in evoking ECG responses in 105 patients; the 29 failures were in the presence of prolonged hypoxia or severe discomfort. The NTP was clinically useful in 82 patients: 43 of 86 were resuscitated from emergency or expected arrest, 38 of 40 were maintained in standby readiness for up to 1 month, but did not require stimulation, and 1 of 8 patients with tachycardia obtained some clinical benefit. The NTP was especially useful in 25 patients with complications or contraindications to endocardial pacing and in 57 patients in whom insertion of an endocardial electrode was avoided. These investigators believe the NTP has proved of major clinical benefit in buying time for the subsequent placement of a temporary endocardial electrode or in avoiding that procedure altogether, in emergency resuscitation from bradycardia or asystole, and suppression of VT, and in standby monitoring in emergency readiness for pacing when bradycardia or asystole appears likely.

Reviews and related topics

It is estimated that 500,000 patients in the United States have a permanent pacemaker and that about 100,000 new pacing systems were implanted in 1985. It has been suggested that pacemaker malfunction (Table 3-4) can be detected by history and electrocardiogram in 99% of patients with a permanent pacemaker. In a review article, Bhatia and Goldschlager[119] from San Francisco, California, focused on the basic office evaluation of patients with permanent pacemakers using equipment readily available in the internist's office.

A superb review on the present status of pacemakers was presented by Shively and Goldschlager.[120,121]

Recent work has questioned the safety of combined therapy with β-blockers and verapamil and occasional reports have described catastrophic results. Maisel and associates[122] from La Jolla, California, described 3 patients who became hypotensive after receiving oral quinidine and intravenous verapamil. They found no previous reports documenting such serious drug interaction. They proposed that this interaction may be due to an addi-

TABLE 3-4. *Categories of pacemaker malfunction. Reproduced with permission from Bhatia and Goldschlager.*[119]

No pacing stimulus observed when generator is not inhibited by native rhythm
    Power source depletion (end of life)
    Pulse generator component failure
    Incomplete circuit (such as lead fracture)
    Improper (loose) connection of lead to generator
    Oversensing
Failure to capture (myocardial tissue nonrefractory)
    Electrode displacement (dislodgment, refraction, myocardial penetration)
    Power source depletion (end of life)
    Increased myocardial stimulation threshold
    Lead fracture
    Insulation break
    Inappropriate (subthreshold) programmed energy output
Failure to sense (undersensing)
  Inadequate intracardiac signal
  Power source depletion (end of life)
  Pulse generator component failure
  Lead fracture
  Poor electrode-myocardial interface
  Inappropriate programmed sensitivity
Pacemaker oversensing
  Physiologic intracardiac signals
    T-wave sensing (VVI mode)
    P-wave sensing (VVI mode)
    QRS sensing (AAI mode)
  Extracardiac myopotentials
    Pectoral muscles
    Diaphragm
  Electromagnetic interference
    Magnetic resonance imaging
    Microwave transmission
    Electrocautery
    Arc welding
  Pacing system source of signals
    Afterpotential sensing (sensing of generator voltage output decay)
    False signals
      Partial lead fracture
      Intermittent contact of pacemaker metal parts (such as two leads)
      Incomplete lead-generator circuit (loose connection)
      Magnet application (positioning or removal leading to changing magnetic fields)
      Electrolysis of dissimilar metals
  Crosstalk (sensing by an electrode of the output stimulus of the other electrode
    in DVI and DDD systems)

---

tive blockade of α-adrenergic receptors by quinidine and verapamil. The interaction of quinidine and verapamil suggest that these agents also may produce drug reactions, such as hypotension, in patients who have heightened adrenergic tone or who are receiving other α-blockers, calcium channel blockers, or vasodilators.

The natural history of patients with asymptomatic prolonged ventricular pauses and the indications for permanent pacing in them are controversial. To examine this problem, Hilgard and associates[123] from Chicago, Illinois, reviewed 6,470 consecutive 24-hour Holter recordings between 1979 and

1983 for the presence of ventricular pauses of ≥3 seconds. Fifty-two patients (0.8% of the total), 22 men and 30 women, were identified with an average longest pause duration of 4.1 seconds. Holter recordings were requested to evaluate syncope in 14 patients (27%), dizziness in 9 (17%), and other reasons in 29 (56%). Causes of the pauses were sinus arrest in 22 patients, AF with slow ventricular response in 18 patients, and AV block in 12. Holter recordings also were evaluated for the presence of tachyarrhythmias. Six patients had nonsustained VT and 7 had SVT. Five of the 52 patients (10%) had dizziness or syncope during pauses. Twenty-six patients received permanent pacemakers. The paced and unpaced groups were similar in the length and cause of pause, associated tachyarrhythmias, presence of bradycardia-related symptoms, prevalence of organic heart disease, medications, and length of follow-up. Four patients in the paced group and 2 in the unpaced group died, yielding 3-year actuarial survival probabilities of 78 and 85%, respectively. It is concluded that ventricular pauses of ≥3 seconds are uncommon, these pauses usually do not cause symptoms, and the presence of these pauses does not necessarily portend a poor prognosis or the need for pacing in asymptomatic patients.

Robertson and associates[124] from Durham, North Carolina, compared 2-D echo and RV angiographic findings in 10 patients with arrhythmogenic RV dysplasia. Diagnosis was based on accepted ECG and angiographic criteria. Nine patients underwent invasive electrophysiologic study, which confirmed RV source of VT in 7. Two-D echo and angiography corresponded closely when diffuse RV enlargement and hypokinesia were present. Such diffuse findings were not invariably present. Localized abnormalities consisting of bulging or sacculation of the RV wall were noted by both techniques, even in the absence of diffuse changes. Echo evidence of localized disease predicted the presence of similar lesions at angiography, but agreement as to specific location was poor. Subjectivity in interpreting subtle RV abnormalities by either technique and the inherent differences in information provided by the 2 methods probably account for the inconsistencies. In the patient with suspected arrhythmogenic RV dysplasia, 2-D echo evidence of diffuse RV enlargement, otherwise unexplained, strongly supports the diagnosis and angiography may be avoided. Isolated local changes seen by echo should increase suspicion of RV dysplasia, but complementary angiographic study is warranted.

Saksena and associates[125] from Newark, New Jersey, examined the economic consequences of invasive electrophysiologic studies for recurrent SVT and VT on a tertiary health care facility during 1980 and 1981. The average cost of hospitalization for electrophysiologic evaluation was substantial (SVT, $6,990; VT, $13,897), as was the length of hospital stay (SVT, 12 ± 8 days; VT, 24 ± 8 days). The cost of a single electrophysiologic procedure in the study period averaged $695 (range, $200 to $1,206). During follow-up (1–3 years), there was substantial improvement in arrhythmia control on electrophysiology-based therapy in SVT and VT compared with prior empirical therapy. Cost:benefit analysis strongly favored electrophysiologic-based therapy over empirical therapy (SVT, 6:1; VT, 18:1) in this follow-up period. Comparison with cost of noninvasive techniques for VT evaluation showed that electrophysiology evaluation had comparable cost. Current prospective reimbursement schedules have no diagnosis related group category for electrophysiology evaluation and do not fairly compensate hospitals for invasive or noninvasive arrhythmia studies. Invasive electrophysiology evaluation is both clinically and cost effective in the management of patients with recurrent SVT and VT.

References

1. KENNEDY HL, WHITLOCK JA, SPRAGUE MK, KENNEDY LJ, BUCKINGHAM TA, GOLDBERG RJ: Long-term follow-up of asymptomatic healthy subjects with frequent and complex ventricular ectopy. N Engl J Med 1985 (Jan 24); 312:193–197.

2. RUSKIN JN: Ventricular extrasystoles in healthy subjects. N Engl J Med 1985 (Jan 24); 312:238–239.

3. DUNNIGAN A, BENSON DW, JR, BENDITT DG: Atrial flutter in infancy: diagnosis, clinical features and treatment. Pediatrics 1985 (April); 75:725–729.

4. CAMPBELL RM, DICK M, II, JENKINS JM, SPICER RL, CROWLEY DC, ROCCHINI AP, SNIDER R, STERN AM, ROSENTHAL A: Atrial overdrive pacing for conversion of atrial flutter in children. Pediatrics 1985 (April); 75:730–736.

5. GARSON A, JR., BINK-BOUKENS M, HESSLEIN PS, HORDOF HA, KEANE JF, NECHES WH, PORTER CJ: Atrial flutter in the young: a collaborative study of 380 cases. J Am Coll Cardiol 1985 (Oct); 6:871–878.

6. BRAND FN, ABBOTT RD, KANNEL WB, WOLF PA: Characteristics and prognosis of lone atrial fibrillation: 30-year follow-up in the Framingham study. JAMA 1985 (Dec); 254:3449–3453.

7. RICH EC, SIEBOLD C, CAMPION B: Alcohol-related acute atrial fibrillation: A case-control study and review of 40 patients. Arch Intern Med 1985 (May); 145:830–833.

8. THEISEN K, HAUFE M, PETERS J, THEISEN F, JAHRMARKER H: Effect of the calcium antagonist diltiazem on atrioventricular conduction in chronic atrial fibrillation. Am J Cardiol 1985 (Jan 1); 55:98–102.

9. HOROWITZ LN, SPIELMAN SR, GREENSPAN AM, MINTZ GS, MORGANROTH J, BROWN R, BRADY PM, KAY HR: Use of amiodarone in the treatment of persistent and paroxysmal atrial fibrillation resistant to quinidine therapy. J Am Coll Cardiol 1985 (Dec); 6:1402–1407.

10. DEAL BJ, KEANE JF, GILLETTE PC, GARSON A JR: Wolff-Parkinson-White syndrome and supraventricular tachycardia during infancy: management and follow-up. J Am Coll Cardiol 1985 (Jan); 5:130–135.

11. LEVINE JH, MICHAEL JR, GUARNIERI T: Multifocal atrial tachycardia: a toxic effect of theophylline. Lancet 1985 (Jan 5); 1:12–14.

12. WALDECKER B, BRUGADA P, DULK K, ZEHENDER M, WELLENS HJJ: Arrhythmias induced during termination of supraventricular tachycardia. Am J Cardiol 1985 (Feb 1); 55:412–417.

13. BENSON DW JR, DUNNIGAN AN, BENDITT DG, THOMPSON TR, NARAYAN A, BOROS S: Prediction of digoxin treatment failure in infants with supraventricular tachycardia: role of transesophageal pacing. Pediatrics 1985 (Feb); 75:288–293.

14. DIMARCO JP, SELLERS D, LERMAN BB, GREENBERG ML, BERNE RM, BELARDINELLI L: Diagnostic and therapeutic use of adenosine in patients with supraventricular tachyarrhythmias. J Am Coll Cardiol 1985 (Aug); 6:417–425.

15. BRUGADA P, WELLENS HJJ: Effects of oral amiodarone on rate-dependent changes in refractoriness in patients with Wolff-Parkinson-White syndrome. Am J Cardiol 1985 (Nov 15); 56:863–866.

16. MANZ M, STEINBECK G, LUDERITZ B: Usefulness of programmed stimulation in predicting efficacy of propafenone in long-term antiarrhythmic therapy for paroxysmal supraventricular tachycardia. Am J Cardiol 1985 (Oct 1); 56:593–597.

17. LEVINE JH, MICHAEL JR, GUARNIERI T: Treatment of multifocal atrial tachycardia with verapamil. N Engl J Med 1985 (Jan 2); 312:21–25.

18. GRAYBOYS TB: The treatment of supraventricular tachycardias. N Engl J Med 1985 (Jan 2); 312:43–45.

19. ABRAMS J, ALLEN J, ALLIN D, ANDERSON J, ANDERSON S, BLANSKI L, CHADDA K, DIBIANCO R, FAVROT L, GONZALEZ J, HOROWITZ L, LADDU A, LEE R, MACCOSBE P, MORGANROTH J, NARULA O, SINGH B, SINGH J, STECK J, SWERDLOW C, TURLAPATY P, WALDO A: Efficacy and safety of esmolol vs propranolol in the treatment of supraventricular tachyarrhythmias: a multicenter double-blind clinical trial. Am Heart J 1985 (Nov); 110:913–922.

20. OTT DA, GILLETTE PC, GARSON A JR, COOLEY DA, REUL GJ, MCNAMARA DG: Surgical management of refractory supraventricular tachycardia in infants and children. J Am Coll Cardiol 1985 (Jan); 5:124–129.

21. HOLMES DR, DANIELSON GK, GERSH BJ, OSBORN MJ, WOOD DL, MCLARAN C, SUGRUE DD, PORTER CJ, HAMMILL SC: Surgical treatment of accessory atrioventricular pathways and symptomatic tachycardia in children and young adults. Am J Cardiol 1985 (June 1); 55:1509–1512.

22. KRAMER JB, CORR PB, COX JL, WITKOWSKI FX, CAIN ME: Simultaneous computer mapping to facilitate intraoperative localization of accessory pathways in patients with Wolff-Parkinson-White syndrome. Am J Cardiol 1985 (Oct 1); 56:571–576.

23. COX J, GALLAGHER J, CAIN M: Experience with 118 consecutive patients undergoing operation for the Wolff-Parkinson-White syndrome. J Thorac Cardiovasc Surg 1985 (Oct); 90:490–501.

24. DANCY M, CAMM AJ, WARD D: Misdiagnosis of chronic recurrent ventricular tachycardia. Lancet 1985 (Aug 10); 2:320–323.

25. MORADY F, BAERMAN JM, DICARLO L, DEBUITLEIR M, KROL RB, WAHR DW: A prevalent misconception regarding wide-complex tachycardias. JAMA 1985 (Nov 15); 254:2790–2792.

26. DONGAS J, LEHMANN MH, MAHMUD R, DENKER S, SONI J, AKHTAR M: Value of preexisting bundle branch block in the electrocardiographic differentiation of supraventricular from ventricular origin of wide QRS tachycardia. Am J Cardiol 1985 (Mar 1); 55:717–721.

27. WREN C, CAMPBELL RW, HUNTER S: Role of echocardiography in differential diagnosis of broad complex tachycardia. Br Heart J 1985 (Aug); 54:166–172.

28. KATZ C, MARTIN RD, LANDA B, CHADDA KD: Relationship of psychologic factors to frequent symptomatic ventricular arrhythmia. Am J Med 1985 (Apr); 78:589–594.

29. BOEHNERT MT, LOVEJOY FH: Value of the QRS duration versus the serum drug level in predicting seizures and ventricular arrhythmias after an acute overdose of tricyclic antidepressants. N Engl J Med 1985 (Aug 22); 313:474–479.

30. SALZMAN C: Clinical use of antidepressant blood levels and the electrocardiogram. N Engl J Med 1985 (Aug 22); 313:512.

31. GOLDBERG RJ, CAPONE RJ, HUNT JD: Cardiac complications following tricyclic antidepressant overdose: issues for monitoring policy. JAMA 1985 (Oct 4); 254:1772–1775.

32. PRATT CM, SLYMEN DJ, WIERMAN AM, YOUNG JB, FRANCIS MJ, SEALS AA, QUINONES MA, ROBERTS R: Analysis of the spontaneous variability of ventricular arrhythmias: consecutive ambulatory electrocardiographic recordings of ventricular tachycardia. Am J Cardiol 1985 (July 1); 56:67–72.

33. PRATT CM, DELCLOS G, WIERMAN AM, MAHLER SA, SEALS AA, LEON CA, YOUNG JB, QUINONES MA, ROBERTS R: The changing base line of complex ventricular arrhythmias: a new consideration in assessing long-term antiarrhythmic drug therapy. N Engl J Med 1985 (Dec 5); 313:1444–1449.

34. BRUGADA P, WELLENS HJJ: Comparison in the same patient of two programmed ventricular stimulation protocols to induce ventricular tachycardia. Am J Cardiol 1985 (Feb 1); 55:380–383.

35. MCPHERSON CA, ROSENFELD LE, BATSFORD WP: Day-to-day reproducibility of responses to right ventricular programmed electrical stimulation: implications for serial drug testing. Am J Cardiol 1985 (Mar 1); 55:689–695.

36. MORADY F, DICARLO LA, LIEM B, KROL RB, BAERMAN JM: Effects of high stimulation current on the induction of ventricular tachycardia. Am J Cardiol 1985 (July 1); 56:73–78.

37. GRADMAN AH, BATSFORD WP, RIEUR EC, LEON L, VAN ZETTA AM: Ambulatory electrocardiographic correlates of ventricular inducibility during programmed electrical stimulation. J Am Coll Cardiol 1985 (May); 5:1087–1093.

38. SPIELMAN SR, GREENSPAN AM, KAY HR, DISCIGIL KF, WEBB CR, SOKOLOFF NM, RAE AP, MORGANROTH J, HOROWITZ LN: Electrophysiologic testing in patients at high risk for sudden cardiac death. I. Nonsustained ventricular tachycardia and abnormal ventricular function. J Am Coll Cardiol 1985 (July); 6:31–39.

39. TORRES V, FLOWERS D, SOMBERG J: The clinical significance of polymorphic ventricular tachycardia provoked at electrophysiologic testing. Am Heart J 1985 (July); 110:17–24.

40. SCHOENFELD MH, MCGOVERN B, GARAN H, KELLY E, GRANT G, RUSKIN JN: Determinants of the outcome of electrophysiologic study in patients with ventricular tachyarrhythmias. J Am Coll Cardiol 1985 (Aug); 6:298–306.

41. VELTRI EP, PLATIA EV, GRIFFITH LSC, REID PR: Programmed electrical stimulation and long-term follow-up in asymptomatic, nonsustained ventricular tachycardia. Am J Cardiol 1985 (Aug 1); 56:309–314.

42. PLATIA EV, REID PR: Nonsustained ventricular tachycardia during programmed ventricular stimulation: criteria for a positive test. Am J Cardiol 1985 (July 1); 56:79–83.

43. SWERDLOW CD, PETERSON J: Prospective comparison of Holter monitoring and electrophysiologic study in patients with coronary artery disease and sustained ventricular tachyarrhythmias. Am J Cardiol 1985 (Oct 1); 56:577–580.

44. RAE AP, GREENSPAN AM, SPIELMAN SR, SOKOLOFF NM, WEBB CR, KAY HR, HOROWITZ LN: Antiarrhythmic drug efficacy for ventricular tachyarrhythmias associated with coronary artery disease as assessed by electrophysiologic studies. Am J Cardiol 1985 (June 1); 55:1494–1499.

45. TORRES V, FLOWERS D, SOMBERG JC: The arrhythmogenicity of antiarrhythmic agents. Am Heart J 1985 (May); 109:1090–1097.

46. POSER RF, PODRID PJ, LOMBARDI F, LOWN B: Aggravation of arrhythmia induced with antiarrhythmic drugs during electrophysiologic testing. Am Heart J 1985 (July); 110:9–16.

47. KERIN NZ, BELVINS RD, FRUMIN H, FAITEL K, RUBENFIRE M: Intravenous and oral loading versus oral loading alone with amiodarone for chronic refractory ventricular arrhythmias. Am J Cardiol 1985 (Jan 1); 55:89–91.

48. HOROWITZ LN, GREENSPAN AM, SPIELMAN SR, WEBB CR, MORGANROTH J, ROTMENSCH H, SOKOLOFF NM, RAE AP, SEGAL BL, KAY HR: Usefulness of electrophysiologic testing in evaluation of amiodarone therapy for sustained ventricular tachyarrhythmias associated with coronary heart disease. Am J Cardiol 1985 (Feb 1); 55:367–371.

49. DICARLO LA, MORADY F, SAUVE MJ, MALONE P, DAVIS JC, EVANS-BELL T, WINSTON SA, SCHEINMAN MM: Cardiac arrest and sudden death in patients treated with amiodarone for sustained ventricular tachycardia or ventricular fibrillation: risk stratification based on clinical variables. Am J Cardiol 1985 (Feb 1); 55:372–374.

50. VELTRI EP, REID PR, PLATIA EV, GRIFFITH SC: Results of late programmed electrical stimulation and long-term electrophysiologic effects of amiodarone therapy in patients with refractory ventricular tachycardia. Am J Cardiol 1985 (Feb 1); 55:375–379.

51. MARCHLINSKI FE, BUXTON AE, FLORES BT, DOHERTY JU, WAXMAN HL, JOSEPHSON ME: Value of Holter monitoring in identifying risk for sustained ventricular arrhythmia recurrence on amiodarone. Am J Cardiol 1985 (Mar 1); 55:709–712.

52. VELTRI EP, REID PR, PLATIA EV, GRIFFITH LSC: Amiodarone in the treatment of life-threatening ventricular tachycardia: role of Holter monitoring in predicting long-term clinical efficacy. J Am Coll Cardiol 1985 (Oct); 6:806–813.

53. KENNEDY EE, ROSENFELD LE, MCPHERSON CA, BATSFORD WP: Evaluation by serial electrophysiologic studies of an abbreviated oral loading regimen of amiodarone. Am J Cardiol 1985 (Nov 15); 56:867–871.

54. ADAMS PC, HOLT DW, STOREY GCA, MORLEY AR, CALLAGHNAN J, CAMPBELL RWF: Amiodarone and its desethyl metabolite: tissue distribution and morphologic changes during long-term therapy. Circulation 1985 (Nov); 72:1061–1075.

55. ELLENBOGEN KA, O'CALLAGHAN WG, COLAVITA PG, SMITH MS, GERMAN LD: Cardiac function in patients on chronic amiodarone therapy. Am Heart J 1985 (Aug); 110:376–381.

56. RAEDER EA, PODRID PA, LOWN B: Side effects and complications of amiodarone therapy. Am Heart J 1985 (May); 109:975–983.

57. SOMBERG J, TORRES V, FLOWERS D, MIURA D, BUTLER B, GOTTLIEB S: Prolongation of QT interval and antiarrhythmic action of bepridil. Am Heart J 1985 (Jan); 109:9–27.

58. DUMOULIN P, JAILLON P, KHER A, POIRIER J-M, CHEYMOL G, VALTY J, FLAMMANG D, COUMEL P, MEDVEDOWSKY J-L, BARNAY C, WARIN J-F, BLANCHOT P, FRANK R, GROSGOGEAT Y: Long-term efficacy and safety of oral encainide in the treatment of chronic ventricular ectopic activity: relationship to plasma concentrations—a French multicenter trial. Am Heart J 1985 (Sept); 110:575–581.

59. DUFF HJ, RODEN DM, CAREY EL, WANG T, PRIMM K, WOOSLEY RL: Spectrum of antiarrhythmic response to encainide. Am J Cardiol 1985 (Nov 15); 56:887–891.

60. FLOWERS D, O'GALLAGHER D, TORRES V, MIURA D, SOMBERG JC: Flecainide: long-term treatment using a reduced dosing schedule. Am J Cardiol 1985 (Jan 1); 55:79–83.

61. JOSEPHSON MA, KAUL S, HOPKINS J, KVAM D, SINGH BN: Hemodynamic effects of intravenous flecainide relative to the level of ventricular function in patients with coronary artery disease. Am Heart J 1985 (Jan); 109:41–45.

62. PLATIA EV, ESTES M, HEINE DL, GRIFFITH LSC, GARAN H, RUSKIN JN, REID PR: Flecainide: electrophysiologic and antiarrhythmic properties in refractory ventricular tachycardia. Am J Cardiol 1985 (Apr 1); 55:956–962.

63. LAL R, CHAPMAN PD, NACCARELLI GV, TROUP PJ, RINKENBERGER RL, DOUGHERTY AH, RUFFY R: Short- and long-term experience with flecainide acetate in the management of refractory life-threatening ventricular arrhythmias. J Am Coll Cardiol 1985 (Oct); 6:772–779.

64. Dubner SJ, Elencwajg BD, Palma S, Mendelzon R, Ramos A, Bertolasi CA: Efficacy of flecainide in the management of ventricular arrhythmias: comparative study with amiodarone. Am Heart J 1985 (Mar); 109:523–528.

65. Rutledge JC, Harris F, Amsterdam EA, Skalsky E: Clinical evaluation of oral mexiletine therapy in the treatment of ventricular arrhythmias. J Am Coll Cardiol 1985 (Oct); 6:780–784.

66. Nademanee K, Feld G, Hendrickson J, Intarachot V, Yale C, Heng MK, Singh BN: Mexiletine: double-blind comparison with procainamide in PVC suppression and open-label sequential comparison with amiodarone in life-threatening ventricular arrhythmias. Am Heart J 1985 (Nov); 110:923–931.

67. Greenspan AM, Spielman SR, Webb CR, Sokoloff NM, Rae AP, Horowitz LN: Efficacy of combination therapy with mexiletine and a type 1A agent for inducible ventricular tachyarrhythmias secondary to coronary artery disease. Am J Cardiol 1985 (Aug 1); 56:277–284.

68. Echt DS, Shapiro M, Trusso J, Mason JW, Winkle RA: Treatment with oral lorcainide in patients with sustained ventricular tachycardia and fibrillation. Am Heart J 1985 (Jan); 109:28–33.

69. Somberg J, Butler B, Flowers D, Keefe D, Torres V, Miura D: Long-term lorcainide therapy in patients with ventricular tachycardia. Am Heart J 1985 (Jan); 109:33–40.

70. Anastasiou-Nana M, Anderson JL, Hampton EM, Nanas JN, Lutz JR: Initial and long-term outpatient experience with lorcainide for suppression of malignant and potentially malignant ventricular arrhythmias. Am Heart J 1985 (Dec); 110:1168–1175.

71. Mead RH, Keefe DL, Kates RE, Winkle RA: Chronic lorcainide therapy for symptomatic premature ventricular complexes: Efficacy, pharmacokinetics and evidence for norlorcainide antiarrhythmic effect. Am J Cardiol 1985 (Jan 1); 55:72–78.

72. Benson DW, Dunnigan A, Green TP, Benditt DG, Schneider SP: Periodic procainamide for paroxysmal tachycardia. Circulation 1985 (July); 72:147–152.

73. Rae AP, Sokoloff NM, Webb CR, Spielman SR, Greenspan AM, Horowitz LN: Limitations of failure of procainamide during electrophysiologic testing to predict response to other medical therapy. J Am Coll Cardiol 1985 (Aug); 6:410–416.

74. Oseran DS, Gang ES, Rosenthal ME, Mandel WJ, Peter T: Electropharmacologic testing in sustained ventricular tachycardia associated with coronary heart disease: Value of the response to intravenous procainamide in predicting the response to oral procainamide and oral quinidine treatment. Am J Cardiol 1985 (Nov 15); 56:883–886.

75. Wynn J, Miura DS, Torres V, Flowers D, Keefe D, Williams S, Somberg JC: Electrophysiologic evaluation of the antiarrhythmic effects of N-acetylprocainamide for ventricular tachycardia secondary to coronary artery disease. Am J Cardiol 1985 (Nov 15); 56:877–881.

76. Dinh H, Murphy ML, Baker BJ, Desoyza N, Franciosa JA: Efficacy of propafenone compared with quinidine in chronic ventricular arrhythmias. Am J Cardiol 1985 (June 1); 55:1520–1524.

77. Brodsky MA, Allen BJ, Abate D, Henry WL: Propafenone therapy for ventricular tachycardia in the setting of congestive heart failure. Am Heart J 1985 (Oct); 110:794–799.

78. Naccarella F, Bracchetti D, Palmieri M, Cantelli I, Bertaccini P, Ambrosioni E: Comparison of propafenone and disopyramide for treatment of chronic ventricular arrhythmias: placebo-controlled, double-blind, randomized crossover study. Am Heart J 1985 (Apr); 109:833–840.

79. Duff HJ, Wyse DG, Manyari D, Mitchell LB: Intravenous quinidine: relations among concentration, tachyarrhythmia suppression and electrophysiologic actions with inducible sustained ventricular tachycardia. Am J Cardiol 1985 (Jan 1); 55:92–97.

80. Morganroth J, Hunter H: Comparative efficacy and safety of short-acting and sustained release quinidine in the treatment of patients with ventricular arrhythmias. Am Heart J 1985 (Dec); 110:1176–1181.

81. Morganroth J, Horowitz LN: Incidence of proarrhythmic effects from quinidine in the outpatient treatment of benign or potentially lethal ventricular arrhythmias. Am J Cardiol 1985 (Oct 1); 56:585–587.

82. Kim SG, Seiden SW, Matos JA, Waspe LE, Fisher JD: Combination of procainamide and quinidine for better tolerance and additive effects for ventricular arrhythmias. Am J Cardiol 1985 (July 1); 56:84–88.

83. Nademanee K, Feld G, Hendrickson J, Singh PN, Singh BN: Electrophysiologic and antiarrhythmic effects of sotalol in patients with life-threatening ventricular tachyarrhythmias. Circulation 1985 (Sept); 72:555–564.

84. LIDELL C, REHNQVIST N, SJÖGREN A, YLI-UOTILA RJ, RØNNEVIK PK: Comparative efficacy of oral sotalol and procainamide in patients with chronic ventricular arrhythmias: a multicenter study. Am Heart J 1985 (May); 109:970–975.

85. MORGANROTH J, OSHRAIN C, STEELE PP: Comparative efficacy and safety of oral tocainide and quinidine for benign and potentially lethal ventricular arrhythmias. Am J Cardiol 1985 (Oct 1); 56:581–585.

86. WOELFEL A, FOSTER JR, McALLISTER RG, SIMPSON RJ, GETTES LS: Efficacy of verapamil in exercise-induced ventricular tachycardia. Am J Cardiol 1985 (Aug 1); 56:292–297.

87. MANN DL, MAISEL AS, ATWOOD JE, ENGLER RL, LeWINTER MM: Absence of cardioversion-induced ventricular arrhythmias in patients with therapeutic digoxin levels. J Am Coll Cardiol 1985 (Apr); 5:882–888.

88. ECHT DS, ARMSTRON K, SCHMIDT P, OYER PE, STINSON EB, WINKLE RA: Clinical experience, complications, and survival in 70 patients with the automatic implantable cardioverter/defibrillator. Circulation 1985 (Feb); 289–296.

89. HERRE JM, GRIFFIN JC, NIELSEN AP, MANN DE, LUCK JC, MAGRO SA, SCHEUNEMEYER T, WYNDHAM CRC: Permanent triggered antitachycardia pacemakers in the management of recurrent sustained ventricular tachycardia. J Am Coll Cardiol 1985 (July); 6:206–212.

90. SAKSENA S, CHANDRAN P, SHAH Y, BOCCADAMO R, PANTOPOULOS D, ROTHBART ST: Comparative efficacy of transvenous cardioversion and pacing in patients with sustained ventricular tachycardia: a prospective, randomized, crossover study. Circulation 1985 (July); 72:153–160.

91. HOLT PM, SMALLPEICE C, DEVERALL PB, YATES AK, CURRY PVL: Ventricular arrhythmias: A guide to their localization. Br Heart J 1985 (Apr); 53:417–430.

92. MILLER JM, MARCHLINSKI FE, HARKEN AH, HARGROVE WC, JOSEPHSON ME: Subendocardial resection for sustained ventricular tachycardia in the early period after acute myocardial infarction. Am J Cardiol 1985 (Apr 1); 55:980–984.

93. MILLER JM, HARKEN AH, HARGROVE CW, JOSEPHSON ME, ORISHIMO TF: Pattern of endocardial activation during sustained ventricular tachycardia. J Am Coll Cardiol 1985 (Dec); 6:1280–1287.

94. NEUSPIEL DR, KULLER LII: Sudden and unexpected natural death in childhood and adolescence. JAMA 1985 (Sept 13); 254:1321–1325.

95. RITCHIE JL, HALLSTROM AP, TROUBAUGH GB, CALDWELL JH, COBB LA: Out-of-hospital sudden coronary death: rest and exercise radionuclide left ventricular function in survivors. Am J Cardiol 1985 (Mar 1); 55:645–651.

96. GOLDSTEIN S, LANDIS JR, LEIGHTON R, RITTER G, VASU M, WOLFE RA, ACHESON A, VANDERBRUG MEDENDORP S: Predictive survival models for resuscitated victims of out-of-hospital cardiac arrest with coronary heart disease. Circulation 1985 (May); 71:873–880.

97. STEVENSON WG, BRUGADA P, WALDECKER B, ZEHENDER M, WELLENS HJ: Clinical, angiographic, and electrophysiologic findings in patients with aborted sudden death as compared with patients with sustained ventricular tachycardia after myocardial infarction. Circulation 1985 (June); 71:1146–1152.

98. MILNER PG, PLATIA EV, REID PR, GRIFFITH LSC: Ambulatory electrocardiographic recordings at the time of fatal cardiac arrest. Am J Cardiol 1985 (Oct 1); 56:588–592.

99. CUMMINS RO, EISENBERG MS: Prehospital cardiopulmonary resuscitation: is it effective? JAMA 1985 (Apr 26); 253:2408–2412.

100. KEENAN RL, BOYAN CP: Cardiac arrest due to anesthesia: a study of incidence and causes. JAMA 1985 (Apr 26); 253:2373–2377.

101. VANDAM LD: Cardiac arrest: signal of anesthetic mishap. JAMA 1985 (Apr 26); 253:2415.

102. BEDER SD, COHEN MH, RIEMENSCHNEIDER TA: Occult arrhythmias as the etiology of unexplained syncope in children with structurally normal hearts. Am Heart J 1985 (Feb); 109:309–313.

103. HYSING J, GRENDAHL H: Ambulatory 24 hour ECG in patients with a history of syncope. A retrospective follow-up study over 2 years. Eur Heart J 1985 (Feb); 6:120–122.

104. OLSHANSKY B, MAZUZ M, MARTINS JB: Significance of inducible tachycardia in patients with syncope of unknown origin: a long-term follow-up. J Am Coll Cardiol 1985 (Feb); 5:216–223.

105. DOHERTY JU, PEMBROOK-ROGERS D, GROGAN EW, FALCONE RA, BUXTON AE, MARCHLINSKI FE, CASSIDY DM, KIENZLE MG, ALMENDRAL JM, JOSEPHSON ME: Electrophysiologic evaluation and follow-up characteristics of patients with recurrent unexplained syncope and presyncope. Am J Cardiol 1985 (Mar 1); 55:703–708.

106. TEICHMAN SL, FELDER SD, MATOS JA, KIM SG, WASPE LE, FISHER JD: The value of electrophysio-

logic studies in syncope of undetermined origin: report of 150 cases. Am Heart J 1985 (Aug); 110:469–479.

107. REIFFEL JA, WANG P, BOWER R, BIGGER JT JR, LIVELLI F JR, FERRICK K, GLIKLICH J, ZIMMERMAN J: Electrophysiologic testing in patients with recurrent syncope: are results predicted by prior ambulatory monitoring? Am Heart J 1985 (Dec); 110:1146–1153.

108. EAGLE KA, BLACK HR, COOK EF, GOLDMAN L: Evaluation of prognostic classifications for patients with syncope. Am J Med 1985 (Oct); 79:455–460.

109. MOSS AJ, SCHWARTZ PJ, CRAMPTON RS, LOCATI E, CARLEEN E: The long QT syndrome: a prospective international study. Circulation 1985 (Jan); 71:17–21.

110. BHANDARI AK, SHAPIRO WA, MORADY F, SHEN EN, MASON J, SCHEINMAN MM: Electrophysiologic testing in patients with the long QT syndrome. Circulation 1985 (Jan); 71:63–71.

111. BHARATI S, DREIFUS L, BUCHELERES G, MOLTHAN M, COVITZ W, ISENBERG HS, LEV M: The conduction system in patients with a prolonged QT interval. J Am Coll Cardiol 1985 (Nov); 6:1110–1119.

112. SCHNEIDER JF, THOMAS E, MCNAMARA PM, KANNEL WB: Clinical-electrocardiographic correlates of newly acquired left bundle branch block: the Framingham study. Am J Cardiol 1985 (May 1); 55:1332–1338.

113. VASEY C, O'DONNELL J, MORRIS S, MCHENRY P: Exercise-induced left bundle branch block and its relation to coronary artery disease. Am J Cardiol 1985 (Nov 15); 56:892–895.

114. KAFKA H, BURGGRAF GW, MILLIKEN JA: Electrocardiographic diagnosis of left ventricular hypertrophy in the presence of left bundle branch block: an echocardiographic study. Am J Cardiol 1985 (Jan 1); 55:103–106.

115. SHAW DB, KEKWICK CA, VEALE D, GOWERS J, WHISTANCE T: Survival in second degree atrioventricular block. Br Heart J 1985 (June); 53:587–593.

116. COUNCIL ON SCIENTIFIC AFFAIRS: The use of cardiac pacemakers in medical practice: excerpts from the report of the advisory panel. JAMA 1985 (Oct 11); 254:1952–1954.

117. ALBIN G, HAYES DL, HOLMES DR: Sinus node dysfunction in pediatric and young adult patients: treatment by implantation of a permanent pacemaker in 39 cases. Mayo Clin Proc 1985 (Oct); 60:667–672.

118. ZOLL PM, ZOLL RH, FALK RH, CLINTON JE, EITEL DR, ANTMAN EM: External noninvasive temporary cardiac pacing: clinical trials. Circulation 1985 (May); 71:937–944.

119. BHATIA S, GOLDSCHLAGER N: Office evaluation of the pacemaker patient: Detection of normal and abnormal pacemaker function. JAMA 1985 (Sept 13); 254:1346–1352.

120. SHIVELY B, GOLDSCHLAGER N: Progress in cardiac pacing: part I. Arch Intern Med 1985 (Nov); 145:2103–2106.

121. SHIVELY B, GOLDSCHLAGER N: Progress in cardiac pacing: part II. Arch Intern Med 1985 (Dec); 145:2238–2244.

122. MAISEL AS, MOTULSKY HJ, INSEL PA: Hypotension after quinidine plus verapamil: possible additive competition at alpha-adrenergic receptors. N Engl J Med 1985 (Jan 17); 312:167–170.

123. HILGARD J, EZRI MD, DENES P: Significance of ventricular pauses of three seconds or more detected on twenty-four-hour Holter recordings. Am J Cardiol 1985 (Apr 1); 55:1005–1008.

124. ROBERTSON JH, BARDY GH, GERMAN LD, GALLAGHER JJ, KISSLO J: Comparison of two-dimensional echocardiographic and angiographic findings in arrhythmogenic right ventricular dysplasia. Am J Cardiol 1985 (June 1); 55:1506–1508.

125. SAKSENA S, GREENBERG E, FERGUSON D: Prospective reimbursement for state-of-the-art medical practice: the case for invasive electrophysiologic evaluation. Am J Cardiol 1985 (Apr 1); 55:963–967.

4

Systemic
Hypertension

Atrial natriuretic peptide

Frohlich[1] from New Orleans, Louisiana, in an editorial entitled, "The Heart, An Endocrine Organ (Revisited)", discussed the "third factor" responsible for the excretion of sodium in water. The first 2, of course, are the glomerular filtration rate and aldosterone. The "third factor" has been sought for years because the total amount of sodium excreted cannot be accounted for by glomerular filtration or aldosterone. The "third factor" has been postulated for years to eminate from the brain and to be digitalis-like in its structure, and it has been measured in blood by some investigators. The "third factor" discussed by Frohlich is the atrial natriuretic peptide (ANP), which is now the center of rapidly developing investigation. The fundamental observations providing the impetus for these investigations concerned the identification of ultrastructural granules within the atrial myocytes as far back as 1956. In 1979 these atrial granules were extracted biochemically from the atrial tissue and their profound natriuretic and diuretic properties were demonstrated. It is now clear that the ANP most likely acts in the distal renal tubule to promote the natriuresis that is unassociated with a marked kaliuresis. It might be inferred that whatever potassium excretion is demonstrated, it conceivably results from a stimulation of aldosterone secretion secondary to the marked sodium and water loss. Other studies have demonstrated that this ANP might be 6 or more polypeptides whose molecular weights vary from 2,000–30,000. Biochemically, ANP is a distinct chemical moiety. It is not digitalis-like in structure. It is a polypeptide. It does not inhibit Na-K-ATPase, and therefore promotes sodium excretion by a mechanism independent of sodium transport and cotransport enzymes. If the ANP hormone or hormones exist, the clinical implications are obvious. Cardiologists have known for years that after episodes of paroxysmal atrial tachycardia there is a profound diuresis. This diuresis may be related to a temporarily expanded cardiopulmonary volume that is associated with paroxysmal atrial tachycardia. With remission of the tachycardia, natriuresis results after the factor is released. Perhaps the substance is depleted from atrial stores in CHF. It may also provide an explanation for the exaggerated natriuresis phenomenon in essential hypertension. At any rate, the heart no longer can be considered a passive organ responding to hemodynamic challenges by adaptive means until its structural responses are exhausted. The heart may also respond by the active production of substances that are released in response to the functional circulating volume. Recognition of the endocrine role of the heart is at hand and a direct chemical link between cardiac and renal function is at long last available for study.

Laragh[2] from New York City provided a superb review on ANP. Other articles on this subject were by Tikkane and associates[3] from Helsinki, Finland, and by Sagnella and colleagues[4] from London, UK.

Effect of cigarette smoking

Baer and Radichevich[5] from New York City, studied the BP and endocrine responses to cigarette smoking in 19 patients with systemic hypertension to determine whether smoking activates the renin-aldosterone axis. BP increased from $140 \pm 7/99 \pm 3$ (mean $\pm$ SEM) to $151 \pm 5/108 \pm 2$ mmHg within 10 minutes after smoking, and pulse rate increased significantly (69 ± 2–96 ± 4 beats/min). Plasma renin activity did not change but increased 15 minutes after ambulation. In contrast, plasma aldosterone and plasma cortisol levels increased significantly after smoking and peaked at 20 minutes: 14 ± 1–20 ± 2 ng/dl and 10 ± 1–22 ± 2 μg/dl, respectively. These responses were closely correlated, suggesting a pituitary-adrenal mechanism is activated during smoking. Total plasma catecholamine levels increased from 468 ± 60–624 ± 73 pg/ml 10 minutes after smoking and to 724 ± 69 pg/ml 15 minutes after ambulation. In hypertensive smokers, cigarette smoking is associated with an increase in BP, pulse rate, and plasma cortisol, aldosterone, and plasma catecholamine levels. The long-term significance of these acute hormonal changes in regard to BP homeostasis and vascular disease in cigarette smokers remains to be determined. Smoking should be avoided before BP and endocrine determinations.

Effect of alcohol

An association between alcohol consumption and systemic hypertension has been found in several studies of general populations. Some investigators have considered high alcohol intake to be the cause of possibly 25% of cases of so-called essential hypertension. The relation between alcohol intake and BP appears to be independent of age, obesity, amount of physical exercise, and number of cigarettes smoked. Evidence on the acute effects of alcohol on BP in nonalcoholics is conflicting, and few studies have examined the pressor effects of alcohol in hypertensive patients. Malhotra and associates[6] from Jaipur, India, studied the effects of acute alcohol consumption and abstinence on BP in normal healthy subjects and in nondrinking and regular drinking hypertensive patients. All subjects drank alcohol (1 g/kg body weight daily) for 5 days, then abstained for 5 days. There was no significant difference in BP in normal subjects during and after alcohol ingestion. However, in hypertensive nondrinkers both systolic and diastolic pressures when standing were significantly higher during the period of alcohol intake; supine

BP was not significantly higher. In hypertensive patients who drank regularly, standing and supine systolic and diastolic BPs were significantly higher during the period of drinking.

Gruchow and associates[7] from Milwaukee and Wood, Wisconsin, analyzed data from the first Health and Nutrition Examination Survey with multivariate statistical techniques to determine whether there was evidence for a contributory role of alcohol in systemic hypertension and to provide a suitable prospective on the importance of nutrient variables compared with other established risk factors for systemic hypertension (Table 4-1). The results of these analyses reaffirm the importance of alcohol and sodium intakes on BP among US adults. Potassium (inversely) and phosphorus (directly) also were identified as important nutrient predictors of higher systolic BP. Calcium intake was significantly related to systolic BP only among nonwhite men and was not a significant predictor of systolic pressure overall. In addition, the results of the study reemphasized the paramount importance of age, race, and obesity in determining hypertension. Current nutrient intakes, by comparison, are relatively less important.

TABLE 4-1. *Age-standardized comparisons of hypertensive persons (systolic BP $\geq$ 160 mmHg) with normotensive persons in race, gender, body mass index, and average daily nutrient intakes.* Reproduced with permission from Gruchow et al.[7]*

	HYPERTENSIVE PERSONS (N = 1,012)	HORMOTENSIVE PERSONS (N = 8,541)	t STATISTIC	SIGNIFICANCE LEVEL (TWO-TAILED)
% Male	45.0	45.3	($\chi^2 = 0.03$)	NS
% White	70.4	84.4	($\chi^2 = 124.88$)	†
Body mass index	29.3 (7.4)	25.4 (4.6)	16.35	†
Total calories	1,814 (956)	1,907 (997)	2.83	†
Alcohol calories (total study cohort)	71.6 (174.1)	53.5 (150.0)	3.18	†
Alcohol calories‡ (drinkers only)	127.1 (216.2)	89.4 (186.6)	4.00	†
Nonalcohol calories	1,723 (722)	1,834 (778)	4.59	†
Total fat, g	74.2 (40.8)	78.4 (41.0)	3.01	†
Total protein, g	71.8 (36.0)	75.1 (37.4)	2.65	†
Total carbohydrate, g	193.1 (84.5)	208.2 (94.8)	5.30	†
Cholesterol, mg	357.1 (233.3)	351.7 (232.9)	0.70	NS
Saturated fat, g	26.8 (15.9)	28.5 (16.9)	3.19	†
Oleic acid, g	28.9 (16.5)	30.1 (17.1)	2.17	†
Linoleic acid, g	8.0 (6.8)	8.3 (7.0)	1.32	NS
Calcium, mg	608.0 (422.6)	722.4 (506.0)	7.96	†
Iron, mg	11.4 (5.5)	11.9 (5.9)	2.88	†
Phosphorus, mg	1,075.1 (532.9)	1,158.3 (577.7)	4.65	†
Potassium, mg	1,995.2 (937.8)	2,217.1 (1,083.8)	7.00	†
Sodium, mg	2,082.6 (1,163.4)	2,166.8 (1,303.2)	2.15	†
Vitamin A, IU	4,892.1 (9,635.5)	5,094.7 (8,794.5)	0.64	NS
Vitamin C, mg	73.1 (81.8)	84.0 (83.6)	3.94	†
Niacin, mg	16.8 (9.9)	17.1 (9.9)	0.80	NS
Riboflavin, mg	1.5 (1.0)	1.6 (1.1)	3.17	†
Thiamine, mg	1.0 (.6)	1.1 (.6)	4.07	†

*Values are means with SD in parentheses except for percentages of males and whites. Values were age standardized by the direct method.
†p <0.01, except for sodium ($p = 0.032$) and oleic acid ($p = 0.030$); NS = p >0.05.
‡For hypertensive persons, n = 570; for normotensive persons, n = 5,105.
χ^2 = chi square.

Relation to blood lead

Heavy lead exposure has been connected to cardiovascular disease, but modest exposures encountered in the general environment have not been associated previously with diseased risk. Harlan and associates[8] from Ann Arbor, Michigan, examined the relation between blood lead levels and BP using data from the Second National Health and Nutrition Examination Survey. A direct relation was found between blood lead levels and systolic and diastolic BP for men and women and for white and black persons aged 12–74 years. Blood lead levels were significantly higher in younger men and women (aged, 21–55 years) with high BP, but not in older men or women (aged 56–74 years). In multiple regression analyses, the relation of blood lead to BP was independent of other variables for men, but not for women. Dietary calcium and serum zinc levels were inversely related to BP.

Effect of snoring

Koskenvuo and associates[9] from Helsinki, Finland, tested by postal questionnaire a population of 3,847 men and 3,664 women aged 40–69 years the association of snoring with systemic hypertension and CAD. Hypertension associated highly significantly with snoring, the relative risk of hypertension between habitual snorers and never snorers being 1.94 in men and 3.19 in women. This association also was found when adjusting for body mass index. A significant association between angina pectoris and habitual snoring was observed in men. In women the relative risk was not significant. An association between habitual snoring and angina pectoris in men also was found after adjusting for hypertension and body mass index. The relative risks for AMI and hospital admission for CAD for habitual snorers were nonsignificant.

Sleep apnea syndrome

More than half of the patients with essential hypertension have sleep apnea. Williams and associates[10] from Los Angeles, California, assessed the incidence of unrecognized sleep apnea in patients with essential hypertension. They studied 23 patients taking antihypertensive medicines. They were evaluated by questionnaire for symptoms of sleep apnea, and during 3 hours of sleep, measurements were made of respiratory patterns using an impedance pneumograph, arterial oxygen saturation with an ear oximeter, and air flow at the mouth or nose with a face mask pneumotacograph. Abnormal sleep apneas (average, 20 seconds) lasting for an average of 19% sleep time were found in 11 patients (48%). Significant arterial oxygen desaturation, defined as a decrease of $\geq 4\%$ and to $<90\%$, was observed in 7 of the 11 (30%), with an average saturation of 87% at the end of the apneic episodes. Thus, almost one-third of patients randomly selected had significant arterial oxygen desaturation during sleep because of sleep apnea, and it was suggested that sleep apnea may play a part in the development of essential hypertension.

Osler's maneuver and pseudohypertension

Messerli and associates[11] from New Orleans, Louisiana, described a simple bedside procedure that they called "Osler's maneuver" that differentiates patients with true systemic hypertension from those whose BP is spuriously elevated because of excessive sclerosis of the large arteries ("pseudohypertension"). The maneuver is performed by assessing the palpability of the pulse-less radial or brachial artery distal to a point of occlusion of the artery manually or by cuff pressure. They classified 24 elderly hypertensive patients as either Osler-positive or Osler-negative, and measured their intra-arterial pressure, arterial compliance, and systemic hemodynamics. Patients with pseudohypertension (Osler-positive) had falsely elevated BP readings, with a difference of 10–54 mmHg between cuff and intra-arterial pressure. Arterial compliance was lower in Osler-positive subjects and correlated with the difference between cuff and intra-arterial pressures, indicating that the stiffer the artery, the more pronounced the degree of pseudohypertension. Pseudohypertension is common in the elderly and becomes more severe as arterial compliance decreases and sclerosis of large arteries progresses.

Hypertensive hypertrophic cardiomyopathy in the elderly

Using echo, Topol and associates[12] from Baltimore, Maryland, identified 21 patients with a syndrome that included severe concentric cardiac hypertrophy, a small LV cavity, and supernormal indexes of systolic function without concurrent medical illness or CAD. Thirteen patients presented with dyspnea or chest pain. All had a history of systemic hypertension and all were compared with normotensive control subjects matched for age and sex. The mean age of the patients was 73 years; 16 were women and 15 were black. The cardiac function was characterized by excessive LV emptying (EF on 2-D echo 79 $^+$ 4 -vs- 59 ± 5% [controls] and abnormal diastolic function as manifested by prolonged early diastolic filling period (279 ± 25 -vs- 160 ± 45 ms) and reduced peak diastolic dimension increase (11 ± 4 -vs- 16 ± 5 cm/s). Despite the clinical presentation of CHF, all 9 patients receiving either β-blocker or calcium channel blocking agents obtained symptomatic relief, whereas 6 of 12 patients receiving vasodilator medications had severe hypotensive reactions, including 1 death.

This article was followed by an editorial by Mangan entitled "The Heart in Hypertension."[13]

Effect on RV wall thickness

Gottdiener and coworkers[14] from Washington, D.C., determined whether RV wall thickness is altered in patients with pressure overload-induced LV hypertrophy. RV wall thickness was measured using M-mode echo with 2-D echo guidance in 65 patients with LV pressure overload; 49 patients had essential hypertension and 16 had AS. Data obtained from these measurements were compared with similar data from 13 patients with "thin-walled" dilated cardiomyopathy and 20 normal volunteers. RV wall thickness in hypertensive patients and patients with AS was significantly greater than in normal subjects and patients with dilated cardiomyopathy who had normal LV wall thickness. Increased RV wall thickness was found in 40 (82%) of 49 patients with hypertension and 10 (63%) of 16 patients with AS. The magnitude of increase in RV wall thickness was linearly related to LV wall thickness, but was not associated with pulmonary hypertension. Thus, these data indicate that increased RV wall thickness is found commonly in patients with LV pressure overload and hypertrophy. Moreover, the increase in wall thickness in these patients appears related to the magnitude of increase in LV wall thickness. These observations suggest that pressure overload in the left ventricle may be the stimulus for increase in wall thickness in the right ventricle.

LV diastolic function

Snider and associates[15] from Ann Arbor, Michigan, studied LV diastolic function by echo in 11 children with systemic hypertension and compared results with 11 normal children. Hypertensive patients were 1–17 years old (mean, 11) and mean duration of hypertension was 2.4 years. Diastolic filling was assessed from digitized continuous tracings of LV cavity as well as Doppler diastolic time intervals, peak velocities, and velocity areas. There were no differences between hypertensive and normal children in terms of heart rate or echo measurements of LV size, wall thickness, or peak filling rates. Hypertensive patients did show abnormalities in terms of diastolic filling velocities, peak A velocity, A area, and A area/total area.

LV systolic function remains normal for many years in patients with mild or moderate systemic hypertension. Papademetriou and associates[16] from Washington, D.C., recorded a high quality M-mode echo in 7 patients with borderline hypertension, 14 patients with mild hypertension, and in 15 normal persons. Measures of systolic and diastolic LV function and the degree of LV hypertrophy were studied with the assistance of a tablet digitizer and dedicated microcomputer. Average BP was $125 \pm 10/77 \pm 7$ mmHg in normal subjects, $146 \pm 18/92 \pm 2$ mmHg in patients with borderline hypertension and $150 \pm 11/102 \pm 4$ mmHg in patients with mild hypertension. Indexes of systolic LV function were similar in all 3 groups. The peak rate of early relaxation of the LV posterior wall was significantly decreased in the group of patients with mild hypertension (4.7 -vs- 6.6 s^{-1}). The mitral valve closure rate was 150 ± 32 mm/s in normal subjects, 119 ± 35 mm/s in patients with borderline hypertension, and 106 ± 26 mm/s in patients with mild hypertension. Mild LV hypertrophy was present in 6 of 7 patients with borderline and 13 of 14 patients with mild hypertension. The degree of hypertrophy and the level of BP correlated poorly. It was concluded that subtle abnormalities of diastolic LV function may be present in patients with mild hypertension at a time when LV systolic function is normal and that the degree of hypertrophy and intermittent measurements of BP at rest correlate poorly, suggesting that additional factors may play a role.

In pregnancy

Lindheimer and Katz[17] in a review article surveyed the problem of systemic hypertension in pregnancy, particularly focusing on preeclampsia and on several controversies remaining (Tables 4-2 and 4-3).

TREATMENT

Nondrug means

Kaplan[18] from Dallas, Texas, reviewed various nondrug therapies for treatment of systemic hypertension. The therapies include weight reduction; sodium restriction; potassium, calcium, and magnesium supplementation; other dietary changes; exercise; relaxation; and moderation of alcohol use. Such therapies have been inadequately used, in part because of a lack of confidence in their effectiveness and overconfidence in the effectiveness and safety of drug therapy. Evidence about the effectiveness, mode of action, safety, and patient acceptance of the various nondrug therapies is reviewed, and practical guidelines to their use are provided. Nondrug therapies may

TABLE 4-2. *Guidelines for treating severe hypertension near term or during labor. Reproduced with permission from Lindheimer and Katz.*[17]

1. The degree to which BP should be decreased is disputed. Levels between 90 and 105 mmHg diastolic are recommended
2. Drug therapy
   a. Parenteral hydralazine is the drug of choice. Use low doses (start with 5 mg, then give 5–10 mg every 20–30 minutes) in order to avoid precipitous decreases. Side effects include tachycardia and headache. Neonatal thrombocytopenia has been reported
   b. Diazoxide is recommended for the occasional patient whose hypertension is refractory to hydralazine. Use 30 mg miniboluses, since maternal vascular collapse and death have been associated with the customary 300 mg dose. Side effects include arrest of labor and neonatal hyperglycemia
   c. Do not use sodium nitroprusside (fetal cyanide poisoning has been reported in animals), ganglion-blocking agents (meconium ileus has been reported), or loop diuretics (such as, furosemide). (However, in the final analysis, maternal well-being will dictate the choice of therapy)
3. Parenteral magnesium sulfate is the drug of choice for preventing impending eclamptic convulsions. Therapy should continue for 12 (and sometimes 24) hours into the puerperium, since one-third of patients with preeclampsia have convulsions after childbirth

TABLE 4-3. *Antihypertensive drugs in pregnancy. Reproduced with permission from Lindheimer and Katz.*[17]

α_2-Receptor agonists	Methyldopa (0.5–3 g/day) is the most extensively used drug of this group in the United States; its safety and efficacy have been supported in randomized trials. Neonatal tremors have been reported; other side effects are the same as in the nongravid population. Trials with clonidine are in progress; embryopathy has been described in animals, and this drug is not currently recommended
β-Receptor antagonists	These agents, currently undergoing extensive testing, appear to be safe and efficacious. Atenolol (50–100 mg/day), metoprolol (50–225 mg/day), and propranolol (40–240 mg/day) are used most frequently to date. Fetal and neonatal bradycardia and hypoglycemia have been reported, and animal data suggest the possibility of a decreased ability of the fetus to tolerate hypoxic stress
α- and β-Receptor antagonists	Labetalol, for example—currently undergoing extensive testing—appears to be as effective as methyldopa. A possible association with retroplacental hemorrhage is under investigation
Arteriolar vasodilators	Hydralazine (50–200 mg/day) is used frequently as adjunctive therapy with methyldopa and β-receptor antagonists. There has only been fragmentary experience with minoxidil, which is thus not recommended at present
Converting enzyme inhibitors	Captopril is associated with fetal death in several animal species. Do not use in pregnancy
Diuretics	Most authorities discourage their use, although some continue these medications if they were prescribed before gestation. We would prescribe diuretics when BP control was poor despite the use of other agents, the fetus was immature, and pregnancy termination was the only alternative
Miscellaneous	Calcium channel blockers and serotonin antagonists (such as ketanserin) are currently under investigation. Do not use ganglion-blocking agents or nitroprusside

provide enough antihypertensive effect to lower BP of many patients with mild hypertension to a safe level without the need for antihypertensive drugs. Kaplan recommended the following as a practical subscription for nondrug therapy of systemic hypertension: 1) for the overweight, weight reduction should be the primary goal; 2) for all hypertensive persons, dietary sodium intake should be restricted to 2 g/day (88 mM/day), with caution not to reduce the consumption of low fat, low sodium milk and cheese products so as to maintain calcium intake; 3) more fiber and less saturated fat are beneficial for other reasons and may also help lower the BP; 4) alcohol should be limited to 2 oz/day; 5) regular isotonic exercise should be encouraged; 6) potassium intake need not be specifically increased because it will increase with a lowered sodium intake; 7) supplemental magnesium and calcium should only be given to those who are deficient until additional evidence of their efficacy is available; 8) those who are willing and able should be encouraged to do some type of relaxation therapy. These recommendations may lower the BP in a significant number of persons with mild hypertension to below 140/90 mmHg in order to eliminate, postpone, or at least minimize the need for drug therapy. Even if it does not lower the BP, this program should do no harm and may provide several other benefits, including a reduction in most other risk factors for premature cardiovascular disease. The intensive incorporation of all these nondrug therapies into management of a given patient could entail considerable expense, far beyond that of 1 or 2 doses a day of antihypertensive drug. However, for most patients, the regimen need only require a few extra visits to a dietician and, for those >40 years of age, perhaps an exercise stress test before beginning a strenuous exercise program. Most follow-up visits, mainly for maintaining the patient's motivation, can be handled by nonphysicians. Overall, the expense may be greater, but the potential for improvement in overall health makes the cost seem trivial. Moreover, the use of drugs to lower BP does not relieve the hypertensive patient of the need to lose weight, exercise regularly, eat a prudent diet, and learn to relax. Therefore, nondrug therapies have a place in the management of all patients with hypertension.

Marzuk[19] wrote this article for the Health and Public Policy Committee of the American College of Physicians on biofeedback for systemic hypertension. The recommendations of this committee were as follows: Biofeedback cannot be recommended as a first-line treatment for essential hypertension. The first nonpharmacologic treatment for hypertensive patients should be life-style counseling on weight reduction, dietary control of sodium, regular exercise, and elimination of cigarette smoking. For patients with mild hypertension or adverse reactions to medication, biofeedback may be a useful adjunct to reduce medication requirements. As with medication or other antihypertensive therapies, the use of biofeedback requires careful monitoring of BP. Current studies indicate that biofeedback is no more effective than various other relaxation therapies, such as yoga, meditation, and autogenic relaxation. Studies using biofeedback for mild to moderate essential hypertension (90–104 mmHg and 105–114 mmHg diastolic, respectively) suggest that some persons are able to achieve moderate decreases in BP (average, 8 mmHg and 6 mmHg). Greater decreases are obtained in systolic pressure than diastolic pressure, but, in general, these decreases are small and of short duration.

Duncan and associates[20] from Dallas, Texas, evaluated the effects of a 16-week aerobic exercise program on BP and plasma catecholamine levels in 56 patients with baseline diastolic BP ranging from 90–140 mmHg. The exercise group significantly improved their physical fitness, and reduced systolic and diastolic BP, compared with controls. To evaluate the relation between exercise, BP, and plasma catecholamine values, the exercise group was further divided into hyperadrenergic and normoadrenergic subgroups. Reductions in systolic pressures were 6.3, 10.3, and 15.5 mmHg for control, normoadrenergic, and hyperadrenergic groups, respectively. Diastolic changes were similar and also significant. Within the hyperadrenergic group, changes in BP were associated with changes in values for plasma catecholamines after training. They concluded that an aerobic exercise program reduces BP, which is at least partially mediated by changes in plasma catecholamine levels.

Diuretics

Changes in potassium balance have been found to have variable effects on the BP of animals and the administration of potassium supplement has been reported to lower the BP of normal kalemic hypertensive patients. To assess the effect of potassium repletion in hypokalemic systemic hypertension, Kaplan and associates[21] from Dallas, Texas, administered either potassium chloride, 60 mM/day, or placebo tablets, each for 6 weeks, in a randomized, double-blind, crossover trial to 16 hypertensive patients who had diuretic-induced hypokalemia and who continued to take a constant amount of diuretic. They selected patients whose control serum potassium levels were <3.5 mM/L. In association with an average increase in the serum potassium concentration of 0.56 mM/L, the mean BP decreased an average of 5.5 mmHg with at least a 4 mmHg decrease observed in 9 of the 16 patients. The decrease in BP correlated with a decrease in plasma renin activity but not with changes in plasma aldosterone levels or other variables. They concluded that short-term potassium supplementation that ameliorates diuretic-induced hypokalemia may induce a significant decrease in BP.

This article was followed by an editorial by Kassirer and Harrington[22] from Boston, Massachusetts, entitled, "Fending off the Potassium Pushers."

Because of evidence suggesting an association of mild hypokalemia with cardiac arrhythmia, Stewart and associates[23] from Christ Church, New Zealand, compared the arrhythmogenic potentials of potassium-losing and po tassium-sparing diuretic treatments in a controlled prospective crossover study of 10 patients with mild systemic hypertension and CAD. Mean plasma potassium of 4.3 ± 0.06 and 3.3 ± 0.07 mM/L after potassium sparing and potassium losing treatments, respectively. BP and volume depletion as assessed by weight change, plasma renin activity, and norepinephrine concentrations did not differ significantly in the 2 treatment periods. The potassium-losing treatment phase was associated with an increased frequency of VPC, a higher Lown grading during ambulatory ECG monitoring, prolonged duration and decreased phase 0 velocity of the monophasic action potential, a prolonged ventricular effective refractory period, and increased myocardial electrical instability as assessed by programmed ventricular stimulation. They concluded that minor changes in plasma potassium concentration are associated with increased ventricular electrical instability in patients with CAD. Mild hypokalemia in such patients may predispose to life-threatening arrhythmias and should be avoided.

Papademetriou and associates[24] from Washington, D.C., used echo as a more sensitive index for the presence of LV hypertrophy. Thirty-one patients with uncomplicated hypertension underwent 48-hour ambulatory ECG monitoring both before any treatment and after 4 weeks of hydrochlorothiazide (HCTZ), 100 mg daily. In 18 patients with LV posterior wall thickness ≥13 mm (average, 14 ± 0.2 mm) on echo, plasma potassium decreased from 4.1 ± 0.3–3.3 ± 0.4 mEq/L with HCTZ. VPC averaged 5.7 ± 9.9/hour at baseline and 7.1 ± 16.6/hour after HCTZ. The total number of couplets was 29 before and 13 after HCTZ, and 4 brief runs of VT occurred only before treatment. In the remaining 13 patients with wall thickness ≤12 mm (average, 11 ± 0.1 mm), plasma potassium decreased from 4.1 ± 0.3–3.4 ± 0.5 mEq/L with HCTZ. The average number of VPC was 4.3 ± 8.0/hour before and 5.2 ± 8.9/hour after HCTZ. One couplet and 1 3-beat run of VT occurred before and 1 3-beat run of VT after HCTZ. Although more complex arrhythmias were noted in the LV hypertrophy group, the differences were not statistically significant. These results indicate that thiazide therapy does not increase ventricular arrhythmias either in patients with or without LV hypertrophy.

Beta blocker

Several drugs used for antihypertensive therapy may interact with lipoproteins and increase associated coronary risk factors. Lehtonen[25] from Turku, Finland, found that β-blocker monotherapy with cardioselective or noncardioselective β-blockers without intrinsic sympathomimetic activity (ISA) usually increased serum triglyceride and decreased the concentration of HDL, especially HDL_2 cholesterol. With the exception of the noncardioselective β-blocker, sotalol, β-blocker therapy had little influence on serum total cholesterol or LDL cholesterol concentrations. The magnitude of these changes in serum lipids did not significantly differ between cardioselective and noncardioselective β-blockers. Two β-blockers possessing ISA, acebutolol and pindolol, did not increase serum triglycerides or serum total cholesterol or LDL cholesterol. Acebutolol produced a nonsignificant decrease in HDL cholesterol level. Pindolol, with marked ISA, had the most favorable lipid profile, increasing serum HDL cholesterol and the ratio of HDL cholesterol to total cholesterol. The concentration of apolipoprotein A-1 increased slightly during pindolol therapy. β-Blockers, with the exception of pindolol, decreased the concentration of serum free fatty acids. β-Blocker therapy had little influence on adipose tissue lipoprotein lipase activity, but lecithin cholesterol acyltransferase activity increased during pindolol therapy. Thus, β-blocking drugs possessing ISA, such as acebutolol and pindolol, appear desirable choices as antihypertensive agents, since they do not produce adverse effects on the lipid profile.

Floras and colleagues[26] from Headington, Oxford, UK, evaluated the ability of cardioselective and nonselective β-blockers with and without partial agonist activity in the control of BP associated with mental and physical activity in 35 patients with systemic hypertension. Direct measurements of BP and radioenzymatic determinations of plasma norepinephrine were obtained before, during, and after various activities and were repeated after random allocation to treatment with atenolol, metoprolol, pindolol, or propranolol. Cardioselective and nonselective drugs modestly reduced the pressor response to reaction time testing, but not to mental arithmetic or isometric exercise. The increase in systolic BP during bicycle exercise was significantly reduced by the cardioselective drugs atenolol (by 23 mmHg, or 38%) and metoprolol (21 mmHg, or 41%), but not by the nonselective blockers, pindolol and propranolol. Only bicycle exercise increased plasma norepinephrine concentration. These data indicate that β-blockers do not attenuate increases in BP during mental or physical activities unless intense sympathoadrenal activation also occurs. Marked elevations in circulating epinephrine, with or without norepinephrine, and peripheral $β_2$-blockade appear necessary for α-mediated vasoconstriction to predominate and for the beneficial effects of cardioselective and nonselective drugs to be evident.

A comparison of once-daily and twice-daily regimens of treatments with a β-adrenoceptor-blocking agent, acebutolol, was carried out in patients with mild to moderate essential hypertension by Weber and Drayer[27] from Long Beach, California. After an initial placebo phase, all patients entered an open 9-week period during which the dose of acebutolol, given on a twice-daily basis to all patients, was titrated to reduce seated diastolic BP to <90 mmHg or to decrease it by ≥10 mmHg. After a further 4-week maintenance period, patients whose BP had been successfully controlled entered a 3-month double-blind study in which they were randomly divided into 3 groups: 47 receiving continuation of twice-daily treatment; 97 receiving once-daily treatment (using the same total daily dose as in the earlier twice-daily phase); and 48 receiving placebo twice daily. By the end of the study, 78% of the once-daily treatment group were still under control, a result similar to that of 72% in the twice-daily treatment group. In contrast, only 39% of the placebo patients remained under control. Moreover, the BP in this group was significantly higher than in the other 2 groups. Acebutolol is an efficacious antihypertensive agent when used on a once-daily basis.

Wahl and associates[28] from Los Angeles, California, in a multicenter double-blind study compared oral acebutolol (n = 186) with propranolol (n = 190) in the treatment of mild to moderately severe essential hypertension (diastolic ≥95–129 mmHg). Both β-blockers produced significant and comparable reductions in diastolic, systolic, and mean arterial BP of 16, 12, and 14% on acebutolol and 15, 12, and 14% on propranolol. At equipotent, antihypertensive doses, acebutolol induced significantly less reduction in resting heart rate than propranolol (13% on acebutolol, 17% on propranolol). The mean effective doses of acebutolol and propranolol were 738 mg and 231 mg, respectively. Significantly fewer acebutolol patients had central nervous system side effects (50 on acebutolol, 75 on propranolol) or withdrew from the study prematurely due to side effects (11 on acebutolol, 29 on propranolol). No clinically significant trends in abnormalities of laboratory parameters were seen. It was concluded that acebutolol is as effective as propranolol in the treatment of hypertension, and acebutolol was better tolerated on the basis of heart rate and central nervous system side effects.

Teit and associates[29] from New York City studied maximal exercise capacity after control of resting BP with labetalol in 9 hypertensive men aged 34–69 years (mean, 52). Subjects exercised to exhaustion on an upright cycle ergometer with workload increased as a step function by 25 W every 3 minutes, both before and after control of BP was obtained. Mean exercise capacity expressed as total time of exercise until exhaustion was 936 seconds before and 884 seconds after control of resting BP with labetalol. Double product at peak exercise decreased from 254×10^2 before to 183×10^2 mmHg beats/minute after control of BP with labetalol. The difference in the means of resting heart rate and both peak BP and heart rate with exercise were all statistically significant after control of BP with labetalol. These findings suggest that labetalol has an ideal exercise profile affording a cardioprotective effect by decreasing double product but without sacrificing exercise capacity.

Some theoretical arguments suggest that added vasodilation could be beneficial in the management of patients with combined systemic hypertension and angina pectoris. Jee and Opie[30] of Cape Town, South Africa, studied in a double-blind crossover trial 10 patients in whom the severity of hypertension and angina pectoris was monitored. The initial run-in period of 2–6 weeks consisted of therapy with fixed-dose atenolol, 100 mg once daily, a thiazide diuretic drug, and any other agents required to control the hypertension. Patients were then randomized for 4 weeks to active atenolol plus 2 tablets of labetalol placebo, or active labetalol (200 mg twice daily) plus atenolol placebo, then crossed over and then changed back to active atenolol without labetalol placebo; the observers were unblinded in the last period. Labetalol and atenolol were equivalent in control of BP at rest, exercise tolerance, and use of nitroglycerin; however, heart rates at rest and during exercise were higher with labetalol, whereas the heart rate-BP product at the end of the exercise test was unchanged with labetalol. The higher heart rates for the same antianginal efficacy may give an advantage to labetalol treatment in some patients. Conversely, atenolol is cardioselective, hydrophilic, and can be given as a single daily dose. Thus, each agent has some advantages in the therapy of patients with hypertension and effort angina.

MacMahon and associates[31] from Sydney, Australia, compared weight reduction with metoprolol (200 mg daily) in a randomized placebo-controlled trial of first-line treatment of mild systemic hypertension (diastolic BP 90–109 mmHg) in 56 overweight patients aged <55 years. After 21 weeks of follow-up the weight-reduction group had lost an average of 7.4 kg. The decrease in the systolic BP of 13 mmHg was significantly greater than that in the placebo group (7 mmHg) but not different from that in the metoprolol group (10 mmHg). The decrease in diastolic pressure (10 mmHg) was greater than that in both the metoprolol (6 mmHg) and placebo (3 mmHg) groups. At the end of the follow-up period, 50% of patients in the weight-reduction group had a diastolic pressure of <90 mmHg. In the metoprolol group, there was a decrease in HDL cholesterol and an increase in the ratio of total to HDL cholesterol; in the weight-reduction group there was a decrease both in total cholesterol and in the ratio of total to HDL cholesterol. Thus, weight reduction produced significant and clinically important reductions in BP without adverse effects on plasma lipids.

This article was followed by an unsigned editorial discussing weight reduction in hypertension.[32] The point of the editorial is that there is sufficient evidence to support the view that every overweight hypertensive person should be encouraged strongly to lower weight. The benefits are directly related to the amount of weight lost.

Angiotensin converting enzyme inhibitor

Edwards and Padfield[33] from Edinburgh, UK, reviewed the use of angiotensin-converting enzyme (ACE) for systemic hypertension and CHF. The review was confined to captopril and enalapril. Since 1979, 1 million patients in the UK and in the United States have been treated with captopril, approximately 70% for systemic hypertension and 30% for CHF. Now that the side effects of ACE inhibitors have been better defined, it would seem inevitable that they will be increasingly prescribed for patients with less severe forms of systemic hypertension and also probably earlier in the treatment of CHF. One major reason for this, apart from their efficacy, is the feeling of well-being reported by many patients on these drugs. Long-term studies of hypertensive patients treated with ACE inhibitors are needed, however, to see whether they decrease the number of cardiovascular deaths more effectively than do other hypotensive agents, possibly by reducing the frequency of ventricular arrhythmias. This is a superb review article.

Ventura and associates[34] from New Orleans, Louisiana, studied systemic and regional hemodynamics in cardiac structural changes in 12 patients with mild to moderately severe essential hypertension before and then 90 minutes and 12 weeks after administration of captopril. Mean arterial BP was reduced from 111–96 mmHg, and this was mediated through a decrease in total peripheral resistance from 26 ± 2–23 ± 2 U. The decreased total peripheral resistance was distributed to all circulations studied: kidney, skeletal muscle, skin, and the splanchnic organs. Furthermore, LV mass index diminished without altering myocardial contractility at rest. Thus, captopril lowered arterial pressure through systemic arteriolar dilation in patients with mild to moderately severe essential hypertension and also reduced LV mass even in patients without evidence of LV hypertrophy.

Jenkins and associates[35] from Princeton, New Jersey, as part of a large multicenter surveillance study of captopril, treated 975 patients aged ≥65 years with severe systemic hypertension. Of the 975 patients, the average sitting BP was 193/105 ± 30/16 mmHg on entry to the study, while receiving an average of 2.5 antihypertensive drugs. Of the 975 patients, 418 received captopril for ≥12 months. Mean BP was lowered from an entry level of 193/105 ± 30/16–159/88 ± 25/12 mmHg and side effects were infrequent. Initial dose of captopril was 25 mg 2 or 3 times a day, increasing to 50 mg 2 or 3 times a day after 2 or 3 weeks, if necessary. The diuretic added after a further 2 or 3 weeks if adequate control of BP had not been achieved. During treatment, renal function was undisturbed in most patients. The frequency of clinically evident hypotensive episodes did not differ from that found in the total study population, suggesting that in this age group, despite the reduction in BP, cerebral profusion was maintained. This study suggests that captopril is useful for treatment of systemic hypertension in the elderly.

Thind and associates[36] from Louisville, Kentucky, gave the ACE inhibitors, enalapril (5–20 mg twice daily) or captopril (25–100 mg thrice daily) and matching ACE inhibitor placebos to 32 moderate to severe essential hypertension patients who were already on 50 mg hydrochlorothiazide daily. α-Methyldopa (250–500 mg twice daily) was given to 16 patients after 6 weeks of ACE inhibitor therapy. Both enalapril and captopril significantly lowered the supine and upright BP (acutely and long-term) without significant reflex heart rate changes. The BP of enalapril patients were, however, significantly lower than those of captopril patients when compared by repeated measures of analysis of variance. Eleven enalapril patients were followed for 1 year with continued BP control. Skin rash occurred in 1 captopril patient and reversible renal insufficiency developed in 2 enalapril patients during the first 16 weeks. It was concluded that although both ACE inhibitors lowered BP, enalapril was more effective than captopril, and twice-daily enalapril was well tolerated during 52 weeks of treatment.

Oren and associates[37] from Philadelphia, Pennsylvania, compared the efficacy of captopril treatment with that of propranolol in a single-blind crossover study in 14 patients with essential hypertension uncontrolled on diuretic alone. Both captopril (37.5–75 mg daily) and propranolol (60–120 mg daily), in combination with hydrochlorothiazide (50 mg daily), caused a significant decrease in sitting systolic and diastolic BP. Heart rate, plasma renin activity, and plasma aldosterone data were consistent with the effects of converting enzyme inhibition or β-blockade. Both drugs were well tolerated. Captopril appeared to be equivalent in efficacy and safety to propranolol when added to hydrochlorothiazide. Thus, captopril may be considered as an alternative step 2 antihypertensive agent, especially in patients having unwanted side effects on β-blockers.

Nitroglycerin or nitroprusside for postoperative hypertension

Fremes and colleagues[38] from Toronto, Canada, treated postoperative hypertension in 33 patients assigned randomly to infusion of either nitroglycerin or nitroprusside in a crossover trial of therapies designed to reduce mean arterial pressure from >95–85 mmHg. Both nitroglycerin and nitroprusside reduced mean BP, although the dose of nitroglycerin required was approximately 10 times greater than the dose of nitroprusside. Nitroglycerin reduced LV stroke work index more than did nitroprusside. Both agents increased LVEF and decreased LV end-diastolic volume index. Coronary sinus blood flow decreased with both drugs but myocardial lactate flux increased with nitroglycerin and decreased with nitroprusside. Cardiac index decreased with nitroglycerin and increased slightly with nitroprusside because of greater venodilatation, RV unloading, and greater reduction in LV preload with nitroglycerin. Because of its greater reduction of LV end-diastolic volume index, nitroglycerin decreased oxygen demand and myocardial oxygen consumption more than did nitroprusside. Lactate extraction and, thus, myocardial lactate flux increased with nitroglycerin so only nitroglycerin improved myocardial metabolism. Either nitroglycerin or nitroprusside may be used after routine operation; however, nitroglycerin is preferred for patients with suspected perioperative ischemia.

Major clinical trials

During 1985, the results of 3 major multicenter trials, each of which has taken over a decade to carry out, were reported.[39–43] One trial was concerned with whether a particular group should be treated, mainly >60.[40] Another specifically examined the possible beneficial effects of regimens containing a β-blocker[43] and the largest of the 3, the Medical Research Council (MRC) trial,[42] examined both the potential benefits of treating mild systemic hypertension and also the relative advantages of diuretics and β-blockers. Although the objectives of these trials overlap, the patients differed in several important ways. The European Working Party on Hypertension in the Elderly (EWPHE) recruited patients >60 years of age for the diastolic BP entry of 90–119 mmHg: patients were selected from a clinic population. The MRC workers recruited patients as a result of screening 500,000 healthy individuals aged 35–64 years: the BP criterion for entry was 90–109 mmHg diastolic. The MRC patients were thus younger, had milder hypertension, and were more representative of a healthy symptom-free population, so it is not surprising that cardiovascular events were much less frequent in the MRC population. The prevalence of fatal strokes in the placebo group of the MRC study, for instance, was 0.6/1,000 patient-years, whereas the prevalence in the EWPHE was 15/1,000 patient-years. The EWPHE included 840 patients and the MRC trial included 17,354 patients. Both studies showed a significant reduction in the overall rate of cardiovascular events. In the MRC study the difference between the placebo and treated groups was 1.6 events/1,000 patient-years: the difference in the EWPHE trial was 29 events/1,000 patient-years. The proportionate reduction, however, was similar. Events were reduced by about one-fifth in the MRC study and by one-fourth in the EWPHE study. The 2 investigations showed a remarkably similar proportionate reduction in the stroke rate. In the MRC study this reduction was 45% (1.2 strokes/1,000 patient-years), and in the EWPHE study the nonfatal stroke rate was reduced by 52% (11 strokes/1,000 patient-years). The reduction in fatal strokes was not statistically significant in either study. The treatment group in the MRC study had an almost identical AMI rate to the placebo group. Similarly, in the EWPHE study nonfatal AMI was not influenced by treatment. The consistent finding between the 2 trials was a significant reduction in fatal AMI in the EWPHE trial. Two of the 3 major trials sought answers to the relative merits of the 2 most widely used first-line agents and the patterns are reasonably consistent. The International Prospective Primary Prevention Study in Hypertension (IPPPSH)[43] examined outcome in 6,357 patients randomly allocated to antihypertensive regimens that included the β-blocker oxprenolol and regimens that included no β-blocker. The 2 groups had a similar prevalence of AMI, cerebrovascular accident, and sudden death. Since diuretics were used in about a third of the patients in each group, this trial could not show the relative merits of β-blockers and diuretics. Fortunately, the MRC study included β-blocker and diuretic-treated groups and placebo groups for each. This study likewise showed no advantage for β-blockers as far as outcome was concerned; indeed, bendroflumethiazide (in higher doses than are now generally recommended) had a significantly more favorable effect on stroke rate. In their search for subgroups of patients who might respond particularly well to β-blockers, the IPPPSH workers examined smoking habits and concluded that there was a significant interaction between smoking and cardiac events in men. The use of β-blockers in nonsmoking men was associated with a particularly low prevalence of cardiac events. Such retrospective subgroup analyses have to be treated with great caution. Independently, the MRC workers also observed a lower rate of cardiovascular events in nonsmokers taking propranolol, whereas the cardiovascular event rate was not affected by smoking habit in the diuretic-treated group or in smokers taking propranolol. In the MRC study, however, the difference in responsiveness to the 2 drugs among smokers and nonsmokers was due to differences in both coronary events and strokes rather than in coronary events alone. Thus, patients and doctors can be reassured that the arguments in favor of β-blockers and against diuretics as first-line agents have not been supported by hard fact, although there is a possibility that β-blockers are preferable in nonsmoking men.

Amery and other investigators[40] from multiple centers in Europe conducted a double-blind randomized placebo-controlled trial of antihypertensive treatment in patients >60 years old. Entry criteria included both a sitting diastolic BP on placebo treatment in the range 90–119 mmHg and a systolic pressure in the range 160–239 mmHg; 840 patients were randomized either to active treatment (hydrochlorothiazide plus triamterene) or to matching placebo. If the BP remained high, methyldopa was added to the active regimen and matching placebo in the placebo group. An overall intention-to-treat analysis, combining the double-blind part of the trial and all subsequent follow-up, revealed a nonsignificant change in total mortality rate (−9%), but a significant reduction in cardiovascular mortality rate (−27%). The latter was due to a reduction in cardiac mortality (−38%) and a nonsignificant decrease in cerebrovascular mortality (−32%). In the double-blind part of the trial, total mortality rate was not significantly reduced (−26%). Cardiovascular mortality was reduced in the actively treated group (−38%), owing to a reduction in cardiac deaths (−47%) and a nonsignificant decrease in cerebrovascular mortality (−43%) (Fig. 4-1). Deaths from AMI were reduced (−60%). Study-terminating morbid cardiovascular events were significantly reduced by active treatment (−60%). Nonterminating cerebrovascular events were reduced (−52%), but the nonterminating cardiac events were not (+3%). In the patients randomized to active treatment there were 29 fewer cardiovascular events and 14 fewer cardiovascular deaths per 1,000 patient-years during the double-blind part of the trial.

This article was followed by an editorial entitled "Treatment of Hypertension in the Over 60s."[41] In this unsigned editorial it was concluded that the EWPHE trial presented useful but by no means final information. It seems likely that treating hypertension in the elderly according to the criteria now applied to younger age groups will at least help some patients. At the same time the likelihood of adverse effects and difficulties in compliance is much greater than in the younger patients.

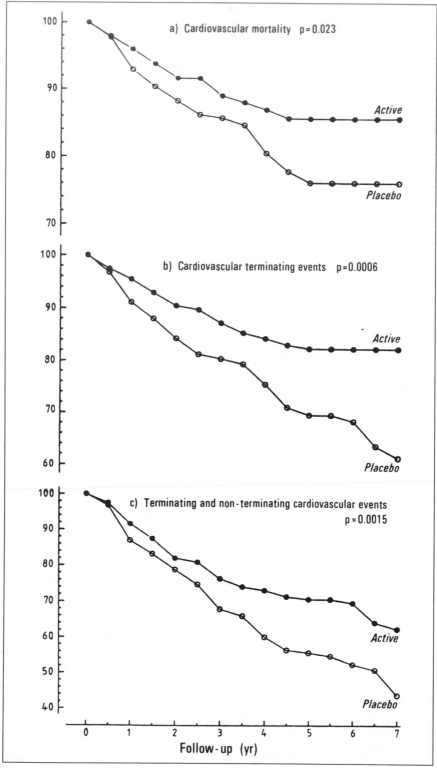

Fig. 4-1. Cumulative percent of survivors without events calculated for the patients on randomized treatment by life-table method. Reproduced with permission from Amery et al.[40]

The main aim of the MRC Trial[42] was to determine whether drug treatment of mild systemic hypertension (diastolic BP 90–109 mmHg) reduced the rates of stroke, of death due to systemic hypertension, and of coronary events in men and women aged 35–64 years. Subsidiary aims were: to compare the course of BP in 2 groups, 1 taking bendroflumethiazide and 1 taking propranolol, and to compare the incidence of suspected adverse reactions to these 2 drugs. The study was single blind and based almost entirely in general practices; 17,354 patients were recruited, and 85,572 patient-years of observation were accrued. Patients were randomly allocated at entry to take bendroflumethiazide or propranolol or placebo tablets. The stroke rate was reduced on active treatment: 60 strokes occurred in the treated group and 109 in the placebo group, giving rates of 1.4 and 2.6/1,000 patient-years of observation, respectively. Treatment made no difference, however, to the overall rates of coronary events: 222 events occurred on active treatment and 234 in the placebo group (5.2 and 5.5/1,000 patient-years, respectively). The incidence of all cardiovascular events was reduced on active treatment: 286 events occurred in the treated group and 352 in the placebo group, giving rates of 6.7 and 8.2/1,000 patient-years, respectively. For mortality from all causes, treatment made no difference; 248 deaths in the treated group and 253 in the placebo group (rates 5.8 and 5.9/1,000 patient-years, respectively). Several post hoc analyses of subgroup results were also performed but they require cautious interpretation. The all-cause mortality was reduced in men on active treatment (157 -vs- 181 deaths in the placebo group; 7.1 and 8.2/1,000 patient-years, respectively) but increased in women on active treatment (91 -vs- 72 deaths; 4.4 and 3.5/1,000 patient-years, respectively). The difference between the sexes in their response to treatment was significant. Comparison of the 2 active drugs showed that the reduction in stroke rate on bendroflumethiazide was greater than that on propranolol. The stroke rate was reduced in both smokers and nonsmokers taking bendroflumethiazide, but only in nonsmokers taking propranolol (Fig. 4-2). This difference between the responses to the 2 drugs was significant. The coronary event rate was not reduced by bendroflumethiazide, whatever the smoking habit, nor was it reduced in smokers taking propranolol, but it was reduced in non-

Fig. 4-2. Incidence of stroke per 1,000 person-years of observation according to randomized treatment regimen and cigarette smoking status at entry to trial. Reproduced with permission from the Medical Research Council Working Party.[42]

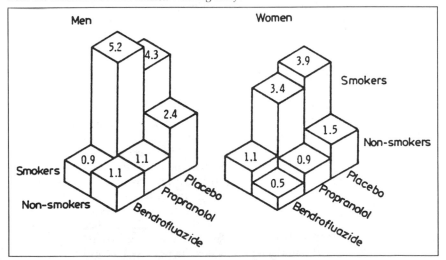

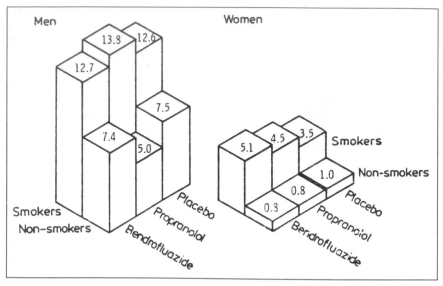

Fig. 4-3. Incidence of coronary events per 1,000 person-years of observation according to randomized treatment regimen and cigarette smoking status at entry to trial. Reproduced with permission from the Medical Research Council Working Party.[42]

smokers taking propranolol (Fig. 4-3). The rate of all cardiovascular events was not reduced by bendroflumethiazide, whatever the smoking habit, or in smokers taking propranolol, but was reduced in nonsmokers taking propranolol. The difference between the 2 drugs in this respect was significant. The trial has shown that if 850 mildly hypertensive patients are given active antihypertensive drugs for 1 year, about 1 stroke will be prevented. This is an important but an infrequent benefit. Its achievement subjected a substantial percentage of the patients to chronic side effects, mostly but not all minor. Treatment did not appear to save lives or substantially alter the overall risk of CAD. More than 95% of the control patients remained free of any cardiovascular event during the trial. Neither of the 2 drug regimens had any clear overall advantage over the other. The diuretic was perhaps better than the β-blocker in preventing stroke, but the β-blocker may have prevented coronary events in nonsmokers. For all categories of events, and in both treated and placebo groups, rates were lower in nonsmokers than in smokers, adding to previous evidence that smoking considerably increases the risk of cardiovascular disease. For stroke and also for all cardiovascular events, the difference between rates in smokers and nonsmokers was greater than the effect of drug treatment.

AMI, sudden coronary death, cerebrovascular accidents, BP control, and treatment tolerability were studied in a randomized double-blind trial conducted in 6,357 men and women aged 40–64 years with uncomplicated essential hypertension (diastolic BP 100–125 mmHg).[43] At the start of the trial 3,185 patients received treatment based on a β-blocker (oxprenolol), and the remaining 3,172 received placebo. Supplementary drugs, excluding β-blockers, were used as necessary in both treatment groups, with the aim of reducing diastolic pressure to ≤95 mmHg. Patients were followed for 3–5 years, a total of 25,651 patient-years at risk. In most respects the 2 groups fared equally well; sudden death and cerebrovascular accident rates were similar (Fig. 4-4). β-Blocker therapy was associated with significantly lower average BP, earlier ECG normalization, less hypokalemia, and fewer with-

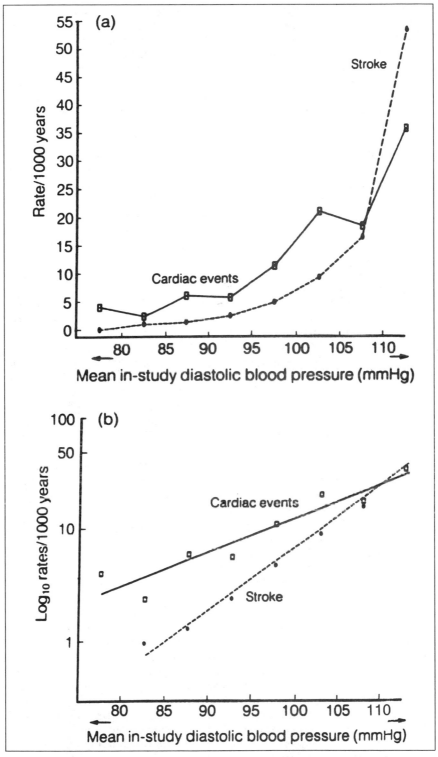

Fig. 4-4. Cardiac events and stroke rates related to diastolic BP during antihypertensive treatment: (a) absolute risk; (b) relative risk. The extremes of the diastolic pressure scale include all values at or <80 and >110 mmHg. Reproduced with permission from the IPPPSH Collaborative Group.[43]

drawals from double-blind treatment for uncontrolled hypertension. Doctor-elicited and patient-assessed unwanted effects demonstrated overall good tolerability. In smokers the cardiac event rate was doubled. The investigators proposed that β-blocker treatment effects depend on smoking status, with a significant interaction benefiting nonsmoking men. Lower BP during treatment was associated with substantially lower rates for both cardiac and cerebrovascular events. Proportional hazards analysis also underlines the importance of other cardiovascular risk factors. The IPPPSH stresses the need for a comprehensive approach to the management of BP and other risk factors in hypertensive patients.

The Multiple Risk Factor Intervention Trial (MRFIT)[44] was a randomized primary prevention trial that tested the effect of a multifactor intervention program on mortality from CAD in 12,866 men aged 35–57 years, selected on the basis of elevated serum cholesterol level, or high diastolic BP, or cigarette smoking, or a combination of these factors. The previously reported mortality results of the MRFIT showed a nonsignificant 7% lower CAD mortality rate in the special intervention (SI) compared with the usual care (UC) group. An explanation for these findings, that risk factor reduction is simply ineffective, was noted as unlikely given the weight of findings from other studies. Two other explanations are plausible. First, CAD and total death rates were considerably lower than had been anticipated in both SI and UC participants, and this reduction reduced the power to test the principal hypothesis. The inconclusive result may therefore represent a false negative finding due to chance. Second, the mortality comparison between all SI and UC participants represented an average of differential responses in important subgroups. For example, there were 35 SI and 45 UC deaths from CAD among men who were not hypertensive at baseline, whereas there were 80 SI and 79 UC CAD deaths among those who were hypertensive. Within the hypertensive subgroup, SI death rates from CAD and all causes were lower than UC death rates for men free of baseline ECG abnormalities at rest. These findings support the interpretation that the MRFIT total experience represents the sum of substantially different findings in various subgroups. The CAD mortality findings for nonhypertensive and hypertensive men with and without ECG abnormalities at rest were examined further. The association between diuretic use and CAD mortality was studied and possible explanations considered. Further analysis in baseline defined subgroups indicated that 1) the most common ECG abnormalities at rest were high R waves and ST-T changes; 2) the CAD mortality differential (SI/UC) was similar in the subgroup with these abnormalities and in the subgroup with other abnormalities at rest; 3) the apparent excess CAD mortality among hypertensive SI men with ECG abnormalities at rest was manifested chiefly as sudden death within 1 hour; and 4) the association between ECG abnormalities at rest and the CAD mortality rate among hypertensive men was independent of the baseline level of BP or the findings on the exercise ECG. CAD mortality in those with abnormalities on the ECG both at rest and during exercise were lower in the SI than the UC group. A possible explanation for the difference in outcome in the baseline-defined subgroup was an unexpectedly low UC mortality rate. Within-group analysis revealed an interaction between ECG abnormalities at rest and diuretic treatment in the SI group, with the risk of CAD death for men prescribed diuretic drugs relative to men not prescribed diuretic drugs estimated as 3.34 among men with baseline ECG abnormalities at rest and as 0.95 among men without such abnormalities. No such effect was found in the UC group, in which men generally were prescribed lower doses of hydrochlorothiazide and chlorthalidone than SI men. However, analyses do not suggest an effect of diuretic dose or of hypokalemia on the CAD mortality rate in treated SI participants. Although subgroup analyses must be interpreted with caution, these findings pose hypotheses for investigation by other researchers in systemic hypertension and may have implications for therapy.

Grimm and associates[45] from Minneapolis, Minnesota, determined the effects on BP and selected biochemical measures of reducing the dosage of chlorthalidone from 100–50 mg. Within the larger study (MRFIT), 140 SI hypertensive men taking 100 mg of chlorthalidone daily were randomly assigned to either a continuation of 100 mg or a dosage reduction to 50 mg daily. Men were followed monthly for 4 months. Measures were made of BP, serum potassium, serum uric acid, serum glucose, serum cholesterol, and triglycerides. BP change from baseline to 4 months revealed a significantly higher diastolic BP in the group continued on the 100 mg dose compared with the dose-reduction group. However, analysis of covariance, which took into account baseline differences in BP, resulted in a nonsignificant difference in follow-up BP (systolic and diastolic) between groups. Serum potassium increased significantly in the dose-reduction group, especially in those taking supplemental potassium chloride. The results of this study demonstrate that a reduced dose of 50 mg chlorthalidone over the 4-month period was as effective as the 100 mg dose in long-term, well-controlled hypertensive men.

In a MRFIT study by Grimm and colleagues[46] from Minneapolis, Minnesota, men randomly assigned to SI were seen frequently and underwent intensive intervention initially followed by maintenance intervention in 22 different clinical centers. Hypertension intervention in SI men primarily consisted of a stepped-care pharmacologic approach designed to lower BP. After 6 years, 52% of SI men and 47% of UC men were receiving antihypertensive medicines. In both study groups, mean systolic and diastolic BP decreased from baseline, diastolic BP being 3.2 mmHg lower in SI men compared with UC men. In antihypertensive men (diastolic BP ≥ 90 mmHg or those taking antihypertensive medicines at baseline), diastolic BP was 4.4 mmHg lower in the SI group compared with the UC group. Use of specific antihypertensive agents differed substantially between the 2 groups, but self-reported complaints were minimal in both. This is a major article on MRFIT and contains 11 tables of data on this multicenter study. These results indicate that long-term BP lowering in a high risk population of middle-aged men was feasible. BP was substantially and significantly lowered in SI men compared with UC men and the difference was largely maintained through 6 years. The BP in the UC group, however, also decreased substantially during this period, which was not anticipated in the original design of the study. The average difference in BP over 6 years between groups was three-fourths of the original design expectation. Results of intervention once again underlined the importance of weight loss in maximizing BP lowering, although it remains unclear as to why the benefit was greater for men not taking antihypertensive medicines. Men in the SI group with resting ECG abnormalities at the start of the study (predominately tall R-waves and T-wave abnormalities) and who were hypertensive had 65% more deaths from CAD compared with the UC group (36 -vs- 21) with the same ECG abnormalities. The corresponding group of SI hypertensive men without these resting ECG abnormalities had 24% fewer CAD deaths than the UC group (44 -vs- 58). A greater number of deaths were present even though the diastolic BP was approximately 4.0 mmHg lower after 72 months in the SI group compared with the UC group for both ECG subgroups.

The Systolic Hypertension in the Elderly Program (SHEP) is a randomized, blinded test of the efficacy of antihypertensive drug treatment. In a large feasibility trial, Hulley and associates[47] from multiple medical centers administered chlorthalidone (25–50 mg/day) or matching placebo as the step 1 drug to 551 men and women with isolated systolic hypertension. All patients were ≥60 years old. After 1 year, 83% of the chlorthalidone group and 81% of the placebo group was still taking SHEP medications. Of those still taking chlorthalidone, 88% had reached goal BP without requiring a step II drug, and most had responded to the lower dose (25 mg/day). The BP response was similar in all age, sex, and race subgroups, with an overall mean difference between randomized groups of 17 mmHg for systolic BP and 6 mmHg for diastolic BP. The only common adverse effects were asymptomatic changes in the serum levels of potassium (0.5 mEq/L lower in the chlorthalidone group, uric acid (0.9 mg/dl higher), and creatinine (0.08 mg/dl higher). This study indicates that chlorthalidone is effective for lowering BP in elderly patients with systolic hypertension and sets the stage for a larger trial of the effects of such treatment on the incidence of cardiovascular disease.

Lewin and associates[48] from Bethesda, Maryland, reviewed data describing the 5,485 participants in the stepped-care group of the Hypertension Detection and Follow-up Program (HDFP) to determine the apparent prevalence of renal parenchymal and reversible, secondary hypertension. The investigation was limited and was not designed to identify all cases of secondary hypertension. Baseline prevalence of proteinuria was 3.6%, pyuria, 7.1%, hematuria, 5.1%, and elevated serum creatinine level (≥1.7 mg/dl), 2.7%. The combined occurrence of an elevated serum creatinine level plus ≥1 urinary abnormality was noted in 0.95%. Initial review of case reports revealed 6 participants with hypertension secondary to use of birth control pills and 3 participants with hypertension that was proved to be secondary to renovascular disease. Specific laboratory or historical criteria were used as indications for more intensive investigation in an additional 65 participants. Among these, 1 participant with renovascular disease and 3 with possible primary hyperaldosteronism were identified. A rapid-sequence intravenous urogram or radionuclide scan was performed on another subgroup of 62 participants whose hypertension was "poorly" controlled (diastolic BP, ≥95 mmHg). Fifty-nine studies were negative, 1 was positive, and 2 were equivocal. These results suggest that the frequency of clinically relevant cases of reversible, secondary hypertension, at least among those with mild to moderate elevation of BP, is low.

Calcium channel blocker

A symposium on calcium channel blockers in systemic hypertension was published in the October *American Journal of Medicine*.[49]

References

1. FROHLICH ED: The heart: an endocrine organ (revisited). Arch Intern Med 1985 (May) 145:809–811.
2. LARAGH JH: Atrial natriuretic hormone, the renin-aldosterone axis, and blood pressure-electrolyte homeostasis. N Engl J Med 1985 (Nov 21); 313:1330–1340.
3. TIKKANE I, METSARINNE K, FYHRQUIST F, LEIDENIUS R: Plasma atrial natriuretic peptide in cardiac disease and during infusion in healthy volunteers. Lancet 1985 (July 13); 2:66–68.
4. SAGNELLA GA, SHORE AC, MARKANDU ND, MACGREGOR GA: Effects of changes in dietary sodium intake and saline infusion on immunoreactive atrial natriuretic peptide in human plasma. Lancet 1985 (Nov 30); 2:1208–1210.

5. BAER L, RADICHEVICH I: Cigarette smoking in hypertensive patients: Blood pressure and endocrine responses. Am J Med 1985 (Apr); 78:564–568.

6. MALHOTRA H, MATHUR D, MEHTA SR, KHANDELWAL PD: Pressor effects of alcohol in normotensive and hypertensive subjects. Lancet 1985 (Sept 14); 2:584–586.

7. GRUCHOW HW, SOBOCINSKI KA, BARBORIAK JJ: Alcohol, nutrient intake, and hypertension in US Adults. JAMA 1985 (Mar 15); 253:1567–1570.

8. HARLAN WR, LANDIS JR, SCHMOUDER RL, GOLDSTEIN NG, HARLAN LC: Blood lead and blood pressure: relationship in the adolescent and adult US population. JAMA 1985 (Jan 25); 253:530–534.

9. KOSKENVUO M, PARTINEN M, SARNA S, KAPRIO J, LANGINVAINIO H, HEIKKILA K: Snoring as a risk factor for hypertension and angina pectoris. Lancet 1985 (Apr 20); 1:893–895.

10. WILLIAMS AJ, HOUSTON D, FINBERG S, LAM C, KINNEY JL, SANTIAGO S: Sleep apnea syndrome and essential hypertension. Am J Cardiol 1985 (Apr 1); 55:1019–1022.

11. MISSERLI FH, VENTURA HO, AMODEO C: Osler's maneuver and pseudohypertension. N Engl J Med 1985 (June 13); 312:1548–1551.

12. TOPOL EJ, TRAILL TA, FORTUIN NJ: Hypertensive hypertrophic cardiomyopathy of the elderly. N Engl J Med 1985 (Jan 31); 312:277–283.

13. MANGAN KF: The heart in hypertension (editorial). N Engl J Med 1985 (Jan 31); 312:306–307.

14. GOTTDIENER JS, GAY JA, MARON BJ, FLETCHER RD: Increased right ventricular wall thickness in left ventricular pressure overload: echocardiographic determination of hypertrophic response of the "nonstressed" ventricle. J Am Coll Cardiol 1985 (Sept); 6:550–555.

15. SNIDER AR, GIDDING SS, ROCCHINI AP, ROSENTHAL A, DICK M, CROWLEY DC, PETERS J: Doppler evaluation of left ventricular diastolic filling in children with systemic hypertension. Am J Cardiol 1985 (Dec); 56:921–926.

16. PAPADEMETRIOU V, GOTTDIENER JS, FLETCHER RD, FREIS EDD: Echocardiographic assessment by computer-assisted analysis of diastolic left ventricular function and hypertrophy in borderline or mild systemic hypertension. Am J Cardiol 1985 (Sept 15); 56:546–550.

17. LINDHEIMER MD, KATZ AI: Hypertension in pregnancy. N Engl J Med, 1985 (Sept 12); 313:675–680.

18. KAPLAN NM: Non-drug treatment of hypertension. Ann Intern Med 1985 (Mar); 102:359–373.

19. MARZUK PM: Biofeedbak for hypertension. Ann Intern Med 1985 (May); 102:709–715.

20. DUNCAN JJ, FARR JE, UPTON SJ, HAGAN RD, OGLESBY ME, BLAIR SN: The effects of aerobic exercise on plasma catecholamines and blood pressure in patients with mild essential hypertension. JAMA 1985 (Nov 8); 254:2609–2613.

21. KAPLAN NM, CARNEGIE A, RASKIN P, HELLER JA, SIMMONS M: Potassium supplementation in hypertensive patients with diuretic-induced hypokalemia. N Engl J Med 1985 (Mar 21); 312:746–749.

22. KASSIRER JP, HARRINGTON JT: Fending off the potassium pushers (editorial). N Engl J Med 1985 (Mar 21); 312:785–787.

23. STEWART DE, IKRAM H, ESPINER EA, NICHOLLS MG: Arrhythmogenic potential of diuretic-induced hypokalemia in patients with mild hypertension and ischemic heart disease. Br Heart J 1985 (Sept); 54:290–297.

24. PAPADEMETRIOU V, PRICE M, NOTARGIACOMO A, GOTTDIENER J, FLETCHER RD, FREIS ED: Effect of diuretic therapy on ventricular arrhythmias in hypertensive patients with or without left ventricular hypertrophy. Am Heart J 1985 (Sept); 110:595–599.

25. LEHTONEN A: Effect of beta blockers on blood lipid profile. Am Heart J 1985 (May); 109:1192–1196.

26. FLORAS JS, HASSAN MO, JONES JV, SLEIGHT P: Cardioselective and nonselective beta-adrenoceptor blocking drugs in hypertension: a comparison of their effect on blood pressure during mental and physical activity. J Am Coll Cardiol 1985 (July); 6:186–195.

27. WEBER MA, DRAYER JIM: Once-daily administration of acebutolol in treatment of hypertension. Am Heart J 1985 (May); 109:1175–1178.

28. WAHL J, TURLAPATY P, SINGH BN: Comparison of acebutolol and propranolol in essential hypertension. Am Heart J 1985 (Feb); 109:313–321.

29. FEIT A, HOLTZMAN R, COHEN M, EL-SHERIF N: Effect of labetalol on exercise tolerance and double product in mild to moderate essential hypertension. Am J Med 1985 (June); 78:937–941.

30. JEE LD, OPIE LH: Double-blind trial comparing labetalol with atenolol in the treatment of systemic hypertension with angina pectoris. Am J Cardiol 1985 (Sept 15); 56:551–554.

31. MacMahon SW, Bernstein L, MacDonald GJ, Andrews G, Blacket RB: Comparison of weight reduction with metoprolol in treatment of hypertension in young overweight patients. Lancet 1985 (June 1); 1:1233–1236.

32. Editorial: Weight reduction in hypertension. Lancet 1985 (June 1); 1:1251.

33. Edwards CRW, Padfield PL: Angiotensin-converting enzyme inhibitors: past, present, and bright future. Lancet 1985 (Jan 5); 1:30–34.

34. Ventura HO, Frohlich ED, Messerli FH, Kobrin I, Kardon MB: Cardiovascular effects and regional blood flow distribution associated with angiotensin converting enzyme inhibition (captopril) in essential hypertension. Am J Cardiol 1985 (Apr 1); 55:1023–1026.

35. Jenkins AC, Knill JR, Dreslinski GR: Captopril in the treatment of the elderly hypertensive patient. Arch Intern Med 1985 (Nov); 145:2029–2031.

36. Thind GS, Johnson A, Bhatnagar D, Henkel TW: A parallel study of enalapril and captopril and 1 year of experience with enalapril treatment in moderate-to-severe essential hypertension. Am Heart J 1985 (Apr); 109:852–858.

37. Oren A, Rotmensch HH, Vlasses PH, Riley LJ Jr, Tadros SS, Koplin JR, Ferguson RK: Crossover comparison of captopril and propranolol as step 2 agents in hypertension. Am Heart J 1985 (Mar); 109:554–557.

38. Fremes SE, Weisel RD, Mickle DAG, Teasdale SJ, Aylmer AP, Christakis GT, Madonik MM, Ivanov J, Houle S, McLaughlin PR, Baird RJ: A comparison of nitroglycerin and nitroprusside: I. Treatment of postoperative hypertension. Ann Thorac Surg 1985 (Jan); 39:53–60.

39. Editorial: Treatment of hypertension: the 1985 results. Lancet 1985 (Sept 21); 2:645–647.

40. Amery A, Brixko P, Clement D, De Schaepdryver A, Fagard R, Forte J, Henry JF, Leonetti G, O'Malley K, Strasser T, Birkenhager W, Bulpitt C, Deruyttere M, Dollery C, Forette F, Hamdy R, Joossens JV, Lund-Johansen P, Petrie J, Tuomilehto J, Williams B: Mortality and morbidity results from the European working party on high blood pressure in the elderly trial. Lancet 1985 (June 15); 1:1349–1354.

41. Editorial: Treatment of hypertension on the over-60s. Lancet 1985 (June 15); 1:1369–1370.

42. Medical Research Council Working Party: MRC trial of treatment of mild hypertension: principal results. Br Med J 1985 (July 13); 291:97–104.

43. The Ipppsh Collaborative Group: Cardiovascular risk and risk factors in a randomized trial of treatment based on the beta-blocker oxprenolol: The International Prospective Primary Prevention Study in Hypertension (IPPPSH). J Hypertension 1985 (Oct); 3:379–392.

44. Multiple Risk Factor Intervention Trial Research Group: Baseline rest electrocardiographic abnormalities, antihypertensive treatment, and mortality in the Multiple Risk Factor Intervention Trial. Am J Cardiol 1985 (Jan 1); 55:1–15.

45. Grimm RH Jr, Neaton JD, McDonald M, Case J, McGill E, Allen R, Bailey-Hoffman G, Kousch D, Childs J, Hulley SB: Beneficial effects from systematic dosage reduction of the diuretic, chlorthalidone: a randomized study within a clinical trial. Am Heart J 1985 (Apr); 109:858–864.

46. Grimm RH, Cohen JD, Smith WM, Falvo-Gerard L, Neaton JD, Multiple Risk Factor Intervention Trial Research Group: Hypertension management in the Multiple Risk Factor Invervention Trial (MRFIT): six-year intervention results for men in special intervention and usual care groups. Arch Intern Med 1985 (July); 145:1191–1199.

47. Hulley SB, Furberg CD, Gurland B, McDonald R, Perry HM, Schnaper HW, Schoenberger JA, Smith WM, Vogt TM: Systolic Hypertension in the Elderly Program (SHEP): antihypertensive efficacy of chlorthalidone. Am J Cardiol 1985 (Dec 1); 56:913–920.

48. Lewin A, Blaufox D, Castle H, Entwisle G, Langford H: Apparent prevalence of curable hypertension in the Hypertension Detection and Follow-up Program. Arch Intern Med 1985 (Mar); 145:424–427.

49. Frohlich ED: Calcium-channel blockers in the management of hypertension. Am J Med 1985 (Oct 11); 79 (Suppl 4A):1–43.

Valvular Heart Disease

Long-term follow-up

Nishimura and associates[1] from Rochester, Minnesota, determined the long-term prognosis for patients with MVP documented by echo by following 237 minimally symptomatic or asymptomatic patients from 1–10 years (mean, 6). The actuarial 8-year probability of survival was 88%, a percent similar to that of a matched control population (Fig. 5-1). An initial LV diastolic dimension >60 mm was the best echo predictor of the subsequent need for MVR (17 patients) (Fig. 5-2). Of the 97 patients with redundant mitral valve leaflets identified by echo, 10 (10%) died suddenly, developed infective endocarditis, or had a cerebral embolic event; in contrast, of the 140 patients without redundant mitral valves, only 1 (1%) had such complications. Most patients with echo evidence of MVP therefore have a benign course, but subsets at high risk for the development of progressive MR, sudden death, cerebral embolic events, or infective endocarditis can be identified by echo.

With ruptured chordae tendineae

To determine the cause of ruptured chordae tendineae and to determine how frequent is MVP in patients with ruptured chordae tendineae, Jeresaty and associates[2] from Hartford, Connecticut, examined operatively excised mitral valves that had ruptured chordae in 25 consecutive patients. Of the 25 patients, MVP was the underlying condition in 23. Infective endocarditis was the cause of the ruptured chordae in 1 patient. The diagnosis of MVP in the 23 patients was made on the basis of redundancy and marked hooding of the mitral leaflets and on the basis of histologic changes. Thus, this study dem-

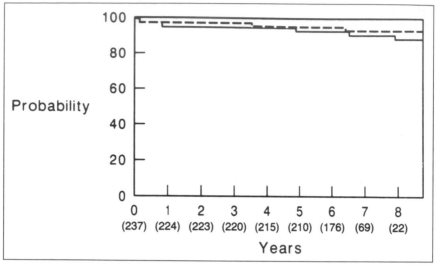

Fig. 5-1. Actuarial 8-year probability (percent) of survival in patients with MVP (———) compared with that for an age- and sex-matched control population (— — — —). The number of surviving patients at each interval is shown in parentheses. Reproduced with permission from Nishimura et al.[1]

onstrates that MVP is the most common underlying morphologic abnormality in patients with ruptured chordae tendineae who have enough MR to warrant MVR.

With infective endocarditis

Hickey and colleagues[3] from Sydney, Australia, investigated the association between MVP and bacterial endocarditis in a case control study of 56 patients with bacterial endocarditis and 168 age- and sex-matched control subjects who had had echo. Patients and control subjects were selected from patients without other known cardiovascular risk factors for bacterial endocarditis: 20% of the bacterial endocarditis cases (11 of 56) and 4% of the control subjects (7 of 168) had MVP; the odds ratio of 5.3 indicated a signifi-

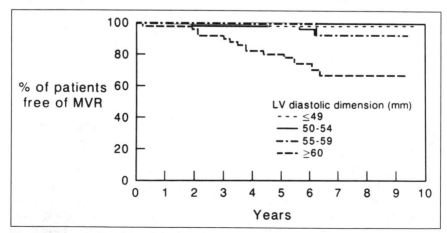

Fig. 5-2. Association of initial LV diastolic dimension with eventual MVR. Reproduced with permission from Nishimura et al.[1]

cantly greater risk of bacterial endocarditis in patients with MVP. This increased risk was only present in those who had preexisting systolic murmurs (9 of 11). Exposure to repeated vascular instrumentation also increased the risk of bacterial endocarditis; this was independent of the risk associated with MVP. Based on these data and the incidence of bacterial endocarditis in New South Wales, Australia, in 1980, the investigators estimated that 14 of every 100,000 adult patients with MVP would develop bacterial endocarditis over a 1-year period, compared with 3 in every 100,000 persons without other known risk factors for bacterial endocarditis in the general population. Thus, although the risk of bacterial endocarditis is 5 times greater in patients with MVP, the absolute risk remains small. This indicates that antibiotic prophylaxis is unnecessary for most patients with MVP. Routine antibiotic prophylaxis should be advised only for those with systolic murmurs.

In drug addicts

Stringer and associates[4] from Syracuse, New York, examined the frequency of MVP in a 2-year period in patients who abused psychoactive drugs and seek detoxification. Of 101 consecutive patients admitted to the substance abuse detoxification unit, 56 had systolic clicks with or without mid to late systolic murmurs by auscultation in supine or standing positions. Of the 56 patients, 48 were then studied by 2-D and M-mode echo: 56 patients had physical signs of MVP (mid to late systolic click with or without systolic murmur) and 38 of these 56 patients had echo confirmation of the diagnosis. The occurrence of echo-confirmed MVP in 37% of the patients admitted to the detoxification unit is substantially greater than the 5–10% prevalence of MVP expected in a randomly selected population. MVP was slightly less prevalent in the alcoholic patients than those admitted for abuse of other drugs (nonalcoholic sedatives, cocaine or amphetamines, opiates, and multiple drug abuse).

Secondary to RV enlargement

A high incidence of MVP has been reported in various entities that produce important RV enlargement with normal or decreased LV volume. To evaluate the importance of RV enlargement in the genesis of MVP in these cases, Garcia-Dorado and associates[5] from Madrid, Spain, analyzed echo studies from 176 patients with pulmonary hypertension after toxic rapeseed oil ingestion. All patients underwent M-mode, cross-sectional and pulsed Doppler examination because of the suspicion of having dietary-induced pulmonary hypertension, a complication that occurred in almost 20% of patients with this epidemic poisoning and that showed a course of gradual resolution in most. RV size was classified according to the RV/LV maximal short-axis dimension ratio as normal, borderline, moderately enlarged and severely enlarged. MVP was diagnosed according to standard M-mode and cross-sectional echo criteria. A second echo was obtained in 38 patients 13 ± 5 months after the first one. The incidence of MVP was 9.3% in 107 patients with normal RV size, 9.5% in 23 patients with borderline RV size, 30% in 30 patients with moderate RV enlargement, and 56% in 16 patients with severe RV enlargement. Fourteen (78%) of the 18 patients with MVP and moderate or severe RV enlargement had holosystolic MVP. At pulsed Doppler examination, no patient showed signs of MR. Of the 38 patients with serial studies, 6 had moderate or severe RV enlargement and MVP; in the last study 3 of them had normal RV size and did not show MVP but the other 3, with persistent moderate or severe RV enlargement, had MVP. These data confirm

that important RV enlargement may produce secondary MVP in some patients without left-sided cardiac abnormalities.

Relation to LV size in the Marfan syndrome

Sporadic reports have suggested that MVP disappears with progressive LV
dilation. To test this hypothesis, Lima and associates[6] from Baltimore, Maryland, determined if an inverse relation existed between MVP and LV cavity
size on M-mode echo in 83 patients with the Marfan syndrome: 46 patients
had MVP. Of patients with an LV end-diastolic dimension ≤5 cm, 90% had
MVP; only 19% of the 32 patients with abnormally large (>5.8 cm) end-
diastolic dimension had MVP. The prevalence of MVP in patients with an LV
end-diastolic dimension of 5.1–5.8 cm was 69%. Thus, the prevalence of
MVP was inversely related to LV cavity size. To determine whether appearance or disappearance of MVP was associated with decrease or increase in LV
cavity size, serial echoes from 67 patients (mean follow-up, 42 months;
range, 3–99) were examined. These patients were separated into 3 groups
based on changes in the LV end-diastolic dimension of >1 cm over time.
Group 1 consisted of 9 patients, all of whom had MVP and normal LV cavity
size on their initial study. With subsequent increase in LV end-diastolic dimension (mean, 1.42 ± 0.3), MVP disappeared in 6. Conversely, group 2
consisted of 4 patients, all of whom had a dilated left ventricle on the initial
echo and no evidence of MVP. After AVR, the LV cavity size decreased (mean,
2.3 ± 0.7) and MVP appeared on follow-up studies. Group 3 consisted of 54
patients with little or no change in LV end-diastolic dimension (≤1 cm;
mean, 0.4 ± 0.2 cm). In this group, MVP status remained unchanged
throughout the follow-up period. Thus, in patients with the Marfan syndrome, serial increase or decrease in LV size is associated with disappearance
or appearance of MVP, respectively.

With atrial flutter

To establish the electrophysiologic determinants of provoked atrial flutter
in patients with MVP, Dobmeyer and associates[7] from Columbus, Ohio, performed studies in 4 groups of patients: group 1, patients with MVP and atrial
flutter; group 2, patients without MVP but with atrial flutter; group 3, patients with MVP but without atrial flutter; and group 4, patients without
MVP and without atrial flutter. P-wave duration, interatrial conduction and
effective refractory periods for the right atrium were longer in group 2 than
in group 1. The effective refractory period of the low right atrium was longer
in group 3 than in group 1. The interatrial conduction interval was longer in
group 2 than in group 4. Thus, in patients without MVP, atrial conduction
delay is the predominant determinant of atrial flutter, whereas differences in
RA refractoriness appear to be most important to the provocation of atrial
flutter in the patient with MVP.

With Wolff-Parkinson-White syndrome

The association of MVP and WPW was examined using simultaneous 2-D
and M-mode echo in a study by Drake and associates[8] from Louisville, Kentucky, and Augusta, Georgia. Twelve-lead ECG and 2-D echo were recorded
in 24 patients with WPW. The location of the accessory pathway was predicted from the ECG as being in 1 of 10 possible sites correlating the delta
wave polarity with epicardial mapping. Nineteen of the 24 patients had conduction via the accessory pathway and 5 were conducting normally during

the echo recording. MVP was found in 13 of the 19 patients conducting via the accessory pathway. The only WPW patient with MVP during normal conduction had a chest deformity that has an independent association with MVP. No association was found between the prediction of the accessory pathway and the presence of MVP. It was concluded that consideration should be given to the possibility that some patients having MVP do so as the result of the altered sequence of ventricular activation, rather than as the result of a structural abnormality.

Ventricular arrhythmias

A high-risk subset of MVP patients and a predisposition to sudden cardiac death has been proposed. Rosenthal and colleagues[9] from Los Angeles, California, analyzed the results of programmed ventricular stimulation in 20 patients with MVP and ventricular arrhythmias (VPC in 6, ventricular couplets in 2, nonsustained VT in 7, VF in 5) and in 12 normal control subjects. With the use of an identical stimulation protocol from the RV apex (twice diastolic threshold, 3 extrastimuli), 9 of 20 MVP patients and 1 of 12 normal subjects had inducible ventricular arrhythmias. When more aggressive attempts at ventricular stimulation were used, an additional 5 MVP patients had positive responses to stimulation, whereas no normal subjects did. In the MVP group, the following arrhythmias were induced: nonsustained polymorphic VT in 10, VF in 3, and ventricular flutter in 1. In all but 2 patients, triple ventricular extrastimuli were required to elicit this response. Two of the 10 MVP patients undergoing electropharmacologic testing had a successful antiarrhythmic region identified, whereas 13 patients were discharged on empiric antiarrhythmic therapy. At a follow-up of 20 ± 13 months, all 19 MVP patients who could be contacted were alive. Five patients had symptomatic recurrences at follow-up, including 2 cardiac arrest survivors (VT in 1 and VF in 1). In conclusion, it was found that most MVP patients with ventricular arrhythmias have inducible ventricular tachyarrhythmias during programmed ventricular stimulation and are more susceptible to this than patients without structural heart disease. No relation between the response to ventricular stimulation and subsequent patient prognosis in the MVP group could be demonstrated. Therefore, programmed ventricular stimulation appears to be of limited clinical utility in certain MVP patients.

Safety of labor and delivery

Shapiro and associates[10] from Baltimore, Maryland, evaluated the records of labor and delivery in 23 patients with auscultatory and echo evidence for MVP detected before the onset of labor after 1981. Labor and delivery are safe in MVP. Their study provided no evidence for an advantage acting through joint laxity or distensible connective tissue during childbirth.

Sickle-cell anemia

To determine the prevalence of MVP in sickle cell disease, Lippman and associates[11] from Torrance, California, performed M-mode echo in 57 patients with sickle-cell disease and in 35 patients with chronic anemia of end-stage renal disease (anemic control group). In 25% (14 of 57) of patients with sickle cell disease, unequivocal MVP was diagnosed by echo; all patients had a mobile systolic click, late systolic murmur, or both. This figure was significantly greater than the reported 5% prevalence in the general adult population, the 1–3% prevalence in the black population, and the 3.0% prevalence (1 of 35) in the anemic control group. The association of MVP and sickle cell disease could not be explained on the basis of LV size, systolic function, ischemic LV or papillary muscle dysfunction, or chronic anemia.

Hyperthyroidism

Brauman and associates[12] from Zerifin, Israel, investigated the prevalence of MVP in 126 patients with hyperthyroidism due to Graves' disease or toxic nodular goiter and that of hyperthyroidism in 64 patients with MVP. The control group consisted of 111 asymptomatic healthy subjects. The patients with hyperthyroidism were divided into those with Graves' disease and those with toxic nodular goiter. Of the group as a whole, 12 (10%) patients had MVP compared with 6 (5%) in the control group, but the difference was not statistically significant. The prevalence of MVP in the patients with toxic goiter was also not significantly different compared with that in the control group (16 -vs- 5%). Only 1 patient with MVP had hyperthyroidism.

In an editorial review-type article Malcolm[13] from West Yorkshire, UK, reviewed the multiple conditions in which MVP has been associated.

Operative therapy

MVP is the most commonly known morphologic entity leading to pure MR. Reconstruction of the mitral valve rather than replacement is particularly applicable to this type morphologic defect but is not often performed in the United States. Penkoske and associates[14] from Boston, Massachusetts, reviewed their experience with reconstruction of the mitral valve for MR secondary to MVP during the period January 1970 to January 1984. A total of 474 patients with mitral valve disease underwent operation during this period, 82 (17%) of whom had MR secondary to MVP. Thirty-one patients (7%) had valve reconstruction by a technique of leaflet plication and posteromedial anuloplasty. Eleven of these patients had associated cardiac disease requiring correction: 2 having AVR and 9, CABG. One hospital death (3%) and 6 late deaths (19%) occurred, of which only 3 were related to cardiac factors. Major complications included recurrent MR in 5 patients and cerebral embolus in 1 patients. The adjusted 5-year survival rate was 89 ± 6 (mean ± SEM), and the overall survival rate of patients free of cardiac-related complications was 73 ± 9%. Thus, reconstruction of the mitral valve is a highly effective surgical approach to the management of symptomatic patients with MR secondary to MVP, and its use in them is favored over replacement.

Tresch and associates[15] from Milwaukee, Wisconsin, described clinical, hemodynamic, surgical, and morphologic findings in 30 patients who required mitral valve surgery because of MVP. The mean age of the patients was 60 years; 28 were >45 years of age; 20 were men. A long history of a precordial systolic murmur was common, whereas symptoms of CHF had abrupt onset. At surgery, a local holosystolic murmur typical of MR was present, although a mid to late systolic click was not heard in any patient. ECG abnormalities were present in all patients; 13 had AF. Only 4 patients had a normal-sized heart radiographically. All 29 patients having cardiac catheterization and angiography had MVP with severe MR. Surgical and morphologic examination revealed findings characteristic of a myxomatous valve, with 19 also having ruptured chordae tendineae.

From 1974–1983 in 37 patients with MVP (Barlow's syndrome only), Cooley performed mitral valve repair operations (mitral anuloplasty using a collar prosthesis in 33 patients and commissural plication in 4 patients.[16] Preoperatively, only 11 (30%) of the 37 had MR and it was minor; 32 patients

(86%) had chest pain, 20 had an arrhythmia (54%) but in only 5 was it a serious one, and 20 patients had dyspnea as their major symptom. There were no operative deaths or late cardiac-related deaths at a follow-up ranging from 1–10 years (mean, 4.7). Of the patients with MVP alone without significant MR, 62% improved by at least 1 New York Heart Association functional class, and of those with associated MR, 91% improved by at least 1 functional class. Only 60% of the 37 patients obtained relief of 1 or more symptoms. This article is presented simply to point out that some surgeons will perform a mitral valve operation in minimally symptomatic patients with MVP who do not have significant MR. That does not mean, however, that that is the correct therapy for these patients, and, indeed, the outcome of the patients without significant MR was not good (WCR). Of the 37 patients, 26 were women and 11 were men. The diagnosis preoperatively of MVP was made "clinically" and confirmed on preoperative cardiac catheterization in all patients. MVP was demonstrated by echo in only 19 of the 37 patients (51%). Of the 19 women with MVP alone (meaning, I believe, insignificant or minor MR), the mean age was 48 years and for the 7 men with MVP without significant MR, 41 years; for the 7 women with significant MR the average age at operation was 38 years and for the 4 men with significant MR, 55 years. I (WCR) have serious doubts on the need for operative therapy in the patients described in this article.

MITRAL REGURGITATION

Forward EF

Previous studies have shown that a normal LVEF is not a reliable index of LV function in MR. Clancy and colleagues[17] from Philadelphia, Pennsylvania, hypothesized that the forward EF, which is the forward stroke volume (measured by Fick or thermodilution) divided by end-diastolic volume (measured by contrast ventriculography) may be a useful index of LV function, since it represents LV emptying into the aorta. This index was examined in 54 patients with chronic MR who had normal EF ($\geq$50%). There were significant correlations between the forward EF and the end-diastolic volume index, end-systolic volume index, cardiac index, and the ratio of systolic pressure to end-systolic volume. Patients were divided into 2 groups according to the forward EF: group 1 (n = 34) had forward EF $\leq$35%; group 2 (n = 20) had forward EF >35%. Of the 32 patients who subsequently underwent MVR, 24 patients were in group 1 and 8 patients were in group 2. At a mean follow-up of 35 months, 4 patients died; all of them were in group 1. Improvement in functional class occurred in 75% of surgical survivors (80% in group 1 and 63% in group 2. These data suggest that forward EF may be a useful index of LV performance in patients with MR who have normal EF.

Ventricular arrhythmias

Kligfield and associates[18] from New York City characterized atrial and ventricular arrhythmias by ambulatory ECG in 31 patients with nonischemic MR, 17 of whom had echo evidence of MVP and 14 had other causes of MR. Frequent and complex arrhythmias were common and equally prevalent in each MR subgroup, whether or not MVP was present (Fig. 5-3). Multiform ventricular ectopic activity was found in 77% (24 of 31), ventricular couplets in 61% (19 of 31), and ventricular salvos or VT in 35% (11 of 31) of patients

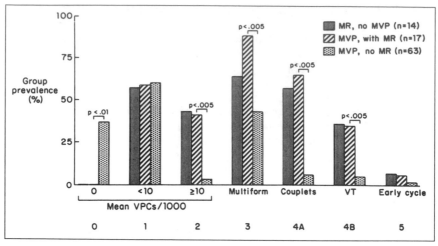

Fig. 5-3. Group prevalence of ventricular arrhythmias in patients with MR without MVP, MR with MVP, and MVP without MR. Each patient must be represented once in the appropriate mean VPC density category and may also be represented in as many VPC complexity categories as are applicable. The numbers along the horizontal axis refer to the corresponding Lown complexity category. However, in this display arrhythmias are represented according to actual prevalence rather than according to mutually exclusive hierarchy of complexity.

with MR. Arrhythmias in patients with MR were significantly more prevalent than in 63 patients with MVP who had no evidence of MR. Among patients with MVP, excess arrhythmias associated with MR were most striking with respect to frequent VPC (41% with MR -vs- 3% without MR), multiform ventricular ectopic activity (88 -vs- 43%), ventricular couplets (65 -vs- 6%), and ventricular salvos or VT (35 -vs- 5%). These data demonstrate that complex arrhythmias are common in patients with nonischemic MR irrespective of etiology, and that these arrhythmias are more strongly associated with hemodynamically important MR than with MVP alone.

Secondary to ruptured chordae tendineae

From 1958 to 1980, 131 patients had repair of ruptured tendineae of the mitral valve at the Mayo Clinic. Orszulak and colleagues[19] from Rochester, Minnesota, reviewed this group and compared their early and late survival to 106 patients having MVR for ruptured chordae during the same interval. In the mitral valve repair group, chordae to the anterior mitral leaflet were ruptured in 44 patients (34%), to the posterior mitral leaflet in 85 (65%), and to both leaflets in 2 patients (1%). The mitral valve was repaired by leaflet plication without resection in 116 patients, plication after wedge resection of the unsupported leaflet in 6, Ivalon buttress of the posterior leaflet in 3, resuspension of chordae in 2, and anuloplasty alone in the remaining 4. Mitral anuloplasty was performed in addition to leaflet repair in 115 patients. Operative mortality was 6.1%. Survival rate of repair patients dismissed from the hospital was 92% at 5 years and 73% at 10 years. Survival for repair patients was significantly better than it was for replacement patients (5-year survival rate 92 -vs- 72%). The incidence of thromboembolism after repair was 1.8 episodes/100 patient-years compared with 8 episodes/100 patient-years after replacement. These data suggest that valvuloplasty is the procedure of choice for most patients with MR due to ruptured chordae tendineae, including selected patients with ruptured chordae to the anterior leaflet.

MITRAL STENOSIS

Effects of atenolol on exercise capacity

Exercise capacity is frequently impaired in patients with MS and sinus rhythm. The resulting increased heart rate, which shortens the diastolic filling period, and the increased cardiac output lead to further elevations of LA pressure and subsequent pulmonary congestion. Klein and associates[20] from Johannesburg, South Africa, assessed the effect of the β-receptor blocking agent, atenolol, 100 mg/day, in 13 patients with MS and sinus rhythm. Exercise performance was assessed using a modified multistage Bruce protocol after 2 weeks of placebo and after 2 weeks therapy with atenolol in a single-blind, crossover, placebo-controlled, randomized study. Atenolol resulted in significant decreases in mean heart rates at rest and during exercise and a significant increase in total exercise time. Maximal exercise capacity was also significantly improved. All patients were both objectively and subjectively improved by atenolol. Thus, β-blockade with atenolol improves exercise capacity in patients with MS and sinus rhythm and may be of benefit to most such patients. The improved effort tolerance is attributed to reduction of the exercise-associated sinus tachycardia by β-blockade, allowing a longer diastolic filling period and better LA decompression.

Percutaneous catheter mitral commissurotomy

Lock and associates[21] from Minneapolis, Minnesota, attempted percutaneous transcatheter-balloon mitral commissurotomy in 8 patients aged 9–23 years with rheumatic MS. The atrial septum was traversed by needle puncture, and an 8 mm angioplasty balloon was advanced over a guide wire. The atrial septal perforation was then dilated to allow passage of the valvuloplasty balloon catheter (18–25 mm) across the mitral anulus. Inflation of the transmitral balloon decreased the end-diastolic transmitral gradient temporarily in all patients (from 21 ± 4–10 ± 6 mmHg [mean, ± SD]) (Fig. 5-4). The immediate decrease in the gradient was associated with increases in cardiac output (from 3.8 ± 1.0–4.9 ± 1.3 L/min/m² body-surface area; and in the calculated mitral valve area index (from 0.73 ± 0.29–1.34 ± 0.32 cm²/m². Murmur intensity diminished immediately after commissurotomy in all patients. The greatest reduction in pressure gradient (76–95%) occurred when the largest balloon (inflated diameter, 25 mm) was used in the smallest patients (0.9–1.2 m²). The balloon commissurotomy produced minimal MR in only 1 child. Follow-up catheterization (at 2–8 weeks) demonstrated persistence of hemodynamic improvement with evidence of partial restenosis in 1 patient. These early results indicate that balloon mitral commissurotomy can be a safe and effective treatment for children and young adults with rheumatic MS.

Open mitral valve reconstruction

Cohn and associates[22] from Boston, Massachusetts, performed open mitral reconstruction for rheumatic MS in 120 patients, 101 women and 19 men, aged 22–75 years (mean, 49). Nine patients were functional class II,

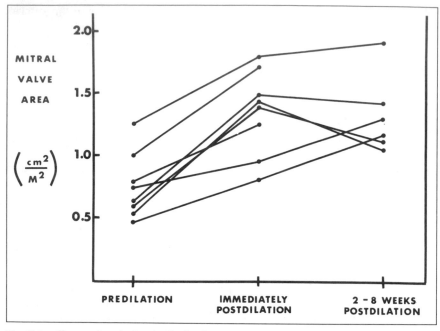

Fig. 5-4.   Changes in calculated mitral valve area immediately after dilation and 2–8 weeks later. Reproduced with permission Lock et al.[21]

106, class III, 5, class IV; 13 underwent noninvasive studies, including echo, before surgery, and 107 had preoperative cardiac catheterization studies. The latter had a mean valve area of 1.09 cm^2 and a PA wedge to LV mean diastolic gradient of 14 mmHg. Cardiopulmonary bypass was used in all patients for open reconstruction under direct vision. Superior commissurotomy was done in 115 patients, inferior, in 114; papillary muscles were incised and chordae lengthened in 39, and calcium was excised from valve leaflets in 23. Suture or ring anuloplasty was not done in any patient. These operations were begun January 1972 and terminated in January 1984. Personal follow-up was conducted in July 1984. There were no operative deaths in the 120 patients. There were 5 late deaths, all from noncardiac causes. The mean follow-up was 53 months. The actuarial probability of survival at 10 years was 95 ± 2%. Thromboemboli occurred in 9 patients; the probability of freedom from thromboemboli at 10 years was 91 ± 3%, and the linearized rate was 1.8%/patient-year of follow-up. Reoperation was required in 9 patients, an absolute incidence of 1.7%/patient-year. At 10 years, the probability of freedom from reoperation was 84 ± 5%.

MITRAL ANULAR CALCIUM

Doppler echo is useful for detecting and quantifying MR and MS. To determine the prevalence of these abnormalities in patients with mitral anular calcium (MAC), Labovitz and associates[23] from St. Louis, Missouri, examined by Doppler ultrasound 51 consecutive patients who had an echo diagnosis of MAC. Transmitral flow was evaluated to determine the presence of MR or LV inflow obstruction (MS) by continuous and pulsed wave Doppler echo. The severity of these hemodynamic abnormalities was quantitated. Eleven patients (22%) had mild MR, 17 (33%) had moderate to severe MR, and 4 (8%) had significant MS. Clinical findings, such as a systolic murmur, evidence of CHF, and exertional dyspnea, were not helpful in distinguishing patients with no or mild MR from those who had moderate to severe MR. M-mode measured LA size was significantly larger in patients with moderate to severe MR. This study suggests that MR is often associated with MAC, that MS is not a rare finding with MAC, and that Doppler echo can quantitate these lesions in the elderly when symptoms are not specific and physical findings are inconclusive or absent.

AORTIC VALVE STENOSIS

Morphologic features of operatively excised valves

Subramanian and associates[24] from Rochester, Minnesota, reviewed gross morphologic features of operatively excised stenotic and incompetent aortic valves in 213 patients who had clinically combined AS and AR and AVR at the Mayo Clinic during the years 1965, 1970, 1975, and 1980. The causes of the combined AS and AR are listed in Table 5-1.

Peterson and associates[25] from St. Paul, Minnesota, described morphologic features of 109 operatively excised stenotic aortic valves. They encountered 5 types of valves in order of decreasing frequency of types as follows (Figs. 5-5, 5-6): 1) Calcium deposits in congenitally bicuspid aortic valves (47%); 2) calcium deposits in normally tricuspid aortic valves without commissural fusion, the so-called senile type of AS (28%); 3) calcium deposits of acquired bicuspid aortic valves (13%); 4) the fibrous rheumatic-type valve (10%); and 5) calcium deposits in congenitally unicuspid valves (1%). The male to female ratio was 3:2. The senile type, however, occurred more often in women than men.

TABLE 5-1. *Number of cases of surgical aortic valve disease. Reproduced with permission from Subramanian et al.*[24]

CLASSIFICATION	PURE AS	PURE AI*	AS + AI[+]	TOTAL
Postinflammatory	130	103	148	381
Bicuspid	171	45	40	256
Aortic dilation	0	48	0	48
Degenerative	38	0	0	38
Unicommissural	21	0	13	34
Endocarditis	0	21	5	26
Tricuspid[‡]	0	4	3	7
Quadricuspid	0	2	1	3
Indeterminate	14	2	3	19
Total	374	225	213	812

*AI = aortic insufficiency.
[+]Current study.
[‡]Tricuspid aortic valve, either congenitally abnormal or associated with VSD.

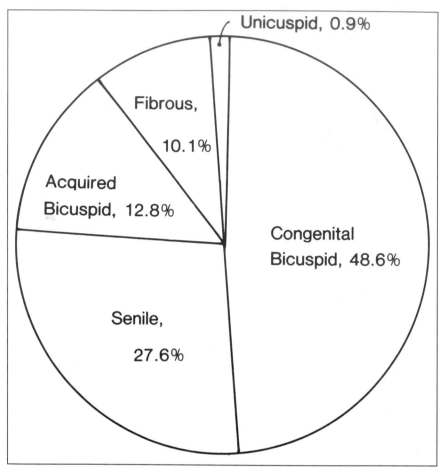

Fig. 5-5.   Percent distribution of background for aortic stenosis in 109 aortic valves removed surgically. In each category, except fibrous type, there was calcific aortic stenosis. Reproduced with permission from Peterson et al.[25]

Determining severity by echo

Williams and associates[26] from St. Louis, Missouri, evaluated 52 adults referred for possible AS by continuous wave and pulsed Doppler echo. Three windows were used to determine which approach (apical, right parasternal, or suprasternal) yielded optimal results. Doppler-derived peak aortic valve gradients were compared with the peak gradients measured at cardiac catheterization in 23 patients. High velocity jets were best recorded from the cardiac apex and less frequently from the right parasternal and suprasternal areas. However, gradients from the right parasternal area correlated best with cardiac catheterization findings, although recordings could be made from this window in only 49% of the patients. Velocities from the suprasternal window were significantly lower than those from the apex or right parasternal areas. Gradient underestimation from the suprasternal window tended to increase with age of the patient. When the maximal Doppler-derived gradient from any window was compared with catheterization measurements, the correlation coefficient was 0.86. Gradients derived from Doppler velocities accurately predicted severe (>50 mmHg) gradients at

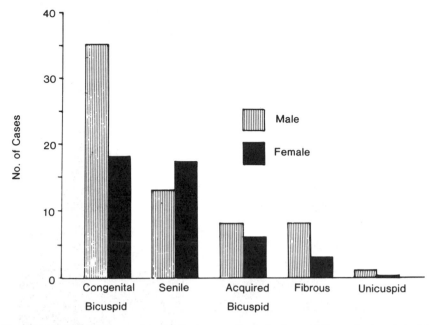

Fig. 5-6.   Distribution by gender of patients according to background for aortic stenosis in this study. Reproduced with permission from Peterson et al.[25]

catheterization. Thus, Doppler echo is useful in evaluating AS when several windows are used for optimal assessment of aortic valve gradient.

Agatston and associates[27] from Miami Beach, Florida, performed continuous wave Doppler echo followed by cardiac catheterization in 25 consecutive elderly patients with suspected AS. Doppler-derived calculations of peak and mean aortic valve gradients were compared with catheterization-derived values of peak to peak, peak, and mean gradients. The best correlation was found between Doppler- and catheterization-derived mean gradients (Figs. 5-7, 5-8). A Doppler-derived measure of the timing of peak aortic flow velocity (modified time to peak velocity/modified LV ejection time) successfully separated those with gradients > or <50 mmHg and also helped to avoid over- or underestimation of aortic valve gradients by Doppler.

Currie and coworkers[28] from Rochester, Minnesota, obtained simultaneous Doppler echo and catheter measurements of pressure gradients in 100 consecutive patients aged 50–89 years: 46 patients also underwent an outpatient Doppler study ≤7 days before catheterization. Simultaneous pressure waveforms and Doppler spectral velocity profiles were analyzed at 10 ms intervals and maximum, mean, and instantaneous gradients (mmHg) were derived for each. The correlation between the Doppler-determined gradient and the simultaneously measured maximum catheter gradient was r = 0.92, that between the Doppler-determined and mean catheter gradient was r = 0.93, and that between the Doppler and peak to peak catheter gradient was r = 0.91 (Fig. 5-9). The correlation between the nonsimultaneously Doppler-determined gradient and the maximum gradient measured by catheter was not as strong (r = 0.79). The continuous wave Doppler echo velocity profile represents the instantaneous transaortic pressure gradient throughout the cardiac cycle. The best correlation with continuous wave Doppler-determined gradient was obtained with maximum and mean gradients measured

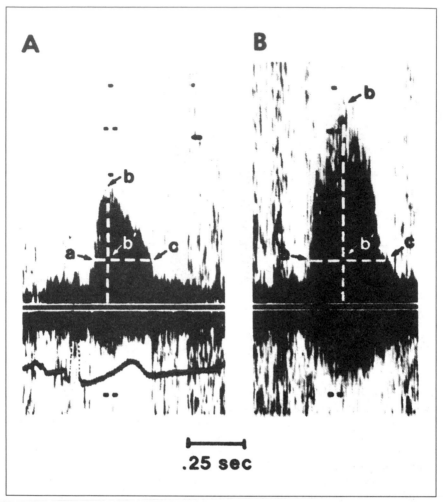

Fig. 5-7. Continuous wave spectrums from a patient with an early peak and insignificant AS (A) and from a patient with a later peaking velocity and critical AS (B). Maximal velocity was taken at point b. The modified time to peak/modified left ejection time is the ratio ab'/ac.

by the catheter. Continuous wave Doppler echo can be used to predict reliably the pressure gradient in adults with calcific AS.

To define further the clinical role of continuous wave Doppler echo for determining aortic valve gradient, Krafchek and colleagues[29] from Durham, North Carolina, studied 60 consecutive adult patients (age range, 22–81 years; mean, 63) with suspected AS within 24 hours of catheterization. Blind comparisons of Doppler peak and mean gradients by the simplified Bernoulli equation were made with catheterization peak to peak, peak, and mean gradients in a double-blind fashion. Despite these favorable correlations, Doppler peak gradient generally overestimated catheterization peak to peak gradient (1–53 mmHg), making it impractical for clinical use. Doppler and catheterization correlations of peak and mean gradients were more favorable, with the least scatter noticed for mean gradient. The results of analysis of pooled data indicated that mean gradient also may be most specific for differentiating severe from less severe AS. In this consecutive series in which

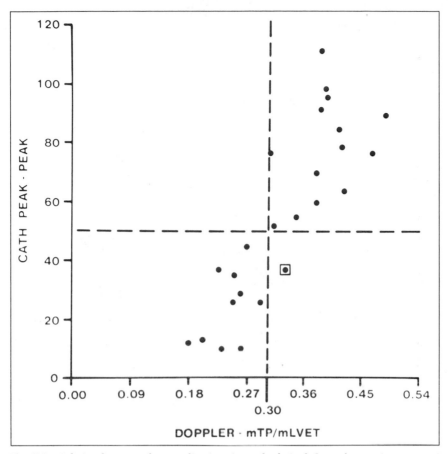

Fig. 5-8. Relation between the systolic time intervals derived from the continuous wave spectrum, modified time to peak/modified LV ejection time (mTP/mLVET) and the catheterization peak to peak gradient. The ratio of 0.30 successfully separates those with gradients of > 50 mmHg from those with < 50 mmHg.

a full range of catheterization gradients was encountered, 7 patients with predicted Doppler gradients were found to have none, which is best explained by the use of the simplified Bernoulli equation in patients with AR. These data indicate that prudence should be maintained when Doppler gradients alone are used for the assessment of AS.

Rubler and associates[30] from New York City devised a system for estimating the degree of aortic valve calcium using echo and tested 153 men who had basal precordial murmurs. The degree of calcium estimated from echo correlated well with LV hypertrophy in patients having no systemic hypertension or CAD. Thirty-one patients had cardiac catheterization (Table 5-2). Those with minimal aortic valve calcific deposits had insignificant gradients, whereas 11 of 14 patients with heavy calcific deposits had gradients >50 mmHg. Those with intermediate size calcific deposits who had LV ejection times >433 ms and LV mass >300 g also had significant obstruction. Noninvasive techniques therefore distinguish aortic valve sclerosis from significant AS, identifying those individuals who need cardiac catheterization.

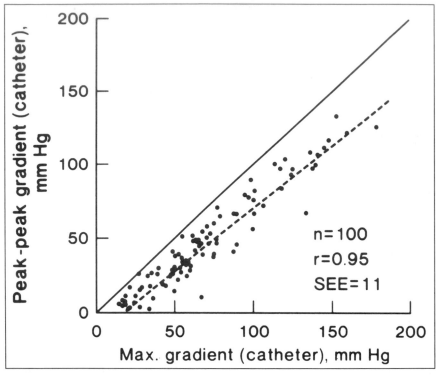

Fig. 5-9. Correlation of the maximum catheter pressure gradient with the peak to peak catheter gradient in the 100 patients. The regression equation is peak to peak gradient = 0.84 × max gradient − 13.7. The dotted line represents the regression line and the solid line, the line of identity. Reproduced with permission from Currie et al.[28]

Usefulness of echo in predicting proper prosthetic valve size

The size of the aortic root is an important factor in determining outcome after AVR, and therefore information regarding the size of the aortic root preoperatively might be useful. Mackay and associates[31] from Edinburgh, UK, performed LV angiography, parasternal long axis cross-sectional echo of the LV outflow tract and proximal ascending aorta, and M-mode echo of the aortic root on 43 patients who underwent AVR for AS with or without AR to predict aortic root size and therefore prosthetic valve size. Cross-sectional echo measurements and angiographic measurements of the aortic root correlated well with the prosthetic size, with >66% of the indirect measurements being within 2 mm of the prosthetic diameter. M-mode echo did not yield useful predictive information. Thus, noninvasive preoperative evaluation of patients likely to require AVR is useful in predicting aortic root dimensions.

H-V conduction

MacMillan[32] from Brown Mills, New Jersey, performed in 48 patients with predominant AS His bundle electrography (HBE) at the time of diagnostic catheterization. Patients were divided into 4 groups based upon severity of calcium of the aortic valve fluoroscopically as judged independently by 3 angiographers. Of 48 patients, 3 had no calcium, 11 had mild, 18 had moderate, and 16 had severe aortic valve calcium. No correlation was found be-

TABLE 5-2. *M-mode and 2-D echo and catheterization data from 31 patients. Degree valve calcification is graded from minimal (1 +) to severe (3 +). Reproduced with permission from Rubler et al.[30]*

PATIENT	CALCIFICATION GRADE M-MODE	CALCIFICATION GRADE 2-D	LV MASS (g)	LV MASS INDEX (g/m²)	LV EJECTION TIME INDEX (ms)	GRADIENT (mmHg)	AORTIC VALVE AREA (cm²)
1	3+	3+	292	161	429	14	1.5
2	3+	2+	378	244	499	71	1.2
3	1+	1+	158	378	378	0	—
4	2+	1+	296	137	404	11	—
5	2+	—	130	76	401	30	4.4
6	3+	3+	548	235	460	108	0.5
7	3+	3+	355	177	461	80	0.7
8	1+	—	261	144	376	0	—
9	2+	—	190	106	378	0	—
10	3+	—	266	164	438	75	0.4
11	2+	2+	498	243	437	60	0.8
12	1+	1+	162	86	393	0	—
13	1+	1+	244	120	414	0	3.3
14	2+	2+	213	131	372	0	3.2
15	2+	2+	292	109	391	0	—
16	1+	1+	189	103	—	0	—
17	1+	1+	215	123	432	0	—
18	2+	2+	190	70	402	0	4.7
19	3+	1+	277	136	402	23	1.2
20	2+	3+	517	296	442	75	—
21	3+	—	432	223	—	50	—
22	1+	—	276	143	441	10	2.3
23	3+	3+	296	144	—	70	0.5
24	3+	3+	324	174	434	—	0.6
25	3+	3+	330	168	492	70	0.7
26	2+	2+	356	185	464	0	—
27	3+	—	488	260	469	136	—
28	3+	2+	342	199	447	72	0.6
29	2+	1+	261	123	413	15	1.8
30	3+	—	324	158	445	105	0.6
31	3+	2+	328	186	433	44	1.2
Mean ± SD			306.0 ± 104.9	162.2 ± 56.5	426.4 ± 35.0	37.3 ± 40.4	1.59 ± 1.36
Grade 3+			355.7 ± 81.6	190.5 ± 37.9	450.6 ± 27.4	70.6 ± 33.6	0.8 ± 0.4
Grade 2+			294.4 ± 129.7	153.6 ± 71.9	410.4 ± 29.2	19.1 ± 27.5	3.0 ± 1.7
Grade 1+			229.7 ± 51.0	121.7 ± 31.8	405.7 ± 27.6	1.4 ± 3.8	2.8 + 0.7

tween H-V interval and severity of aortic valve calcium. Significant correlation was found between H-V interval prolongation and aortic valve area, history of CHF, and increasing LV end-diastolic pressure. LVEF <45% had greater likelihood of H-V interval prolongation. No correlation was established between H-V interval and age, aortic valve gradient, LV peak systolic pressure, syncope, and CAD. Aortic valve area was the most significant independent predictor of H-V prolongation, with history of CHF second. It was concluded that H-V interval prolongation in AS with calcified valves is best predicted by evidence of declining LV function rather than severity of aortic valve calcium.

Coronary luminal diameter

Abdulali and associates[33] from Leeds, UK, compared coronary artery luminal diameter in 32 patients with AS with those of 24 control subjects without LV hypertrophy by means of a derived index. Patients with AS had significantly larger coronary arteries than the control subjects. The increase in coronary luminal diameter had a weak correlation to LV wall thickness and LV mass. Among 21 patients with AS and normal coronary angiograms, those with angina had higher peak LV pressures (224 ± 8 -vs- 196 ± 7 mmHg) and greater peak systolic gradients (103 ± 9 -vs- 74 ± 10 mmHg) than those without angina. However, there was no significant difference in CAD, peak LV stress, or LV tension at rest between patients with and without angina.

Significance of angina as predictor of degree of coronary arterial narrowing

Green and associates[34] from Manhasset, New York, retrospectively analyzed 103 patients with isolated severe AS to determine the relation of angina pectoris to angiographically significant CAD. All patients underwent coronary angiography regardless of the presence or absence of angina. Angina was significantly associated with CAD, with a sensitivity of 78% and a specificity of 53%. However, 25% of the patients without angina had angiographically significant CAD, and in these patients there was a 70% prevalence of 1-vessel CAD. Patients with isolated, severe AS should undergo coronary angiography to identify coexistent CAD accurately.

AORTIC REGURGITATION

Idiopathic etiology

Lakier and coworkers[35] from Detroit, Michigan, evaluated 27 consecutively removed aortic valves from patients with AR to establish the etiology of isolated aortic valve regurgitation. In 12 patients, the AR was due to rheumatic or syphilitic valvular disease or a congenitally bicuspid aortic valve. In the remaining 15, no etiology was apparent. Among the latter 15 patients, the histologic features were similar, consisting of increased and disorganized elastic and collagen fibers. Small foci of myxomatous stroma were present, but the amounts did not differ substantially from those observed in age-matched competent aortic valves removed at necropsy. Thus, idiopathic degeneration of the aortic valve cusps appears to be a common cause of isolated AR.

Allen and associates[36] from Los Angeles, California, reviewed clinical and morphologic data in 55 patients who had AVR for pure AR during a 6-year period. The clinical histories established the cause of the AR in 35 cases: 11 rheumatic, 13 infective endocarditis, 4 congenital, 4 associated with aortic aneurysms, and 2, the Marfan syndrome. In the valves from the other 21 patients, 13 had myxoid degeneration, defined as significant disruption of the valve fibrosa and its replacement by acid mucopolysaccharides and cystic change. Myxoid degeneration was also the primary pathologic abnormality in the 2 patients with the Marfan syndrome, in 3 patients with a history of rheumatic disease, and in 1 patients with a history of infective endocarditis. The patients with myxoid degeneration of uncertain origin were predominantly elderly (average age, 63 years), had a long-standing history of systemic hypertension (77%), and had CAD (46%); 85% were male. In these patients the replacement valves were not larger than those of the other groups studied, indicating that dilation of the aortic "anulus" was not a significant factor in the pathogenesis of the valve disease. These findings indicate that "myxoid degeneration" of the aortic valve is common (36% of all valves examined) and, in many cases, may be secondary to long-standing systemic hypertension.

Ankylosing spondylitis and variants

Qaiyumi and associates[37] from Richmond, Virginia, evaluated 100 consecutive cases of pure AR for the prevalence of seronegative spondyloarthropathies. Four patients had ankylosing spondylitis and 3 had Reiter's syndrome. Six of these 7 patients had cardiac conduction abnormalities, 4 of which required permanent pacemaker insertion. All 7 had the HLA-B27 antigen, whereas of 89 patients tested with no evidence of spondylitis, only 5 had the antigen. The seronegative spondyloarthropathies apparently are associated frequently with lone AR. The HLA-B27 antigen is not specifically associated with lone AR in the absence of spondylitis.

LaBresh and associates[38] from Providence, Rhode Island, described 2-D echo findings of subaortic fibrous ridging, aortic cuspal thickening, and aortic root dilation and thickening in 36 patients with rheumatoid variant diseases. The group consisted of 25 patients with ankylosing spondylitis, 9 patients with Reiter's syndrome, and 2 patients with inflammatory bowel disease and spondylitis. No patients had clinical or laboratory evidence of AR or heart block. Subaortic fibrous ridging or marked leaflet thickening was noted in 11 of 36 patients; in contrast, no such changes were found in an age-matched control group of 29 men. The subgroup of patients with subaortic fibrous ridging or leaflet thickening (11 patients) had significantly longer disease duration (28 -vs- 18 years) and higher incidence of aortic root echo density (82 -vs- 36%) than the remaining patients. It was concluded that a significant portion of patients with ankylosing spondylitis or Reiter's syndrome have echo evidence of aortic root involvement before the clinical onset of AR.

ECG findings

Roberts and Day[39] from Bethesda, Maryland, described certain ECG findings in 30 necropsy patients with clinically isolated pure, chronic, severe AR. They were 19–65 years old (mean, 45). The hearts of the 22 men ranged in weight from 430–1,110 g (mean, 717) and of the 8 women, from 375–950 g (mean, 638). Four had grossly visible LV scars. All but 1 patient was in sinus rhythm. The P-R interval was >0.20 second in 8 patients (28%) and the QRS duration was ≥0.12 second in 6 patients (20%). Only 5 patients (17%) had ≥1 VPC recorded on the resting ECG. The mean QRS amplitude for each of the 12 leads averaged 23 mm. The highest mean QRS voltage occurred in leads V_2 and V_3 (each, 38 mm), and the lowest in lead aVR (11 mm). The mean QRS voltage in V_5 was higher than in V_6 (33 -vs- 28 mm), and in 22 patients (73%) the QRS voltage in V_5 was higher than in V_6. The sum of the S wave in V_1 plus the larger of the R wave in V_5 or V_6 (Sokolow-Lyon index) averaged 51 mm and in only 22 patients (73%) was it >35 mm (Table 5-3). The Romhilt-Estes voltage criteria for LV hypertrophy was fulfilled even less frequently, despite the severe degrees of LV hypertrophy in the patients studied. The total 12-lead QRS amplitude in the 30 patients ranged from 109–428 mm (mean, 272) (10 mm = 1 mV), and in 27 patients (90%) it was >175 mm. The ratio of total 12-lead QRS voltage to heart weight in the 30 patients with AR was 0.42, only slightly higher than that in previously studied

TABLE 5-3. *Recommended or modified ECG criteria for determining LV hypertrophy as applied to 30 necropsy patients with severe cardiomegaly from chronic, pure, severe AR.*

NO.	QRS COMPLEX MEASURED	VALUE CONSIDERED UPPER LIMIT OF NORMAL (MM)	NO. (%) of 30 PATIENTS ABOVE NORMAL LIMIT
1a	$SV_1 + RV_5$ or V_6 (larger)	35	22(73)
b	$SV_1 + RV_5$ or V_6 (larger)	40	18(60)
2a	SV_1 or V_2 (larger) + RV_5 or V_6 (larger)	35	26(87)
b	SV_1 or V_2 (larger) + RV_5 or V_6 (larger)	40	22(73)
3a	SV_1 or V_2 (larger) + RV_6	35	25(83)
b	SV_1 or V_2 (larger) + RV_6	40	21(70)
4a	$SV_2 + RV_5$	35	24(80)
b	$SV_2 + RV_5$	40	22(73)
5a	Deepest $SV_1 - V_3$ + tallest $RV_4 - V_6$	35	26(87)
b	Deepest $SV_1 - V_3$ + tallest $RV_4 - V_6$	40	25(83)
c	Deepest $SV_1 - V_3$ + tallest $RV_4 - V_6$	45	22(73)
d	Deepest $SV_1 - V_3$ + tallest $V_4 - V_6$	50	21(70)
6a	Tallest R + deepest S in any V lead	35	19(63)
b	Tallest R + deepest S in any V lead	40	16(53)
7a	Deepest $SV_1 - V_3$	25	23(77)
b	Deepest $SV_1 - V_3$	30	19(63)
8a	Tallest $RV_4 - V_6$	25	19(63)
b	Tallest $RV_4 - V_6$	30	14(47)
9a	Deeper SV_1 or V_2	25	19(63)
b	Deeper SV_1 or V_2	30	17(57)
10a	Tallest RV_5 or V_6	25	26(87)
b	Tallest RV_5 or V_6	30	14(47)
11	$RV_6 > RV_5$	<1	9(30)
12a	Tallest limb-lead R + deepest limb-lead S	15	27(90)
b	Tallest limb-lead R + deepest limb-lead S	20	17(57)
13a	$R_1 + S_3$	15	20(67)
b	$R_1 + S_3$	20	14(47)
14a	Tallest limb-lead R	10	21(70)
b	Tallest limb-lead R	15	13(43)
15a	Deepest limb-lead S	10	18(60)
b	Deepest limb-lead S	15	11(37)
16	R_1	10	15(50)
17	S_3	10	13(43)
18a	Total 12-lead QRS voltage	175	27(90)
b	Total 12-lead QRS voltage	200	23(77)

adults with severe AS (0.39), an observation indicating that cavity dilation does not magnify the QRS voltage generated by a given mass of myocardium (Fig. 5-10).

E-point septal separation

Separation between the mitral E-point and left side of the ventricular septum on M-mode echo has been shown to be a practical index of LV performance in adults and children with unrestricted motion of the mitral valve. Patients with AR are usually excluded from studies of E point septal separation (EPSS) because of the possibility of abnormal mitral valve motion, and

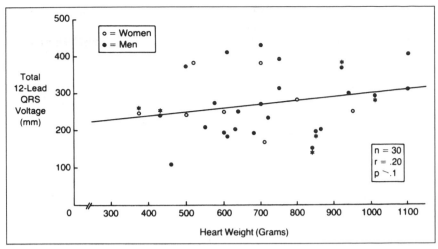

Fig. 5-10. Relation of the total 12-lead QRS voltage (mm) to heart weight (g) in the 30 patients with severe, pure AR. *Widths of the QRS complexes were at least 0.12 second.

echo performed on a few of these patients has revealed no significant relation to contractile function. To evaluate the significance of EPSS in patients with AR, Rosoff and Cohen[40] from New York City retrospectively examined M-mode echoes of 56 patients who underwent cardiac catheterization for AR. Fifty-six patients with moderate or severe AR had technically adequate angiograms and echoes and no evidence of other significant valvular lesions. EPSS 1 exceeded EPSS 2 by 4–7 mm in 9 patients. In all other patients EPSS 1 was 0–3 mm greater than EPSS 2. Nineteen of 56 patients (34%) had an EF >55% with EPSS >10 mm. Thus, although increased EPSS appears to be associated with larger ventricles and poorer systolic function in patients with AR, correlation is poor for individual patients, and therefore EPSS is not a useful predictor of LV function or dilation in individual patients with AR.

LV end-systolic dimension

Criteria for the optimal timing of surgical intervention in chronic AR remain controversial. Henry and colleagues in 1980 reported that preoperative echo data could be used to predict the likelihood of a good or poor postoperative result. But subsequent studies have questioned the validity of these observations. Daniel and coinvestigators[41] from Hannover, West Germany, evaluated retrospectively the prognostic significance of a preoperative echo LV end-systolic dimension (ESD) >55 mm and/or fractional shortening (FS) of ≤25% in 84 patients who had undergone AVR for isolated chronic AR due to various causes. Preoperative survival, improvement in symptoms, and echo evidence of regression of LV dilation and hypertrophy were compared between patients with a preoperative ESD >55 mm (category 1) and those with an ESD of ≤55 mm (category 2) and between patients with FS of ≤25% (category 3) and those with FS >25% (category 4; Fig. 5–11). Patients in categories 1 and 3 had a higher preoperative LV end-diastolic dimension (EDD) and cross-sectional area than those in categories 2 and 4, respectively; but their preoperative functional impairment (New York Heart Association [NYHA] class) was similar. There were 13 deaths, only 2 of which could be attributed to LV dysfunction. In both patients, FS was ≤25%, and in 1, ESD was >55 mm. There was a weak association without useful positive predic-

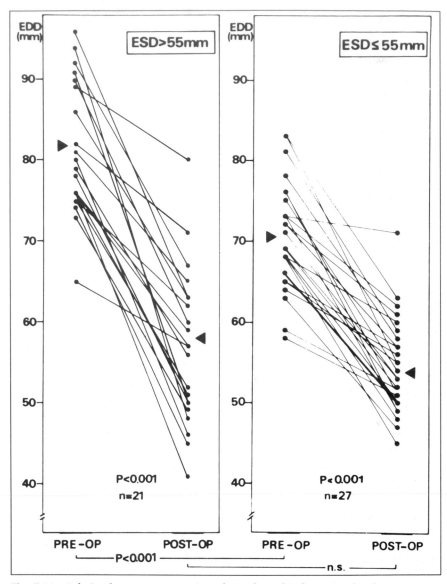

Fig. 5-11. Relation between preoperative echo end-systolic dimension (ESD) >55 mm or ≤55 mm and end-diastolic dimension (EDD) in 48 survivors of aortic valve replacement for chronic AR who had high quality echo tracings before and after operation. Preoperative EDD was greater when preoperative ESD was >55 mm but postoperative EDD decreased to the same degree as when preoperative ESD was ≤55 mm. Reproduced with permission from Daniel et al.[41]

tive value between the echo variables and postoperative death due to all causes. Among 42 patients with a preoperative ESD >55 mm and/or FS of ≤25%, 33 (79%) were alive at a mean follow-up of 30 months. Symptoms improved in all categories of survivors, with the postoperative NYHA class being similar between categories 1 and 2 and between categories 3 and 4. Among 48 survivors with high quality echo both before and after surgery, EDD decreased in all groups but decreased to a lesser extent in category 3 than in category 4. Postoperative cross-sectional area decreased to the same level in all categories. Follow-up intervals were similar in all categories. The investigators concluded that in patients undergoing AVR for chronic AR, a preoperative ESD >55 mm or an FS of ≤25% does not reliably predict early or late death, does not correlate with lack of improvement in symptoms, and does not preclude postoperative regression of LV dilation and hypertrophy. Thus, these echo criteria alone cannot be used for the timing of surgical intervention in these patients.

Impact of preoperative LV function on operative result

Recent studies suggest that preoperative LV function may no longer be an important determinant of survival or functional results after operation for AR because of improved operative techniques. To evaluate the effect of LV function on prognosis in the current surgical era, Bonow and coworkers[42] from Bethesda, Maryland, performed echo and RNA studies in 80 consecutive patients undergoing AVR from 1976–1983. No patients had associated CAD. For all patients, 5-year survival was 83%, significantly better than the 62% 5-year survival in patients operated on from 1972–1976. Preoperative resting LVEF, fractional shortening, and end-systolic dimension were the most significant predictors of survival (Fig. 5-12). Five-year survival was 63% in patients with subnormal EF compared with 96% in those with normal EF. Patients with subnormal LVEF and poor exercise tolerance or prolonged duration of LV dysfunction (−18 months) comprised the high risk subgroup (5-year survival, 52%). Patients in this subgroup also had persistent LV dysfunction after operation, with greater LV end-diastolic dimensions and reduced EF compared with patients with normal preoperative LVEF or a brief duration of LV dysfunction (−14 months). Cold hyperkalemic cardioplegia was used for myocardial preservation in 46 patients. Survival was not influenced by cardioplegia, nor did cardioplegia alter the influence of LV function

Fig. 5-12. Preoperative echo and RNA data for 69 patients surviving after AVR and the 11 patients who died after operation. Significance values indicate the ability of each variable to predict subsequent mortality by life-table analysis rather than direct differences between the 2 groups. Cause of death is indicated by different symbols: ● = LV dysfunction, ○ = sudden death; △ = valve-related deaths. Reproduced with permission from Bonow et al.[42]

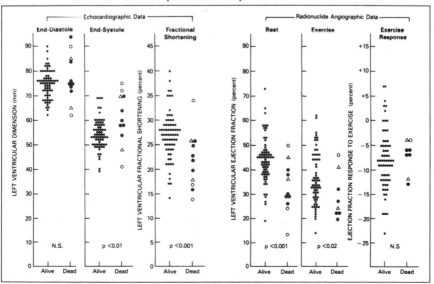

on postoperative prognosis. Hence, despite improved operative techniques and better long-term survival compared with earlier results, preoperative resting LV dysfunction continues to identify patients with AR at risk of death or persistent LV dysfunction after AVR.

Exercise EF response

Since patients with AR may remain asymptomatic for many years even with significant LV dysfunction, Shen and associates[43] from Sydney, Australia, examined the relation between myocardial contractile state and LV functional response to exercise in 14 asymptomatic patients with isolated moderate to severe AR and 6 control subjects. The slope of the systolic BP-LV end-systolic volume (pressure-volume) relation determined by radionuclide ventriculography during angiotensin infusion was used as an indirect measure of myocardial contractility and was compared with LVEF at rest and during both isometric handgrip and dynamic bicycle exercise (Fig. 5-13). The slope of the pressure-volume relation was significantly lower in patients with AR than in the control subjects (1.75 ± 0.57 -vs- 2.78 ± 0.42). The slope correlated exponentially with resting EF and was linearly related to changes in LVEF during both handgrip and bicycle exercise. In patients with AR, resting EF may overestimate myocardial function. The slope of the pressure-

Fig. 5-13.   Examples of determination of systolic BP/LV end-systolic volume relation in a control subject (●) and a patient with AR (○). Reproduced with permission from Shen et al.[43]

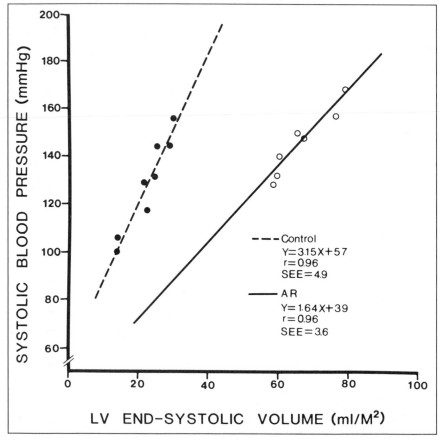

volume relation measured during afterload stress and LVEF response to exercise intervention more reliably reflect the degree of LV dysfunction. Since LV dilation due to the volume overload of AR can maintain the resting EF, this study nicely demonstrates that an increase in preload can diffiantiate the contractile reserve in the normally functioning LV and chronic dilation created by AR.

Although some patients with chronic AR demonstrate an increase in EF during exercise, others may show little change or even a reduction after exertion. Greenberg and coworkers[44] from San Francisco, California, studied the exercise EF response in 56 patients with chronic AR. All patients had LV dilation but preserved resting EF and minimal or no symptoms. Exercise EF increased ≥0.05 U in 18 (32%) patients (group I), remained within 0.05 U of the resting value in 18 patients (group II), and decreased by ≥0.05 U in 20 (36%) patients (group III). No significant differences were noted among the groups in LV end-diastolic dimension, end-systolic dimension, or fractional shortening by echo or in resting LV volumes and EF by RNA. LV end-systolic wall stress was significantly higher in group III than either group I or II. At peak exercise, there were no differences among groups in systolic BP. End-systolic volume increased in group III and decreased in group I. Thus, at peak exercise, end-systolic volume was nearly 3 times greater in group III than in group I. A highly significant inverse correlation was present between the EF response and the change in end-systolic volume. Exercise capacity was significantly lower in group III than in groups I and II. Thus, these data demonstrate that patients with chronic AR whose EF decreases during exercise have elevated resting LV systolic wall stress, suggesting that LV hypertrophy has not been adequate. Although these patients may demonstrate a normal resting EF, LV systolic pump performance cannot be sustained during exercise when wall stress further increases.

Gee and associates[45] from Ann Arbor, Michigan, performed gated equilibrium RNA in 23 patients with hemodynamically significant AR to assess rest and exercise LVEF before and after AVR. Preoperatively, LVEF decreased from 54 + 3% at rest to 45 ± 3% during exercise. Two patients died at operation. Postoperatively, after 5.7 ± 1.6 months, LVEF was 62 ± 5% at rest and 60 ± 4% during exercise (difference not significant). Exercise LVEF improved significantly postoperatively (Fig. 5-14). The patients were followed for a mean of 30 months (range, 1–56), after AVR and during this period, 13 patients were in functional class I, 5 patients were in class II, and 2 patients were in class III. One late death occurred and was unrelated to myocardial failure. Thus, in most patients with AR, exercise LVEF improves after AVR. A preoperative decrease in LVEF during exercise in patients with significant AR does not predict a poor postoperative outcome.

Massie and colleagues[46] from San Francisco, California, studied the relation between simultaneous hemodynamic measurements and supine exercise blood pool scintigraphy in 14 patients with severe, asymptomatic or minimally symptomatic AR. These patients had well-preserved LV function at rest and cardiomegaly. Patients were categorized into groups whose LVEF increased by >0.05 (group 1) and those whose EF decreased by >0.05 (group 2). Echo, radionuclide, and hemodynamic measurements at rest in the 2 patient groups were similar, but patients in group 1 demonstrated a greater increase in cardiac index during supine exercise (2.8 ± 0.4–10.0 ± 1.8 -vs- 2.7 ± 0.5–6.9 ± 1.0 L/min/m^2) and a lesser increase in PA wedge pressure (13 ± 4–19 ± 7 compared with 12 ± 4–31 ± 8 mmHg, respectively). The severity of AR decreased with exercise in all patients, but end-diastolic volume decreased and end-systolic volume decreased or was unchanged in group 1, whereas end-diastolic volume was unchanged and end-systolic vol-

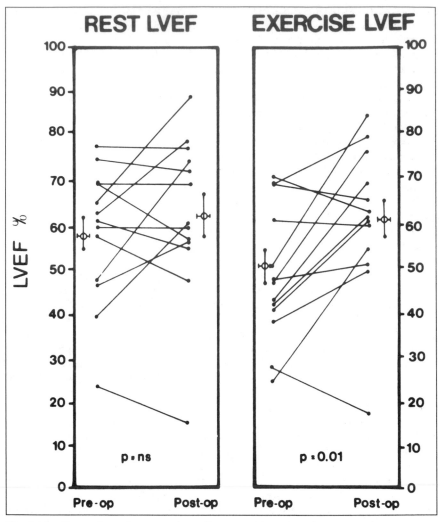

Fig. 5-14. Comparison of preoperative and postoperative rest and exercise LVEF.

ume increased in group 2 patients. Change in LVEF correlated closely with the exercise-induced increase in cardiac index and significantly, but inversely with an increase in PA wedge pressure. Thus, the LVEF response during supine exercise is a useful indicator of LV reserve in patients with AR and correlates well with exercise hemodynamic measurements determined by direct catheter measurement.

INFECTIVE ENDOCARDITIS

Some patients with active infective endocarditis have vegetations that may be identified by echo and this finding has been suggested to indicate a poor prognosis with a high incidence of complications. To confirm or oppose this thesis, Stafford and associates[47] from Queensland, Australia, performed cross-sectional echo in 62 patients with clinical evidence of active infective endocarditis and identified echo densities consistent with vegetations in 45 patients (73%). The sensitivity of this technique in diagnosing vegetations in infective endocarditis was 93% and the specificity 89%. The predictive value of a positive test was 96% and that of a negative test, 80%. Vegetations were detected with a similar frequency on the aortic and mitral valves. The incidence of valvar regurgitation, CHF, and the need for surgical intervention was similar in the patients with and without vegetations. Embolism occurred in 47% of those patients with vegetations and in 12% of those without. The mortality rate was 27% in those with vegetations, and no patient without vegetations died. Thus, cross-sectional echo is accurate in diagnosing vegetations in patients with infective endocarditis, and this finding identifies patients at high risk of embolic complications and death.

Griffin and associates[48] from Rochester, Minnesota, used strict criteria to identify all definite, probable, and possible cases of infective endocarditis in residents of Olmsted County, Minnesota, from 1950 through 1981: 78 episodes of infective endocarditis were identified in 78 Olmsted County residents during the 30-year period. Of these 78 episodes, 40 were labeled definite, 24 probable, and 14 possible. The mean annual age- and sex-adjusted incidence rates per 100,000 person-years were 3.8 for total cases and 3.2 for definite and probable cases only. Total rates were 4.3 for 1950 through 1959, 3.3 for 1960 through 1969, and 3.9 for 1970 through 1981. Rheumatic heart disease was the underlying disorder in 26% of cases, with a shift noted during 1970 through 1981 to involvement of prosthetic rather than natural valves in these patients. MVP was identified in 17% of cases. No source of infection could be identified in 41% of cases, including half of those with rheumatic or congenital heart disease. In cases diagnosed before autopsy, the 60-day fatality decreased from 46% during 1950 through 1959 to 22% and 26% during 1960 through 1969 and 1970 through 1981, respectively.

Cremieux and associates[49] from Paris, France, described clinical and echo data from 12 patients with pulmonic valve endocarditis. Seven patients had isolated pulmonic endocarditis and in 5 patients other valves were infected (aortic, tricuspid, mitral, or all 3). Two patients were heroin addicts and 4 had underlying heart disease (congenital heart disease in 3 and AR in 1). The organisms involved were alpha-streptococci in 3 patients (all with underlying heart disease), *Staphylococcus aureus* in 4, *Streptococcus bovis*, group D, in 1 patient and *Candida guilliermondii* in 1. M-mode and 2-D echo was performed in 10 patients and revealed vegetations in 8. Pulsed Doppler echo was performed in 6 patients and revealed pulmonary regurgitation in all 6. Seven patients had pulmonary emboli. Four patients had surgery. Four patients died, including 1 after cardiac surgery. Five patients, including the patient infected with *C. guilliermondii*, recovered with antibiotic treatment.

Ellis and colleagues[50] from Stanford and San Jose, California, used 2-D echo in 22 patients with perivalvular abscess found at surgery or necropsy compared with 24 patients without abscess in a retrospective blinded study to determine the efficacy of echo in identifying perivalvular abscess. Forty-six valves were examined (31 aortic and 15 mitral, 35 prosthetic and 11 native). Four ± 2.4 days (range, 0–7) elapsed between echo and surgery or necropsy. In this study, patients with perivalvular abscess had a higher incidence of serious complications, including emergency repeat valve replacement or death than did patients with endocarditis alone (63 -vs- 35%, respectively). No single echo finding was found frequently in patients with a perivalvular abscess. A "typical" echo-free abscess was noted in only 1 patient. Prosthetic valve rocking, sinus of Valsalva aneurysm, anterior aortic thickness of ≥10 mm, posterior aortic root thickness of ≥10 mm, or perivalvular density in the septum of ≥14 mm had a positive predictive value of 86% and a negative predictive value of 87% for perivalvular abscess. In 10 patients with documented perivalvular abscess, no valve mass was detected on echo, but 1 of the 5 criteria just mentioned was present. Therefore, these echo findings should be sought in patients with endocarditis and their presence should suggest possible associated perivalvular abscess.

It has been securely established that operative treatment of infective endocarditis usually has a better outcome than nonoperative treatment. There remains an important risk to operation. D'Agostino and colleagues[51] from Stanford, California, examined the influence of 27 variables on operative mortality and late complications using discriminate analysis for 108 patients undergoing valve replacement for native valve endocarditis. CHF was the indication for valve replacement in 86% of the patients; 58% had active and 42% had healed endocarditis. Follow-up included 515 patient-years and extended to a maximum of 19 years. Operative mortality was 15 ± 4% and 17 patients had late complications (linearized rate, 3.3%/patient-year). Seven variables were significantly related to operative mortality in univariant analysis, but only organisms (S. aureus -vs- all others) was a significant independent predictor of operative mortality (Fig. 5-15). For late complications, only 2 of 7 significant univariant covariants proved to be significant independent determinants: organisms on valve culture or Gram's stain and the presence of anular abscess (Figs. 5-16, 5-17). Thus, patients with S. aureus endocarditis not showing prompt response to antibiotic treatment must be considered for early operation. Similarly, timely operative intervention for patients with anular abscesses will be essential in decreasing late valve infections and perivalvular leaks.

TRICUSPID VALVE DISEASE

Curtius and associates[52] from Dusseldorf, West Germany, studied 68 patients with contrast and Doppler echo to evaluate both methods for detecting and grading TR. In all patients RV angiography was performed. The severity of TR was graded on a 4-point scale. Only 68 of 88 patients who underwent RV angiography (77%) could be evaluated, but 65 of 68 patients who under-

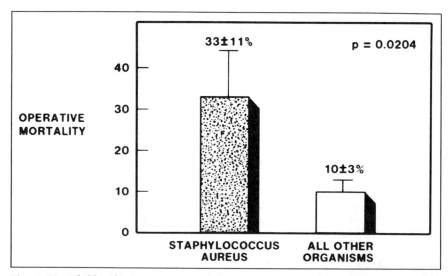

Fig. 5-15. Likelihood of operative mortality with and without *Staphylococcus aureus* endocarditis. The operative mortality is shown as ±SEM. Reproduced with permission from D'Agostino et al.[51]

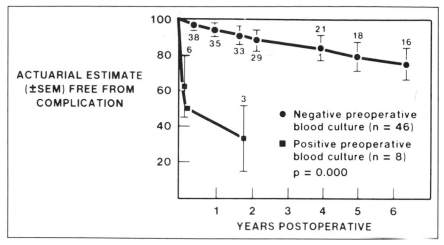

Fig. 5-16. Influence of preoperative blood culture on actuarial complication-free survival. Reproduced with permission from D'Agostino et al.[51]

went contrast echo (96%) and all 68 who underwent Doppler echo could be evaluated. TR was present in 33 patients, as seen on RV angiography. Contrast and Doppler echo correctly diagnosed 27 and 30 patients, respectively, corresponding to a sensitivity of 82% for contrast echo and 91% for Doppler echo. Specificity was 100% for contrast echo and 86% for Doppler echo. Contrast and Doppler echo grading, respectively, of TR -vs- RV angiographic grading showed no difference in 50 and 47 patients, a 1-level difference in 8 and 13 and a 2-level difference in 7 and 5 cases. Thus, contrast echo and Doppler echo are accurate methods for routine diagnosis of TR, with Doppler echo having higher sensitivity and easier grading.

Berger and coworkers[53] from New York City used Doppler echo in 69 patients with different cardiopulmonary disorders to determine the value of this approach in assessing the presence of TR in patients with pulmonary hypertension. TR was detected by Doppler ultrasound in 2 of 20 patients in whom PA systolic pressures were <35 mmHg and in 39 of 49 patients whose PA systolic pressures were >35 mmHg. Twenty-six of 27 patients in whom the PA systolic pressures were >50 mmHg had Doppler evidence of TR. These data indicate that TR may be detected by Doppler ultrasound in patients with moderately severe to severe PA hypertension.

MISCELLANEOUS TOPICS

Morphologic features of operatively excised mitral valves

Hanson and associates[54] from St. Paul, Minnesota, described morphologic features of 100 consecutive operatively excised mitral valves for either MS, MR, or both. The cause of the valve dysfunction are summarized in Table 5-4.

Normal aortic valve anatomy

Silver and Roberts[55] from Bethesda, Maryland, determined in the same patients the area, weight, and 4 linear variables in each aortic valve cusp in

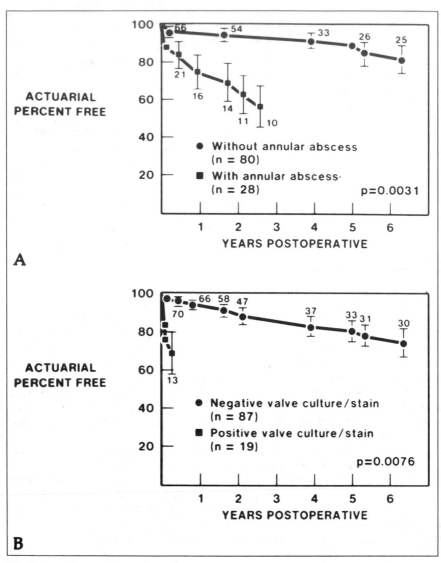

Fig. 5-17. Influence of significant determinants on actuarial complication-free survival. A = anular abscess; B = valve culture or stain. Reproduced with permission from D'Agostino et al.[51]

100 necropsy patients with normally functioning aortic valves and the volume of each sinus of Valsalva and the aortic area at the sinotubular junction in the same patients. The sums of the aortic valve cuspal areas, cuspal weights, and sinus of Valsalva volumes increased with age and with heart weight. These 3 variables also increased with age and heart weight relative to each other. The luminal area of aorta at the sinotubular junction also increased with age and heart weight and it also increased as the sum of the aortic valve cuspal areas and weights and sinus of Valsalva volumes increased. In only 16% of the 100 patients were the 3 aortic valve cusps of similar size (<5% difference in area between cusps); in 51%, 1 cusp was of different size than the other 2, and in 33% of patients, all 3 cusps were of different sizes.

TABLE 5-4. *Disease states identified and incidence of each among 100 valves studied*

TYPE OF DISEASE	# CASES
Rheumatic disease	
Stenosis	39
Insufficiency	0
Stenosis and insufficiency	15
Total	54
Myxomatous (prolapsed) valve	
With ruptured chordae	19
With intact chordae	13
Total	32
Papillary muscle dysfunction	7
Myocardial infarction with ruptured papillary muscle	4
Miscellaneous conditions	2
Subacute bacterial endocarditis	1

The heart in the carcinoid syndrome

Carcinoid heart disease is a morphologically specific type of cardiac disorder that involves the mural and valvular endocardium primarily on the right side of the heart. Ross and Roberts[56] from Bethesda, Maryland, reviewed 21 patients (57%) (Group I) with carcinoid heart disease (Fig. 5-18) and 15 patients (43%) (Group II) without carcinoid heart disease at necropsy. The 2 groups were similar in mean age (54 -vs- 55 years), duration of clinical illness (4.7 -vs- 6.3 years), body weight (50 -vs- 52 kg), mean systemic BP (117/77 -vs- 128/77 mmHg), blood hematocrit levels (37 -vs- 36%), total serum protein levels (6.0 g/dl), and serum albumin levels (2.2 -vs- 2.6 g/dl). The 2 groups were different in the frequency of the presence of precordial murmurs consistent with TR and/or pulmonic stenosis (95 -vs- 13%), cardiomegaly by chest radiography (38 -vs- 0%), low voltage on ECG (47 -vs- 0%), and location of the primary site of the carcinoid tumor. Total ECG 12-lead QRS voltage was similar in each group (105 -vs- 132 mm; 10 mm = 1 mV). Of Group I subjects, 43% died of cardiac causes; none of the Group II subjects died of cardiac causes. Of the 21 subjects with carcinoid heart disease, 7 had left-sided cardiac involvement, but in none was it of functional significance. Thus, although carcinoid heart disease frequently is the cause of death in patients with the carcinoid syndrome, the development of carcinoid heart disease is not related to the duration of symptoms of the carcinoid syndrome.

Echo findings in families with the Marfan syndrome

Pan and coworkers[57] from Taipei, Taiwan, studied 12 patients with the Marfan syndrome and 48 of their first degree relatives (16 males and 22 females; mean age, 30 years) by echo. In the patients with the Marfan syndrome, aortic valve prolapse was present in 1, tricuspid valve prolapse in 4, MVP in 12, and aortic root dilation in 10. Tricuspid valve prolapse was found in 3 patients among the 48 first degree relatives of the 12 patients with the Marfan syndrome, MVP in 15, and aortic root dilation in 12. Aortic valve prolapse was not found in any of the first degree relatives. Overall, cardiac involvement was found in 28 (47%) of the 60 patients studied. Among the 28 with cardiac involvement, aortic valve prolapse was observed in 1, tricuspid

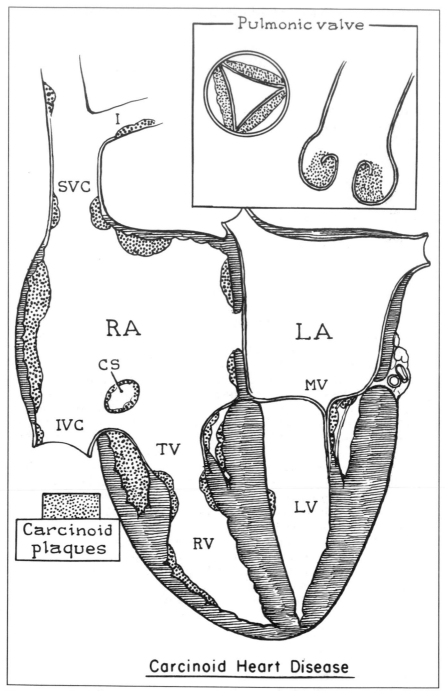

Fig. 5-18. Illustration of location and distribution of carcinoid plaques. CS = ostium of coronary sinus; I = innominate (brachiocephalic) vein; IVC = inferior vena cava; LA = left atrium; LV = left ventricle; MV = mitral valve; RA = right atrium; RV = right ventricle; SVC = superior vena cava; TV = tricuspid valve.

valve prolapse in 7, MVP in 27 (96%), and aortic root dilation in 22, (79%). MVP was also found in 7 individuals with tricuspid valve prolapse and 1 with aortic valve prolapse. At least 1 abnormality of the cardiac, skeletal, or ophthalmologic system was found in 32 of the 60 patients among the 12 families. Nineteen individuals were <18 years of age and all had cardiac involvement associated with the Marfan syndrome. These data indicate a high penetrance of cardiac abnormalities among first degree relatives of patients with the Marfan syndrome. Furthermore, they suggest the need to evaluate carefully first degree relatives, including young family members of patients with the Marfan syndrome. Finally, they indicate that MVP and aortic root dilation are among the most common cardiac abnormalities, but that combined valvular prolapse also is found.

Evaluating mitral valve operations by echo

Present methods for intraoperative detection of MR, primarily hemodynamic measurements and direct palpation, may not detect or underestimate the presence and severity of MR. Mindich and associates[58] from New York City used 2-D echo as a means of improving intraoperative assessment of mitral valve function both before and after repair or replacement. Microbubbles were injected in the left ventricle and the contrast they produced was sensed at the left atrium with a hand-held 5 mHz probe. Forty-three patients (37 with mitral valve disease and 6 additional patients without mitral valve disease) undergoing cardiac operations were evaluated. Four of 5 patients undergoing mitral commissurotomy had varying degrees of MR postoperatively by 2-D echo, but only 2 required an immediate secondary procedure. Of the 19 patients with MR, 8 underwent anuloplasty, 2 of these patients were found by 2-D echo to have significant MR after repair and 1 required MVR. Microbubbles were detected in the left atrium in 3 of these patients. In 1, the needle tip was within the cage of a Starr-Edwards mitral prosthesis. Another patient had a 4-M prothesis, which had some early systolic reflux, and a third had a minor leak. No complications associated with the microbubble technique developed. It was concluded that intraoperative 2-D echo was more sensitive than other techniques for detecting intraoperative MR.

CARDIAC VALVE REPLACEMENT

Determinants of mortality after AVR

Scott and colleagues[59] from Stanford, California, examined the influence of 35 preoperative and intraoperative characteristics on operative mortality after 1,479 isolated AVR procedures from 1967–1981. Physiology was classified as AS (58%), AR (30%), or both (9%). The overall operative mortality rate was $7 \pm 1\%$, but there were substantial differences in operative mortality rates among physiologic subgroups (AR, $10 \pm 2\%$; AS, $6 \pm 1\%$, and AS/AR $5 \pm 2\%$). Independent determinants of operative mortality in AR were functional class, AF, and operative year; for AS, significant determinants were functional class, renal dysfunction, age, prosthetic valve dysfunction, and absence of angina. Concomitant CABG, previous operation, endocarditis, and ascending aortic replacement had no independent predictive effect on operative mortality rate. Cardioplegia was used in combination with topical hypothermia in 26% of patients. Cardioplegia had no influence on operative mortality in the AS or AS/AR subgroups or in the entire group; but a possible saluatory effect was suggested by the univariate analysis for the AR subgroup. Eighty-two percent of patients with angiographic CAD underwent concomitant CABG. This concomitant procedure had no significant effect on operative mortality. This study, like many others, shows that functional class had the strongest independent effect on early mortality for the entire group and in all of the physiologic subgroups. In all subgroups operative intervention earlier predicts a lower operative risk.

Evaluation of MVR

Cohn and associates[60] from Boston, Massachusetts, reported a consecutive series of 706 MVR performed in the 12-year period, 1972–1984. A porcine bioprosthesis was implanted in 528 patients and a prosthetic disk valve in 178 patients. A concomitant operative procedure was done in 253 patients. Operative mortality was 77 of 706 (11%) for the overall group; 34 of 453 (7.5%) for isolated MVR, 30 of 169 (18%) for MVR plus CABG, 49 of 528 (9%) for bioprosthetic valve group, and 28 of 178 (16%) for the prosthetic disk valve group. The long-term survival rate was significantly lower in patients who had an associated procedure, MR rather than MS, who were functional class IV rather than classes I to III, and who received a prosthetic disk valve rather than a bioprosthesis. Thromboembolic rates were higher with prosthetic valves than with bioprosthetic valves (4.6 ± 0.22% -vs- 2.4 ± 0.5%/patient-year of follow-up). Primary valve dysfunction was significantly more common in the bioprosthesis (1.23 -vs- 0.4%/patient-year). The rates of perivalvular leakage and endocarditis were equal in the 2 groups, as was the rate of reoperation. However, all valve-related morbidity and mortality were 5.2 ± 0.5%/patient-year for the bioprosthetic valve group and 8.1 ± 0.26%/patient-year for the prosthetic valve group.

MVR plus CABG

The contemporary risks of MVR with and without CABG were reviewed by Magovern and coworkers[61] from Hershey, Pennsylvania: 130 consecutive patients had MVR without or with CABG using cold crystalloid cardioplegic myocardial protection. Mortality was 7% for 28 patients with MS, 5% for 37 patients with MR, 8% for 37 patients with both MS and MR, 0 for 5 with MS and CAD, and 22% for 23 patients with MR and CAD. Overall mortality was 9%. Eleven patients had emergency operations for cardiogenic shock, with a mortality of 45%. Nineteen additional patients in New York Heart Association functional class IV had MVR or MVR plus CABG with a mortality of 26%. Sixteen patients had intra-aortic balloon pump assistance and only 9 survived. Four patients with MR and CAD had LV assist devices and 3 survived. Thus, factors associated with death were cardiogenic shock, New York Heart Association class IV, LV end-diastolic pressure >15 mmHg (16% mortality) and age >60 years (15% mortality). Actuarial 5-year survival was 75%. Long-term survival was not statistically different among patients grouped by pre-operative diagnosis. Despite a higher operative mortality, late mortality for patients with MR and CABG was not higher than for the other groups.

St. Jude Medical prosthesis

Baudet and colleagues[62] from Bordeaux, France, implanted St. Jude Medical valves in 671 patients aged 9 months to 82 years. Sixteen (2.4%) were <15 years and 82 (12%) were >70 years old. Hospital mortality was 3.6% for aortic, 4.7% for mitral, and 0 for double-valve replacement. Fourteen of 41 late deaths (34%) were considered to be valve related. At 5.5 years, the actuarial survival rate, operative mortality excluded, was 91% for aortic, 90% for mitral, and 95% for double-valve replacement. Valve thrombosis did not occur in the 630 patients having long-term anticoagulation. Thromboembolism occurred 0.34 times/100 patient-years in the AVR group, 0.45 times/100 patient-years in the MVR group, and did not occur in 64 patients with double-valve replacement in those having anticoagulation.

Porcine bioprosthesis

Magilligan and colleagues[63] from Detroit, Michigan, have an extensive experience with porcine bioprosthetic valves: 817 patients with 951 porcine valves were discharged from the hospital and were available for long-term follow-up. Survival rates for patients with aortic valve prostheses were 78% at 5 years and 57% at 10 years. For patients with MVR, survival rates were 80% at 5 years and 69% at 10 years. Freedom from thromboembolism for aortic patients was 93% at 5 years and 88% at 10 years. For mitral valve patients, the freedom from thromboembolism was 89% at 5 years and 84% at 10 years. Freedom from degeneration or primary tissue failure for aortic valves was 97% at 5 years and 71% at 10 years (Fig. 5-19). For mitral valves, the figures were 96% at 5 years and 71% at 10 years. Porcine valves in patients ≤35 years of age had a significantly greater rate of degeneration. For patients >35 years of age the freedom from primary tissue failure was 80% at 10 years.

Ionescu-Shiley bioprosthesis

Gallo and colleagues[64] from Santander, Spain, reported on a retrospective follow-up of 88 patients who received the Ionescu-Shiley bovine pericardial valve in the aortic position between August 1977 and June 1980. Primary tissue degeneration occurred in 7 of the 65 patients with adequate follow-up. Cumulative duration of follow-up was 335 patient-years. Late deaths of unknown cause without autopsy and valve failures resulting from infection, thrombosis, and perivalvular leak were excluded from the analysis. The linearized incidence of primary tissue failure was 3%/patient-year. The actuarial

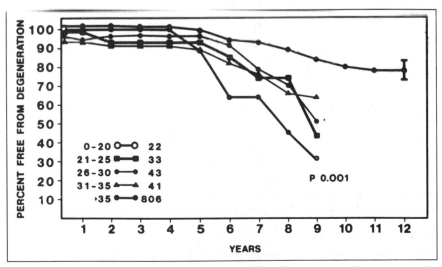

Fig. 5-19.   Freedom from degeneration was similar for all age groups ≤35 years, and the difference between these groups and patients >35 years was significant (p <0.001). Reproduced with permission from Magilligan et al.[63]

rate of freedom from valve failure for patients with an Ionescu-Shiley valve in the aortic position was 79 ± 8% at 7 years of follow-up. This series shows a higher incidence of primary tissue failure with this first generation pericardial valve prosthesis than with the glutaraldehyde-preserved porcine xenograft prosthesis in the aortic position from the same institution.

Doppler echo evaluation of prosthetic and bioprosthetic cardiac valves

Williams and Labovitz[65] from St. Louis, Missouri, investigated 134 patients with prosthetic or bioprosthetic heart valves by Doppler echo to determine normal values for commonly used prosthetic valves and to test the specificity of abnormal Doppler findings. In 70 patients the aortic valves had been replaced and in 64 the mitral valves had been replaced. Gradients across prostheses in the aortic position were calculated from maximal velocity. Peak calculated aortic transvalvular gradients in normal subjects were 22 ± 10 mmHg in 33 Björk-Shiley valves, 23 ± 10 mmHg in 27 porcine valves and 29 ± 13 mmHg in 6 Starr-Edwards valves. Mild AR was seen in 42% of Björk-Shiley valves, 26% of porcine valves, and 2 of 6 Starr-Edwards valves. Mitral valve orifice was calculated by the pressure half-time method. In clinically normal patients with mitral valve prostheses, the effective mitral valve orifice was 2.5 ± 0.8 cm^2 in 35 Björk-Shiley valves, 2.1 ± 0.7 cm^2 in 17 porcine valves, and 2.0 ± 0.3 cm^2 in 10 Starr-Edwards valves. MR was found in 11% of Björk-Shiley valves, 19% of porcine valves, and 30% of Starr-Edwards valves. Repeat studies at 2 weeks to 14 months revealed no difference in 8 aortic and 14 mitral prostheses. Seven aortic and 4 mitral valves functioned abnormally, as determined by Doppler, and the abnormal function was confirmed in each at surgery or by cardiac catheterization. Hemodynamic measurements by Doppler provide noninvasive information similar to that provided by cardiac catheterization that is reproducible and specific for valve dysfunction.

Treatment of right-sided cardiac failure after MVR

D'Ambra and colleagues[66] from Boston, Massachusetts, reported on an innovative use of the pharmacologic treatment of severe pulmonary hypertension and right-sided CHF immediately after bypass after MVR. They observed that such patients have intense pulmonary vasoconstriction and that the markedly increased pulmonary impedance may aggravate right-sided CHF and prevent recovery of RV function in this setting. They reported the effects of high dose prostaglandin E$_1$ (PGE$_1$; 30–150 ng/kg/min) with massive infusion of norepinephrine (up to 1 μg/kg/min) into the left atrium in 5 patients with refractory right-sided CHF and pulmonary hypertension after MVR. Each of the 5 patients had rapid pulmonary vasodilator responses followed by marked improvement in right-sided heart function. All survived operation and none had RV infarction or chronic right-sided CHF postoperatively. The investigators suggest that there is cardiopulmonary bypass-associated depression of RV function coupled with excessive alteration in pulmonary vascular resistance leading to refractory right-sided CHF after MVR. They used PGE$_1$ based on the expectation that the agent would allow afterload reduction therapy for RV failure. Theoretically, dilation engendered by PGE$_1$ might be restricted to the pulmonary vascular bed if it is infused into the right atrium, since it is rapidly metabolized during a single passage through the lung. Experience suggested that this was not the case and that patients required large doses of norepinephrine infused into the left atrium to counteract systemic vasodilatory properties of PGE_1. Right-sided CHF after MVR is an infrequent but devastating occurrence shortly after cardiopulmonary bypass. This pharmacologic therapy may go a long way to alleviate this frequently catastrophic event.

Anatomic analysis of prosthetic or bioprosthetic failure

Schoen and Hobson[67] from Boston, Massachusetts, investigated the causes of failure of 91 substitute cardiac valves, 33 mechanical and 58 bioprostheses obtained at reoperation (83 valves) or at necropsy (8 valves) during a 42-month period from mid-1980 through 1983, 1–264 months (mean, 72) after valve replacement. Paravalvular leak occurred in 15%, prosthetic or bioprosthetic thrombosis in 7%, tissue overgrowth in 8%, bioprosthetic degeneration or mechanical failure in 43%, and prosthetic or bioprosthetic endocarditis in 19%. Infective endocarditis and paravalvular leak were equally frequent with mechanical prostheses and with bioprostheses. Sterile degeneration was the overwhelming cause of failure for bioprostheses, accounting for the failure of 35 to 58 (60%) of those recovered. Sterile degeneration took several forms: calcification, with or without cuspal tears (27 cases, 47% of bioprostheses; mean, 77 months; range, 44–108 months) and cuspal defects without calcium (8 cases, 14%; mean, 59 months; range, 8–122 months). In general, calcium increased with time after implantation, but the propensity for the mineralization of bioprostheses varied widely among patients. Four torn valves that had been in place for >6 years had radiographically undetectable calcific deposits.

Prosthetic valve endocarditis

Calderwood and coworkers[68] from Boston, Massachusetts, analyzed the risk factors for the development of prosthetic valve endocarditis (PVE) in 2,642 patients undergoing initial valve replacement at the Massachusetts General Hospital from 1975–1982. Follow-up was available in 2,608 patients (99%) and the mean length of follow-up was 40 months. PVE developed in 116 patients (4.4%) and the actuarial risk was 3.1% at 12 months and 5.7% at 60 months. A Cox model was employed to identify risk factors for PVE and recipients of multiple valves had a higher risk of PVE than single valve. There was no difference in the risk for PVE for patients receiving aortic valves -vs-those receiving mitral valves. Recipients of mechanical valves had a higher risk of PVE than recipients of porcine valves in the first 3 months after surgery, but the risk of PVE was higher for porcine valve recipients ≥12 months after surgery. Despite the difference in the time course of development of PVE, there was no significant difference in the cumulative risk of PVE by 5 years of follow-up between mechanical and porcine valve recipients. Male sex was a risk factor for PVE within 12 months of AVR but not thereafter. Sex did not influence the risk of PVE after MVR. Older patients had a higher risk of PVE after multiple of MVR, but not after AVR. Thus, this study provides an accurate assessment of the risk for developing PVE at a major cardiovascular surgical center with current techniques.

References

1. NISHIMURA RA, McGOON MD, SHUB C, MILLER FA, ILSTRUP DM, TAJIK AJ: Echocardiographically documented mitral-valve prolapse: Long-term follow-up of 237 patients. N Engl J Med 1985 (Nov 21); 313:1305–1309.

2. JERESATY RM, EDWARDS JE, CHAWLA SK: Mitral valve prolapse and ruptured chordae tendineae. Am J Cardiol 1985 (Jan 1); 55:138–142.

3. HICKEY AJ, MacMAHON SW, WILCKEN DEL: Mitral valve prolapse and bacterial endocarditis: When is antibiotic prophylaxis necessary? Am Heart J 1985 (Mar); 109:431–435.

4. STRINGER JC, OBEID A, O'SHEA E: Mitral valve prolapse and addictions. Am J Cardiol 1985 (Nov 1); 56:808–809.

5. GARCIA-DORADO D, GARCIA EJ, BELLO L, MAROTO E, ALMAZAN A, GOMEZ A, FERNANDEZ-AVILES, GARCIA-DORADO A: Mitral valve prolapse secondary to right ventricular enlargement in patients with pulmonary hypertension after toxic rapeseed oil ingestion. Eur Heart J 1985 (Jan); 6:85–90.

6. LIMA SD, LIMA JAC, PYERITZ RE, WEISS JL: Relation of mitral valve prolapse to left ventricular size in Marfan's syndrome. Am J Cardiol 1985 (Mar 1); 55:739–743.

7. DOBMEYER DJ, STINE RA, LEIER CV, SCHAAL SF: Electrophysiologic mechanisms of provoked atrial flutter in mitral valve prolapse syndrome. Am J Cardiol 1985 (Oct 1); 56:602–604.

8. DRAKE CE, HODSDEN JE, SRIDHARAN MR, FLOWERS NC: Evaluation of the association of mitral valve prolapse in patients with Wolff-Parkinson-White type ECG and its relationship to the ventricular activation pattern. Am Heart J 1985 (Jan); 109:83–87.

9. ROSENTHAL ME, HAMER A, GANG ES, OSERAN DS, MANDEL WJ, PETER T: The yield of programmed ventricular stimulation in mitral valve prolapse patients with ventricular arrhythmias. Am Heart J 1985 (Nov); 110:970–976.

10. SHAPIRO EP, TRIMBLE EL, ROBINSON JC, ESTRUCH MT, GOTTLIEB SH: Safety of labor and delivery in women with mitral valve prolapse. Am J Cardiol 1985 (Nov 1); 56:806–807.

11. LIPPMAN SM, GINZTON LE, THIGPEN T, TANAKA KR, LAKS MM: Mitral valve prolapse in sickle cell disease: presumptive evidence for a linked connective tissue disorder. Arch Intern Med 1985 (Mar) 145:435–438.

12. BRAUMAN A, ALGOM M, GILBOA Y, RAMOT Y, GOLIK A, STRYJER D: Mitral valve prolapse in hyperthyroidism of two different origins. Br Heart J 1985 (Apr); 53:374–377.

13. MALCOLM AD: Mitral valve prolapse associated with other disorders: casual coincidence, common link, or fundamental genetic disturbance? Br Heart J 1985 (Apr); 53:353–362.

14. PENKOSKE PA, ELLIS H, ALEXANDER S, WATKINS E: Results of valve reconstruction for mitral regurgitation secondary to mitral valve prolapse. Am J Cardiol 1985 (Mar 1); 55:735–738.

15. TRESCH DD, DOYLE TP, BONCHECK LI, SIEGEL R, KEELAN MH, OLINGER GN, BROOKS HL: Mitral valve prolapse requiring surgery: clinical and pathologic study. Am J Med 1985 (Feb); 78:245–250.

16. REECE IJ, COOLEY DA, PAINVIN GA, OKEREKE OUJ, POWERS PL, PECHACEK LW, FRAZIER OH: Surgical treatment of mitral systolic click syndrome: results in 37 patients. Ann Thorac Surg 1985 (Feb); 39:155–158.

17. CLANCY KF, HAKKI A-H, ISKANDRIAN AS, HADJIMILTIADES S, MUNDTH ED, HAKKI A-H, BEMIS CE, NESTICO PF, DePACE NL, SEGAL BL: Forward ejection fraction: a new index of left ventricular function in mitral regurgitation. Am Heart J 1985 (Sept); 110:658–664.

18. KLIGFIELD P, HOCHREITER C, KRAMER H, DEVEREUX RB, NILES N, KRAMER-FOX R, BORER JS: Complex arrhythmias in mitral regurgitation with and without mitral valve prolapse: Contrast to arrhythmias in mitral valve prolapse without mitral regurgitation. Am J Cardiol 1985 (June 1); 55:1545–1549.

19. ORSZULAK TA, SCHAFF HV, DANIELSON GK, PIEHLER JM, PLUTH JR, FRYE RL, McGOON DC: Mitral regurgitation due to ruptured chordae tendineae. Early and late results of valve repair. J Thorac Cardiovasc Surg 1985 (Apr); 89:491–498.

20. KLEIN HO, SARELI P, SCHAMROTH CL, CARIM Y, EPSTEIN M, MARCUS B: Effects of atenolol on exercise capacity in patients with mitral stenosis with sinus rhythm. Am J Cardiol 1985 (Oct 1); 56:598–601.

21. LOCK JE, KHALILULLAH M, SHRIVASTAVA S, BAHL V, KEANE JF: Percutaneous catheter commissurotomy in rheumatic mitral stenosis. N Engl J Med 1985 (Dec 12); 313:1515–1518.

22. COHN LH, ALLRED EN, COHN LA, DISESA VJ, SHEMIN RJ, COLLINS JJ: Long-term results of open mitral valve reconstruction for mitral stenosis. Am J Cardiol 1985 (Mar 1); 55:731–734.

23. LABOVITZ AJ, NELSON JG, WINDHORST DM, KENNEDY HL, WILLIAMS GA: Frequency of mitral valve dysfunction from mitral anular calcium as detected by Doppler echocardiography. Am J Cardiol 1985 (Jan 1); 55:133–137.

24. SUBRAMANIAN R, OLSON LJ, EDWARDS WD: Surgical pathology of combined aortic stenosis and insufficiency: a study of 213 cases. Mayo Clin Proc 1985 (Apr); 60:247–254.

25. PETERSON MD, ROACH RM, EDWARDS JE: Types of aortic stenosis in surgically removed valves. Arch Pathol Lab Med 1985 (Sept) 109:829–832.

26. WILLIAMS GA, LABOVITZ AJ, NELSON JG, KENNEDY HL: Value of multiple echocardiographic views in the evaluation of aortic stenosis in adults by continuous-wave doppler. Am J Cardiol 1985 (Feb 1); 55:445–449.

27. AGATSTON AS, CHENGOT M, RAO A, HILDNER F, SAMET P: Doppler diagnosis of valvular aortic stenosis in patients over 60 years of age. Am J Cardiol 1985 (July 1); 55:106–109.

28. CURRIE PJ, SEWARD JB, REEDER GS, VLIETSTRA RE, BRESNAHAN DR, BRESNAHAN JF, SMITH HC, HAGLER DJ, TAJIK AJ: Continuous-wave Doppler echocardiographic assessment of severity of calcific aortic stenosis: a simultaneous Doppler-catheter correlative study in 100 adult patients. Circulation 1985 (June); 71:1162–1169.

29. KRAFCHEK J, ROBERTSON JH, RADFORD M, ADAMS D, KISSLO J: A reconsideration of Doppler assessed gradients in suspected aortic stenosis. Am Heart J 1985 (Oct); 110:765–773.

30. RUBLER S, REITANO J, DOLGIN M, KING ML, TARKOFF DM, SCHREIBER J: Aortic valve calcium as a marker for aortic stenosis. Cardiol Board Rev 1985 (Nov/Dec); 2:78–89.

31. MACKAY A, BEEN M, RODRIGUES E, MURCHISON J, DE BONO DP: Preoperative prediction of prosthesis size using cross sectional echocardiography in patients requiring aortic valve replacement. Br Heart J 1985 (May); 53:507–509.

32. MACMILLAN RM, DEMORIZI NM, GESSMAN LJ, MARANHAO V: Correlates of prolonged HV conduction in aortic stenosis. Am Heart J 1985 (July); 110:56–60.

33. ABDULALI SA, GANESH B, CLAYDEN AD, SMITH DR: Coronary artery luminal diameter in aortic stenosis. Am J Cardiol 1985 (Feb 1); 55:450–453.

34. GREEN SJ, PIZZARELLO RA, PADMANABHAN VT, ONG LY, HALL MH, TORTOLANI AJ: Relation of angina pectoris to coronary artery disease in aortic valve stenosis. Am J Cardiol 1985 (Apr 1); 55:1063–1065.

35. LAKIER JB, COPANS H, ROSMAN HS, LAM R, FINE G, KHAJA F, GOLDSTEIN S: Idiopathic degeneration of the aortic valve: a common cause of isolated aortic regurgitation. J Am Coll Cardiol 1985 (Feb); 5:347–351.

36. ALLEN WM, MATLOFF JM, FISHBEIN MC: Myxoid degeneration of the aortic valve and isolated severe aortic regurgitation. Am J Cardiol 1985 (Feb 1); 55:439–444.

37. QAIYUMI S, HASSAN Z, TOONE E: Seronegative spondyloarthropathies in lone aortic insufficiency. Arch Intern Med 1985 (May) 145:822–824.

38. LABRESH KA, LALLY EV, SHARMA SC, HO G: Two-dimensional echocardiographic detection of preclinical aortic root abnormalities in rheumatoid variant diseases. Am J Med 1985 (June); 78:908–912.

39. ROBERTS WC, DAY PJ: Electrocardiographic observations in clinically isolated, pure, chronic, severe aortic regurgitation: analysis of 30 necropsy patients aged 19 to 65 years. Am J Cardiol 1985 (Feb 1); 55:431–438.

40. ROSOFF MH, COHEN MV: Significance of E point-septal separation by M-mode echocardiography in patients with aortic regurgitation. Am J Cardiol 1985 (Nov 1); 56:809–811.

41. DANIEL WG, HOOD WP, SIART A, HAUSMANN D, NELLESSEN U, OELERT H, LICHTLEN PR: Chronic aortic regurgitation: reassessment of the prognostic value of preoperative left ventricular end-systolic dimension and fractional shortening. Circulation 1985 (Apr); 71:669–680.

42. BONOW RO, PICONE AL, MCINTOSH CL, JONES M, ROSING DR, MARON BJ, LAKATOS E, CLARK RE, EPSTEIN SE: Survival and functional results after valve replacement for aortic regurgitation from 1976 to 1983: impact of preoperative left ventricular function. Circulation 1985 (Dec); 72:1244–1256.

43. SHEN WF, ROUBIN GS, CHOONG CY, HUTTON BF, HARRIS PJ, FLETCHER PJ, KELLY DT: Evaluation of relationship between myocardial contractile state and left ventricular function in patients with aortic regurgitation. Circulation 1985 (Jan); 71:31–38.

44. GREENBERG B, MASSIE B, THOMAS D, BRISTOW JD, CHEITLIN M, BROUDY D, SZLACHCIC J, KRISHNAMURTHY G: Association between the exercise ejection fraction response and systolic wall stress in patients with chronic aortic insufficiency. Circulation 1985 (Mar); 71:458–465.

45. GEE DS, JUNI JE, SANTINGA JT, BUDA AJ: Prognostic significance of exercise-induced left ventricular dysfunction in chronic aortic regurgitation. Am J Cardiol 1985 (Oct 1); 56:605–609.

46. MASSIE BM, KRAMER BL, LOGE D, TOPIC N, GREENBERG BH, CHEITLIN MD, BRISTOW D, BYRD RC:

Ejection fraction response to supine exercise in asymptomatic aortic regurgitation: relation to simultaneous hemodynamic measurements. J Am Coll Cardiol 1985 (Apr); 5:847–855.

47. STAFFORD WJ, PETCH J, RADFORD DJ: Vegetations in infective endocarditis: clinical relevance and diagnosis by cross sectional echocardiography. Br Heart J 1985 (Mar 1); 53:310–313.

48. GRIFFIN MR, WILSON WR, EDWARDS WD, O'FALLON WM, KURLAND LT: Infective endocarditis: Olmsted County, Minnesota, 1950 through 1981. JAMA 1985 (Sept 6); 254:1199–1202.

49. CREMIEUX AC, WITCHITZ S, MALERGUE MC, WOLFF M, VITTECOCQ D, VILDE JL, FROTTIER J, VALERE PE, GIBERT C, SAIMOT AG: Clinical and echocardiographic observations in pulmonary valve endocarditis. Am J Cardiol 1985 (Oct 1); 56:610–613.

50. ELLIS SG, GOLDSTEIN J, POPP RL: Detection of endocarditis-associated perivalvular abscesses by two-dimensional echocardiography. J Am Coll Cardiol 1985 (Mar); 5:647–653.

51. D'AGOSTINO R, MILLER D, STINSON E, MITCHELL R, OYER P, JAMIESON S, BALDWIN J, SHUMWAY N: Valve replacement in patients with native valve endocarditis: what really determines operative outcome? Ann Thorac Surg 1985 (Nov); 40:429–438.

52. CURTIUS JM, THYSSEN M, BREUER HWM, LOOGEN F: Doppler versus contrast echocardiography for diagnosis of tricuspid regurgitation. Am J Cardiol 1985 (Aug 1); 56:333–336.

53. BERGER M, HAIMOWITZ A, VAN TOSH A, BERDOFF RL, GOLDBERG E: Quantitative assessment of pulmonary hypertension in patients with tricuspid regurgitation using continuous wave Doppler ultrasound. J Am Coll Cardiol 1985 (Aug); 6:359–365.

54. HANSON TP, EDWARDS BS, EDWARDS JE: Pathology of surgically excised mitral valves: one hundred consecutive cases. Arch Pathol Lab Med 1985 (Sept); 109:823–828.

55. SILVER MA, ROBERTS WC: Detailed anatomy of the normally functioning aortic valve in hearts of normal and increased weight. Am J Cardiol 1985 (Feb 1); 55:454–461.

56. ROSS EM, ROBERTS WC: The carcinoid syndrome: comparison of 21 necropsy subjects with carcinoid heart disease to 15 necropsy subjects without carcinoid heart disease. Am J Med 1985 (Sept); 79:339–354.

57. PAN CW, CHEN CC, WANG SP, HSU TL, CHIANG BN: Echocardiographic study of cardiac abnormalities in families of patients with Marfan's syndrome. J Am Coll Cardiol 1985 (Nov); 6:1016–1020.

58. MINDICH BP, GOLDMAN ME, FUSTER V, BURGESS N, LITWAK R: Improved intraoperative evaluation of mitral valve operations utilizing two-dimensional contrast echocardiography. J Thorac Cardiovasc Surg 1985 (July); 90:112–118.

59. SCOTT WC, MILLER DC, HAVERICH A, DAWKINS K, MITCHELL RS, JAMIESON SW, OYER PE, STINSON EB, BALDWIN JC, SHUMWAY NE: Determinants of operative mortality for patients undergoing aortic valve replacement. J Thorac Cardiovasc Surg 1985 (Mar); 89:400–413.

60. COHN L, ALLRED E, COHN L, AUSTIN J, SABIK J, DISESA V, SHEMIN R, COLLINS J: Early and late risk of mitral valve replacement. J Thorac Cardiovasc Surg 1985 (Dec); 90:872–881.

61. MAGOVERN JA, PENNOCK JL, CAMPBELL DB, PIERCE WS, WALDHAUSEN JA: Risks of mitral valve replacement and mitral valve replacement with coronary artery bypass. Ann Thorac Surg 1985 (Apr); 39:346–352.

62. BAUDET EM, OCA CC, ROQUES XF, LABORDE MN, HAFEZ AS, COLLOT MA, GHIDONI IM: A 5-1/2 year experience with the St. Jude Medical cardiac valve prosthesis. J Thorac Cardiovasc Surg 1985 (July); 90:137–144.

63. MAGILLIGAN DJ JR, LEWIS JW, TILLEY B, PETERSON E: The porcine bioprosthetic valve. Twelve years later. J Thorac Cardiovasc Surg 1985 (Apr); 89:499–507.

64. GALLO I, NISTAL F, REVUELTA JM, GARCIA-SATUE E, ARTINANO E, DURAN CG: Incidence of primary tissue valve failure with the Ionescu-Shiley pericardial valve. J Thorac Cardiovasc Surg 1985 (Aug); 90:278–280.

65. WILLIAMS GA, LABOVITZ AJ: Doppler hemodynamic evaluation of prosthetic (Starr-Edwards and Bjork-Shiley) and bioprosthetic (Hancock and Carpentier-Edwards) cardiac valves. Am J Cardiol 1985 (Aug 1); 56:325–332.

66. D'AMBRA MN, LARAIA PJ, PHILBIN DM, WATKINS WD, HILGENBERG AD, BUCKLEY MJ: Prostaglandin E_1. A new therapy for refractory right heart failure and pulmonary hypertension after mitral valve replacement. J Thorac Cardiovasc Surg 1985 (Apr); 89:567–572.

67. SHOEN FJ, HOBSON CE: Anatomic analysis of removed prosthetic heart valves: causes of failure of 33 mechanical valves and 58 bioprostheses, 1980 to 1983. Hum Pathol 1985 (June); 16:549–559.

68. CALDERWOOD SB, SWINSKI LA, WATERNAUX CM, KARCHMER AW, BUCKLEY MJ: Risk factors for the development of prosthetic valve endocarditis. Circulation 1985 (July); 72:31–37.

Myocardial Heart Disease

Endomyocardial biopsy in infants and children

Some recent studies in adults with idiopathic dilated cardiomyopathy (IDC) have reported interstitial myocardial inflammation in 5–63% of patients studied by transvascular myocardial biopsy techniques. Lewis and associates[1] from Los Angeles, California, performed transvascular endomyocardial biopsy in 15 infants and children with IDC. The light and electron microscopic findings were reviewed to evaluate the presence of lymphocytes as an indicator of active myocarditis. Both ventricles were biopsied in 13 patients, and the RV wall only, in 2. No endomyocardial specimen contained inflammatory cells. Interstitial fibrosis, myofiber hypertrophy, degeneration, and necrosis were found. Ultrastructural abnormalities of the mitochrondria, T tubules, or Z bands were noted in approximately one-third of patients. Persistent, active myocarditis is an uncommon cause of IDC in children. Immunosuppressive therapy, which may be harmful, should be considered only after myocardial inflammation has been documented by endomyocardial biopsy.

Relation to acute myocarditis

Dec and associates[2] from Boston, Massachusetts, studied clinical features and course (average follow-up, 18 months) of 27 patients with acute idiopathic dilated cardiomyopathy (IDC) (symptoms for <6 months) who were referred for endomyocardial biopsy. Almost 40% of the patients subsequently had an increase in LVEF (on average, from 0.21–0.41) and substantial improvement in CHF; the remainder died or had chronic IDC. Biopsy revealed myocarditis in 18 patients, and this finding was especially common (89%) in patients who had been ill for <4 weeks. The biopsy specimen was negative in

4 patients whose clinical features and later course were diagnostic of myocarditis. Nine patients received immunosuppressive drugs, and 4 improved, a rate that did not differ from the rate of spontaneous improvement. Neither the histologic features of the biopsy specimen nor the clinical features at presentation were clearly correlated with subsequent improvement, whether or not immunosuppressive drugs were given. It was concluded that many cases of IDC result from myocarditis. Definitive histologic confirmation depends on the duration of illness. The efficacy of immunosuppressive treatment must still be established.

Correlation of myocardial ultrastructural findings to myocardial function

Although hemodynamic status has been assessed by invasive and noninvasive techniques in idiopathic dilated cardiomyopathy (IDC), a longitudinal hemodynamic study has not been published. Figulla and coworkers[3] from Goettingen, West Germany, investigated the hemodynamic courses of 56 patients with IDC: 14 patients died within 24 months after diagnosis (25% mortality). The hemodynamic courses of the remaining 42 patients were investigated in subsequent examinations by determination of LVEF, mean PA pressure at maximal workload, and peak systolic pressure/end-systolic volume index. During the study interval of 32 months, the conditions of 20 patients (48%) deteriorated, according to their hemodynamic status, and at least 5 of these died of CHF. Surprisingly, the conditions of 22 patients (52%) improved or stabilized; 1 died of leukemia. Seven of the 22 patients with an initial LVEF of ≤0.30 experienced an average increase from 0.22–0.51. Age, alcohol intake, exercise capacity, and hemodynamic status were not helpful in predicting the course of the disease. In 38 patients, endomyocardial biopsy samples were obtained at diagnosis. Reduced myofibril volume fraction (<60%) had prognostic significance for both hemodynamic deterioration and death (sensitivity, 23 of 24, 96%), whereas 14 of 15 patients whose conditions improved or stabilized had a myofibril volume fraction of ≥60% (specificity, 14 of 15, 93%) (Fig. 6-1). A relation between hemodynamic status and the myofibril volume fraction could not be found. Individual patients with IDC differ significantly with respect to course of the disease. A distinct separation of the patients by means of morphologic criteria is possible, which makes it more likely that the pathogenesis of the disease is not unique.

Prevalence in 2 regions in England

Williams and Olsen[4] from Norfolk and London, UK, assessed the prevalence of idiopathic dilated cardiomyopathy in 2 regions in England from 420 replies to 771 questionnaires sent to general practitioners. Overall point prevalence was 8.3/100,000 population in areas covering a total sample of nearly 914,000 inhabitants.

Familial aggregation

The role of genetic factors in the pathogenesis of idiopathic dilated cardiomyopathy (IDC) is unknown. Although IDC usually is sporadic, families with >1 affected member have been observed. Michels and associates[5] from Rochester, Minnesota, determined the proportion of familiar cases of IDC in a retrospective series of 169 patients <50 years of age at diagnoses and seen at the Mayo Clinic from 1976 through 1982. Of the 169 patients, 11 (6.5%) had familial IDC. Two patients were brothers. Four percent of the male

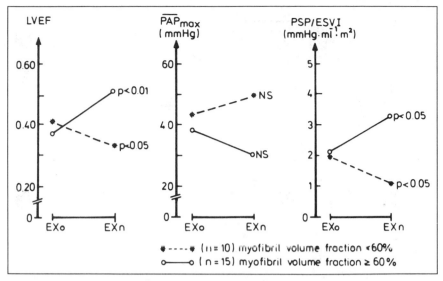

Fig. 6-1. Hemodynamic courses, as determined by the parameters LVEF, PA pressure at maximal workload, and peak systolic pressure/end-systolic volume index (PSP/ESVI) in the patients with myofibril volume fractions of <60% and those with fractions ≥60%. The patients with myofibril volume fractions of <60% had a significant decrease in LVEF and PSP/ESVI over the study interval, and the opposite was true in patients with myofibril volume fractions of ≥60%. Ex_0 = time of diagnosis; Ex_n = time of reexamination. Reproduced with permission from Figulla et al.[3]

patients and 12% of the female patients had familial IDC. The mean age of both male and female patients with familial IDC was 32 years. Of the 53 patients who were ≤35 years of age, 6 (11%) had familial disease. In contrast, of the 116 patients who were 36–50 years of age, only 5 (4%) had familial IDC. The pedigrees of the 10 familial cases are shown in Figure 6-2.

Effect of Valsalva maneuver

Little and colleagues[6] from San Antonio, Texas, studied the effect of the Valsalva maneuver (40 cm H_2O for 15 s) on LV volume in 12 normal subjects with a mean LVEF of 0.65 and in 8 patients with idiopathic dilated cardiomyopathy (IDC), evidence of pulmonary congestion, and a mean LVEF of 0.23. LV volume and RV area were determined by apical 2-D echo. In both groups the RV end-diastolic area decreased during the late strain phase of the Valsalva maneuver. In normal subjects it decreased from 9.3–5.6 cm^2 and in patients it decreased from 13–10 cm^2. In normal subjects, LV end-diastolic volume decreased from the control level during the Valsalva maneuver and this was apparent in both the 4-chamber and 2-chamber views. In the patients, LV end-diastolic volume was not significantly different from control in either view. In normal subjects, a decrease in stroke volume from control during the Valsalva maneuver was evident in both views, but in the patients there was no change in stroke volume in either view during the Valsalva maneuver. Thus, these investigators concluded that in patients with pulmonary congestion and reduced LVEF, LV stroke volume does not decrease during the strain phase of the Valsalva maneuver because LV end-diastolic volume is maintained.

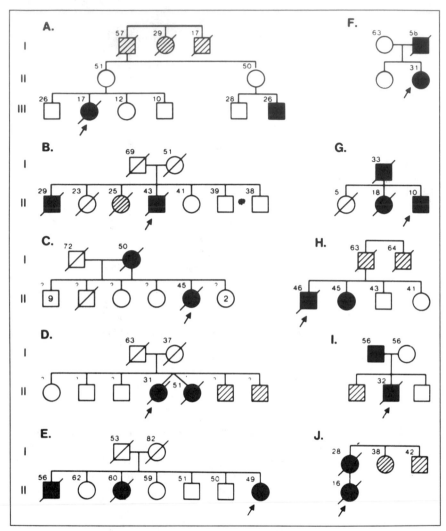

Fig. 6-2. Pedigrees of 10 families in this study with familial idiopathic cardiomyopathy. Superscript numbers give age at presentation or at time of death (slashed line). ■ = males and ● = females of confirmed cases. Hatched lines = suspected cases; arrows = index cases.

Prognosis

To define prognosis in patients with idiopathic dilated cardiomyopathy (IDC), Costanzo-Nordin and associates[7] from Hines, Illinois, performed radionuclide ventriculagraphy, echo, 12-lead ECG, and 24-hour ambulatory monitoring in 55 patients. Over 14 ± 8 months, 11 patients died, all suddenly. Univariate analysis showed that patients with more severe functional impairment, lower cardiac index, lower EF, and higher PA wedge pressure had greater mortality risk. Age, duration of symptoms, 12-lead ECG abnormalities, and atrial arrhythmias were not predictive of higher mortality. The number of VPC/hr, the occurrence of couplets, the degree of VPC prematurity, and the presence, frequency, rate, and duration of VT did not have prognostic significance. A stepwise discriminant analysis identified functional class, cardiac index, and presence or absence of multiform VPC as the group of variables that together could more accurately predict outcome. Using a formula derived from the results of this analysis, the outcomes of 36 of 49 patients (74%) was correctly predicted, with a specificity of 100% and a sensitivity of 70%.

Meinertz and associates[8] from Mainz, West Germany, prospectively assessed the incidence and prognostic significance of electrically induced ventricular arrhythmias in 42 patients with IDC. All patients underwent 24-hour, long-term ECG (Holter) monitoring and 30 were analyzed by a signal-averaging vectorcardiographic procedure at entry into the study. Their response to programmed electrical stimulation during basic RV pacing was investigated using 1 and 2 ventricular extrastimuli. A monomorphic tachycardia was not induced in any patient. In 36 patients (86%) polymorphic ventricular arrhythmias were initiated: ≥3 induced consecutive VPC occurred in 9 patients (21%), nonsustained polymorphic VT in 2 (4.8%), and VF in 1 patient (2.4%). There was no association between electrically induced polymorphic ventricular arrhythmias and the degree of impairment of LV function. Furthermore, the incidence of induced ventricular arrhythmias was not related to the Lown grade or to the total number of VPC during Holter monitoring. A late potential was detected by the averaged vectorcardiogram in only 1 of the 30 patients. During follow-up (mean, 16 ± 7 months) 7 patients died, 5 from CHF and 2 suddenly. No patient had an electrically induced arrhythmia of ≥3 VPC. Thus, in most patients with IDC, programmed electrical stimulation of the RV with up to 2 extrastimuli fails to reproduce an electrophysiologic correlate to the frequent ventricular arrhythmias.

Effects of digoxin

Ribner and associates[9] from Chicago, Illinois, correlated the hemodynamic and hormonal effects of digoxin in 11 normotensive men in sinus rhythm with CHF due to idiopathic dilated cardiomyopathy. Patients were evaluated at rest and during submaximal exercise before and 6 hours after the intravenous infusion of 1.0 mg of digoxin (mean serum concentration, 1.7 ng/ml). With digoxin therapy, heart rate, PA wedge pressure, and RA pressure declined and cardiac output increased. Although vasopressin was unchanged, both plasma norepinephrine concentrations and plasma renin activity decreased, the reduction in norepinephrine correlating with the increase in cardiac output. Despite these hemodynamic and hormonal effects, there was no change in total SVR at rest or during exercise. It was concluded that the improvement in cardiac function with digoxin in this patient group was a result of the inotropic properties of the drug, without an associated reduction in impedance.

Effects of hydralazine

Smucker and associates[10] from Dallas, Texas, assessed the effects of intravenous hydralazine in 8 patients with severe idiopathic dilated cardiomyopathy (IDC). Hydralazine increased stroke volume index (from 24 ± 8–40 ± 9 ml/m^2) and decreased systemic vascular resistance (from 1,603 ± 619–810 ± 317 dynes s cm^{-5}) and peak LV wall stress (from 476 ± 118–410 ± 68 kdynes/cm^2). Two groups were defined by normal or high LV wall stress. Patients with high LV stress had higher LV end-diastolic pressure (38 ± 12 -vs- 17 ± 8 mmHg), LV end-diastolic volume index (184 ± 24 -vs- 149 ± 7 ml/m^2) and systemic vascular resistance (1,423 ± 686 -vs- 846 ± 293 dynes s cm^{-5}). Hydralazine decreased stress more in these patients (-101 ± 57 -vs- -6 ± 9 kdynes/cm^2), LV end-diastolic pressure (-12 ± 7 -vs- 2 ± 2 mmHg), systolic pressure (-15 ± 13 -vs- 3 ± 4 mmHg) and systemic vascular resistance ($-1,053 \pm 247$ -vs- -363 ± 83 dynes s cm^{-5}) than in patients with normal LV stress. Decreased LV stress was caused by decreased systolic and diastolic pressures and/or volumes. Late systolic pressure-volume relations in patients with normal LV stress suggested increased myocardial contractility, but this was not confirmed by LV dp/dt. Hydralazine improves LV function in patients with IDC by reducing elevated LV wall stress, with little inotropic effect.

Metoprolol therapy

β-blockade therapy to improve survival in idiopathic dilated cardiomyopathy (IDC) has been both advocated and criticized. Randomized studies have not been performed until Anderson and associates[11] from Salt Lake City, Utah, randomized 50 patients with IDC in pairs to standard therapy (C) alone or with β-blockade (BB). β-blockade therapy with metoprolol was titrated from 12.5–50 mg twice daily as tolerated (final average dose, 61 mg/day). Groups were comparable in age (C, 50 ± 15 years; BB, 51 ± 13 years), gender (C, 76% male; BB, 56% male), entry functional class (C, 2.8 ± 0.8; BB, 2.7 ± 0.7), and LVEF (C, $27 \pm 12\%$; BB, $29 \pm 10\%$). Follow-up averaged 19 months (range, 1–38). One subject in each group was lost to follow-up. There were 3 early BB dropouts (within 2 days) due to low output syndrome (2 patients) or fatigue (1 patient). Eleven patients died. By intention to treat, 5 BB and 6 C patients died (difference not significant). By actual treatment, 3 BB patients died, including 2 late dropouts (at 0.2, 10, and 17 months), and 8 C patients died (at 2, 9, 15, 18, 24, 29, and 32 months) (Fig. 6-3). In addition, functional evaluation on follow-up (functional class, San Diego questionnaire, and exercise time) all tended to favor those receiving BB. Low-dose BB is tolerated in 80% of IDC patients on a long-term basis. Those continuing to take BB have a good prognosis. Mortality in C patients, however, is less than in some retrospective studies. The improved survival trend in the BB group may be due to selection of less ill patients and to possible protective effects of BB.

Engelmeier and coinvestigators[12] from Maywood, Illinois, tested the long-term effect of metoprolol on 8 patients in a double-blind, randomized protocol and 12 patients in an unblinded, crossover protocol who were treated for 12 months and compared them with 6 similar subjects who were treated with placebo for 10 months in a double-blind, randomized protocol. Patients were followed by serial clinical assessment, treadmill testing, radionuclide ventriculography, and echo. Metoprolol-treated patients had an improvement in exercise capacity by 3 mets while experiencing a significant improvement in functional class during both the double-blind and open-label crossover studies and had an improved EF during the double-blind study. These improvements were not seen in matched control subjects receiving placebo. Seven of 20 patients receiving long-term metoprolol therapy had resolution of all symptoms of CHF, doubled their exercise capacity, and had progressive improvement in resting radionuclide LVEF (13–27%) and echo LV end-diastolic dimension (7.7–6.5 cm). Only 1 of 21 patients treated was intolerant of metoprolol. The investigators concluded that metoprolol can be given safely to a select group of patients with IDC in doses that substantially reduce both resting and exercise heart rates. Long-term BB improved functional class and exercise capacity in 14 of 20 patients while producing an

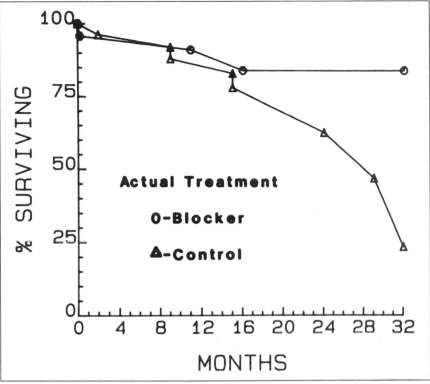

Fig. 6-3. Survival curves by actual treatment method for control and β-blockade groups. The difference in curves is not significant.

exceptional clinical response in 7 that was accompanied by improved resting parameter of LV function.

Nifedipine

Miller and associates[13] from Jacksonville, Florida, studied 9 patients with chronic severe CHF secondary to idiopathic dilated cardiomyopathy (IDC) to determine the acute effects of 10 mg of sublingual nifedipine on LV function. Hemodynamic and echo data were obtained at rest and 30 minutes, 1, 2, 4, and 6 hours after nifedipine. Measurements at rest reflected LV dysfunction with elevation of end-diastolic volume index (102 ± 46 m/m^2), PA wedge pressure (17 ± 8 mmHg), systemic vascular resistance ($1,547 \pm 439$ dynes s cm^{-5}) and reduction of cardiac index (2.8 ± 0.5 L/min/m^2). There were no adverse effects noted with administration of sublingual nifedipine. Initial changes through 1 hour reflected an unloading effect of nifedipine with reduction in PA wedge pressure (11 ± 5 mmHg), systemic vascular resistance ($1,179 \pm 289$ dynes s cm^{-5}), end-diastolic volume index (91 ± 37 ml/m^2 [difference not significant]) and an increase in cardiac index (3.6 ± 0.7 ml L/min/m^2). Subsequently, the cardiac index, systemic vascular resistance, and end-diastolic volume index returned toward baseline. Only the PA wedge and PA pressures had a sustained reduction through the 6-hour study period, suggesting an effect of nifedipine on LV relaxation. Thus, sublingual nifedipine administered acutely to patients with CHF from IDC is safe and efficacious.

Myocardial ischemia

Chest pain is a frequent symptom of patients with HC and commonly occurs in the setting of angiographically normal epicardial coronary arteries. To study the mechanism and hemodynamic significance of myocardial ischemia in HC, Cannon and coworkers[14] from Bethesda, Maryland, examined 20 patients with resting LV outflow tract obstruction >30 mmHg, a history of angina pectoris, and angiographically normal coronary arteries. Patients underwent a pacing study with measurement of great cardiac vein flow, lactate and oxygen content, and LV filling pressure. Compared with 28 control subjects without HC, the resting coronary blood flow was higher and the coronary resistance was lower. LV end-diastolic pressure and PA wedge pressure were significantly higher in patients with HC. During pacing, coronary flow increased in both groups, although coronary and myocardial hemodynamics differed greatly. In contrast to the linear increase in flow in control subjects up to a heart rate of 150 beats/min, patients with HC had an initial increase in flow to 133 ml/min at an intermediate heart rate of 130 beats/min. At this point, 12 of 20 patients developed their typical chest pain. With continued pacing to a rate of 150 beats/min, mean coronary flow decreased to 114 ml/min, with 18 of 20 patients having typical chest pain and metabolic evidence of myocardial ischemia. This decrease in coronary flow was associated with a substantial increase in LV end-diastolic pressure. In the 14 patients whose coronary flow actually decreased from intermediate to peak pacing, the increase in LV end-diastolic pressure in the same interval was greater than that of the 6 patients whose flow remained unchanged or increased. In addition, despite metabolic and hemodynamic evidence of myocardial ischemia, the arteriovenous oxygen difference actually narrowed at peak pacing. Thus, most patients with HC achieved maximum coronary vasodilation and flow at modest increases in heart rate. Elevation in LV filling pressure, probably related to ischemia-induced changes in ventricular compliance, was associated with a decline in coronary flow. These investigators conclude that the paradoxical narrowing of the arteriovenous oxygen difference, despite apparent limitation of coronary flow, may also be of pathogenetic importance to myocardial ischemia in HC.

Doppler flow observations

Maron and coworkers[15] from Bethesda, Maryland, determined whether true obstruction to LV ejection exists in patients with HC and a subaortic gradient. They used pulsed Doppler echo to analyze the patterns of LV emptying in 50 patients with HC (20 with and 30 without evidence of obstruction) and in 20 normal volunteers. In the patients with obstructive HC, LV ejection was characterized by early and rapid emptying. The proportion of forward blood flow velocity occurring before initial mitral-septal contact was variable, but averaged 58%. However, the proportion of forward flow velocity occurring after mitral valve-septal contact was considerable, averaging >40%. Midsystolic obstruction to LV outflow was suggested by the rapid deceleration in aortic flow velocity occurring with mitral-septal complex and premature partial AV closure. LV ejection was prolonged and the left ventricle continued to empty and shorten during the period when both the pressure gradient and increased intraventricular pressure were present. Sixteen of 20 patients had a relatively small second peak in flow velocity in late systole. In contrast, patients with nonobstructive HC had no evidence of resistance to LV forward flow. Aortic flow velocity waveforms were similar to those in normal volunteers and flow persisted to AV closure. These data indicate that in patients with HC: 1) systolic anterior motion of the mitral valve produces a mechanical obstruction to LV emptying; 2) the subaortic gradient appears to be of pathophysiologic importance because the LV continues to contract in the presence of markedly increased intraventricular pressure; and 3) LV ejection characteristics differ between patients with and without mitral systolic anterior motion or subaortic gradient.

Some investigators have found that LV ejection is completed much earlier than normal in patients with HC, whether or not an LV outflow gradient is present, and they have concluded that LV ejection is not impeded in HC but merely ends early because of early completion of LV emptying. Gardin and associates[16] from Irvine, California, examined this possibility using pulse Doppler echo to record ascending aortic flow velocity in 20 patients with HC, 12 with evidence of LV outflow gradient at rest (obstructed HC), and 8 without evidence of significant resting gradient (nonobstructed HC). Peak aortic flow velocity was similar in patients with nonobstructed HC (92 ± 26 cm/s) and those with obstructed HC (94 ± 26 cm/s) and in 20 normal subjects (92 ± 11 cm/s). However, mean ejection time measured from the aortic flow velocity tracing or aortic echogram was longer in those with obstructed HC (345 ± 30 ms) than in those with nonobstructed HC (296 ± 24 ms) and in normal subjects (294 ± 19 ms). Furthermore, a rapid decrease in aortic flow velocity in midsystole was seen in 11 of 12 patients with obstructed HC, but in none of the patients with nonobstructed HC or normal subjects. Doppler LA flow velocity recordings, obtained in 11 patients, demonstrated MR in 4 of 5 patients with obstructed HC but in none of 6 patients with nonobstructed HC. The temporal relation between the decrease in Doppler aortic flow velocity, the peaking of Doppler mitral regurgitant flow, and the onset of mitral valve-septal contact in midsystole—and observations regarding LV internal dimensional changes—suggest that the early deceleration of aortic blood flow in obstructed HC is not merely a result of early completion of mechanical systole by a hyperdynamic LV. Rather, midsystolic aortic flow deceleration is at least in part a result of the anterior mitral leaflet impeding LV outflow and causing ejection of blood by an alternate route into the left atrium.

Diastolic abnormalities

To investigate the relation between diastolic abnormalities and LV hypertrophy, Spirito and coworkers[17] from Pavia, Italy, studied 52 patients with HC and 22 normal subjects with digitized M-mode and 2-D echo. Echo indexes of diastolic function were compared in patients with different extent of LV hypertrophy. Time interval from minimum LV internal dimension to mitral valve opening and time to peak rate of increase in LV internal dimension were significantly prolonged in patients with HC and the most extensive LV hypertrophy compared with those in patients with mild LV hypertrophy. Furthermore, peak rate of posterior wall diastolic excursion was significantly reduced in those patients with HC and posterior wall hypertrophy compared with that in patients with HC but normal posterior wall thickness. Abnormal M-mode echo indexes of diastolic function also were identified in a substantial proportion of patients with HC and only mild LV hypertrophy. In these patients, time interval from minimum LV internal dimension to mitral valve opening, peak rate, and time to peak rate of increase in LV internal dimension were significantly different from normal. Furthermore, in 32 patients with HC who had normal posterior wall thickness, peak rate of posterior wall diastolic excursion was significantly reduced compared with normal. These findings demonstrate a relation in patients with HC between magnitude of LV hypertrophy and extent of diastolic wall motion abnormalities.

Magnetic resonance imaging

A distinct advantage of gated magnetic resonance imaging (MRI) in cardiac disease is the sharp discrimination of the endocardial and epicardial interfaces of the myocardial walls. This technique therefore would potentially be useful in patients with HC. Higgins and associates[18] from San Francisco, California, performed gated MRI using a 0.35 Tesla cryogenic system in 14 patients with HC to define the site and extent of abnormal wall thickness. These studies were compared with 2-D echo. Gated MRI studies in 12 normal volunteers were used for comparison. In normal subjects and in patients with HC, the sharp demarcation of the myocardial wall permitted measurement of wall thickness. The thickness of the septal and posterolateral walls in normal subjects was 10.2 ± 0.4 mm ($\pm$SD) and 10.8 ± 0.5 mm, respectively, whereas septal thickness in all but 1 patient with HC was ≥ 15.0 mm. In patients with HC, septal and posterolateral wall thicknesses were 2.2 ± 0.8 cm and 1.3 ± 0.17 cm, respectively, by MRI. The 2-D echo measurements for septal and posterolateral walls were 2.4 ± 0.6 cm and 1.4 ± 0.7 cm, respectively. The severity and distribution of abnormal wall thickness were comparable on 2-D echo and MRI. Gated MRI is an effective and completely noninvasive technique for demonstrating the presence, site, and extent of abnormal wall thickness in HC.

Comparison of ventricular emptying with and without outflow pressure gradient

Controversy has existed for a long time about the importance of intraventricular pressure gradients in patients with HC. Systolic anterior motion of the anterior mitral leaflet with apposition of the anterior mitral leaflet with the ventricular septum has generally been accepted as the anatomic basis for the pressure gradient and for an impediment to egress of blood from the left ventricle. The ability of the ventricle to empty rapidly in the presence of outflow tract obstruction has been attributed to late systolic MR. An alternative nonobstructive basis for the intracavitary pressure gradient in HC derives its theoretical premise from gradients recorded within hyperkinetic and hypovolemic left ventricles in experimental animals during hemorrhagic shock and during the application of negative gravitational forces. This nonobstructive mechanism (cavitary obliteration or elimination) has been shown to be responsible for intracavitary LV gradients in experimental animals and in man during various conditions that increase the contractile force or diminish the filling volume and peripheral resistance or both (catecholamines, septic shock, amyl nitrite inhalation combined with the Valsalva maneuver, or postextrasystolic potentiation). In the Gauer (*Aerospace Medicine* 1964; 35:533–544) a pressure gradient develops within a hyperdynamic ventricle. The outflow tract shares the same systolic pressure as the aorta beyond because they are in free communication. The LV body generates a higher pressure as it progressively separates itself from the outflow tract while obliterating its cavities. These diametrically opposed explanations of the pressure gradient in HC have not been satisfactorily resolved. Siegel and Criley[19] from Los Angeles and Torrence, California, used LV angiography in patients with HC to study

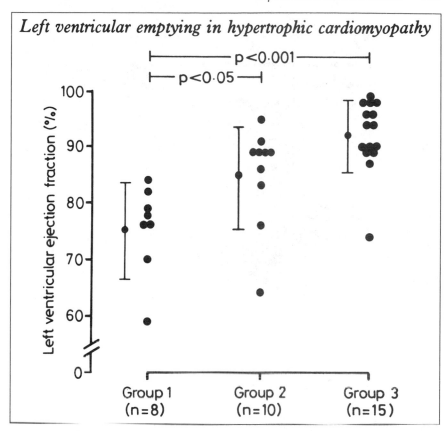

Left ventricular emptying in hypertrophic cardiomyopathy

Fig. 6-4.   Angiographic LVEF in 33 patients with HC with no gradient (group 1), an inducible gradient (group 2), and a resting gradient (group 3). Reproduced with permission from Siegel and Criley.[19]

the relation between the pressure gradient and the ability of the ventricle to empty itself. They studied 33 patients, mean age 55 years, 18 men and 15 women, and divided them into 3 groups: Group 1 included 8 patients without a pressure gradient; group 2, 10 patients with a provocable gradient; and group 3, 15 patients with a resting gradient. Patients with resting gradients had a higher mean LVEF ($92 \pm 6\%$) than patients without a resting or inducible pressure gradient ($75 \pm 9\%$) (Fig. 6-4). The rate and degree of emptying increased when gradients >85 mmHg were induced in 2 patients with insignificant MR. The investigators reasoned that if the induced gradients had been the result of obstruction that a decrease in the rate or degree of ventricular emptying would be expected. The higher EF in patients with intracavitary pressure gradients and enhanced rate and degree of LV emptying with induced gradients are inconsistent in their view with outflow obstruction. These findings in their view support the concept that cavity obliteration is responsible for the pressure gradient in HC.

Anesthetic risk for noncardiac surgery

Thompson and associates[20] from Boston, Massachusetts, reviewed the records of 35 patients with HC diagnosed by cardiac ultrasound and/or catheterization who underwent general (52 patients) or spinal (4 patients) anesthesia, a total of 56 major surgical procedures, to determine their periopera-

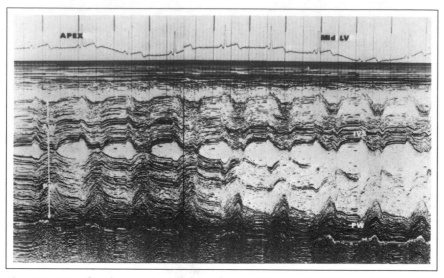

Fig. 6-5. M-mode echo scan from the apex of the left ventricle (LV) through the mid left ventricle and mitral area. The severe hypertrophy in the apical region and the typical pattern of contraction in this region are obvious. AW = anterior wall; PW = posterior wall; IVS = interventricular septum. Reproduced with permission from Keren et al.[21]

tive risk. There was no operative or related perioperative deaths. Intraoperative or postoperative complications included: AMI with CHF in 1 patient who also had CAD and was 1 of 3 patients who had spinal anesthesia, arrhythmia requiring therapy in 8, and angina during SVT in 1. It was concluded that the risk of general anesthesia and major noncardiac surgery is low in patients with HC.

"Apical" variety

In a 3-year period Keren and coworkers[21] from Tel Aviv, Israel, evaluated 23 patients with apical HC by noninvasive and invasive methods. Sixteen patients had chest pain, but the cardiovascular examination was normal in 17 individuals. The ECG showed precordial inverted T waves in all patients and these were of mild-to-moderate amplitude in 18 and giant (>10 mm) in 5. M-mode echo demonstrated a typical pattern of contraction and relaxation in the apical region of the LV that was associated with significant hypertrophy (Fig. 6-5). Systolic anterior motion of the mitral valve was not observed nor was there evidence of obstruction to the LV outflow tract. Doppler echo studies of the mitral and aortic flow were normal in all patients except 1 who had mild MR. RNA studies of 14 patients revealed a mean LVEF of 66 ± 6% with normal LV contraction in all patients but 2 who had apical hypokinesis. In all 6 patients who had catheterization, a characteristic appearance of the LV at end-systole and abnormal end-diastolic contour were noted on the LV angiogram, but the "ace of spades" configuration was seen in only 1 patient.

Frequency of epicardial CAD

Cokkinos and associates[22] from Houston, Texas, analyzed 85 consecutive patients with HC who also had coronary angiography. A basal gradient >20 mmHg was present in 51 patients and a gradient <20 mmHg was present in 31 patients. All patients had LV hypertrophy and evidence of LV cavity obliteration on angiography. Sixteen of the 85 patients (19%) had a fixed narrowing of the luminal diameter of >60% in ≥1 coronary artery. In 5 patients with CAD who had severe obstruction (>90%) of the LAD artery, there was no evidence of collateral vessels to this branch. The mean age of the patients with CAD was 64 years and that of the patients without CAD, 42 years. Ninety-four percent of the patients with and 43% of those without CAD were >45 years of age. The frequency of angina in patients with CAD was 81% and in patients without CAD, 46%. In 5 of the 13 patients with CAD and angina, there was recent worsening of the symptoms, whereas in the group without CAD, angina was unchanged. Two patients with and 1 patient without CAD had had a previous AMI. The patients with CAD had a lower LV end-diastolic pressure (17 -vs- 23 mmHg). These investigators concluded that all patients >45 years, especially when angina pectoris is present, should undergo coronary angiography in addition to the other hemodynamic evaluation. They also concluded that the presence of significant CAD in patients with HC does not significantly increase the operative mortality. Thus, patients with combined HC and CAD undergoing corrective surgery for HC concurrently with CABG usually continued to have symptomatic improvement and a low risk of death after relatively long-term follow-up.

Amiodarone

McKenna and associates[23] from London, UK, assessed the effect of amiodarone on survival in patients with HC and VT in a drug trial with historical controls. During 1976 and 1977, 24-hour (7 patients) or 48-hour (79 patients) ECG monitoring was performed in 86 consecutive patients; 24 had VT and received conventional antiarrhythmic agents. Nineteen clinical, echo, and hemodynamic features were assessed. Seven patients died suddenly during follow-up of 3 years; of these, 5 had continued to have VT and 2 had no documented VT. During 1978 and 1979, VT was detected during 48-hour ECG monitoring in 21 of the next 82 consecutive patients with HC. They received amiodarone (150–400 mg/day; median, 300); VT was suppressed in all during repeat 48 hour ECG examination. Two patients died suddenly during a 3-year follow-up, but neither belonged to the amiodarone treated group with VT. The clinical and hemodynamic variables were similar in patients taking amiodarone and conventional agents. The fact that control of ventricular arrhythmia with amiodarone is significantly associated with improved survival suggests that amiodarone may prevent or delay sudden death in patients with HC and VT.

Nifedipine

Although several studies have demonstrated that verapamil is an effective therapeutic agent for patients with HC, about one-third of patients started on this agent do not find the drug beneficial either because of inability to reduce symptoms or because of adverse drug effects. Betocchi and colleagues[24] from Bethesda, Maryland, examined the hemodynamic effects of sublingual nifedipine in 36 patients with HC: 21 patients were initially given 20 mg and 15 patients were given 10 mg of the drug; 30 minutes after this first dose, 26 patients received 10 mg and 1 patient 20 mg as a second dose. Hemodynamic findings in patients who received different doses of the drug were similar. Peak effects included an increase in heart rate from 79–91 beats/min and a decrease in mean BP from 89–77 mmHg. Cardiac index increased from 2.8–3.3 L/min/m^2; stroke volume index did not change. Peripheral vascular resistance index decreased significantly from 822–610 dynes/sec/cm^{-5}. Overall, LV outflow tract gradient did not change in patients with significant basal gradients, but it increased significantly in those 6 patients in whom peripheral vascular resistance decreased by ≥25%. PA wedge pressure increased significantly in patients with normal basal values and in patients with significant basal gradients. In 10 patients, systolic and diastolic function were studied simultaneously by a nonimaging scintillation probe. No changes in systolic or diastolic function were detected when determinations obtained at the time of the peak nifedipine effect were compared with control values recorded at similar heart rates obtained by atrial pacing. The pattern of change in the pressure-count loops after administration of nifedipine was not consistent; in only 3 of 10 patients was an improvement in the diastolic pressure-volume relation observed. These results indicate that in patients with HC, sublingual nifedipine induces a marked reduction in afterload without any beneficial effect on outflow obstruction and diastolic function. Moreover, in patients with normal PA wedge pressures and/or significant gradients, nifedipine seems to be detrimental because it increases filling pressure, with these changes being exaggerated in patients with more marked decreases in peripheral vascular resistance.

Verapamil

To investigate the association between changes in LV filling and exercise tolerance after verapamil, Bonow and coworkers[25] from Bethesda, Maryland, studied 55 patients with HC by RNA and graded treadmill testing before and after 1–4 weeks of therapy with orally administered verapamil, 320–640 mg/day. The verapamil-induced increase in peak LV filling rate at rest was associated with an increase in exercise tolerance; exercise capacity increased in 34 of 43 patients (79%) manifesting an increase in peak filling rate, but only 1 of 12 patients (8%) was unchanged or decreased peak filling rate. This initial trend persisted in 25 patients studied after 1 year of therapy; 11 of 16 patients (69%) with a persistent increase in peak filling rate had persistent improvement in exercise tolerance relative to pre-verapamil values, compared with only 1 of 9 patients in whom peak filling rate was unchanged or decreased relative to pre-verapamil levels. Verapamil withdrawal after 1–2 years in 24 patients resulted in reduction in peak filling rate and was associated with deterioration in exercise tolerance in 17 patients (71%). Thus, verapamil-induced changes in LV peak filling rate were associated significantly with objective symptomatic improvement. These data support the concept that enhanced LV diastolic filling is an important mechanism contributing to the clinical improvement in many patients with HC during therapy with verapamil.

CARDIAC AMYLOIDOSIS

Cueto-Garcia and colleagues[26] from Rochester, Minnesota, evaluated 132 patients with biopsy-proved systemic amyloidosis to determine the utility of echo in identifying the extent of cardiac involvement. Patients were grouped according to LV wall thickness as follows: Group I had LV mean wall thickness of ≤12 mm; group II had a mean wall thickness >12 mm, but <15 mm; group III had LV mean wall thickness ≥15 mm; and group IV had segmental wall motion abnormalities or LV dilation. Those patients with the greatest LV wall thickness had a higher frequency of associated echo abnormalities, including LA enlargement and granular sparkling appearance on 2-D echo and, more often, reduced systolic global LV function. The presence of CHF clinically was strongly correlated with greater wall thickness and additional echo abnormalities. Survival was negatively influenced both by greater wall thickness and reduced global LV systolic function. For patients in this study, the median survival was 1.1 years. These data indicate that the echo examination can be an important tool in establishing the presence of substantial cardiac infiltration by amyloid and may be useful in estimating prognosis.

ASSOCIATION WITH A CONDITION AFFECTING PRIMARILY A NONCARDIAC STRUCTURE(S)

Myotonic muscular dystrophy

Moorman and associates[27] from Durham, North Carolina, and Hanover, New Hampshire, studied 46 patients with muscular dystrophy in whom the diagnosis was established by demonstration of myotonia by physical examination or electromyography or by the presence of characteristic lenticular opacities by slit-light examination. All had other family members with muscular dystrophy. Although symptomatic cardiac illness in myotonic muscular dystrophy is infrequent, subclinical cardiac involvement is common and was found in 42 of the 46 subjects studied. ECG abnormalities were present in 72% of the 46 patients, LV dysfunction in 70%, MVP in 37%, and 4% died suddenly. These investigators did not find ominous bradyarrhythmias or AV block, evidence of CHF, noninvasive evidence of CAD, or any correlation of type or amount of cardiac involvement with any clinical parameter, such as age, sex, or severity of the systemic dystrophy. The investigators pointed out that the most important problem in the clinical management of myotonic muscular dystrophy is sudden death, and the solution does not appear to be empiric ventricular pacing.

Thalassemia major

Wolfe and associates[28] from Boston, Massachusetts, and Toronto, Canada, examined the efficacy of long-term subcutaneous deferoxamine therapy in the prevention of iron-related cardiac disease in patients with thalassemia major who began treatment after the age of 10 years. Of 36 such patients without preexisting cardiac disease, 19 did not comply with the program of chelation therapy. Over the course of treatment (1977–1983) serum ferritin and aspartate aminotransferase levels decreased in the compliant group, from mean values ($\pm$SD) of 4,765 $\pm$ 2,610–2,950 $\pm$ 1,850 ng/ml and 58 $\pm$ 22–30 $\pm$ 20 IU/L, respectively, but increased in the noncompliant group, from 5,000 $\pm$ 2,316–6,040 $\pm$ 2,550 ng/ml and 57 $\pm$ 20–90 $\pm$ 35 IU/L, respectively. Only 1 patient in the compliant group acquired CAD and died of fulminant CHF. In contrast, 12 noncompliant patients acquired cardiac disease and 7 died. In addition, the mean age of the compliant population (19 $\pm$ 5 years) now approaches the mean age of acquisition of cardiac disease in the noncompliant group (19 $\pm$ 4). These data demonstrate that compliance with treatment with deferoxamine may protect patients from cardiac disease induced by iron overload.

References

1. LEWIS AB, NEUSTEIN HB, TAKAHASHI M, LURIE PR: Findings on endomyocardial biopsy in infants and children with dilated cardiomyopathy. Am J Cardiol 1985 (Jan 1); 55:143–145.

2. DEC GW, PALACIOS IF, FALLON JT, ARETZ HT, MILLS J, LEE DCS, JOHNSON RA: Active myocarditis in the spectrum of acute dilated cardiomyopathies: clinical features, histologic correlates, and clinical outcome. N Engl J Med 1985 (Apr 4); 312:885–890.

3. FIGULLA HR, RAHLF G, NIEGER M, LUIG H, KREUZER H: Spontaneous hemodynamic improvement or stabilization and associated biopsy findings in patients with congestive cardiomyopathy. Circulation 1985 (June); 71:1095–1104.

4. WILLIAMS DG, OLSEN EGJ: Prevalence of overt dilated cardiomyopathy in two regions of England. Br Heart J 1985 (Aug); 54:153–155.

5. MICHELS VV, DRISCOLL DJ, MILLER FA: Familial aggregation of idiopathic dilated cardiomyopathy. Am J Cardiol 1985 (Apr 15); 55:1232–1233.

6. LITTLE WC, BARR WK, CRAWFORD MH: Altered effect of the Valsalva maneuver on left ventricular volume in patients with cardiomyopathy. Circulation 1985 (Feb); 71:227–233.

7. COSTANZO-NORDIN MR, O'CONNELL JB, ENGELMEIER RS, MORAN JF, SCANLON PJ: Dilated cardiomyopathy: functional status, hemodynamics, arrhythmias, and prognosis. Cathet Cardiovasc Diagn 1985; 11:445–453.

8. MEINERTZ T, TREESE N, KASPER W, GEIBEL A, HOFMANN T, ZEHENDER M, BOHN D, POP T, JUST H: Determinants of prognosis in idiopathic dilated cardiomyopathy as determined by programmed electrical stimulation. Am J Cardiol 1985 (Aug 1); 56:337–341.

9. RIBNER HS, PLUCINSKI DA, HSIEH AM, BRESNAHAN D, MOLTENI A, ASKENAZI J, LESCH M: Acute effects of digoxin on total systemic vascular resistance in congestive heart failure due to dilated cardiomyopathy: a hemodynamic-hormonal study. Am J Cardiol 1985 (Nov 15); 56:896–904.

10. SMUCKER ML, SANFORD CF, LIPSCOMB KM: Effects of hydralazine on pressure-volume and stress-volume relations in congestive heart failure secondary to idiopathic dilated cardiomyopathy. Am J Cardiol 1985 (Oct 1); 56:690–695.

11. ANDERSON JL, LUTZ JR, GILBERT EM, SORENSEN SG, YANOWITZ G, MENLOVE RL, BARTHOLOMEW M: A randomized trial of low-dose beta blockade therapy for idiopathic dilated cardiomyopathy. Am J Cardiol 1985 (Feb 1); 55:471–475.

12. ENGELMEIER RS, O'CONNELL JB, WALSH R, RAD N, SCANLON PJ, GUNNAR RM: Improvement in symptoms and exercise tolerance by metoprolol in patients with dilated cardiomyopathy: a double-blind, randomized, placebo-controlled trial. Circulation 1985 (Sept); 72:536–546.

13. MILLER AB, CONETTA DA, BASS TA: Sublingual nifedipine: acute effects in severe chronic congestive heart failure secondary to idiopathic dilated cardiomyopathy. Am J Cardiol 1985 (May 1); 55:1359–1362.

14. CANNON RO, ROSING DR, MARON BJ, LEON MB, BONOW RO, WATSON RM, EPSTEIN SE: Myocardial ischemia in patients with hypertrophic cardiomyopathy: contribution of inadequate vasodilator reserve and elevated left ventricular filling pressures. Circulation 1985 (Feb); 71:234–243.

15. MARON BJ, GOTTDIENER JS, ARCE J, ROSING DR, WESLEY YE, EPSTEIN SE: Dynamic subaortic obstruction in hypertrophic cardiomyopathy: analysis by pulsed Doppler echocardiography. J Am Coll Cardiol 1985 (July); 6:1–15.

16. GARDIN JM, DABESTANI A, GLASGOW GA, BUTMAN S, BURN CS, HENRY WL: Echocardiographic and Doppler flow observations in obstructed and nonobstructed hypertrophic cardiomyopathy. Am J Cardiol 1985 (Oct 1); 56:614–621.

17. SPIRITO P, MARON BJ, CHIARELLA F, BELLOTTI P, TRAMARIN R, POZZOLI M, VECCHIO C: Diastolic abnormalities in patients with hypertrophic cardiomyopathy: relation to magnitude of left ventricular hypertrophy. Circulation 1985 (Aug); 72:310–316.

18. HIGGINS CB, BYRD BF, STARK D, McNAMARA M, LANZER P, LIPTON MJ, SCHILLER NB, BOTVINICK E, CHATTERJEE K: Magnetic resonance imaging in hypertrophic cardiomyopathy. Am J Cardiol 1985 (Apr 1); 55:1121–1126.

19. SIEGEL RJ, CRILEY JM: Comparison of ventricular emptying with and without a pressure gradient in patients with hypertrophic cardiomyopathy. Br Heart J 1985 (Mar); 53:283–291.

20. THOMPSON RC, LIBERTHSON RR, LOWENSTEIN E: Perioperative anesthetic risk of noncardiac surgery in hypertrophic obstructive cardiomyopathy. JAMA 1985 (Nov 1); 254:2419–2421.

21. KEREN G, BELHASSEN B, SHEREZ J, MILLER HI, MEGIDISH R, BERENFELD D, LANIADO S: Apical hypertrophic cardiomyopathy: evaluation by noninvasive and invasive techniques in 23 patients. Circulation 1985 (Jan); **71:45–56.**

22. COKKINOS DV, KRAJCER Z, LEACHMAN RD: Coronary artery disease in hypertrophic cardiomyopathy. Am J Cardiol 1985 (May 1); **55:1437–1438.**

23. MCKENNA WJ, OAKLEY CM, KRIKLER DM, GOODWIN JF: Improved survival with amiodarone in patients with hypertrophic cardiomyopathy and ventricular tachycardia. Br Heart J 1985 (Apr); **53:412–416.**

24. BETOCCHI S, CANNON RO III, WATSON RM, BONOW RO, OSTROW HG, EPSTEIN SE, ROSING DR: Effects of sublingual nifedipine on hemodynamics and systolic and diastolic function in patients with hypertrophic cardiomyopathy. Circulation 1985 (Nov); **72:1001–1007.**

25. BONOW RO, DILSIZIAN V, ROSING DR, MARON BJ, BACHARACH SL, GREEN MV: Verapamil-induced improvement in left ventricular diastolic filling and increased exercise tolerance in patients with hypertrophic cardiomyopathy: short- and long-term effects. Circulation 1985 (Oct); **72:853–864.**

26. CUETO-GARCIA L, REEDER GS, KYLE RA, WOOD DL, SEWARD JB, NAESSENS J, OFFORD KP, GREIPP PR, EDWARDS WD, TAJIK AJ: Echocardiographic findings in systemic amyloidosis: spectrum of cardiac involvement and relation to survival. J Am Coll Cardiol 1985 (Oct); **6:737–743.**

27. MOORMAN JR, COLEMAN RE, PACKER DL, KISSLO JA, BELL J, HETTLEMAN BD, STAJICH J, ROSES AD: Cardiac involvement in myotonic muscular dystrophy. Medicine (Baltimore) 1985; **64:371–387.**

28. WOLFE L, OLIVIERI N, SALLAN D, COLAN S, ROSE V, PROPPER R, FREEDMAN MH, NATHAN DG: Prevention of cardiac disease by subcutaneous deferoxamine in patients with thalassemia major. N Engl J Med 1985 (June 20); **312:1600–1603.**

Congenital Heart Disease

Transatrial velocity by Doppler echo

Marx and associates[1] from Tucson, Arizona, studied RA velocities measured perpendicular to the atrial septum by Doppler echo in 17 patients with ASD. For control subjects, the mean RA velocity was 15 ± 4 cm/s and that for ASD patients was 41 ± 11 cm/s. Mean transatrial septal velocity in ASD patients correlated with both catheterization and simultaneous Doppler Qp:Qs ratios. The highest RA velocity in control subjects was 21 cm/s and the lowest velocity in the ASD patients was 22 seconds in a patient with a small shunt. These investigators present a useful technique that can confirm the presence of a left-to-right atrial shunt. However, several notes of caution are provided. Firstly, superior vena caval velocities are in the range of the ASD patients' RA velocities and should be carefully differentiated. This can be a particular problem in patients with sinus venosus ASD. Secondly, patients with restrictive ASD may have high velocities. With these precautions, however, the technique can be useful in documenting the presence of atrial shunting.

Spontaneous closure in infancy

The incidence and timing of spontaneous closure of isolated secundum ASD are unknown. Thus, in a study by Ghisla and associates[2] from Cincinnati, Ohio, 29 consecutive infants <12 months of age with clinical evidence of significant left-to-right shunting through an ASD were evaluated by M-mode and 2-D echo. All had RV hypertrophy by ECG. Spontaneous closure of the defect in 4 infants was suggested by normalization of clinical examination and ECG and was documented by 2D and M-mode echo at 15–31 months of age. All remaining patients, who had suitable 2D echo and in whom the defects did not spontaneously close, had enlarged RV and RA areas. LA areas were normal in the 4 whose defects closed spontaneously, and were large in all but 3 whose defects did not close. The mean diameter of the defect was similar for all patients. The 14% incidence reported here may underestimate the true incidence of spontaneous closure, since 7 patients had surgical closure, all before 30 months of age, the oldest age at which spontaneous closure was documented. An atrial septal flap, found in all 4 patients who closed spontaneously but only in 4 of the 16 patients who did not close spontaneously, may contribute to spontaneous closure. Since spontaneous closure may occur up to 30 months, it seems clear that surgical closure should not be performed before that age unless medical management has failed to control symptoms.

ATRIOVENTRICULAR CANAL DEFECT

Effect of Down's syndrome on management

Bull and associates[3] from London, UK, explored the proposition that children with Down's syndrome should be treated differently from normal children with complete AV canal defect by reviewing the outcome of these anomalies after surgical or medical treatment. Since 1970, 75 patients with the Down's syndrome and complete AV canal defect were seen at their hospital. When first seen, 25 patients had inoperable pulmonary vascular disease and the remaining 50 were considered suitable for surgery because pulmonary vascular resistance was <8 U (mmHg/L/m^2 body surface area) or because they were aged <2 years. Of the 50 patients considered suitable for operation, 8 had undergone PA banding or primary correction with partition of the common AV valve and closure of the ASD and VSD. The remaining 67 children had no operation. All 67 patients who had no operation were followed and an actuarial survival curve was created (Figs. 7-1 and 7-2). Of the 67 unoperated children, 8 died in infancy from consequences of excessive pulmonary blood flow.

Left AV valve replacement

Narrowing of the LV outflow tract is an intrinsic characteristic of patients with AV canal defects. Prosthetic replacement of a severely incompetent left AV valve may result in the creation of subaortic stenosis. This is particularly true when an oversized prosthetic valve is used. McGrath and associates[4] from Birmingham, Alabama, developed a technical modification to prevent this complication. They employed a crescent-shaped Dacron cuff attaching it to the superior aspect of the anulus in order to lengthen the area of aortic-mitral continuity. The valve prosthesis was then sutured to this cuff superiorly and to remnants of the valve tissue inferiorly, tilting the prosthesis into the left atrium and away from the LV outflow tract. This method was used in 5 patients aged 8 months to 19 years, 3 with the complete form and 2 with the partial form of the defect. Each survived operation, and at follow-up from 35–348 days (mean, 152) each patient was in functional class I and without episodes of thromboembolism, prosthetic valve endocarditis, or re-operation.

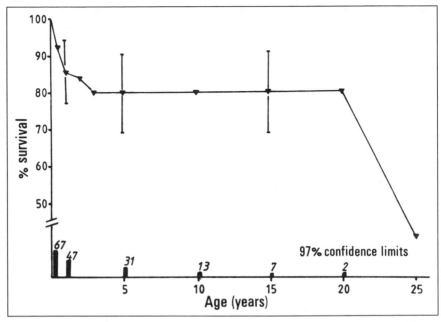

Fig. 7-1. Actuarial survival of 67 patients with Down's syndrome and complete AV canal defect managed medically. Reproduced with permission from Bull et al.[3]

VENTRICULAR SEPTAL DEFECT

Standardized echo nomenclature

In a superb article, Hagler and associates[5] from Rochester, Minnesota, reviewed certain aspects of the anatomy of the ventricular septum and classified VSD on the basis of position and the presence or absence of septal malalignment. The investigators presented a standardized nomenclature for the various types of VSD and also the usefulness of this classification for 2-D echo (Figs. 7-3–7-7).

Localization by superimposed Doppler and cross-sectional echo

Ortiz and associates[6] from London, UK, used superimposed color Doppler on cross-sectional echo images in 23 patients with unoperated VSD, 8 after closure of VSD, and 12 children with normal hearts. A color-coded blood flow jet entering the right ventricle during systole was identified in all 23 unoperated patients, in 11 of whom the defect was too small to be visualized by conventional echo. The Doppler technique precisely located 19 perimembraneous and 5 trabecular defects. Five postoperative patients without clinical evidence of significant shunt had pansystolic murmurs and in all 5 shunt flow was demonstrated, whereas in only 3 of 5 was the defect visualized by conventional echo. Three postoperative patients with no murmur showed no residual shunt on color imaging. Thus, color Doppler studies are spectacular and may well prove to be useful clinically in a number of different situations. These investigators demonstrate their precision in diagnosing

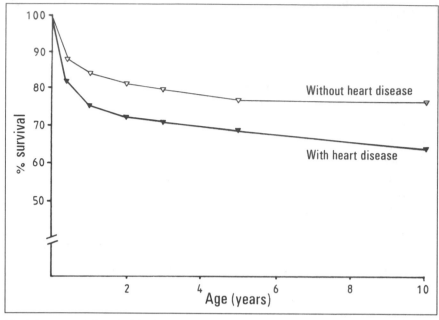

Fig. 7-2.   Actuarial survival for first 10 years of life of children with Down's syndrome with and without congenital heart disease. Reproduced with permission from Bull et al.[3]

small VSD. It is seldom a problem, however, to diagnose a small VSD for a clinician with experience and expertise in congenital heart disease. Lesions that occasionally are confusing, such as MR or subaortic stenosis, can be differentiated by standard echo Doppler study. Color Doppler may have important clinical uses, but diagnosing small VSD is probably not one of them.

Fig. 7-3.   Normal anatomy of ventricular septum. APM = anterior papillary muscle (tricuspid); AVS = AV septum; CS = coronary sinus; IL = inferior limb (of SB); IS = infundibular septum; L = left cusp; MB = moderator band; MPM = mitral papillary muscle (tricuspid); MS = membraneous septum; P = posterior cusp; PB = parietal band; PT = pulmonary trunk; R = right cusp; SB = septal band; SL = superior limb (of SB). Reproduced with permission from Hagler et al.[5]

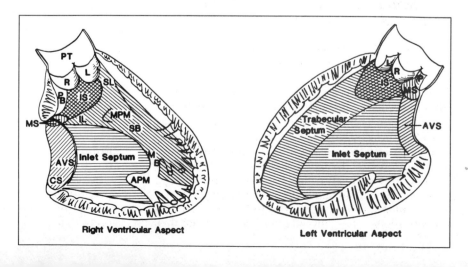

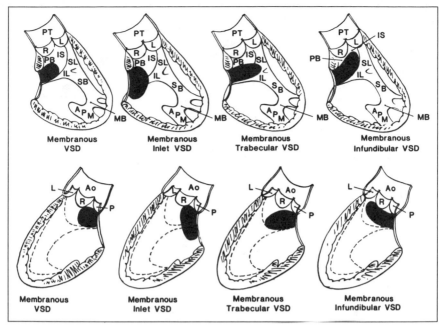

Fig. 7-4. Membraneous VSDs, viewed from the RV aspect (upper panel) and LV aspect (lower panel). Ao = aorta; for other abbreviations, see Figure 7-3. Reproduced with permission from Hagler et al.[5]

Isolated in adults

Otterstad and coworkers[7] from Oslo, Norway, restudied 52 patients with isolated congenital VSD an average of 16 years after they had been studied for the first time at age ≥10 years. Of the 52 patients, 17 had been operated on an average of 19 years earlier (group 1), and 35 with a smaller VSD were not operated on (group 2). Although more pronounced findings were made in group 1, a similar pattern was observed in group 2: 1) In most subjects in both groups a subnormal working capacity was observed; 2) a subnormal LV fractional shortening and circumferential shortening velocity were noted in a higher proportion at echo; 3) a number of hemodynamic aberrations were observed in a high proportion of patients during exercise but not at rest. Thus, a subnormal increase in LV and RV cardiac output was found in addition to abnormal increase in RV and LV end-diastolic, PA, and PA wedge pressures. In group 1, elevated PA pressures before operation and small residual VSD were associated with a poor hemodynamic outcome. In neither group could significant correlations be observed between hemodynamic aberrations, shunt size, or age. Among patients who underwent surgery, the earlier surgical trauma might have contributed to the functional aberrations, but in group 2 the only likely explanation for the findings seems to be the VSD itself.

With aneurysm of the membranous ventricular septum

Beerman and associates[8] from Pittsburgh, Pennsylvania, retrospectively studied the clinical and catheterization data from 87 patients with VSD and aneurysm of the membranous septum. Initial evaluation was made at a

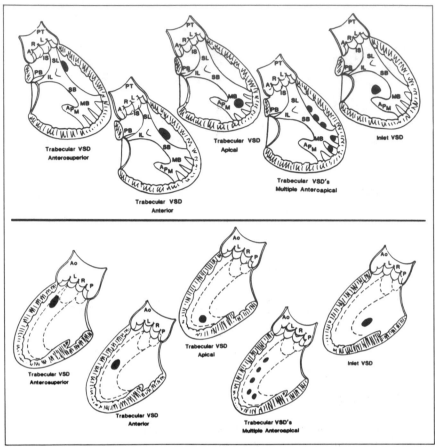

Fig. 7-5. Muscular VSDs involving the trabecular and inlet septa, viewed from the RV aspect (upper panel) and LV aspect (lower panel). A = anterior cusp; Ao = aorta; for other abbreviations, see Figure 7-3. Reproduced with permission from Hagler et al.[5]

Fig. 7-6. AV canal VSD (a basal inlet defect). A = anterior cusp; Ao = aorta; for other abbreviations, see Figure 7-3. Reproduced with permission from Hagler et al.[5]

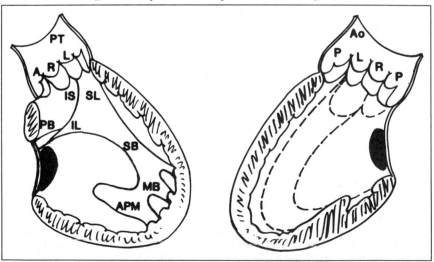

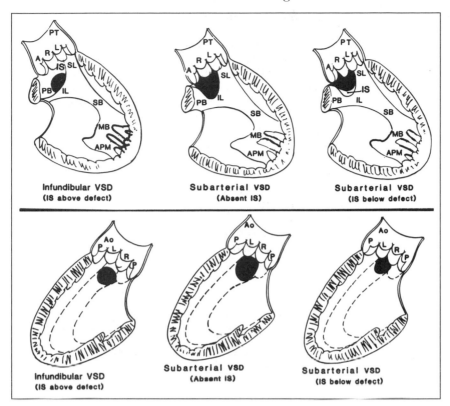

Fig. 7-7.   Infundibular VSD, viewed from RV aspect (upper panel) and LV aspect (lower panel). Such defects may be muscular (left) or subarterial (center and right). A = anterior cusp; Ao = aorta; for other abbreviations, see Figure 7 3. Reproduced with permission from Hagler et al.[5]

median age of 0.3 years (range, 0.1–11), with the final evaluation at a median age of 10 years (1.5–20) and a median duration of follow-up of 8.6 years (range, 1.2–18.8). Approximately 75% had a small or no left to right shunt via the "VSD" at last evaluation. There was no significant change in defect size in 55% and 45% showed improvement. Only 4 patients had spontaneous VSD closure. Of the 49 patients who presented with a large left to right shunt with or without CHF, 47% had persistence of a shunt large enough to warrant surgery. When spontaneous improvement occurred, it did so by 6 years of age. These investigators present an interesting study regarding the natural history of perimembranous VSD associated with what has been called aneurysm of the ventricular septum. As they point out, the anatomic substrate for the tissue around the VSD is usually derived from the tricuspid valve, either accessory tags or adherence of leaflets. The study demonstrates that the rate of diminution in size and spontaneous closure of this type of defect is no greater than that reported for VSD in general. In addition, when spontaneous improvement occurred in patients with a large shunt, it did so by 6 years of age. Thus, these patients do not, as previously suspected, have a high rate of spontaneous closure, although they do in general have a relatively small shunt when seen at any age. This study does alert the clinician to careful follow-up of patients with VSD and septal "aneurysm" who have a large or moderate shunt, since spontaneous closure seems less likely to occur than has previously been suspected.

Pulmonary arterial development in infants

Juaneda and associates[9] from London, UK, and Leiden, The Netherlands, used quantitative morphometric techniques to study the pulmonary vascular bed in 13 patients with large VSD, 12 of whom died between age 2 days and 9 months. All patients had a large VSD that was approximately equal to aortic root size. In patients aged 2 months to 4 years, there was an increase in arterial medial thickness and extension of muscle, whereas the intra-acinar arteries were larger than normal in size and normal in number. Intimal thickening was seen in 1 case at 4.5 months, but it caused significant obstruction only in 1 child aged 4 years. These data emphasize the rapidity with which structural adaptation to extrauterine life can occur in a patient with large communications between the left and right sides of the heart with excessive pulmonary blood flow. A rapid increase in muscularity can be seen by 2 months of age. The investigators further speculate that in patients with complex conditions in which the Fontan repair may eventually be performed, banding of the PA when required should be carried out by 2 months of age to prevent the development of increased pulmonary vascular resistance.

PULMONIC VALVE STENOSIS

Lange and associates[10] from Kiel, West Germany, studied the natural history of RV function and pressure gradient in 5 infants and 13 children at 2 cardiac catheterizations performed at intervals of 2–12 years. There was no change in the pressure gradient between RV cavity and PA when the initial gradient was <50 mmHg, but a mean increase of 8.6 mmHg/year occurred in those with a higher initial gradient. End-diastolic and stroke volume were normal, and end-systolic volume was smaller and EF above normal in these children. There were no patients with impaired ventricular function. Data are compatible with past studies indicating that relatively mild pulmonic stenosis stays mild, whereas patients with moderate gradients in infancy or early childhood can show a marked increase in gradient. As shown previously by other investigators, hypertrophy is in general adequate to produce a normal or increased EF and instances of RV dysfunction in children are rare.

PULMONIC VALVE ATRESIA

Trowitzsch and associates[11] from Boston, Massachusetts, studied RV size and function by echo in 15 infants, age 1–30 days with severe RV outflow tract obstruction. All patients with a normalized RV end-diastolic volume <5 ml/m^2 and a normalized tricuspid anulus <1 cm/m$^{2/3}$ required a shunt operation. Only 1 patient with a volume >6 ml/m^2 and a normalized tricuspid anulus >1.4 cm/m$^{2/3}$ required more than relief of RV outflow obstruction. One patient with a volume >6 ml/m^2 had a anulus diameter <1.4 cm/m$^{2/3}$, and 1 patient with an anulus diameter >1.4 cm/m$^{2/3}$ had a volume <6 ml/m^2; both required shunt procedures. Wall thickness, area change, and EF measurements were not significantly correlated with RV volume or postoperative outcome. Data are presented regarding the ability to use tricuspid anulus and RV area and volume measurements to predict whether or not a small RV will be able to pump a normal cardiac output after relief of outflow tract obstruction. These data should be useful in initial assessment of this condition. Further data on the usefulness of this methodology to follow these patients in terms of need for further RV outflow tract reconstruction and the results of such procedures would be a welcome addition to this important clinical problem.

Patients with pulmonic atresia and intact ventricular septum have been classified according to their RV morphology as type 1 when inlet, trabecular, and infundibular portions are present, type 2, when the trabecular portion is absent, and type 3 when both the trabecular and infundibular portions are absent. Cobanoglu and colleagues[12] from Portland, Oregon, reviewed their experience with 35 patients, 32 <7 days of age, who underwent operation between 1964 and 1983. Two patients with type 2 and 8 with type 3 received a shunt alone with 6 hospital and 3 late survivors. Of the remaining 25, 17 had type 1 and 8, type 2, and 18 underwent valvotomy alone with 6 hospital deaths and 1 late death; 7 underwent valvotomy plus shunt with 2 hospital deaths and 3 late deaths. Since the availability of prostaglandin E_1 in 1977, no patient with a type 1 ventricle has died as a result of operation. Thus, overall hospital mortality since 1977 was 16% as opposed to 56% for those operated on earlier. Overall hospital mortality was 34%, and in patients >3 kg, it was 18% compared with 62% for those <3 kg. Since 1977, there were no deaths among 14 patients >3 kg at operation. The probability of reoperation for operative survivors was 100% by the age of 6 years. A synthetic patch to enlarge the RV outflow tract was used successfully in 9 of 10 patients with type 1 ventricles who received valvotomy alone and in 1 type 2 ventricle initially treated by valvotomy and shunt. Each of 2 patients with a type 3 ventricle, initially treated by shunt alone, died during late RV reconstruction. One patient with type 2 RV, initially treated by shunt alone, survived valvotomy at 1 year, but has had failure of RV growth. There was no correlation between RV type and angiographic measurement of tricuspid valve anulus diameter. It was concluded that primary valvotomy without shunt is the operation of choice for patients with pulmonic atresia and intact ventricular septum and type 1 ventricle. Concomitant shunt may be required for some patients with type 1 and most patients with type 2, selected preoperatively by angiography or after valvotomy by clinical necessity. Delayed RV reconstruction is essentially necessary in all because of persistent or recurrent RV outflow obstruction and elevated RV pressure. Delayed RV reconstruction after shunt alone is not an acceptable approach when an outflow tract is present.

Premature obstruction and degeneration of porcine valved-Dacron extracardiac conduits have led some surgical groups to abandon their use in favor of nonvalved tubes. Kay and colleagues[13] from London, UK, reported their experience with 97 patients with pulmonic atresia who underwent RV outflow tract reconstruction using a homograft conduit. In 82, the length of the conduit was increased by suturing the homograft to a tube fashioned from autologous pericardium (25 patients) or a preclotted Dacron tube (57 patients). There were 46 hospital deaths (47%), which were significantly related to persistent pulmonary hypertension and thoracotomy for ligation of bronchial collaterals. Operations were performed between 1966 and 1984, and the actuarial survival at 10 years was 37 ± 7%. There were 11 late deaths during the follow-up period, 6 sudden, 2 from bacterial endocarditis, and 1 each from reoperation, pulmonary infarction, and childbirth. There was no evidence of conduit obstruction at necropsy. Sixteen patients had postoperative cardiac catheterization between 3 and 10 years (mean, 6), demonstrating a mean transconduit gradient of 24 ± 15 mmHg. There were 3 who had gradients >50 mmHg and at reoperation the main obstruction was related to a fibrinous peel within the Dacron tube. Two patients had severe calcium in the wall of the homograft, but in only 1 of the 3 was there calcium in the valve cusps. The actuarial incidence of conduit obstruction requiring replacement was 13 ± 8% at 10 years. Thirty-eight (95%) of the 40 survivors are asymptomatic, leading normal lives, and 2 have had normal pregnancies. The investigators believe the fresh, antibiotic-sterilized aortic homograft is the conduit of choice for RV outflow tract reconstruction. The valve leaflets are more resistant to calcification than the porcine valve, and obstruction has been related to the use of Dacron tubular extensions that have been abandoned in favor of autologous pericardial tubes.

Liao and associates[14] from Rochester, Minnesota, studied the heart and lung specimens in 31 cases of pulmonic atresia and VSD at necropsy. Three types of natural arterial blood supply were identified: PDA (12 of 31), major systemic collateral arteries (20 of 31), and a few small pleural arterial plexus (17 of 31). PDA and major collateral arteries did not coexist in the same lung. Confluent central pulmonary arteries were present in 22 of 31 involving 7 of 12 patients with PDA, 20 of 31 with major collateral arteries, and 1 of 31 with an aorticopulmonary window. A patent or atretic pulmonary trunk was identified in 24 of 31. A lung or lungs that connected to a ductus or ligamentum had a complete and unifocal intrapulmonary arterial distribution without arborization abnormalities. Major collateral blood supply was frequently multifocal and associated with arborization abnormalities. The size of the central pulmonary arteries was not related to the type of blood source but to the amount of blood flow reaching the vessels. These data confirm previous demonstrations of the complex nature of pulmonary blood supply in many of these patients and the need for complete and careful angiographic demonstration of the multiple sources of blood supply before surgery is contemplated.

TETRALOGY OF FALLOT

With absent pulmonic valve

McCaughan and coworkers[15] from Rochester, Minnesota, reviewed their experience between 1957 and 1983 with 35 patients with TF and absent pulmonic valve. Group A consisted of 21 patients who had absent or minimal symptoms and were operated on between 3 and 42 years of age (mean, 10 ± 9). Group B consisted of 14 markedly symptomatic patients who were operated on between 1 day and 9 years (mean, 4 years) of age. Operation consisted of closure of the VSD and relief of infundibular and anular pulmonic stenosis. Pulmonic cuspal remnants were resected. In 5 patients (2 in group A, 3 in group B) transanular patch enlargement of the outflow tract was performed; in 9 patients (7 in group A and 2 in group B), a porcine heterograft valve was orthotopically inserted in the RV outflow tract and main PA. In 5 patients, aneurysmally dilated pulmonary arteries were plicated or partially resected (4 in group A and 1 in group B). The mean postrepair RV-PA gradient was 23 ± 13 mmHg. There was 1 hospital death (4.8%) among 21 group A patients from an early postoperative neurologic deficit. In this group, 1 late death occurred 3.5 years postoperatively in the 1 patient who developed surgically induced complete heart block. Each of the remaining 19 late group A survivors were well without physical limitation; 1 required re-replacement of the pulmonic heterograft valve because of degeneration 8 years after repair. Of the 14 group B patients, 5 (36%) died within 30 days of operation. Nine survivors were followed between 1 and 22 years (median, 12) and 4 additional deaths occurred during this period. One of these was related to the complication of complete heart block, and 3 additional deaths were associated with persistent respiratory difficulties. It was concluded that pulmonic valve replacement is tolerated well in minimally symptomatic patients, and for those with severe symptoms, results may be improved if repair includes establishment of pulmonic valvular competence and reduction of size and length of aneurysmally dilated branch pulmonary arteries. The latter was performed in 4 group A patients and 1 group B patient. The best management of the stenotic and incompetent pulmonary anulus in this group of patients, however, remains controversial. I (ADP) prefer orthotopic insertion of a cryopreserved homograft valve in most patients at the time of complete repair. Management of the seriously ill neonate with this malformation is difficult and experience with various management programs has been associated with high mortality and morbidity. The suggestion of the investigators that complete repair, including orthotopic pulmonic valve replacement and simultaneous reduction of size and length of aneurysmally dilated pulmonary arteries, is the procedure of choice seems sound, but awaits confirmation by additional surgical experience.

Operative repair

Zhao and associates[16] from Stanford, California, reported the early and late results of repair of TT in 309 patients operated on between 1960 and 1982. Early (within 30 days of operation) mortality was $5 \pm 1\%$ and in 9 of the 15 patients it was from low cardiac output. Multivariate analysis showed young age, long cardiopulmonary bypass time, and extent of RV outflow patch (transanular > none > separate RV or PA patch) as independent determinants of early death. Forty-two (14%) had transient third degree AV block with return of normal sinus rhythm within 7 days. Two had permanent complete heart block and required permanent pacemakers, and 119 (39%) had transient SVT that required treatment in the hospital. Actuarial survival at 16 years was 85% and older age at operation, absence of hypoxic spells, and need for reoperation were independently related to the probability of late death; 97% of survivors were in New York Heart Association functional class I; $15 \pm 3\%$ required late reoperation by 13 years postoperatively, and multivariate analysis showed the extent of RV outflow tract patch, longer ischemic arrest time, previous palliative shunt, and primary suture closure of VSD as incremental risk factors. It was concluded that repair of TF is a durable procedure for upward of 20 years and that high risk subsets of patients can be identified who have increased risk of reoperation and early and late death. Additional information is needed to define the electrophysiologic status of these patients and to elucidate mechanisms of late postoperative arrhythmias.

The trend toward earlier repair of TF is based on the risk of 2 operative procedures, the potential complications of a right to left intracardiac shunt, and the possibility that earlier repair will result in better ventricular function. Earlier repair, however, is associated with a higher incidence of transanular patching, which is >50% in most series for infants <12 months. In an effort to minimize early mortality and the need for transanular patching, Rittenhouse and colleagues[17] from Seattle, Washington, based the decision to perform a shunt rather than primary repair on the angiographic appearance of the pulmonary anulus and distal tree and clinical judgment irrespective of the patient's age or size: 124 patients underwent surgical treatment between 1976 and 1983 with 1 (0.8%) hospital death in an infant during a repeat shunting procedure. Primary repair was performed in 61, shunt and later repair in 30, and an initial shunt alone in 33. The mean ratio of pulmonary anulus to descending thoracic aorta increased from 0.8 ± 0.25 before the shunt to 1.22 ± 0.26 before the repair, which was similar to 1.23 ± 0.25 in the primary repair group. A transanular patch was necessary in only 6 (6.6%) of 91 patients, 1 of 30 having repair after a shunt, and in 5 of 61 undergoing initial primary repair. Postrepair RV/LV pressure ratio averaged 0.50 ± 0.11 in the shunt plus repair group and 0.43 ± 0.12 in the primary repair group. The investigators confirmed that a small pulmonary anulus can enlarge after an initial shunting procedure and demonstrated that selective staged management of patients with TF can result in minimal hospital mortality and frequent avoidance of a transanular patch. This is a superb surgical series, soundly analyzed, and provocative. Since significant data are accumulating to indicate that transanular patching will ultimately result in RV dilation and failure and the need for orthotopic pulmonary valve replacement, preservation of the native pulmonic valve during repair of TF is therefore an important surgical goal. Accurate measurement of the pulmonic valve anulus by angiography and intraoperatively can minimize the need for transanular patching. Whether or not this should be the basis for primary repair or a 2-stage management program as practiced by these investigators requires integration of many factors and awaits collection of more information regarding the late results after repair of TF.

Abdulali and colleagues[18] from Leeds, UK, reported their experience with a bovine pericardial monocusp patch used for RV outflow tract reconstruction in 21 patients, 17 during repair of TF, 2 with double-outlet right ventricle and 2 with other defects. There were 2 early postoperative deaths and 1 late death unrelated to monoscusp patch function. Survivors were followed between 29 and 141 months (mean, 113) and all were asymptomatic. Eleven patients were reinvestigated with sequential postoperative hemodynamic and angiographic studies at mean periods of 16, 48, and 100 months. The mean peak systolic RV-PA pressure gradient was 13 ± 2 mmHg at 16 months and without significant change at intervals up to 124 months postoperatively. In each of the 11, the monocusp valve was visualized by angiography and was freely mobile. The degree of estimated pulmonic regurgitation by angiography was mild in 9 and moderate in 2. Eleven (61%) of the 18 survivors had a short diastolic murmur of pulmonic regurgitation. There was no evidence of primary tissue failure, tissue ingrowth, or calcification. The investigators believe that bovine pericardium induces less host reaction than various synthetic materials and that this contributes significantly to the maintenance of long-term pliability in the monocusp patches. They believe that this type of monocusp patch effectively reduces or abolishes pulmonic regurgitation when a transanular patch is required.

Bove and colleagues[19] from Syracuse, New York, studied RV function by radionuclide ventriculography and M-mode echo before and after pulmonic valve replacement in 11 patients to treat residual pulmonic regurgitation in 8 or stenosis in 3. All but 1 had initial repair of TF, associated with absent pulmonic valve in 2, and the remaining patient had initial repair of VSD after previous PA banding. Three patients had stenotic extracardiac RV-PA conduits and the remaining 8 had pulmonic regurgitation after the placement of a transanular patch in 6, pulmonic valvotomy in 2, and the use of a nonvalved extracardiac conduit in 1. Reoperation was performed between 1 and 12 years postoperatively (mean, 8). Indications for pulmonic valve replacement were conduit stenosis with a gradient >75 mmHg in 3, symptoms in 2, progressive cardiomegaly in 3 and new onset of tricuspid regurgitation in 3. Before pulmonic valve replacement, RVEF was 0.29 ± 0.12 and increased to 0.35 ± 0.10 (mean, 11 ± 2 months) after operation. RVEF increased >0.05 in 7 patients and was unchanged in 4. LVEF before operation was 0.55 ± 0.12 and remained unchanged postoperatively. M-mode echo demonstrated significant reduction in RV dilation and RV/LV end-diastolic dimension decreased from 1.03 ± 0.30–0.73 ± 0.13 after operation. Subjective improvement in exercise tolerance was noted in each of the 7 patients who showed a postoperative increase in RVEF. Of the remaining 4, 2 had no improvement, 1 was symptomatically improved, and 1 was too young for evaluation. The investigators demonstrated objective improvement in RV function after pulmonic valve replacement in most patients. They indicated that serial measurement of RVEF with RNA techniques may allow early detection of patients with worsening function before the onset of symptoms, and this may warrant earlier pulmonic valve replacement to preserve RV function.

Electrophysiologic findings after operative repair

Deanfield and associates[20] from London, UK, studied 22 patients 5 to 24 years after repair of TF. Electrophysiologic studies were performed without the use of provocative tests. Local RV electrograms were fractionated or delayed in 55% at ≥1 RV site, reflecting disordered depolarization, but LV recordings were normal in all. Ventricular arrhythmia out of hospital was more common and more severe in patients with depolarization abnormalities than in those with normal findings. In contrast, there was no association between ventricular arrhythmia and conduction disturbances. Abnormalities of RV repolarization consisting of low frequency signals after the T wave were observed in 17 patients but were not associated with arrhythmia.

COMPLETE TRANSPOSITION OF THE GREAT ARTERIES

Tricuspid valve abnormalities

Deal and associates[21] from Boston, Massachusetts, used subziphoid echo to examine tricuspid valve morphology in 39 infants aged ≤2 years who had TGA and VSD. Age-matched control groups were 21 patients with simple TGA, 30 patients with VSD and normal great arteries, and 15 normal subjects. Valve abnormalities consisting of chordal attachments to the infundibular septum or ventricular septal crest, straddling, overriding, or some combination of these were identified in 25 of 39 (64%) of patients with TGA and VSD. No patients with simple TGA were abnormal and only 6 of 30 (20%) patients with isolated VSD had similar abnormalities. Intra-atrial baffle repair was performed in 27 of 39 patients with TGA and VSD at a median age of 3.5 months and in 19 of 21 patients with simple TGA at a median age of 4 months. After repair, TR was present in 9 of 17 patients with TGA and VSD and 0 of 8 simple TGA patients who underwent angiography. This study provides echo demonstration of anomalous attachment of the tricuspid valve in approximately two-thirds of all patients with TGA and VSD, a frequency that is considerably higher than that previously reported. The 2-D analysis was confirmed by surgery or autopsy in most patients, illustrating that echo was relatively precise in defining subtle details of valve attachments. The high morbidity and mortality for intra-atrial baffle in patients with TGA and VSD may well be partially due to abnormalities of the tricuspid valve. These can either cause major difficulties in proper VSD closure or may result in damage to the tricuspid valve apparatus during repair, and postoperative TR then can contribute to poor results.

Ventricular function after corrective operations

Okuda and associates[22] from Tokyo, Japan, studied RV and LV volume characteristics in patients with TGA after Senning and Jatene procedures; 15 patients had Senning repair and were studied from 25 days to 2 years after repair; 9 patients had the Jatene operation and were studied from 28–64 days after repair. RV end-diastolic volume was 181 ± 74% of normal and RVEF, 0.48 ± 0.09 in 15 patients with Senning repair. Nine patients with Jatene repair, LV end-diastolic pressure was 152 ± 27% of normal and LVEF was 0.61 ± 0.09. Three patients had LV wall hypokinesia after the Jatene repair with AR present in 2. Pulmonary ventricular volumes and EF were within normal ranges except in patients with persistent PA hypertension, regardless of the type of repair. In regard to resting measurements of ventricular pump function, these early results indicate that the patients fare better after arterial repair. Data with afterload stress after Jatene repair have been reported only by Borow, (*Circulation* 1984; 69: 106–112), who found a normal LV response in 10 of 12 patients.

Hurwitz and associates[23] from Indianapolis, Indiana, estimated RVEF and TR by radionuclide ventriculography to quantitate systemic ventricular function in "simple" TGA. Mean RVEF was 0.52 ± 0.07 for 18 infants before the Mustard operation, 0.54 ± 0.07 for 23 patients operated on <1 year before, and 0.57 ± 0.08 for 14 patients operated on >3 years earlier. Eight patients were evaluated before and after the Mustard operation: EF increased in 3, decreased in 3, and remained constant in 2. Mean RVEF was not different between groups nor when compared with normal. The LV:RV stroke volume ratio of the postoperative patients was compatible with TR in 4 patients. This radionuclide study suggests that after surgery for TGA: 1) mean RVEF remains at levels consistent with values usually found for the normal right ventricle; 2) group RV function does not deteriorate in the years after surgery; and 3) TR may be detected in the early postoperative years.

Results of Mustard-type venous switch and insertion of conduit from LV to PA

Direct resection or bypass using an LV-PA extracardiac conduit are the 2 surgical alternatives for management of severe LV outflow tract obstruction in patients with TGA and intact ventricular septum, small VSD or large VSD removed from the subarterial area. Crupi and associates[24] from Bergamo, Italy, and London, UK, reported their experience with 16 patients who underwent repair by a Mustard-type of venous switch and the placement of a conduit from LV to PA between 1976 and 1983. Mean age was 5.3 years, and 10 patients had intact ventricular septum and 6 had a VSD. The LV outflow obstruction consisted of a fibrous shelf in 5, a tunnel-type in 10, and an aneurysm of the membranous septum in 1. No patient was <1 year of age at operation. Porcine heterograft valved conduits were used in 6, homograft valved conduits in 7, and nonvalved Dacron tubes in 3. There were 3 deaths within 30 days of operation. Preoperative LV-PA gradients ranged from 36–109 mmHg. Postoperative cardiac catheterization was performed in 10 of 13 early survivors at a mean interval of 45 days after operation, and peak LV-PA gradients decreased from a mean of 66 to a mean of 8.5 mmHg. Follow-up ranged from 7 months to 6 years (mean, 5 years) and 9 of the 10 patients who had early postoperative catheterization were restudied at a mean interval of 48 months after repair. The mean increase in peak systolic LV-PA gradient compared with the initial post-repair gradient was 6 mmHg (range, 0–45). The patient with the 45 mmHg gradient had stenosis of a porcine valve. In 4 patients, the LV outflow obstruction had become remarkably less severe by angiographic appearance. At late follow-up, 8 patients were in New York Heart Association class I and 4 were in class II.

Arrhythmias after the Mustard procedure

Earlier reports have suggested that the incidence of arrhythmias after the Mustard procedure can be reduced if the sinus node is protected during surgery. To determine if these initial differences continue after longer follow-up, Duster and associates[25] from Houston, Texas, examined all ECGs available for 3 groups of patients operated on from January 1965 through December 1977. Group A included 37 patients who survived the operation before January 1972, when surgical modifications were initiated to protect the sinus node; group B included 44 patients available for follow-up who were operated on from 1972 through 1974; and group C consisted of the 39 patients available for follow-up operated on from 1975 to 1977. Arrhythmias were classified as passive (failure of initiation or propagation of the sinus node impulse), active (atrial flutter or SVT), or AV conduction defects. Results were expressed as the incidence per number of different rhythms during follow-up intervals. The incidence of sinus rhythm in groups B and C (80%) was much greater than in group A (27%) during the first 2 years. After 8 years, <50% of the rhythms were sinus. Both brady- and tachyarrhythmias were common. Seven patients (6%) required pacemaker insertion for symptomatic sick sinus syndrome. Therefore, despite efforts to protect the sinus node, late-occurring arrhythmias remain a significant problem in patients after the Mustard procedure.

Arterial switch operation

Arensman and colleagues[26] from Kiel, West Germany, and Harefield, UK, performed 1 or 2 cardiac catheterization studies on 25 children from 1–53 months (mean, 19) after the arterial switch operation for TGA. Early studies (mean, 12 months) were made in 23 patients and late studies (mean, 30 months) in 13 patients. Age at repair ranged from 2–168 months (mean, 26) and 15 patients were <1 year of age. Measurements were made of the aortic anulus and of multiple areas of the ascending aorta, including the anastomotic site. They were compared with measurements made in a control population of 21 patients between 1 and 196 months of age (mean, 102). The diameter of the aortic anulus and of the multiple levels of ascending aorta studied were larger than normal in the 15 patients who had simple TGA and the 10 children who had complex TGA. There were no differences between early and late measurements even at the anastomotic site. No pressure gradients were identified across the aortic anastomosis. Subjective evaluation of the coronary artery anastomoses showed no kinking or obstruction. The data indicate that over the medium term, no progression of aortic dilation occurs after arterial switching, and although growth of the anastomotic site was not demonstrated, narrowing and gradients were absent. Coronary arterial anastomoses were unobstructed. The potential for long-term appropriate growth of these sites seems to be preserved.

LEFT VENTRICULAR OUTFLOW OBSTRUCTION

Aortic valve stenosis

Kveselis and associates[27] from Ann Arbor, Michigan, studied 12 patients with valvar AS who had treadmill-induced ST-segment depression and compared data with 5 patients without treadmill exercise-induced ST depression. Both groups had a mean age of 13 years and were studied with maximal supine exercise during cardiac catheterization. The LV systolic pressure at rest (177 ± 25 -vs- 138 ± 8 mmHg) and during maximal supine exercise (248 ± 37 -vs- 189 ± 17 mmHg) were both significantly greater in patients with treadmill-induced ST depression. The LV/oxygen supply demand ratio during supine exercise was significantly less (6.4 ± 2.7 -vs- 11.8 ± 0.7) in patients with exercise-induced ST depression. An LV/oxygen supply demand ratio <11 was 100% sensitive and specific in predicting treadmill-induced ST depression. These investigations provide an excellent correlation between ST-segment abnormalities induced by treadmill exercise and the relation during exercise of LV/oxygen supply demand ratio, which has been used to estimate the adequacy of LV subendocardial blood flow. This type of exercise evaluation may be useful in the frequent clinical problem of whether or not to operate in the young patient with AS who has borderline hemodynamic variables for surgery at rest.

Fifer and associates[28] from Boston, Massachusetts, studied 16 children and 25 adults with AS using echo-derived rates of LV early diastolic filling and wall thinning. Data were compared with 48 normal children and adults. LV early diastolic filling and wall thinning rates were significantly depressed in both children and adults with AS compared with normal subjects. Filling and thinning rates correlated negatively with LV peak systolic pressure and wall thickness in all subjects. Furthermore, the effect of age on diastolic function appeared to be mediated by age-related increases in systolic pressure and wall thickness. In adults, early diastolic filling abnormalities were depressed to a similar extent in subjects with normal and abnormal systolic function. Thus, diastolic dysfunction does not appear to be a manifestation of abnormal systolic loading and ejection performance. These results suggest that the extent of hypertrophy itself plays a dominant role in the mechanism of impaired LV diastolic filling in pressure overload due to AS.

Subaortic stenosis

Freedom and associates[29] from Toronto, Canada, reported serial catheterization studies on 22 patients with fixed subaortic stenosis. Patients with HC were excluded from this study. Age at initial catheterization was from 1 month to 11 years and the second study was from 4 months to 15 years. Most patients, 17 of 22 (77%) had a shelf-like fixed obstruction, with the remainder having a diffuse fibromuscular obstruction or tunnel malformation. The peak systolic LV outflow gradient increased from 22 ± 20–67 ± 22 mmHg between the 2 studies. Nineteen patients with associated VSD also were studied with age at initial investigation ranging from 2 days to 11 years and at subsequent study, from 10 months to 17 years. The mean LV outflow gradient at the initial catheterization was 9 mmHg, ranging from 0–90 mmHg, and at the second study it was 35 mmHg, ranging from 0–110 mmHg. The investigators provide an excellent documentation of the progressive nature of subaortic stenosis in children. New concepts evolving about this malformation include the fact that in most instances it is probably an acquired lesion and not congenital in nature. The question as to when to intervene in the patients who have mild gradients remains unresolved. Fortunately with echo and Doppler studies available, clinical follow-up will be much easier, and intervention before myocardial dysfunction or significant AR occurs should be feasible in most patients.

AORTIC ISTHMIC COARCTATION REPAIR

Repair of aortic coarctation in the first 3 months of life continues to have high hospital mortality. To determine if a correlation is present between the coarctation anatomy and the surgical procedure performed, Pellegrino and colleagues[30] from London and Liverpool, UK, studied 42 autopsy specimens from patients <3 months of age. They found the anatomy more complex than simply a discrete lesion at the site of coarctation. In some, a shelf of ductal tissue was present within the aortic lumen; others had hypoplasia of a segment of the arch; others had a "waist" lesion. In this group, the wall of the aorta itself was constricted to form the obstruction. These "waist" lesions coexisted with discrete shelves and isthmic narrowing.

Although controversy persists regarding the best technique of repair of aortic coarctation in infants, most surgical groups currently prefer the use of the subclavian flap arterioplasty. Some, however, continue to prefer the use of resection with end-to-end anastomosis. Cobanoglu and coworkers[31] from Portland, Oregon, reported their experience with 134 infants <3 months of age at the time of repair; 90 (67%) <1 month. Twenty-seven had profound low cardiac output that necessitated preoperative intubation and ventilation, 13 of them had severe acidosis requiring inotropic support. Associated congenital cardiac lesions were present in 117 patients: PDA in 63%, VSD in 53%, and ASD in 23%. Subclavian flap arterioplasty was used in 67, resection with end-to-end anastomosis in 55, and other procedures in 12. The 2 major groups were similar in age and weight at the time of repair, and hospital mortality was 29% for those with end-to-end anastomosis, 19% for those with subclavian flap arterioplasty. Follow-up information was obtained in all survivors for a mean period of 5 years in the end-to-end anastomosis group and 2 years in the subclavian flap group. The reoperation-free rate at 5 years for the end-to-end anastomosis group was 92 ± 5% and for the subclavian flap arterioplasty, 75 ± 7%. Eight of the 10 patients who had reoperation after arterioplasty had early recurrence with continued involution of the periductal tissue and growth of the posterior aortic ridge. It was concluded that resection with end-to-end anastomosis is the preferred operation for infants less than 3 months of age.

The choice of operation for symptomatic aortic coarctation during infancy remains controversial. Korfer and associates[32] from Dusseldorf, West Germany, reported their experience over a 9-year period with 55 infants who underwent resection and end-to-end anastomosis during the first 120 days of life. There were 27 infants <1 month, 11 <2 months, 9 <3 months, and 8 <4 months of age at operation. Associated congenital cardiac defects were present in 48 infants; a VSD in 37 and TGA in 7. After division of PDA, the coarctated segment was resected and end-to-end anastomosis performed with interrupted 6–0 polypropylene suture. No patient had an intraoperative systolic pressure gradient >6 mmHg or a mean pressure gradient >2 mmHg. In those with VSD, the pressure in the PA was measured through the ductal stump and in those with a nonrestrictive VSD, an additional banding of the PA was performed (19 patients with VSD) to reduce distal PA pressure to 50–60% of systemic. There were 2 early deaths (3.6%). Twenty-seven were recatheterized between 5 months and 7 years (mean, 3.2 years) after operation. The mean pressure gradient at the site of the anastomosis was 7 mmHg (range, 0–33). Only 3 survivors had a systolic pressure gradient >20 mmHg. There were no operations for recoarctation. The investigators emphasize the need to remove not only the area of maximal constriction, but the surrounding aortic tissue that may consist partially or totally of ductal material. In addition, they stress the importance of circumferencial interrupted sutures to allow future anastomotic growth.

Although the subclavian flat aortoplasty is commonly used for repair of aortic coarctation in neonates, there have been few reports of follow-up data in this subset. Thus, Metzdorff and coworkers[33] from Portland, Oregon, reviewed their experience with 83 patients having this operation between 1976 and 1983. Among 60 patients <8 weeks of age at operation (mean, 2.6 weeks), operative and late mortality were 18% and 14%, respectively. Ten patients in this group developed recurrent coarctation requiring reoperation after a mean follow-up of 26 months. Thus, 75% of those <8 weeks of age at repair were free of recoarctation at 2 years. In contrast, operative and late mortality among 23 patients >8 weeks of age at operation was 13% and 10%, respectively, after a mean follow-up of 16 months. There were no recurrent coarctations in this group. The investigators believe the difference in recurrence rates may be related to age-dependent involution of residual coarctation tissue unavoidably left in place during subclavian flat aortoplasty. They conclude that although subclavian flap aortoplasty is effective for repair of coarctation in infants, patients <8 weeks of age have a significant risk of early recurrence. In this subset, they prefer the use of resection with end-to-end anastomosis when technically feasible.

A major disadvantage of the subclavian flap arterioplasty for repair of aortic coarctation is the requirement for division of the subclavian artery and its resultant ischemic consequences to the upper extremity. Thus, Teles de Mendonca and colleagues[34] from Aracaju-Sergipe, Brazil, developed a new surgical technique that has the advantages of the classic Waldhausen subclavian flap arterioplasty with maintenance of patency of the subclavian artery itself. The method consists of removing the subclavian artery from its aortic origin, longitudinally incising the aorta from this opening through the coarctate segment, making a longitudinal incision in the subclavian artery, and after mobilization suturing its margins to the margins of the aortic incision. The technique is reported in a 6-year-old patient who postoperatively was shown angiographically to have absence of residual coarctation and unobstructed flow into the subclavian artery. This ingenious technique is particularly useful when the left subclavian artery is large and the site of coarctation reasonably close to its origin.

Brown and coworkers[35] from Indianapolis, Indiana, described their results with a new technique to repair coarctation of the aorta using an isthmus flap aortoplasty in 4 patients <3 months of age (mean, 36 days) operated on between 1980 and 1984. Each had a long segment coarctation of the aorta and CHF. Preoperative prostaglandin E_1 was used in 2 infants <1 week of age. A short segment of aorta, including the ductal entrance and coarctation web, was resected. The posterior wall of the long isthmus was opened longitudinally to the transverse portion of the aortic arch just inferior to the origin of the left subclavian artery. The descending aorta was mobilized and advanced to the level of the aortic arch where the posterior half was sutured. The attached isthmus was used as an anterior flap and sutured into a longitudinal incision made in the anterior wall of the descending aorta. Each patient survived and hemodynamic and angiographic measurements were made in each at a mean follow-up of 42 months. Gradients were 0 at rest and 7.0 ± 0.93 mmHg after angiography, which demonstrated that the reconstructed area had grown in diameter and attained a normal caliber in each child. The investigators believe that this technique of isthmus flap aortoplasty provides good repair of the coarctation without sacrificing the subclavian artery. They believe the technique is not suitable for all neonates and that the precise repair should be dictated by the individual anatomic considerations present. The method described, however, eliminates all of the ductal tissue and the coarctation web and may result in a lower incidence of recurrent coarctation than other currently used methods to repair long segment coarctation in infancy.

To determine whether altered vascular reactivity could contribute to systemic hypertension after repair of coarctation, Gidding and coinvestigators[36] from Ann Arbor, Michigan, measured the change in forearm and calf vascular resistances to small intra-arterial infusions of norepinephrine in 6 patients who had undergone surgical correction of aortic coarctation but still had upper extremity hypertension and compared them with similar measurements made in 5 normotensive patients with mild heart disease. Only the upper extremity pressure was significantly greater in the group that underwent repair of coarctation (102 -vs- 83 mmHg for mean arm pressures and 96 -vs- 83 mmHg for mean leg pressures in patients who had coarctation -vs- normotensive patients, respectively). Forearm and calf BP were measured in the right arm and leg with a mercury-in-plastic strain-gauge plethysmograph. Forearm and calf vascular resistance was calculated by dividing mean arterial pressure of the appropriate extremity by the blood flow of that extremity. Norepinephrine was infused into the right brachial and femoral arteries of the patients in increasing doses. Resting forearm and calf vascular resistances were similar in both groups of patients. The norepinephrine dose-response curves showed that control patients required more than 3 times the norepinephrine to produce the same percent increase in forearm vascular resistance (after 0.2 μg/minute forearm vascular resistance increased by 55% in the coarctation group, but the resistance in the control group increased by only 3%). There was no difference between the 2 groups with regard to the dose-response curves for calf vascular resistance. These data suggest the presence in the resistance vessels anatomically positioned above the coarctation of abnormal vascular reactivity that may have persisted despite successful repair.

Patients undergoing repair of aortic isthmic coarctation often have self-limited but severe systemic hypertension in the first week after surgery (paradoxical hypertension). Gidding and associates[37] from Ann Arbor, Michigan, conducted a controlled trial of treatment with propranolol before repair of aortic coarctation in 14 children to determine whether the drug would prevent paradoxical hypertension. Seven patients were randomly assigned to receive propranolol for 2 weeks before surgery and throughout the first postoperative week, and 7 patients were assigned to receive standard postoperative care. Both groups had a similar significant increase in the plasma norepinephrine level in response to surgery; however, when compared with no treatment, treatment with propranolol reduced not only the increase in systolic and diastolic BP but also the postoperative increase in plasma renin activity (Fig. 7-8). It was concluded that prophylactic propranolol can prevent paradoxical hypertension and should therefore become a routine part of the operative care of patients with coarctation of the aorta.

Sweeney and coworkers[38] from Houston, Texas, reported their experience with 53 patients who underwent operation for repair of recurrent thoracic

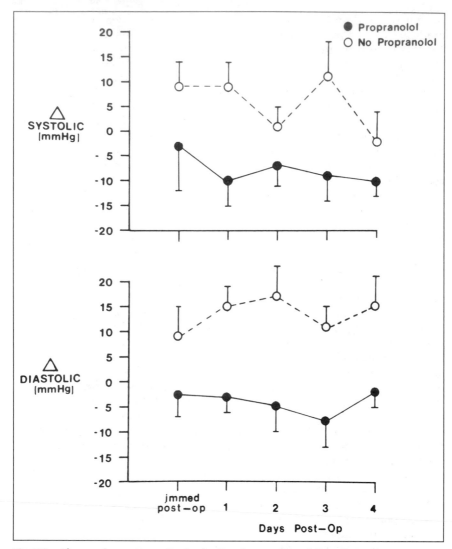

Fig. 7-8. Changes from preoperative levels of resting systolic and diastolic BP after coarctation repair. The propranolol-pretreated group (●) had a significant decline in systolic BP after surgery (p = 0.02). The increase in diastolic BP in the control group was significant (p = 0.05). Pretreatment with propranolol blunted the hypertensive response to coarctation repair. Reproduced with permission from Gidding et al.[37]

aortic coarctation between 1961 and 1983. The previous procedures performed were resection with end-to-end anastomosis in 27 patients, patch graft aortoplasty in 12, subclavian flap angioplasty in 2, prosthetic graft interposition in 8, and bypass in 4. At initial repair, patients ranged in age from 1 day to 44 years (mean, 3 years) and 29 were <3 years of age. At the time of reoperation, systemic hypertension was present in 94%, reduced peripheral pulses in 76%, exertional fatigue in 32%, severe headaches in 25%, epistaxis in 19%, and CHF in 6%. Preoperative angiography was performed in all patients. The type of reoperation included a Dacron patch graft angioplasty in 26, local bypass graft in 12, ascending-descending aortic bypass graft in 4, resection and interposition grafting in 8, and resection and end-to-end anastomosis in 3. Mean age at reoperation was 18 years, and among 11 patients whose initial operation was in the first month of life, 5 required reoperation before the age of 4 years. Patients older at the initial procedure showed no correlation between age and time to reoperation, the average interval being 9 years. All survived the reoperative procedure and the 3 perioperative complications (6%) were left recurrent laryngeal nerve paralysis in 1, anastomotic bleeding in 1, and postoperative chylothorax in another. All but 1 was available for late follow-up and were well and without subsequent reoperation an average of 7 years postoperatively. Only 2 (4%) were hypertensive and neither had an arm-leg BP gradient at rest or with exercise. These gradients were measured in 44 of the 53 patients and were <10 mmHg in 41, and 10–20 mmHg in 3. It was concluded that operative management of severe recurrent coarctation is safe and effective and that several techniques of reconstruction have a place in this therapy. In the 4 patients who had been operated on twice previously, severe scarring was considered prohibitive for safe local dissection and each underwent an ascending-descending aortic bypass and were satisfactory at follow-up between 2 and 9 years postoperatively.

MISCELLANEOUS TOPICS IN PEDIATRIC CARDIOLOGY

The newborn transitional circulation

Mahoney and associates[39] from Iowa City, Iowa, studied the transitional circulation of 11 normal newborns using echo and Doppler. Initial examination was performed within 10 hours after delivery and serial studies were performed for 3 days. Diastolic PA velocities indicative of a PDA were detected in 10 infants on day 1, 2 infants on day 2, and none on day 3. Localized retrograde systolic flow proximal to the septal leaflet of the tricuspid valve and consistent with TR was detected in 6 of 10 on day 1, 8 of 10 on day 2, 7 of 10 on day 3. Maximal Doppler velocities were derived for PA, aorta, tricuspid, and mitral orifices in all patients. There appears to be mild TR by Doppler even in normal newborns.

Aortic valve regurgitation and nonimmune hydrops

Silverman and associates[40] from San Francisco, California, and New Haven, Connecticut, used echo and Doppler studies in 466 fetuses and found 12 cases of AV valve regurgitation and nonimmune hydrops. Death occurred in 11 of the 12, all of whom had structural heart disease. The 1 surviving fetus had SVT and all abnormalities disappeared on treatment; 7 additional fetuses had AV valve regurgitation but did not develop hydrops. All survived pregnancy and the early neonatal period. This study verifies the extremely poor prognosis of AV valve regurgitation associated with nonimmune hydrops and structural heart disease in the fetus. The hydrops is believed to reflect fetal cardiac failure related to venous hypertension and low colloid oncotic pressure.

Congenital heart disease in offspring of affected parents

Rose and associates[41] from Toronto, Canada, determined the prevalence of congenital heart disease in children of 219 parents with 1 of 4 selected defects: ASD, aortic coarctation, AS, or complex dextrocardia. A prevalence of 8.8% of substantial cardiac defects was found in their children. This recurrence risk is considerably higher than the 2.9% previously reported by Nora (*Teratology* 1970; 3: 325–330). The risk of recurrence was significantly greater in children if the mother was affected than if the father was. In particular, mothers who had an ASD were found to be 3.5 times as likely to have a significant cardiac defect as children whose father had this condition. These data are similar to those previously published by Whittemore et al (*Am J Cardiol* 1982; 50: 641–651) showing a much higher prevalence of congenital heart disease in offspring of affected mothers than was previously suspected. There was a particularly high recurrence with mothers with ASD or AS and indicates the need to revise current counseling for prospective parents who have congenital heart disease.

Absent right superior vena cava and conduction tissue abnormalities

Lenox and associates[42] from Pittsburgh, Pennsylvania, studied the conduction tissue of 8 hearts with abnormal caval drainage. Ages ranged from 2 days to 2.7 years and all had 4-chambered hearts and normal atrial situs. Four patients had absence of the right superior caval vein and 3 of these had persistent left superior caval vein. The coronary sinus varied in size from normal to markedly enlarged. In all cases the sinus node was in its usual location. The AV node and bundle were normal in all but 1 case, in which the node was hypoplastic but normal cellular elements were present and the bundle was normally distributed. In contrast, in 3 of 4 hearts with absent right superior caval view, the sinus node tissue was markedly hypoplastic. The investigations shed some light on the clinical syndrome of atrial rhythm abnormalities and the frequent occurrence of a LA rhythm pattern on ECG in patients with absence of the right superior caval vein.

Straddling AV valve

Rice and associates[43] from Rochester, Minnesota, reviewed echoes in 56 patients with a known diagnosis of 66 straddling AV valve without knowledge of surgical or pathologic findings. They classified patients into 3 groups on the basis of site of chordae insertion into a contralateral ventricle: A) chordae inserting into the contralateral ventricle near the crest of the ventricular septum, B) chordae inserting along the contralateral ventricular septum, C) chordae inserting into the free wall or papillary muscles of the contralateral ventricle. In 60 of 66 straddling AV valves the diagnosis and the degree of straddling were identified correctly by echo. Major associated defects included double-outlet right ventricle, TGA, congenitally corrected TGA, and double-inlet ventricle. In 41 patients, straddling AV valve had a major impact on the type of surgery or surgical outcome. Of the valves inspected, 52% were type A, 26%, type B, and 22%, type C.

Criss-cross heart

Robinson and associates[44] from London, UK, reported echo and angiographic correlates in 8 patients aged 6 weeks to 12 years with criss-cross heart. Complete anatomic diagnosis was achieved with echo in all patients, but identification of ventricular morphology was easier using angiograms. With the transducer held in either a precordial or subcostal position and rocked anteriorly and posteriorly, the characteristic crossing of the ventricular inflows could be seen. In no plane was there complete parallel arrangement of ventricular inflows.

LV mechanics in combined AS and aortic isthmic coarctation

Borow and associates[45] from Chicago, Illinois, and Boston, Massachusetts, used echo to compare myocardial mechanics in 11 patients with AS (aged 6–41 years) and 11 with aortic coarctation who were matched for age, body surface area, and peak systolic ejection gradient. Data were compared with 22 normal subjects. No differences for LV diameters, heart rate, or peak wall stress were present among the 3 groups. Peak LV pressure and wall mass were higher for patients than for normal subjects, but these parameters did not differ between the patient groups. Patients with AS had higher shortening fraction than either coarctation or normal groups. Afterload as quantified by end-systolic stress was 41% lower than normal for AS patients and 13% higher than normal for coarctation patients. LV contractility as assessed by load independent indicies was depressed in 3 of 11 patients with coarctation, all of whom were >20 years of age. In contrast, the increased systolic performance in AS patients was caused by reduced afterload rather than altered contractile state. The investigators have shown that the altered systolic performance in young patients with AS is most likely related to a reduced afterload secondary to their marked increase in wall thickness. In addition, they showed a decreased in contractile state in older patients with aortic coarctation, indicating the potential damaging effects of long-standing pressure overload.

Combined subaortic stenosis and VSD

Smith and associates[46] from London and Newcastle, UK, presented data on 15 children, aged 3–11 months with fixed subaortic stenosis and VSD. Evidence of congenital heart disease was noted within the first year of life and in 13 within the first 3 months. All patients had a pansystolic murmur, maximal at the left sternal border, and in 5 patients an early diastolic murmur was present. Echo in each case showed a subaortic ridge identified together with a VSD. The stenosis was best identified using a left parasternal and apical long axis view of the LV outflow tract and aortic root. These investigators provide a good demonstration of the necessity of looking for subaortic stenosis in patients with known or suspected VSD. The diagnosis usually can be made by echo and surgical relief of the obstruction performed at the time of VSD closure.

Doppler PA pressure estimate

Marx and associates[47] from Tucson, Arizona, estimated PA pressure using Doppler echo in 25 patients with either a VSD or a single ventricle. Pressure drops estimated by Doppler studies were referenced to systolic systemic arterial pressure. The PA pressure measurement at cardiac catheterization ranged from 15–100 mmHg and that measured by Doppler ranged from 9–100 ± 9.2 mmHg. These investigators show excellent results in estimation of PA pressure using careful and meticulous Doppler techniques. These techniques should be helpful in the follow-up of patients with ventricular communications.

LV function before and after the Fontan operation for tricuspid valve atresia

Nakae and associates[48] from Tokyo, Japan, studied 6 patients with tricuspid valve atresia before and 1 month after Fontan repair. Age at operation ranged from 6–19 years. LV end-diastolic volume decreased from 166 ± 45–120 ± 51% of normal. LVEF also decreased from 0.61 ± 0.1–0.48 ± 0.1. Cardiac index was low at a mean value of 2.2 ± 0.2 L/min/m^2. These data again document partial relief of the LV volume overload in tricuspid atresia with the Fontan operation. Pump function measurements appeared depressed 1 month after operation, but multiple factors may be involved, including effects of the surgery itself as well as the loading conditions of the ventricle.

MISCELLANEOUS TOPICS IN PEDIATRIC CARDIAC SURGERY

Blalock-Taussig shunt

Interposition of polytetrafluoroethylene (PTFE) tubes between the ipsilateral subclavian artery and PA has become the preferred shunt of many surgical groups. Early experience reported by de Leval indicated a 67% 2-year failure rate for the 4 mm prosthesis, significantly higher than that of larger sizes. More recently, Kay and colleagues showed no significant difference in the 2-year patency rate between 4 and 6 mm grafts using aspirin and dipyridamole for 3 months after operation. In an effort to define the effectiveness of PTFE interposition shunts, Karpawich and colleagues[49] from Newark, New Jersey, reviewed their experience with 19 patients. Four mm conduits were used in 9 patients and 5 and 6 mm conduits, in the remainder. Two of the 9 (22%) 4 mm prostheses failed after a mean of 12.5 months, whereas the other 7 grafts (2 patients on aspirin) remained patent. Occlusion of the subclavian artery distal to the anastomotic site occurred in 2 patients who received 4 mm prostheses. This study supports the use of PTFE grafts >4 mm when possible. Patients with 4 mm grafts must be followed closely, and if they have shunt-dependent circulations, either a second shunt or a complete repair should be considered within 1 year.

Repair of congenital pulmonary venous stenosis

Previous experience with congenital stenosis of pulmonary veins has been associated with rapid and progressive restenosis in most patients. These disappointing results led Pacifico and coworkers[50] from Birmingham, Alabama, to devise a repair using living autologous atrial tissue in the hopes of providing lasting relief of obstruction. The tip of the LA appendage was opened and used as an onlay patch to widen the stenotic area of the left pulmonary veins, leaving a double pathway for venous return. A flap of atrial septum was evaginated through an incision in the right side of the left atrium and used as an onlay patch to widen the stenotic area of the right pulmonary veins. Effective relief of obstruction was demonstrated by nearly normal postrepair PA pressure in each of 2 patients and early postoperative angiography in 1. These 2 patients remain well 21 and 24 months after repair.

Repair of total anomalous pulmonary venous connection to right superior vena cava

Total anomalous pulmonary venous connection (TAPVC) to the right superior vena cava (SVC) is an uncommon malformation usually repaired by construction of a pericardial or Dacron tunnel joining the site of connection with a preexisting or created ASD. Vargas and colleagues[51] from Buenos Aires, Argentina, described a new surgical technique that uses living autologous atrial tissue for correction of this anomaly. The right SVC was divided above the site of drainage and its proximal end oversewn. The azygous vein was closed. A J-shaped right atriotomy was made to the right of the base of the appendage, the ASD enlarged, and the superior edge of the atriotomy incision sutured to the anterior and inferior walls of the ASD. This procedure diverted pulmonary venous return to the left atrium. The distal end of the right SVC was then anastomosed to the incised RA appendage and the remaining atriotomy closed primarily. This method was successfully used in 3 patients, 2 months, 7 and 16 years of age with variations of this anomaly. Postoperative clinical, radiologic, and echo evaluation in each, and cardiac catheterization in 1, between 4 months and 4 years postoperatively, confirmed the adequacy of repair.

Prostaglandin E_1 in ductus-dependent neonates

To improve the results of systemic-PA shunting operations in infants with cyanotic heart disease and hypoplastic pulmonary arteries, Yokota and co-workers[52] from Shizuoka, Japan, infused prostaglandin E_1 (PGE_1) for 26–65 days (mean, 47). Thirteen of 16 infants were <4 days old when PGE_1 was begun and had a variety of defects that included severe pulmonic valve stenosis or atresia. Side effects of PGE_1 included apneic episodes in 2, seborrheic dermatitis, edematous protrusion of the orbita, and periosteal thickening of the long bones and ribs. Histologic study of the PA was done in 9 patients and showed thinning of the media in 1. Pretreatment PA size (determined by 2D echo) ranged from 2.2–4.0 mm (mean, 2.9) and increased to 2.6–7.2 mm (mean, 4.5) at the time of operation. At operation, a 4 mm polytetraflouroethylene (PTFE) graft was used in 15 patients and a 5 mm graft in 1, interposed between the subclavian artery and PA. The PDA was disected in 9 and ligated in 4. There was 1 early death from infection and 2 sudden late deaths 5 and 9 months postoperatively in patients known to have patent shunts immediately before death. The remaining survivors, followed between 1 and 39 months (mean, 22), continued to have patent shunts and good palliation. The investigators believe that long-term low dose (0.02–0.03 μg/kg/min) PGE_1 provides good preoperative palliation, results in increased PA size, and may permit a better systemic-PA shunt operation. They present an alternative to the more classic management of these patients. Despite this, I (ADP) continue to prefer short-term administration of PGE_1 to permit a semiurgent, but not emergent, shunt operation and believe this can be accomplished with similar success and a considerably shorter period of hospitalization.

Normothermic caval inflow occlusion

Jonas and colleagues[53] from Boston, Massachusetts, reviewed their experience using the technique of normothermic caval inflow occlusion to accomplish a variety of surgical procedures in 140 patients. There were no deaths among 94 children who underwent pulmonic valvotomy, 13 of whom were <1 week of age, 14 between 1 month and 1 year, and 67 >1 year of age. In this group there were no late deaths and no reoperations for recurrent pulmonic stenosis over a mean follow-up time of 45 months (1–117). There were 4 hospital deaths (19%) among 21 patients who underwent aortic valvotomy. Seven of them were <1 month of age, 11 between 1 and 6 months, and 3 >1 year. Two (29%) deaths occurred among the 7 patients <1 month of age, and 2 (18%) among 11 infants between 1 and 6 months. There were 10 patients with pulmonic valve atresia and intact septum with 5 deaths, 1 of 3 who underwent placement of an RV outflow patch, 3 of 5 who had pulmonic valvotomy and 1 in the single patient who had a Brock procedure. Hospital mortality was 9% among 11 patients who had an atrial septectomy and 50% among 4 patients who had miscellaneous procedures. The investigators concluded that the technique of inflow occlusion is a safe and effective method for patients with pulmonic stenosis and AS and in the critically ill neonate is preferable to valvotomy on cardiopulmonary bypass. The technique can be applied to a variety of other procedures and represents a considerable financial saving over operations performed with cardiopulmonary bypass.

Cavopulmonary shunt

Hopkins and associates[54] from Durham, North Carolina, reported their experience in 21 patients who underwent a modified Glenn shunt by connecting the divided end of the superior vena cava (SVC) to the side of the undivided right PA. This allowed bilateral PA distribution from the SVC. Twelve patients underwent this type of shunt before a planned Fontan operation, which was later performed in 5; 8 had construction of this shunt at the time of a Fontan procedure, and in 1 patient it was constructed 4 months after an atriopulmonary connection because of restricted RA outflow. There were 2 hospital deaths and the remaining 19 patients were followed between 2 months and 9 years. One sudden late death occurred at 9 years. The shunts were evaluated by postoperative angiography in 8 patients and by RNA in 7. SVC blood flow had a bilateral pulmonary distribution in all but 1 patient, but tended to be greater to the right lung. The investigators concluded that this modified shunt provides excellent relief of cyanosis, allows bilateral PA distribution of both SVC return and also RA blood flow after atriopulmonary connection. It may be constructed before, concomitant with, or after a Fontan procedure and is compatible with all currently recommended modifications. This type of procedure will probably have limited application in the group of patients currently managed by a Fontan-type procedure, but may be useful in some and should remain in the surgeon's armamentarium. In some whose malformation includes a dilated ascending aorta which is rightward and posterior, reducing the amount of space for a usual type of atrial pulmonary connection, concomitant use of this procedure might be beneficial.

Intracardiac repair without blood transfusion

Henling and coworkers[55] from Houston, Texas, reported their experience with 110 children of members of the Jehovah's Witness faith who underwent 112 operations for repair of congenital heart defects using cardiopulmonary bypass (CPB). Thirty-nine (35%) patients weighed <15 kg and 36 (33%) were polycythemic preoperatively. Operations were performed during normothermic CPB with a glucose crystaloid prime. No patient received blood or blood products during the perioperative period, and only 1 of the 6 deaths was attributed to blood loss. Hemoglobin levels declined maximally immediately after CPB and frequently exceeded 50% in the 8 patients between 5 and 10 kg in weight. Pre-bypass values were nearly restored within 6 hours as a consequence of active diuresis. Hemoglobin levels remained >8 g/dl with few exceptions during the remaining period of hospitalization. Hemoglobin values during CPB were 4.5 g/dl in the 8 patients between 5 and 10 kg in weight, 5.5 in the 14 between 10 and 15 kg, and progressively higher in larger subjects. CPB time was shortest in smaller subjects, being 26 ± 14 minutes in those between 5 and 10 kg. The investigators believe that cardiac operations can be safely performed in children denied blood transfusion and suggest that hemodilution techniques without blood transfusion might be extended to repair of congenital cardiac defects in children of families with other religious beliefs.

Results of operations for Ebstein's anomaly

Oh and associates[56] from Rochester, Minnesota, reported on perioperative and postoperative arrhythmias in 52 consecutive patients who underwent operation for Ebstein's anomaly. There were 25 male and 27 female patients, with a mean age of 18 years (range, 11 months to 64 years). Preoperative arrhythmia occurred in 34 of 52: 28 with supraventricular and 13 with ventricular arrhythmia. During the perioperative and early postoperative period 14 had atrial and 8 ventricular arrhythmia. There were 7 deaths between 1 day and 27 months postoperatively and 5 were sudden, with 4 of 5 having a history of perioperative VT or VF; 22% of patients with preoperative SVT and 33% with preoperative AF continued to have symptomatic tachycardia postoperatively. Nine patients without preoperative documentation or symptoms or arrhythmia were followed for a mean of 31 months and none died suddenly or developed symptomatic arrhythmia.

These data indicate the prevalence and severity of both supraventricular and ventricular arrhythmias in patients with Ebstein's anomaly. Younger patients were less likely to have preoperative or postoperative arrhythmia. Less than one-third of patients with preoperative SVT continued to have symptomatic arrhythmias after surgical repair. Patients with perioperative ventricular arrhythmia were at increased risk for sudden death

Repair of double-orifice mitral valve

Double-orifice mitral valve is present in about 5% of patients with AV canal defects. Its presence has been thought to complicate surgical repair and increase the risk of residual MS. Lee and colleagues[57] from Rochester, Minnesota, reviewed their experience with 25 patients, 16 with the partial form and 9 with the complete form, who ranged in age from 3 months to 56 years (mean, 8 years). The classic repair using a 1-patch technique for the complete form and closure of the so-called mitral valve cleft was used and continues to be recommended by these investigators. There was 1 hospital death (4%), which occurred in 1967 in a patient in whom the tissue bridge separating the minor and major orifices was divided, leaving severe MR. In the remaining 24 patients the tissue bridge was left intact. No patient had clinically significant MS during a follow-up of 1–14 years (mean, 4.9), 2 (8%) developed progressive MR and required MVR at 3 and 11 years postoperatively. One of these patients died and a second late death occurred suddenly 2 years after repair. The remaining survivors are in New York Heart Association class I or II. The investigators indicate that the minor orifice is usually competent and does not require closure. They recommend measuring the major and minor orifices intraoperatively and relating their combined area to normal. They believe that repair of AV canal associated with double-orifice mitral valve can be achieved with low operative mortality and the incidence of late development of MR is similar to that of the usual type of AV canal. This is a selected surgical experience, since the mean age at operation was 8 years. Currently, elective repair of complete AV canal defects is advised in infancy (3–6 months) and the presence of a double-orifice mitral valve probably is an incremental risk factor for increased hospital mortality and residual MS. Measurement of each orifice and relating their combined area to normal, as these investigators advise, is especially important.

Repair with discordant AV connection

McGrath and colleagues[58] from Birmingham, Alabama, reviewed their experience with 99 patients who underwent operation for a variety of congenital cardiac defects in the presence of a discordant AV connection. Atrial situs was solitus in 98, inversus in 9, and the ventriculoarterial (VA) connection was discordant (corrected transposition) in 77, double-outlet right ventricle (DORV) in 18, double-outlet left ventricle in 4, concordant in 3, and single outlet RV in 5: 92% of patients had a VSD, 17%, an ASD, and 2%, an AV canal defect. Tricuspid valve anomalies were frequent, and 17% of patients had important TR that required repair in 1 and replacement in 16. MR was present in only 1%, and 56% had at least moderate pulmonary outflow obstruction. Actuarial survival after reparative surgery at 1 month, 1 year, and 10 years was 86, 75, and 68%, respectively. Risk factors for premature death included DORV, complete heart block preoperatively or developing perioperatively, very young or older (>25 years) age, higher hematocrit valves, and earlier date of operation; 26% of 88 patients at risk developed complete heart block perioperatively and patients with corrected transposition had a lesser probability of this than did those with other VA connections. Eight patients developed important TR after repair of additional intracardiac defects and the presence of an Ebstein-like anomaly of the tricuspid valve was among the risk factors for this. Fifty-seven (81%) of 70 surviving patients were in New York Heart Association class I and 12 (17%), in class II. The overall hospital mortality in the largest subset, corrected transposition, was 9%, and solution of the multivariate equation showed that in this subset, the current estimated 10-year survival rate of patients subjected to repair was 92%. The increased risk associated with repair at an older age indicates that every effort should be made to perform the repair before the age of about 5 years. The advantages of near routine repair in infancy of patients with these malformations are reduced by the fact that nearly half will require a valved extracardiac conduit that will be outgrown and require later replacement and also by the greater incidence of surgically induced complete heart block and the requirement for a permanent pacemaker.

Baffle obstruction after the Mustard operation

Kron and colleagues[59] from Charlottesville, Virginia, followed 33 patients who underwent the Mustard procedure between 1970 and 1982. Each was >1 year postoperative and baffle obstruction of either the superior (SVC) or inferior (IVC) vena cava or both was documented in 11 (33%). Of these, 8 were symptomatic and underwent reoperation, which included the placement of separate pericardial patches at the sites of SVC and IVC obstruction in 1 patient in whom recurrent obstruction later developed and death occurred at reoperation. Of the remaining 7, 1 had a polytetrafluoroethylene

(PTFE) patch placed at the site of SVC obstruction with a good long-term result and the remaining 6 underwent enlargement of the entire baffle and the atriotomy by the placement of a large PTFE patch. There was 1 death in this group (overall mortality, 2 of 8) and the 6 survivors had no evidence of reobstruction after a mean follow-up of 18 months (range, 6–48 months). The study confirms a higher incidence of late baffle obstruction in children who undergo the Mustard operation within the first year of life. Of those with baffle obstruction, the average age at initial operation was 9.5 ± 5.4 months compared with 19.6 ± 15.2 months for those without obstruction. Obstruction occurred an average of 8 ± 6 months after the initial procedure (range, 3–18). One baffle revision was required in 9 patients with a dumb-bell-shaped Dacron patch, 7 in 17 patients with a trousers-shaped Dacron baffle, and none in 7 patients with a pericardial baffle. This experience confirms a higher incidence of late baffle obstruction in children who are <1 year of age at the time of the initial operation, shows no difference according to the shape of the baffle, and confirms a lesser incidence of obstruction when parietal pericardium is used as the baffle material. The investigators believe that at the time of reoperation it is safer to enlarge the entire baffle with 1 long strip of PTFE than to use localized patches at the site of obstruction.

Operation for double-outlet right ventricle

Mazzucco and colleagues[60] from Padua, Italy, reported their experience with 32 consecutive patients who underwent surgical treatment of double-outlet right ventricle (DORV). In each, both great arteries arose entirely from the RV, and patients having fibrous continuity between the mitral and semilunar valves were excluded. Twenty patients had a palliative operation, which included a systemic-PA shunt in 10, a Brock procedure in 2, and PA banding in 8. Subsequently, 10 of these and 12 additional patients without previous palliation underwent intracardiac correction. A subaortic VSD was present in 16, a doubly committed VSD in 1, and each of these survived intraventricular tunneling. Of this group, 7 had pulmonic valve stenosis (PS) and 5 required reconstruction of the RV outflow using a patch in 3 or an extracardiac conduit in 2; enlargement of the VSD also was required in 5. In 3 patients with a subpulmonic VSD and in 1 with a noncommitted VSD, each without PS, repair was achieved using an intraventricular tunnel and Senning operation in 2, a Mustard operation in 1, and an arterial switch repair in 1. The latter patient died of intrapulmonary hemorrhage 7 days later, yielding a hospital mortality of 4.5%. Recurrent VSD occurred in 1 and late progression of pulmonary vascular disease in another. There were no late deaths and all but 1 was asymptomatic and complication-free 2–84 months after operation. The investigators indicate that surgical repair of DORV can be accomplished with gratifying early and late results and a low hospital mortality. Early intervention is recommended.

Arterial switch for TGA and for double-outlet right ventricle

The arterial switch operation is being increasingly used for patients with TGA and related malformations. Kanter and colleagues[61] from London, UK, reviewed their experience with 30 patients ranging in age from 18 hours to 6 years (mean, 11 months) who underwent arterial switching between 1981 and 1984. There was one death (12.5%) among 8 patients with TGA and intact ventricular septum, 6 (40%) among 15 patients with TGA and VSD, and 1 (14%) among 7 patients with double-outlet right ventricle (DORV). There were no late deaths during a mean follow-up period of 17 months, and 95% of the survivors were in New York Heart Association class I. Postoperative cardiac catheterization in 13 showed normal LV function, absence of coronary artery stenoses, and AR. The Lecompte maneuver to establish RV-PA continuity was successfully used in 12 of 13 with anteroposterior great vessels, but in none of those with side-by-side great arteries. Seven patients developed subvalvar RV outflow tract obstruction recognized at operation in 5 and postoperatively in 2. This was responsible for death in 3 patients, was noted in all subsets, but in only 1 of 16 with anteroposterior great arteries compared with 6 of 14 with side-by-side great arteries. Severe supravalvar pulmonic stenosis was identified 9 months postoperatively in 1 patient with anteroposterior great arteries in whom the Lecompte maneuver was employed. The investigators concluded that arterial switching can be performed in this group of patients with acceptable mortality, which will probably decline with further experience. The optimal method of establishing continuity between the RV and PA remains to be demonstrated. They favor a direct anastomosis without use of the Lecompte maneuver or a conduit. They have serious concern regarding the development of subvalvar pulmonic stenosis postoperatively and believe that this may limit the application of this procedure in patients with side-by-side great arteries.

Assessment of ventricular function after Fontan procedure

Del Torso and associates[62] from Melbourne, Australia, evaluated 18 patients at a mean of 2.6 years after Fontan repair for tricuspid atresia (9 patients) or single ventricle (9 patients). RNA studies were performed at rest and during exercise. Abnormally low LVEF at rest was present in 8 of 18 by an equilibrium technique and 6 of 13 by first-pass studies. An abnormal response to exercise was found in 10 of 16 by gated and 8 of 12 by first-pass techniques. Only 2 patients by each RNA technique had both normal EF at rest and with exercise. There were 6 patients with an AV connection who were compared with 12 patients with an atrio-PA connection. Patients with an AV connection were similar in all respects except for a higher exercise EF value during exercise. These investigators present further evidence of abnormalities of LV function in patients after the Fontan procedure. The patients in the study did have repair at a mean age of 9.2 years. Further investigations are warranted to determine if an earlier age at repair with less duration of LV volume overload and chronic cyanosis and improved surgical techniques may improve these postoperative results.

Permanent pacing after Fontan procedure

Taliercio and colleagues[63] from Rochester, Minnesota, evaluated 15 patients who underwent a Fontan procedure between 4 and 31 years of age (mean, 16.5). Tricuspid atresia was present in 3, double-outlet right ventricle in 3, and univentricular heart in 9. Permanent pacing was instituted because of preexisting heart block in 6 (congenital in 5), postoperative heart block in 7, and postoperative sick sinus syndrome in 2. Pacemakers were implanted immediately postoperatively in 11 patients and between 12 and 57 months later in 4. All ventricular leads were epicardial, 4 atrial leads were transvenous endocardial and 1 was epicardial; a variety of pulse generators were employed. There were 3 late deaths at 4, 9, and 69 months postoperatively from CHF, in the presence of normally functioning pacing systems. The remaining 12 survivors were followed between 1 and 107 months (mean, 34) and there were 3 episodes of loss of ventricular capture because of chronic increased thresholds. When the indication for permanent pacing is present at the conclusion of a Fontan procedure, the investigators recommend intraoperative attachment of permanent ventricular epicarial leads, postoperative insertion of transvenous atrial electrodes if dual-chamber pacing is indicated, and the use of programmable pulse generators with high output capability.

Repair of truncus arteriosus

Di Donato and coworkers[64] from Rochester, Minnesota, reported their results with surgical repair of truncus arteriosus in 167 patients operated on between 1965 and 1982. Mean age at repair was 6 years and included 11 patients <1 year of age and 16 between 1 and 2 years. Moderate or severe truncal valve regurgitation was present in 62 (37%), and 59 (35%) had previous banding of either the main or branch pulmonary arteries. Factors related to hospital mortality were: age <2 years, postrepair PA/LV pressure ratio >0.5 for patients with 2 pulmonary arteries and >0.6 for patients with a single PA, and a postrepair RV/LV pressure ratio >0.8. Actuarial survival at 5 years was 84% and at 10 years, 69%. Reduced late survival was correlated with older age at operation, the presence of moderate or severe truncal valve regurgitation, lower QP/QS, and unilateral absence of a PA. Reoperation was required in 36 (30%) patients primarily for replacement of the RV-PA extracardiac conduit or for truncal valve replacement. The experience showed that truncal valve regurgitation progressed even after corrective operation, worsening in 28 (40%) of 70 patients recatheterized postoperatively. The investigators concluded that this anomaly should be electively repaired during the first 6 months of life. They recommended the use of an extracardiac conduit with a fresh antibiotic-sterilized aortic homograft valve. Improved late results remain dependent on development of methods to control or repair truncal valve incompetence and better extracardiac valved conduits.

Sharma and coworkers[65] from Melbourne, Australia, reviewed their experience with 23 patients who underwent repair of truncus arteriosus between 1979 and 1983. Nineteen had primary repair and 4, secondary repair after PA banding. Heterograft valved conduits were used in 21 patients and valveless tubes in 2 patients <1 month of age at repair. There were 4 hospital deaths, 2 among 3 patients <1 month, 0 among 9 between 1 and 6 months, 1 among 4 between 7 and 12 months, and 1 among 7 >12 months. Eight infants received ventilatory and inotropic support preoperatively because of their rapid deterioration due to cardiorespiratory failure and required semiurgent total corrections. The remaining 8 infants were electively ventilated preoperatively for 24 hours. PA pressure was monitored postoperatively and any patient who showed signs of a pulmonary hypertensive crisis was hyperventilated to keep the oxygen tension >100 mmHg and the carbon dioxide tension <30 mmHg. The 19 survivors were clinically well between 4 months and 4 years follow-up (mean, 29 months). Eight had postoperative cardiac catheterization studies and 2 had mild truncal valve regurgitation, which was present preoperatively; 1 with severe conduit stenosis underwent reoperation 12 months after initial repair. The investigators concluded that patients with truncus arteriosus who present with severe CHF during the first few days of life should be vigorously treated with inotropic support, diuretics, and ventilation, and after stabilization should undergo total correction. Those who have controllable CHF should undergo elective total correction at 2–3 months of age. They believe that preoperative ventilation with positive end-expiratory pressure (5–8 mmHg) is useful.

Repair of single ventricle with subaortic stenosis

Spontaneous narrowing or closure of the VSD in hearts with single- or double-inlet ventricle occurs with significant frequency and results in sub-pulmonic stenosis when the nondominant ventricle supports the PA, and subaortic stenosis, when it supports the aorta. In the latter group, pulmonic stenosis is usually absent and PA banding has been the most common initial procedure used to control CHF and to prevent the development of increased pulmonary vascular resistance. PA banding has been associated with acceler-ation of the development of subaortic obstruction, and this has worsened the results after either a modified Fontan procedure or a septation operation. Jonas and colleagues[66] from Boston, Massachusetts, described 3 patients, 1 with tricuspid atresia and TGA, 1 with mitral atresia, and 1 with double-inlet left ventricle. Each underwent PA banding at 3 days, 16 days, and 7 weeks of age. Repeat catheterization studies 10 days, 7 weeks, and 13 days postoperatively demonstrated the development of subaortic stenosis. A modi-fied Norwood procedure consisting of atrial septectomy, debanding, and transection of the main PA, end-to-side anastomoses of the proximal PA to the ascending aorta, and placement of a 4 mm systemic-PA shunt was suc-cessfully performed in each. The investigators believe it may be preferable to perform a modified Norwood procedure as the primary reoperation in any infant in whom it is suspected that a restrictive VSD may develop, which would result in subaortic stenosis. Although it is not precisely known how to predict which patients will have subaortic stenosis, the presence of coarcta-tion certainly increases the probability. If a PA band is placed, the child should be closely followed for the development of subaortic stenosis. Serial Dopplor echo studies and early catheterization should be performed at a maximum of 6 months in the absence of symptoms. If high pulmonary vas-cular resistance is present, the modified first stage Norwood procedure should be performed with debanding. If normal pulmonary resistance is present, a single stage physiologically corrective procedure should be done. They believe the modified Norwood operation is a viable surgical option for the management of subaortic obstruction in infants with single ventricle type malformations in whom primary performance of a Fontan-type procedure or septation operation are prohibited.

References

1. Marx GR, Allen HD, Goldberg SJ, Flint CJ: Trans-atrial septal velocity measurement by Doppler echocardiography in atrial septal defect: correlation with Qp:Qs ratio. Am J Cardiol 1985 (Apr); 55:1162–1167.
2. Ghisla RP, Hannon DW, Meyer RA, Kaplan S: Spontaneous closure of isolated secundum atrial defects in infants: an echocardiographic study. Am Heart J 1985 (June); 109:1327–1333.
3. Bull C, Rigby ML, Shinebourne EA: Should management of complete atrioventricular canal defect be influenced by coexistent Down syndrome? Lancet 1985 (May 18); 1:1147–1149.
4. McGrath LB, Kirklin JW, Soto B, Bargeron LM Jr: Secondary left atrioventricular valve re-placement in atrioventricular septal (AV canal) defect: a method to avoid left ventricular outflow tract obstruction. J Thorac Cardiovasc Surg 1985 (Apr); 89:632–635.

5. HAGLER DJ, EDWARDS WD, SEWARD JB, TAJIK AJ: Standardized nomenclature of the ventricular septal defect with applications for two-dimensional echocardiography. Mayo Clin Proc 1985 (Nov); 60:741–752.

6. ORTIZ E, ROBINSON PJ, DEANFIELD JE, FRANKLIN R, MACARTNEY FJ, WYSE RKH: Localisation of ventricular septal defects by simultaneous display of superimposed colour Doppler and cross sectional echocardiographic images. Br Heart J 1985 (July); 54:53–60.

7. OTTERSTAD JE, SIMONSEN S, ERIKSSEN J: Hemodynamic findings at rest and during mild supine exercise in adults with isolated, uncomplicated ventricular septal defects. Circulation 1985 (Apr); 71:650–662.

8. BEERMAN LB, PARK SC, FISCHER DR, FRICKER FJ, MATTHEWS RA, NECHES WH, LENOX CC, ZUBER-BUHLER Jr: Ventricular septal defect associated with aneurysm of the membranous septum. J Am Coll Cardiol 1985 (Jan); 5:118–123.

9. JUANEDA E, GITTENBERGER DE GROOT A, OPPENHEIMER, DEKKER A, HAWORTH SG: Pulmonary arterial development in infants with large perimembranous ventricular septal defects associated with overriding of the aortic valve. Int J Cardiol 1985 (Mar); 7:223–230.

10. LANGE PE, ONNASCH DW, HEINTZEN PH: Valvular pulmonary stenosis. Natural history and right ventricular function in infants and children. Eur Heart J 1985 (Aug); 6:706–709.

11. TROWITZSCH E, COLAN SD, SANDERS SP: Two dimensional echocardiographic evaluation of right ventricular size and function in newborns with severe right ventricular outflow tract obstruction. J Am Cardiol 1985 (Aug); 6:388–393.

12. COBANOGLU A, METZDORFF MT, PINSON CW, GRUNKEMEIER GL, SUNDERLAND CO, STARR A: Valvotomy for pulmonary atresia with intact ventricular septum. A disciplined approach to achieve a functioning right ventricle. J Thorac Cardiovasc Surg 1985 (Apr); 89:482–490.

13. KAY PH, ROSS DN: Fifteen years' experience with the aortic homograft: the conduit of choice for right ventricular outflow tract reconstruction. Ann Thorac Surg 1985 (Oct); 40:360–364.

14. LIAO T-K, EDWARD DW, JULRESD TR, PUGA FJ, DANIELSON GK, FELDT RH: Pulmonary blood supply in patients with pulmonary atresia and ventricular septal defect. J Am Coll Cardiol 1985 6:1343–1350.

15. MCCAUGHAN BC, DANIELSON GK, DRISCOLL DJ, MCGOON DC: Tetralogy of Fallot with absent pulmonary valve. Early and late results of surgical treatment. J Thorac Cardiovasc Surg 1985 (Feb); 89:280–287.

16. ZHAO HX, MILLER DC, REITZ BA, SHUMWAY NE: Surgical repair of tetralogy of Fallot. Long-term follow-up with particular emphasis on late death and reoperation. J Thorac Cardiovasc Surg 1985 (Feb); 89:204–220.

17. RITTENHOUSE EA, MANSFIELD PB, HALL DG, HERNDON SP, JONES TK, KAWABORI I, STEVENSON JG, FRENCH JW, STAMM SJ: Tetralogy of Fallot: selective staged management. J Thorac Cardiovasc Surg 1985 (May); 89:772–779.

18. ABDULALI SA, SILVERTON NP, YAKIREVICH VS, IONESCU MI: Right ventricular outflow tract reconstruction with a bovine pericardial monocusp patch. Long-term clinical and hemodynamic evaluation. J Thorac Cardiovasc Surg 1985 (May); 89:764–771.

19. BOVE EL, KAVEY RW, BYRUM CJ, SONDHEIMER HM, BLACKMAN MS, THOMAS FD: Improved right ventricular function following late pulmonary valve replacement for residual pulmonary insufficiency or stenosis. J Thorac Cardiovasc Surg 1985 (July); 90:50–55.

20. DEANFIELD J, MCKENNA W, ROWLAND E: Local abnormalities of right ventricular depolarisation after repair of tetralogy of Fallot: a basis for ventricular arrhythmia. Am J Cardiol 1985; 55:522–525.

21. DEAL BJ, CHIN AJ, SANDERS P, NORWOOD WI, CASTANEDA AR: Subziphoid two-dimensional echocardiographic identification of tricuspid valve abnormalities in transposition of the great arteries with ventricular septal defect. Am J Cardiol 1985; 55:1146–1151.

22. OKUDA H, NAKAZAWA M, IMAI Y, KUROSAWA H, TAKANASHI Y, HOSHINO S, TAKAO A: Comparison of ventricular function after Senning and Jatene procedures for complete transposition of the great arteries. Am J Cardiol 1985; 55:530–534.

23. HURWITZ RA, CALDWELL RL, GIROD DA, MAHONY L, BROWN J, KING H: Ventricular function in transposition of the great arteries: evaluation by radionuclide angiocardiography. Am Heart J 1985 (Sept); 110:600–605.

24. CRUPI G, PILLAI R, PARENZAN L, LINCOLN C: Surgical treatment of subpulmonary obstruction in transposition of the great arteries by means of a left ventricular-pulmonary arterial conduit. Late results and further considerations. J Thorac Cardiovasc Surg 1985 (June); 89:907–913.

25. Duster MC, Bink-Boelkens MTE, Wampler D, Gillette PC, McNamara DG, Cooley DA: Long-term follow-up of dysrhythmias following the Mustard procedure. Am Heart J 1985 (June); 109:1323–1326.

26. Arensman FW, H-Sievers H, Lnage P, Radley-Smith R, Bernhard A, Heintzen P, Yacoub MH: Assessment of coronary and aortic anastomoses after anatomic correction of transposition of the great arteries. J Thorac Cardiovasc Surg 1985 (Oct); 90:597–604.

27. Kveselis DA, Rocchini AP, Rosenthal A, Crowley DC, Dick M, Snider R, Moorehead C: Hemodynamic determinants of exercise-induced ST-segment depression in children with valvar aortic stenosis. Am J Cardiol 1985 (Apr); 55:1133–1139.

28. Fifer MA, Borow KM, Colan SD, Lorell BH: Early diastolic left ventricular function in children and adults with aortic stenosis. J Am Coll Cardiol 1985 (May); 5:1147–1154.

29. Freedom R, Pelech A, Brand A, Vogel M, Olley PM, Smallhorn J, Rowe RD: Progressive nature of subaortic stenosis in congenital heart disease. Int J Cardiol 1985 (June); 8:137–143.

30. Pellegrino A, Deverall PB, Anderson RH, Smith A, Wilkinson JL, Russo P, Girod DA, Tynan M: Aortic coarctation in the first three months of life. An anatomopathological study with respect to treatment. J Thorac Cardiovasc Surg 1985 (Jan); 89:121–127.

31. Cobanoglu A, Teply JF, Grunkemeier GL, Sunderland CO, Starr A: Coarctation of the aorta in patients younger than three months. A critique of the subclavian flap operation. J Thorac Cardiovasc Surg 1985 (Jan); 89:128–135.

32. Korfer R, Meyer H, Kleikamp G, Bircks W: Early and late results after resection and end-to-end anastomosis of coarctation of the thoracic aorta in early infancy. J Thorac Cardiovasc Surg 1985 (Apr); 89:616–622.

33. Metzdorff MT, Cabanoglu A, Grunkemeier GL, Sunderland CO, Starr A: Influence of age at operation on late results with subclavian flap aortoplasty. J Thorac Cardiovasc Surg 1985 (Feb); 89:235–241.

34. Teles de Mendonca J, Carvalho MR, Costa RK, Filho EF: Coarctation of the aorta: a new surgical technique. J Thorac Cardiovasc Surg 1985 (Sept); 90:445–447.

35. Brown JW, Fiore AC, King H: Isthmus flap aortoplasty: an alternative to subclavian flap aortoplasty for long-segment coarctation of the aorta in infants. Ann Thorac Surg 1985 (Sept); 40:274–279.

36. Gidding SS, Rocchini AP, Moorehead C, Schork MA, Rosenthal A: Increased forearm vascular reactivity in patients with hypertension after repair of coarctation. Circulation 1985 (Mar); 495–499.

37. Gidding SS, Rocchini AP, Beekman R, Szpunar CA, Moorehead C, Behrendt D, Rosenthal A: Therapeutic effect of propranolol on paradoxical hypertension after repair of coarctation of the aorta. N Engl J Med 1985 (May 9); 312:1224–1228.

38. Sweeney MS, Walker WE, Duncan JM, Hallman GL, Livesay JJ, Cooley DA: Reoperation for aortic coarctation: techniques, results, and indications for various approaches. Ann Thorac Surg 1985 (July); 40:46–49.

39. Mahoney LT, Coryell KG, Lauer M: The newborn transitional circulation: a two-dimensional Doppler echocardiographic study. J Am Cardiol 1985 (Sept); 6:623–629.

40. Silverman NH, Kleinman CS, Rudolph AM, Copel JA, Weinstein EM, Enderlein MA, Golbus M: Fetal atrioventricular valve insufficiency associated with nonimmune hydrops: a two-dimensional echocardiographic and pulse Doppler ultrasound study. Circulation 1985 (Oct); 72:825–832.

41. Rose V, Gold RJM, Lindsay G, Allen M: A possible increase in the instance of congenital heart defects among the offspring of affected parents. J Am Cardiol 1985 (Aug); 6:376–382.

42. Lenox C, Hashida Y, Anderson RH, Hubbard JD: Conduction tissue anomalies in absence of the right superior caval vein. Int J Cardiol 1985 (July); 8:251–260.

43. Rice MJ, Seward JB, Edwards WD, Hagler DJ, Danielson GK, Puga FJ, Tajik AJ: Straddling atrioventricular valve: two dimensional echocardiographic diagnosis, classification and surgical implications. Am J Cardiol 1985 (Feb); 55:505–513.

44. Robinson PJ, Kumpeng V, Macartney FJ: Cross sectional echocardiographic and angiocardiographic correlation in criss-cross heart. Br Heart J 1985 (July); 54:61–67.

45. Borow KM, Colan SD, Neumann A: Altered left ventricular mechanics in patients with valvular aortic stenosis and coarctation of the aorta: effects on systolic performance and late outcome. Circulation 1985 (Sept); 72:515–522.

46. Smith LDR, Charalmbopoulos C, Rigby ML, Pallides S, Hunter S, Lincoln C, Shinebourne E: Discrete sub-aortic stenosis and ventricular septal defect. Arch Dis Child 1985 (Mar); 60:196–199.

47. MARX GR, ALLEN HD, GOLDBERG SJ: Doppler echocardiographic estimation of systolic pulmonary artery pressure in pediatric patients with interventricular communications. J Am Coll Cardiol 1985; 6:1132–1137.

48. NAKAE S, IMAI Y, HARADA Y, SAWATARI K, KAWADA M, TAKANASHI Y, ISHIHARA K, HASHIMOTO A, HAYASHI H, KOYANAGI H, KANAYA M, NAKAZAWA M, TAKAI A: Assessment of left ventricular function before and after Fontan's operation for the correction of tricuspid atresia. Heart Vessels 1985; 1:83–88.

49. KARPAWICH PP, BUSH CP, ANTILLON JR, AMATO JJ, MARBEY ML, AGARWAL KC: Modified Blalock-Taussig shunt in infants and young children. Clinical and catheterization assessment. J Thorac Cardiovasc Surg 1985 (Feb); 89:275–279.

50. PACIFICO AD, MANDKE NV, McGRATH LB, COLVIN EV, BINI RM, BARGERON LM JR: Repair of congenital pulmonary venous stenosis with living autologous atrial tissue. J Thorac Cardiovasc Surg 1985 (Apr); 89:604–609.

51. VARGAS FJ, KREUTZER GO: A surgical technique for correction of total anomalous pulmonary venous drainage. J Thorac Cardiovasc Surg 1985 (Sept); 90:410–413.

52. YOKOTA M, MURAOKA R, AOSHIMA M, NOMOTO S, SHIRAISHI Y, KYOKU I, KITANO M, SHIMADA I, NAKANO H, UEDA K, SAITO A: Modified Blalock-Taussig shunt following long-term administration of prostaglandin E_1 for ductus dependent neonates with cyanotic congenital heart disease. J Thorac Cardiovasc Surg 1985 (Sept); 90:399–403.

53. JONAS RA, CASTANEDA AR, FREED MD: Normothermic caval inflow occlusion. Application to operations for congenital heart disease. J Thorac Cardiovasc Surg 1985 (May); 89:780–786.

54. HOPKINS RA, ARMSTRONG BE, SERWER GA, PETERSON RJ, OLDHAM HN: Physiological rationale for a bidirectional cavopulmonary shunt. A versatile complement to the Fontan principle. J Thoracic Cardiovas Surg 1985 (Sept); 90:391–398.

55. HENLING CE, CARMICHAEL MJ, KEATS AS, COOLEY DA: Cardiac operation for congenital heart disease in children of Jehovah's Witnesses. J Thorac Cardiovasc Surg 1985 (June); 89:914–920.

56. OH JK, HOLMES DR JR, HAYES DL, PORTER CJ, DANIELSON GK: Cardiac arrhythmias in patients with surgical repair of Ebstein's anomaly. J Am Coll Cardiol 1985; 6:1351–1357.

57. LEE CN, DANIELSON GK, SCHAFF HV, PUGA FJ, MAIR DD: Surgical treatment of double-orifice mitral valve in atrioventricular canal defects. Experience in 25 patients. J Thorac Cardiovasc Surg 1985 (Nov); 90:700–705.

58. McGRATH LB, KIRKLIN JW, BLACKSTONE EH, PACIFICO AD, KIRKLIN JK, BARGERON LM JR: Death and other events after cardiac repair in discordant atrioventricular connection. J Thorac Cardiovasc Surg 1985 (Nov); 90:711–728.

59. KRON IL, RHEUBAN KS, JOOB AW, JEDEIKEN R, MENTZER RM, CARPENTER MA, NOLAN SP: Baffle obstruction following the Mustard operation: cause and treatment. Ann Thorac Surg 1985 (Feb); 89:112–115.

60. MAZZUCCO A, FAGGIAN G, STELLIN G, BORTOLOTTI U, LIVI U, RIZZOLI G, GALLUCCI V: Surgical management of double-outlet right ventricle. J Thorac Cardiovasc Surg 1985 (July); 90:29–34.

61. KANTER KR, ANDERSON RH, LINCOLN C, RIGBY ML, SHINEBOURNE EA: Anatomic correction for complete transposition and double-outlet right ventricle. J Thorac Cardiovasc Surg 1985 (Nov); 90:690–699.

62. DEL TORSO S, KELLY MJ, KALFF V, VENABLES AW: Radionuclide assessment of ventricular contraction at rest and during exercise following the Fontan procedure for either tricuspid atresia or single ventricle. Am J Cardiol 1985 (Apr 15); 55:1127–1132.

63. TALIERCIO CP, VLIETSTRA RE, McGOON MD, PORTER CJ, OSBORN MJ, DANIELSON GK: Permanent cardiac pacing after the Fontan procedure. J Thorac Cardiovasc Surg 1985 (Sept); 90:414–419.

64. DI DONATO RM, FYFE DA, PUGA FJ, DANIELSON GK, RITTER DG, EDWARDS WD, McGOON DC: Fifteen-year experience with surgical repair of truncus arteriosus. J Thorac Cardiovasc Surg 1985 (Mar); 89:414–422.

65. SHARMA AK, BRAWN WJ, MEE RBB: Truncus arteriosus. Surgical approach. J Thorac Cardiovasc Surg 1985 (July); 90:45–49.

66. JONAS RA, CASTANEDA AR, LANG P: Single ventricle (single- or double-inlet) complicated by subaortic stenosis: surgical options in infancy. Ann Thorac Surg 1985 (Apr); 39:361–366.

Congestive Heart Failure

Mechanism of fatigue

Since exertional fatigue is a major limiting symptom in patients with CHF, Wilson and coworkers[1] from Philadelphia, Pennsylvania, investigated the metabolic basis of fatigue using gated nuclear magentic resonance (NMR) spectroscopy to compare inorganic phosphate (Pi), phosphocreatine (PCr) and pH levels, and fatigue (1–4+) during mild forearm exercise in 8 normal men and 9 men with CHF. Wrist flexion every 5 seconds for 7 minutes was performed at 1, 2, and 3 J (average power output, 0.2, 0.4, and 0.6 W). In both groups linear relations were noted between power output and Pi/PCr; the slope of this relation was used to compare PCr depletion patterns. At rest, both groups had similar Pi/PCr ratios and pH. In normal subjects exercise resulted in a progressive increase in Pi/PCr, a reduction in pH only at 0.6 W, and moderate fatigue. In patients with CHF exercise resulted in significantly greater fatigue at all workloads. This was associated with twice as rapid an increase in Pi/PCr and greater acidosis. These data suggested exertional fatigue in patients with CHF may result from greater than normal PCr depletion and/or acidosis in the working muscle and thus serial measurements with NMR may provide a unique tool for evaluation of fatigue and oxygen delivery in patients with CHF.

Associated ventricular arrhythmias

Chakko and Gheorghiade[2] from Salem, Virginia, carried out on 43 patients receiving maximal medical therapy for severe chronic CHF from dilated cardiomyopathy (28 ischemic, 15 idiopathic) and VPC on 12-lead ECG a baseline 24-hour ambulatory ECG monitoring. Complex VPC (multiform, repetitive—couplets, R-on-T phenomenon) and asymptomatic, nonsustained VT were present in 38 patients (88%) and 22 patients (51%), respectively. Twenty-three patients (group I) were placed on long-term antiarrhythmic therapy (20 patients received procainamide and the remaining, quinidine); 20 patients (group II) did not receive antiarrhythmic therapy. At baseline, no significant differences between the 2 groups were noted for age, functional class, type of cardiomyopathy, medical therapy for CHF, cardiothoracic ratio, RNA EF, or rate and complexity of ventricular arrhythmias on 24-hour ambulatory ECG tracings. At a mean follow-up period of 16 months (range, 1–37), there were 16 deaths, 10 (63%) of which were sudden and unexpected. No significant differences in the incidence of sudden death and overall mortality were noted between the 2 groups. Among patients with nonsustained VT, those who died suddenly had a lower mean LVEF (0.15 ± 0.01) compared with survivors (0.23 ± 0.02). It was concluded that 1) patients with severe CHF have a high mortality from both sudden and nonsudden cardiac death; 2) incidence of complex VPC is high; 3) sudden death is more common when LV function is severely compromised; and 4) therapeutic plasma levels of conventional antiarrhythmic drugs do not appear to protect this group of patients from dying.

With intact LV function

Clinical CHF is traditionally associated with significant LV systolic dysfunction. Over a 1-year period, Soufer and associates[3] from New Haven, Connecticut, identified 58 patients with CHF and intact systolic function (LVEF 62 ± 11%). An objective clinical-radiographic CHF score was used to document the clinical impression. Based on RNA evaluation of peak filling rate, 38% of these patients were found to have a significant abnormality in diastolic function as measured by peak filling rate (<2.50 end-diastolic volume/s). An additional 24% of the patients had probable diastolic dysfunction with borderline abnormal peak filling rate measurements (2.5–3.0 end-diastolic volume/s). The disease states most frequently associated with CHF and intact systolic function were CAD and systemic hypertension. During a 3-month sampling period, 42% of patients with clinical diagnosis of CHF referred to the nuclear cardiology laboratory were found to have intact systolic function; thus, intact systolic function often occurs in patients with clinical CHF. Abnormal diastolic function is the most frequently encountered mechanism for the occurrence of CHF.

Responses to exercise

Several studies have shown full correlations between exercise tolerance and measurements of LV function during rest in patients with CHF. To evaluate further the determinants of exercise tolerance and their relation to prognosis, Szlachcic and associates[4] from San Francisco, California, performed rest and exercise hemodynamic measurements and blood pool scintigraphy in 27 patients with CHF. All patients were treated with digitalis and diuretic drugs, but not vasodilator drugs. Exercise capacity was assessed by maximal oxygen consumption (VO_2max) during upright bicycle ergometry. Both RV and LVEF were measured by RNA techniques, and arterial, RA and PA pressures, cardiac output, and derived hemodynamic indexes were determined. As a group, patients with severely impaired exercise tolerance (group 1, VO_2max <10 ml/min/kg) had significantly higher rest PA wedge and RA pressures (30 ± 4 -vs- 23 ± 6 and 12 ± 4 -vs- 7 ± 2 mmHg, respectively) than those with a VO_2max of 10–18 ml/min/kg (group 2). They also had a lower LV and RVEF (16 ± 4% -vs- 21 ± 4% and 19 ± 12% -vs- 27 ± 7%, respectively). However, overlap among individual patients was considerable, and only PA wedge pressure at rest correlated significantly with VO$_2$max. During exercise, patients in group 1 had lower heart rates, stroke indexes and cardiac indexes (117 ± 10 -vs- 133 ± 14 beats/min, 25 ± 5 -vs- 31 ± 7 ml/m^2, and 2.8 ± 0.5 -vs- 3.9 ± 0.6 L/min/m^2, respectively), and higher RA pressures (18 ± 4 -vs- 11 ± 5 mmHg). Both exercise heart rate and cardiac index correlated significantly with VO$_2$max. Patients in group 1 had a significantly higher mortality rate during the subsequent year compared with those in group 2 (77 -vs- 21%). Thus, exercise tolerance in CHF appears to be most closely related to the patients' ability to increase their heart rate and cardiac index. Measurements of cardiac function at rest, although worse in patients with severely impaired exercise tolerance as a group, correlate poorly with exercise VO$_2$max in individual subjects. Nonetheless, exercise capacity provided important prognostic information, in that patients with poor tolerance had a significantly higher mortality rate during the first year of follow-up.

To determine what influences the LV volume and EF response to exercise, Shen and associates[5] from Sydney, Australia, studied 24 patients with chronic CHF (13 with dilated cardiomyopathy [DC], CHF-DC group; 11 previous AMI [MI], CHF-MI group), and 6 age-matched control subjects who underwent simultaneous hemodynamic monitoring and radionuclide ventriculography during semiupright bicycle exercise. Both CHF groups had similar hemodynamic values, LV volumes, and EF at rest. Exercise hemodynamics were also similar, but LV volume and EF responses to exercise were different. In the CHF-DC group LV end-diastolic volume increased by 15% during exercise, significantly less than the 44% increase in the CHF-MI group. During exercise, EF increased in the CHF-DC group, but did not change in the CHF-MI group because of a larger increase in end-systolic volume. The slope of mean PA wedge pressure-LV end-diastolic volume relation was steeper in the CHF-DC group than in the CHF-MI group. The study suggests that LV volume and EF response to exercise in patients with CHF depends on the origin of the CHF.

Francis and coworkers[6] from Minneapolis, Minnesota, evaluated 10 healthy normal volunteers and 31 patients with chronic clinical class II and III CHF during upright maximal bicycle exercise to compare response of the sympathetic nervous system to exercise in normal subjects and patients with CHF. Eighteen of the 31 patients had a nonischemic cardiomyopathy and 13 had ischemic cardiomyopathy. The LVEF at rest was 24 ± 10% (+SD) in the group with CHF. Heart rate, systolic BP, myocardial oxygen consumption, and plasma norepinephrine levels were measured at rest and throughout exercise. When the data were evaluated as a function of percent peak maximal myocardial oxygen consumption, patients with CHF had a diminished response of plasma norepinephrine to exercise, indicating a blunting of sympathetic stimulation. The reduction in plasma norepinephrine increases was accompanied by an attenuated heart rate and BP response to exercise in patients with CHF. These data suggest that patients with severe CHF have a relative attentuation of sympathetic drive during exercise. The data are compatible with the hypothesis that patients with CHF have a generalized inability to activate maximally the sympathetic nervous system with stress.

Weber and Janicki[7] from Chicago, Illinois, studied 63 patients (mean age, 53 ± 12 years) having chronic, stable CHF to determine the reproducibility of the response of cardiac output and mixed venous lactate concentration when exercise tests are repeated the same or the next day and to evaluate the influence of the inotropic agent, amrinone, on alterations in lactate concentration. Treadmill exercise was used in this study and recordings of intravascular pressures, cuff BP, heart rate, and cardiac output were obtained. The data obtained demonstrate that 1) cardiac output and mixed venous lactate concentrations with similar degrees of exercise are reproducible when assessed either the same or the next day; 2) when exercise cardiac output is increased by oral amrinone therapy, the increase in lactate concentration is delayed to higher levels of muscular work; and 3) submaximal anaerobic exercise that is symptom limited is associated with an increase in lactate concentration. Thus, the lactate response and anaerobic threshold determined should be useful in patients in assessing the severity of chronic stable CHF and its response to pharmacologic intervention.

RVEF, but not LVEF, correlates with exercise capacity in patients with LV failure, suggesting an important role of the pulmonary circulation. Franciosa and associates[8] from Little Rock, Arkansas, measured hemodynamics at rest and during bicycle exercise to symptomatic maximum in 41 patients with chronic LV failure. Maximal oxygen consumption averaged only 13 ± 5 ml/min/kg. PA wedge pressure increased from 22 ± 8–36 ± 9 mmHg during exercise, whereas PA mean pressure increased from 32 ± 11–50 ± 13 mmHg. Resting cardiac index and resting systemic arterial mean pressure did not correlate with maximal oxygen consumption, which, however, did correlate with PA wedge pressure, PA mean pressure, and total pulmonary resistance. Maximal oxygen consumption did not correlate with resting systemic vascular resistance or resting pulmonary vascular resistance. During exercise, total pulmonary resistance remained unchanged at 6.5 ± 3.8 U, but systemic vascular resistance decreased significantly. The relation between total pulmonary resistance and exercise capacity and the failure of total pulmonary resistance to decrease during exercise suggest that RV afterload may be an important determinant of exercise capacity in patients with chronic LV failure.

Few data are available on the consequences of isometric exercise in patients with chronic advanced CHF in whom both hemodynamic and neurohumoral status is significantly altered. Elkayam and colleagues[9] from Los Angeles, California, evaluated the hemodynamic effects of isometric exercise in 53 patients with CHF and compared them with those found in 10 normal subjects. In both groups, isometric exercise increased heart rate and BP. Systemic resistance increased in patients with CHF but not in normal subjects. Cardiac index and stroke volume increased mildly but not significantly in the normal subjects and had a significant decrease in patients with CHF. Mean PA wedge pressure increased in patients with CHF from 26–30 mmHg. Although no significant change was found in the mean value for stroke work index, the individual changes were variable, with marked decrease (−15%) in 17 of the patients. This hemodynamic deterioration could not be predicted from resting hemodynamics, LVEF, or functional classification. Isometric exercise resulted in no significant change in circulatory catecholamine levels or plasma renin concentration in 10 normal subjects. In the patients with CHF renin and epinephrine also did not change during isometric exercise, but norephinephrine levels increased significantly. No correlation was found between changes in hormonal levels and any of the hemodynamic changes during static exercise. The investigators concluded that in patients with chronic CHF, isometric exercise can lead to a significant increase in LV outflow resistance and filling pressure and to a decrease in cardiac performance. This form of exercise in CHF results in a consistent elevation in norephinephrine levels, but there is no correlation between changes in plasma levels and in hemodynamic values. Finally, there is considerable individual variation in the hemodynamic response, with a significant deterioration in cardiac performance in some patients, which cannot be separated by resting hemodynamic values, LVEF, or clinical status.

TREATMENT

Amrinone

A number of uncontrolled studies have indicated that oral administration of amrinone, a phosphodiesterase inhibitor with potent positive inotropic effects in experimental preparations, may be beneficial in patients with chronic CHF. Massie and colleagues[10] from San Francisco, California, designed a multicenter trial to evaluate prospectively clinical response and change in exercise tolerance during 12-weeks of amrinone therapy in a double-blind, placebo-controlled protocol. Ninety-nine patients with New York Heart Association (NYHA) functional class III or IV CHF on digitalis and diuretics, of whom 31 were also receiving captopril, were enrolled. After baseline clinical assessment and determination of exercise tolerance, radionuclide LVEF, and roentgenographic cardiothoracic ratio, patients were randomly assigned to receive amrinone or placebo, beginning at 1.5 mg/kg 3 times daily and increasing to a maximum dosage of 200 mg 3 times daily. After 12 weeks of therapy or at the last blinded evaluation in patients who did not complete this protocol, there were no significant differences from baseline values between treatment with amrinone or placebo with regard to symptoms, NYHA functional class, LVEF, cardiothoracic ratio, frequency and severity of ventricular ectopic activity, or mortality. Exercise tolerance improved significantly from baseline by 37% in patients on amrinone and 35% in patients on placebo, but there was no significant difference between treatments (Fig. 8-1). Adverse effects were significantly more frequent and more severe on amrinone, occurring in 83% of patients and necessitating withdrawal in 34%. Downward adjustment of amrinone dosage because of side effects was responsible for a significantly lower mean total daily dose of 355 -vs- 505 mg for placebo. These findings indicate that oral administration of amrinone is not clinically effective in patients with chronic CHF, in part because of frequent adverse effects. Of interest was the increase in exercise tolerance in patients continuing on captopril, whether given amrinone or placebo, which was particularly striking and may have represented a further response to captopril, since maximum improvement in exercise tolerance with captopril may take many months to occur.

Captopril and enalapril

Chatterjee and associates[11] in a multicenter cooperative study evaluated the acute hemodynamic effects, long-term clinical efficacy, and safety of the oral angiotensin-converting enzyme inhibitor, captopril, in 124 patients with CHF resistant to digitalis and diuretics. The cardiac status of most patients was deteriorating before study. Favorable acute hemodynamic effects consistently occurred with captopril. Maximal mean percentage increases in cardiac index, stroke index, and stroke work index were, respectively, 35, 44, and 34%. Systemic and pulmonary vascular resistances each were decreased by approximately 40%, as were the filling pressures of the right and left sides of the heart. Infusion of nitroprusside in some of the same patients to an endpoint of a PA wedge pressure of 12–18 mmHg (equivalent to that after capto-

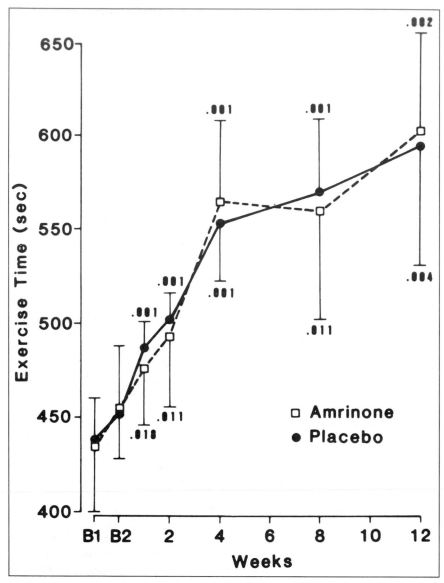

Fig. 8-1.   Mean and SEM for exercise times in the cohort of patients who completed the 12-week blinded trial (41 placebo, 27 amrinone). The 2 baseline values (B1 and B2) and the significance levels refer to changes from the mean of these 2 in both the palcebo- and amrinone-treated groups. There were no significant differences between treatments. Reproduced with permission from Massie et al.[10]

pril) revealed no significant difference in the effect of either drug on the other hemodynamic parameters. Recatheterization after 8 weeks of captopril therapy revealed sustained hemodynamic changes. Significant and sustained improvements in clinical status were observed in most patients as measured by changes in New York Heart Association (NYHA) functional classification and exercise tolerance times. Seventy-nine percent of patients for whom there were adequate NYHA class data improved; 20% remained unchanged and 1% deteriorated. Those patients who had both pretreatment and post-treatment exercise stress testing had a highly significant mean increase in exercise tolerance times of 34% (317 ± 32 seconds pretreatment to 425 ± 34 seconds, final measurement). There was no evidence of tachyphylaxis over an 18-month period. Survival rates at 6, 12, 18, and 24 months were 79, 63, and 58%, respectively. Cardiothoracic ratios showed a significant decrease from a mean of 0.60–0.57 at 2 months. All patients with hypokalemia at entry and all but 1 with hyponatremia attained normal values rapidly on captopril therapy. Captopril was generally well tolerated, although hypotension caused withdrawal of the drug in 6% of patients. The results suggest a useful role for captopril in chronic CHF.

Shaw and associates[12] from Edinburgh, UK, measured plasma free captopril concentrations and hemodynamic responses to captopril in 20 patients with severe chronic CHF secondary to CAD in 13 patients and to cardiomyopathy, type not specified, in 7 patients. A 25 mg oral dose of captopril produced a 36% reduction in systemic vascular resistance, with individual responses bearing from 13–64%. Mean systemic pressure decreased by 20% and cardiac output increased 28%. The absorption of captopril was rapid. Peak plasma free captopril concentration occurred at 45 minutes after the dose and was followed by a smaller second peak. Peak plasma free captopril concentrations varied more than 20-fold but did not correlate with the maximal reduction in systemic vascular resistance. Elimination half-life was 7 hours. Fourteen patients were restudied after 1–2 months of captopril treatment and 12 had symptomatic benefit. There was a sustained improvement in hemodynamic state and in noninvasive indices of myocardial function. During long-term treatment, the predose plasma free captopril concentration correlated well with dosage, but steady state captopril concentrations did not show a significant relation with hemodynamic response. On a dosage regimen of 25–50 mg 3 times daily, the morning predose plasma free captopril concentration correlated well with dosage, but steady state captopril concentrations did not show a significant relation with hemodynamic response. On a dosage regimen of 25–50 mg 3 times daily, the morning predose plasma free captopril concentration and plasma renin activity were relatively low and suggested that maximal inhibition of the renin-angiotensin system was not maintained throughout the dosage interval.

Wilson and colleagues[13] from Philadelphia, Pennsylvania, studied 12 patients with CHF to determine whether inadequate perfusion to working skeletal muscle is due to the accumulation of angiotensin II and subsequent limitation in arteriolar dilation. Captopril was utilized to test these relations, and leg blood flow, leg vascular resistance, leg oxygen consumption, and leg lactate release during maximal upright bicycle were measured. The data obtained demonstrate that captopril decreased leg resistance at rest (258 ± 115–173 ± 67 U) and maximal exercise (68 ± 69–45 ± 29 U) and also decreased systemic vascular resistance. Maximal exercise duration and leg oxygen consumption were unchanged and at identical peak exercise work times, there was no improvement in leg blood flow or leg lactate release. These data indicate that during exercise in patients with CHF, angiotensin II does not interfere importantly with blood flow to working skeletal muscle.

Packer and coworkers[14] from New York City evaluated the efficacy of captopril in 75 patients with severe CHF to test the hypothesis that changes in pulmonary vascular resistance during long-term vasodilator therapy influence exercise capacity in patients with CHF. Patients were grouped according to the relative changes in pulmonary and systemic vascular resistance during long-term therapy. Patients in group I (n = 24) had greater decreases in pulmonary arteriolar resistance than in systemic vascular resistance after captopril therapy. In contrast, patients in group II had predominant systemic vasodilatation. Patients in group I had greater increases in cardiac index, stroke volume index, and LV stroke work index, but less marked decreases in mean systemic arterial pressure than did patients in group II. Patients in group I had greater decreases in mean PA and mean RA pressure than did patients in group II. Plasma renin activity was higher and serum sodium concentration was lower in patients in group II than in group I. Patients in both groups improved clinically after 1–3 months, but symptomatic hypotension occurred more frequently in group II patients (36 -vs- 8%). These data indicate that alterations in the pulmonary circulation influence RV and LV performance during treatment with captopril in patients with severe CHF.

To test the hypothesis that intravenous enalapril is a useful pharmacologic probe of the renin-angiotensin system, Kubo and associates[15] from New York City administered enalapril intravenously to 9 patients with severe chronic CHF. This produced abrupt and complete blockade of converting enzyme, with peak effect occurring at 30 minutes, as reflected by increases of plasma renin activity (from 17 ± 6–87 ± 23 ng/ml/hour) and decreases of plasma aldosterone levels (from 46 ± 14–25 ± 6 ng/dl). With reduction of angiotensin II-mediated vasoconstriction, systemic vascular resistance decreased markedly (from $1,974 \pm 233$–$1,400 \pm 136$ dyne s cm^{-5}) and cardiac index was improved (from 1.88 ± 0.9–2.20 ± 0.21 L/min/m^2). The time course of angiotensin II levels suggested that the lack of a cumulative effect from additive doses of intravenous enalapril was a reflection of complete inhibition of converting enzyme. One patient did not respond to enalapril; despite comparable hemodynamic severity of CHF, the renin-angiotensin system was not activated in this patient. Thus, intravenous enalapril is capable of rapid and complete inhibition of converting enzyme for the accurate assessment of angiotensin II-mediated vasoconstriction in patients with severe CHF.

Franciosa and coworkers[6] from Little Rock, Arkansas, utilized enalapril or placebo with digoxin and diuretic drugs in 17 patients with chronic CHF to determine its efficacy in the treatment of CHF. In randomized, double-blind fashion, 9 patients received enalapril and 8 received placebo. Cardiac dimensions and function improved slightly but insignificantly in both groups. Treadmill exercise duration increased from a mean value of 9.1 ± 3.2–12.0 ± 3.5 minutes during enalapril, but was unchanged during a placebo period (Fig. 8-2). In addition, maximal oxygen consumption also increased during enalapril therapy, but it was unchanged during placebo treatment. Clinical functional class improved during enalapril treatment, but there was no change during the period of placebo administration. No significant side effects from enalapril therapy were observed. These data suggest that enalapril is a clinically effective and relatively safe new angiotensin-converting enzyme inhibitor for the treatment of CHF.

The long-term efficacy of enalapril was studied by Creager et al[17] from Boston, Massachusetts, and San Francisco, California, in 10 patients with CHF during a 12-week placebo-controlled trial. At rest, enalapril decreased mean BP by 13% and systemic vascular resistance by 20% and increased stroke volume by 21%. During maximal exercise, enalapril decreased systemic vascular resistance and increased both cardiac output and stroke volume indexes. Enalapril acutely increased exercise duration and maximal oxygen consumption. During the randomized, placebo-controlled study, these same 10 patients and an additional 13 patients were randomized and followed for 12 weeks. Among the 11 patients given enalapril, 73% considered themselves improved compared with 25% of the patients assigned to placebo treatment. During long-term treatment, exercise capacity increased in patients receiving enalapril but was unchanged in patients receiving placebo. No adverse effects resulting from enalapril occurred. These data suggest that

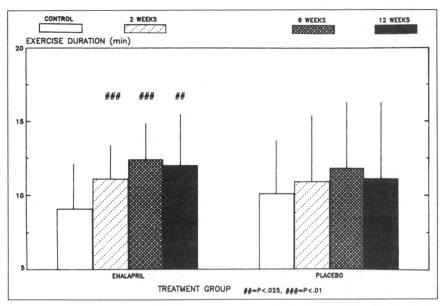

Fig. 8-2. Effects of long-term enalapril administration and placebo on exercise duration in the same 17 patients with CHF. The p values represent comparisons with enalapril control. Mean values ± SD are plotted. Reproduced with permission from Franciosa et al.[16]

enalapril treatment improves cardiac function at rest and during exercise and results in symptomatic improvement and increased exercise capacity in patients with CHF.

Packer and associates[18] from New York City determined the relation between plasma renin activity before treatment and the hemodynamic and clinical responses to either captopril or enalapril in 100 consecutive patients with severe chronic CHF. Initial doses of captopril produced significant increases in cardiac index and decreases in LV filling pressure, mean arterial pressure, mean RA pressure, heart rate, and systemic vascular resistance that varied linearly with the pretreatment value for plasma renin activity. In contrast, there was no relation between the pretreatment activity and the magnitude of hemodynamic improvement after 1–3 months of treatment with the converting enzyme inhibitors, and, consequently, a similar proportion of patients with a high (>6 ng/ml/hour; >4.62 mmol/L/hour), intermediate (2–6 ng/ml/hour; 1.54–4.62 mmol/L/hour), and low (>2 ng/ml/hour; >1.54 mmol/L/hour) pretreatment value improved clinically during long-term treatment (64, 60, and 64%, respectively). Long-term survival after 1, 2, and 3 years was similar in the 3 groups. Estimating the degree of activation of the renin-angiotensin system by measuring pretreatment plasma renin activity fails to predict the long-term hemodynamic or clinical responses to converting enzyme inhibitors in patients with severe CHF, and thus appears to be of limited value in selecting those patients likely to benefit from treatment with these drugs. (The cause of the chronic CHF in the 100 patients was variable, namely CAD in 68, idiopathic dilated cardiomyopathy in 25, and primary MR or AR or both in 7, 4 of whom had undergone valve replacement. In my view (WCR), patient populations with CHF should have similar etiologies of the CHF. Otherwise, evaluation of results is difficult.)

Cleland and associates[19] from Glasgow, UK, assessed the concomitant long-term effects of enalapril, on symptoms, exercise performance, cardiac function, arrhythmias, hormones, electrolytes, body composition, and renal function in a placebo-controlled double-blind crossover trial with treatment periods of 8 weeks. Twenty patients with NYHA functional class II–IV CHF who were clinically stable on digoxin and diuretic therapy were studied. Enalapril treatment significantly improved functional class, symptom score for breathlessness, and exercise tolerance. Systolic BP was significantly lower on enalapril treatment. Echo assessment indicated a reduction in LV dimensions and an improvement in systolic time intervals. In response to enalapril, the plasma concentration of angiotensin II was reduced and that of active renin increased; plasma concentrations of aldosterone, vasopressin, and norepinephrine decreased. There were significant increases in serum potassium and serum magnesium on enalapril. Glomerular filtration rate measured both by isotopic techniques and by creatinine clearance declined on enalapril, whereas serum urea, creatinine and effective renal plasma flow increased. Body weight and total body sodium were unchanged, indicating that there was no overall diuresis. There was a statistically insignificant increase in total body potassium, although the increase was related directly to pretreatment plasma renin. On enalapril the improvement in symptoms, exercise performance, decrease in plasma norepinephrine, and increase in serum potassium coincided with a decline in the frequency of VPC recorded during ambulatory monitoring. Adverse effects were few. In patients with CHF, enalapril had a beneficial effect on symptoms and functional capacity. The decline in glomerular filtration rate on enalapril may not be beneficial in early CHF.

Webster and associates[20] from Christ Church, New Zealand, used 24-hour Holter ECG recordings to measure the effects of enalapril, given for 12 weeks, on the frequency of cardiac arrhythmias in 10 patients with CHF (NYHA functional class II or III) receiving maintenance therapy with digoxin and furosemide. Nine patients were given placebo, and both study groups were conducted in a double-blind, parallel manner. The placebo group had no change in the frequency of arrhythmias, whereas enalapril-treated patients showed a significant decrease in the frequency of VPC, ventricular couplets, and VT. A minor, nonsignificant reduction in atrial premature complexes occurred in patients who received enalapril. Compared with placebo patients, those who received enalapril had an increase in plasma potassium levels of 0.33 mmol/L, a decrease in plasma digoxin, and decreases in PA wedge, mean PA, and RA pressures. However, none of these indexes were correlated with the concomitant decline in cardiac arrhythmias. It was concluded that enalapril reduced the frequency of ventricular arrhythmias in CHF.

McGrath and associates[21] from Melbourne and Prahran, Australia, in a randomized, double-blind trial treated 13 patients with chronic CHF with enalapril and 12 with placebo added to their existing regimen of digoxin and furosemide. Four hours after the first 5 mg dose, the enalapril group had significant decreases in BP, heart rate, and concentrations of plasma angiotensin II, angiotensin-converting enzyme, and norepinephrine. During the 12-week trial CHF became worse in 1 enalapril-treated patient (8%) and in 7 placebo-treated patients (58%). There were no significant changes in cardiac EF or exercise duration in either group. Plasma norepinephrine response to graded exercise and maximum exercise rate-BP product were significantly reduced after 4 and 12 weeks of active treatment but unchanged with placebo treatment. There was a sustained increase in plasma potassium and a slight increase in plasma creatinine in the enalapril group. Plasma concentrations of the active drug, enalaprilat, were dose-related and log enalaprilat correlated significantly with percentage of plasma angiotensin-converging enzyme activity. Enalapril was well tolerated and produced no adverse effects. The drug offers considerable promise for the treatment of CHF.

Captopril -vs- isosorbide dinitrate

Packer and associates[22] from New York City compared the short-term hemodynamic effects of isosorbide dinitrate (40 mg orally) and captopril (25 mg orally) in 18 patients with severe chronic CHF in a randomized, crossover study conducted on consecutive days. Captopril and isosorbide dinitrate produced similar decreases in systemic vascular resistance, but whereas nitrate therapy decreased pulmonary arteriolar resistance significantly, captopril did not; the difference between the 2 drugs was highly significant (−25 -vs- −5%). LV filling pressures declined similarly with both captopril (−10.5 mmHg) and with isosorbide dinitrate (−9.3 mmHg), but because pulmonary arteriolar resistance decreased significantly with nitrate therapy, mean RA pressure decreased more with isosorbide dinitrate than with captopril (−5.4 -vs- −2.8 mmHg, respectively). Although systemic resistance declined similarly with both drugs, cardiac index increased more with nitrate therapy than during converting enzyme inhibition (+0.47 -vs- +0.23 L/min/m² (p <0.01), and therefore mean arterial pressure decreased less with isosorbide dinitrate than with captopril (−10.5 -vs- −16.7 mmHg); 2 patients developed symptomatic hypotension with captopril, whereas none did with the nitrate. The difference in the effects of the 2 drugs on cardiac index was not due to differences in their effects on heart rate, since heart rate decreased similarly with both drugs, and thus both drugs produced similar increases in stroke volume index. These data indicate that, in patients with severe chronic CHF, nitrates exert favorable dilating effects on the pulmonary circulation not shared by captopril.

Dopamine -vs- enalaprilat

The reduced renal blood flow in patients with CHF can be selectively increased by inhibition of the angiotensin II-converting enzyme or stimulation of dopaminergic receptors. Maskin and colleagues[23] from New York City measured renal and systemic hemodynamics during titration of dopamine and serially after intravenous administration of enalaprilat in 9 patients with chronic severe CHF. During titration of dopamine, renal blood flow increased by 99%, from 304–604 ml/minute at a dose of dopamine of 2.1 mg/kg/minute, which produced only a 21% increase in cardiac index, from 2.0–2.4 L/min/m². Cardiac index was increased maximally at a dose of 4.0 mg/kg/minute dopamine; however, renal blood flow was not further augmented. In contrast, after intravenous administration of enalaprilat, peak improvement of renal blood flow and cardiac index occurred concomitantly. Renal blood flow increased by 35%, from 316–427 ml/minute and cardiac index increased by 18%, from 1.99–2.35 L/min/m². At similar increases in cardiac index, dopamine produced a greater increase in renal blood flow than enalaprilat: 604 -vs- 427 L/minute. Mean systemic arterial pressure, however, was greater with dopamine than with enalaprilat (78 -vs- 70 mmHg) at peak effect. Thus, although both drugs appear to be potent renal vasodilators in patients with severe CHF, dopamine may be more effective in augmenting renal blood flow.

Fenoldopam

Young and coworkers[24] from Houston, Texas, evaluated the influence of dopamine receptor stimulation in 10 patients with severe CHF. Fenoldopam, a new, orally available, and selective dopamine-receptor agonist with potent renal vasodilating properties and without positive inotropic or adrenergic activity was used. Placebo produced no change in hemodynamic function. Peak hemodynamic effect was noted 30 minutes to 1 hour after a 200 mg dose of fenoldopam with mean BP decreasing from 96 ± 15–83 ± 8 mmHg (mean ± SD), PA wedge pressure decreasing from 23 ± 6–20 ± 8 mmHg), and mean PA pressure decreasing from 32 ± 9–29 ± 8 mmHg. There was no change in heart rate and RA pressure, but systemic vascular resistance decreased from 1,987 ± 887–1,191 ± 559 dynes · s · cm^{-5} with a 55% increase in cardiac index after fenoldopam therapy. Baseline hemodynamics returned to control values within 3–4 hours. These data indicate that fenoldopam is a short-acting, orally effective drug that decreases systemic vascular resistance and increases cardiac index in patients with important CHF.

Milrinone

Simonton and colleagues[25] from San Francisco, California, and New York City evaluated the influence of milrinone, a new oral inotropic-vasodilator agent in 37 patients with severe CHF. Most patients had not responded to prior vasodilator therapy. All patients had acute hemodynamic improvement with oral milrinone and an optimal maintenance dose was chosen for each patient with an average dose of 48 mg/day of milrinone being administered. Milrinone was discontinued in 12 patients before follow-up hemodynamic study because of worsening CHF in 6, sudden death in 3, arrhythmia in 1, and refusal by 2 patients. The hemodynamic effects of milrinone both acutely and after chronic therapy (average, 37 days) were compared in the remaining 25 patients. Mean cardiac index increased from 1.9 ± 0.5–2.5 ± 0.5 L/min/m^2 and mean PA wedge pressure decreased from 28 ± 9–18 ± 8 mmHg. New York Heart Association functional class improved in 18 of the 25 patients treated with milrinone for a mean of 5.5 ± 2.3 months. No major adverse side effects were observed with chronic therapy, although 23 patients developed fluid retention requiring increased doses of diuretic drugs. The cumulative survival rate at 6 months for the entire group was 34%. These data confirm a sustained and potent inotropic effect of oral milrinone therapy in patients with severe CHF. However, although hemodynamic and clinical improvement is associated with chronic milrinone therapy, it does not appear that there is a major reduction in the risk of overall mortality in these patients.

Milrinone is a potent noncatecholamine, nonglycoside inotropic agent that can improve hemodynamic performance and functional capacity in patients with severe CHF. However, the potential effect of chronic inotropic stimulation on ventricular arrhythmias in patients with CHF requires evaluation. Holmes and colleagues[26] from New York City compared 24-hour ambulatory ECG before and 2–4 weeks after initiation of chronic milrinone therapy in 20 patients with severe CHF (mean cardiac index, 1.79 ± 0.43 L/min/m^2). A >10-fold increase in complex VPC form density, or an increase from 0–5 episodes per 24 hours of any complex VPC form occurred in 35% (7 of 20) of patients. A >10-fold reduction in simple VPC density was noted in 5% (1 of 20), and 60% (12 of 20) of the study group had no significant change in ventricular arrhythmia profile on milrinone. The hemodynamic and functional response to milrinone and entry hemodynamic profiles were unrelated to the change in frequency or complexity of ventricular arrhythmias during therapy. Thus, milrinone therapy in CHF may be associated with the development of VPC complexity and with a significantly increased density of complex VPC forms.

MDL 17,043

Uretsky and coworkers[27] from Pittsburgh, Pennsylvania, evaluated MDL 17,043 (MDL), an agent with both inotropic and vasodilator properties, in 20 patients with severe CHF. Among these patients, MDL increased cardiac output by 28%, and decreased mean PA wedge pressure by 46%. Mean arterial pressure was decreased from 78 ± 9–70 ± 11 mmHg (10%) and hemodynamic improvement was sustained for 8 hours after oral MDL therapy. In these studies, plasma renin activity increased slightly, plasma norepinephrine concentration decreased slightly, and vasopressin concentrations did not change. The elimination half-life for MDL was approximately 20 hours. The improvement in hemodynamic variables was sustained in 6 patients who were restudied at 4 weeks. Initial subjective improvement in all 20 patients occurred in 90% and was sustained at 4 weeks in 50%, but was found at 3 months in only 25% of the patients. Side effects requiring cessation of therapy with MDL occurred in 10% of the patients; 93% of patients on long-term therapy died at a mean interval of 39 days after beginning MDL 17,043. Thus, these data suggest that oral MDL produces acute beneficial hemodynamic changes in patients with severe CHF. Subjective benefit in symptoms may not persist several week after onset of therapy and the frequency of cardiac deaths, including sudden death, remains high in such patients.

Amin and colleagues[28] from Los Angeles, California, compared the acute hemodynamic effect of intravenous nitroprusside (NTP), a pure vasodilator, to those of intravenous MDL in 12 patients with chronic refractory CHF. Intravenous NTP was infused and titrated to achieve optimal hemodynamic effects, whereas MDL was given intravenously in 0.5 mg/kg increments every 10–15 minutes until no further increase occurred in cardiac output or until a maximum cumulative dose of 4.5 mg/kg had been given. Both NTP and MDL reduced PA wedge pressure (27 ± 5–15 ± 6 and 29 ± 3–15 ± 7 mmHg, respectively, systemic vascular resistance (2,173 ± 1,137–1,118 ± 306 and 1,805 ± 425–956 ± 235 dynes sec cm^{-5}, respectively; mean arterial pressure (85 ± 18–69 + 14 and 83 ± 15 75 ± 16 mmHg respectively, and increased cardiac index (1.7 ± 0.4–2.6 ± 0.4 and 1.8 ± 0.2–3.3 ± 0.5 L/min/m^2, respectively) without an overall significant change in heart rate. For comparable reductions of PA wedge pressure and systemic vascular resistance, MDL in comparison to NTP resulted in a significantly higher cardiac index (3.3 ± 0.5 -vs- 2.6 ± 0.4 L/min/m^2), stroke work index (31 ± 17 -vs- 24 ± 10 gm/m^2), and mean arterial pressure (75 ± 16 -vs- 69 ± 14 mmHg). Thus, intravenous MDL is of considerable value in the acute therapy of certain patients with refractory CHF.

Amin and associates[29] from Los Angeles, California, investigated 14 patients with severe CHF due to CAD or idiopathic dilated cardiomyopathy. The hemodynamic response to intravenous infusion of dobutamine (D) was compared to that of MDL administered in incremental intravenous doses. D and MDL produced comparable increases in cardiac index (1.8 ± 0.4–2.9 ± 0.8 and 1.7 ± 0.3–3.3 ± 0.6 L/min/m^2, respectively) and stroke volume index (24 ± 8–35 ± 9 and 22 ± 7–39 ± 11 ml/beat/m^2, respectively). Both D and MDL reduced LV filling pressure (29 ± 5–24 ± 5 and 29 ± 6–17 ± 6 mmHg, respectively) and mean RA pressure (11 ± 4–8 ± 4 and 13 ± 5–6 ± 4 mmHg, respectively). The overall changes in heart rate and mean arterial pressure were small with both D and MDL. MDL in comparison to D resulted in a significantly lower LV filling pressure, mean PA pressure, and mean arterial pressure. The salutary hemodynamic effects of MDL on cardiac index and LV filling pressure were sustained for an average of 9.6 hours, whereas the effects of D dissipated within 30 minutes of stopping the infusion. No serious adverse effects were noted during acute administration with either drug. Therefore intravenous MDL may be a useful substitute for dobutamine in the acute therapy of severe CHF.

Captopril -vs- milrinone

LeJemtel and coworkers[30] from New York City compared the effects of milrinone and captopril on ventricular performance, renal blood flow, and femoral vein oxygen content in 11 patients with severe CHF. The increase in stroke volume index was greater with milrinone than with captopril, whereas PA wedge pressures decreased similarly with both agents. Mean systemic arterial pressure declined significantly with captopril but did not change with milrinone. Neither drug changed heart rate significantly, although milrinone produced a greater improvement in ventricular performance than captopril, renal blood flow increased similarly with both drugs. Femoral vein oxygen content was increased by milrinone but was not changed by captopril. In 7 additional patients, intravenous milrinone, administered at the peak effect of captopril further augmented stroke volume index and tended to reduce PA wedge pressure. The addition of intravenous milrinone to captopril did not reduce mean systemic arterial pressure or significantly increase heart rate compared with captopril alone. Although renal blood flow was not further increased by the addition of intravenous milrinone to captopril, femoral vein oxygen content increased. Thus, the simultaneous administration of captopril and milrinone has synergistic effect on cardiac performance and complementary effects on the peripheral circulation.

Nifedipine

Elkayam and associates[31] from Los Angeles, California, evaluated the acute hemodynamic effects of 20–50 mg of orally administered nifedipine in 31 patients with severe chronic CHF, and the results were analyzed according to the response of the cardiac index. Although this group mean value of cardiac index increased significantly after nifedipine treatment (from 2.1 ± 0.5–2.4 ± 0.8 L/min/m^2), the individual response was variable. Twenty of the patients had ≥15% increase in cardiac index (group A), and 11 patients had <15% increase or a decrease in cardiac index (group B). Marked differences also were noted in the effects of nifedipine on other hemodynamic variables. Stroke volume increased 29 ± 14% in group A and decreased 11 ± 18% in group B. Systemic vascular resistance decreased 34 ± 11% in group A and increased slightly, 2 ± 28%, in group B. LV stroke work index increased 11 ± 19% in group A and decreased markedly in group B (21 ± 20%). Six group B patients had a substantial worsening (≥20%) of ≥1 hemodynamic measurements, including cardiac index, stroke volume index, LV stroke work index, and mean PA wedge pressure. A comparison of control hemodynamic values at rest, LVEF, associated CAD, nifedipine dose, and concomitant diuretic therapy revealed no significant differences between the 2 groups. This study confirms, in a large group of patients with severe CHF, the variable hemodynamic effects of nifedipine. Although cardiac index improved in many patients, in some patients (35%) it did not. Moreover, nifedipine therapy resulted in a significant hemodynamic deterioration in 6 patients. The response to therapy was not dose-related and could not be predicted by baseline hemodynamics, LV function, presence of associated CAD, and concomitant diuretic therapy.

Salbutamol

The long-term efficacy and potential side effects of oral sympathomimetic amines in the treatment of advanced CHF remain controversial. Mettauer and colleagues[32] from Montreal, Canada, studied the acute and chronic hemodynamic and arrhythmogenic effects of the beta$_2$ agonist, salbutamol, 6 mg by mouth 4 times/day, in 20 patients with New York Heart Association classes III–IV CHF. Acutely, salbutamol increased the cardiac index (1.9–2.3 L/min/m^2) and heart rate (92–97 beats/minute) and it decreased PA wedge pressure (35–31 mmHg). Salbutamol increased the number of patients having episodes of VT from 2–6 and increased the number of episodes of VT from 2–27. Once salbutamol was discontinued, no further episodes of VT occurred in these 6 patients. Six patients did not have long-term hemodynamic studies because of serious arrhythmias and 2 died. In the 12 patients who had long-term studies, the initial beneficial hemodynamic effects of salbutamol were maintained. Thus, although salbutamol may have beneficial long-term hemodynamic effects, it may cause serious arrhythmias in patients predisposed to develop arrhythmias.

Sublingual nitroglycerin

Since nitroglycerin (NTG) is used in unloading therapy for patients with CHF, Imaizumi and coworkers[33] from Fukuoka, Japan, examined the effects of sublingually administered NTG on forearm resistance vessels in 9 normal subjects and in 8 patients with CHF. Forearm blood flow was measured with a strain-gauge plethysmograph and forearm vascular resistance was calculated. To evaluate the magnitude of reflex forearm vasconstriction triggered by decreased central venous pressure after NTG, lower body negative pressure (LBNP) was applied to produce a comparable decrease in central venous pressure to that after NTG. The change in forearm vascular resistance during LBNP was comparable with that after NTG. In normal subjects LBNP increased, but the NTG did not change forearm vascular resistance. In patients with CHF, neither the NTG nor LBNP changed forearm vascular resistance. The direct vasodilator effect of NTG on forearm resistance vessels assessed by the difference between the change in forearm vascular resistance produced by NTG and that during LBNP tended to be less in patients with CHF than in normal subjects. There was no difference in changes of forearm vascular resistance with the cold pressor test in normal subjects and in patients with CHF. This study suggests that in normal subjects NTG does not alter forearm vascular resistance because its dilator effect is offset by reflex vasoconstriction. However, in patients with CHF, reflex vasoconstriction is impaired, but the direct vasodilator effect of NTG also tends to be reduced, so that as a net effect forearm vascular resistance is not altered.

Transdermal nitroglycerin

Of the presently available vasodilator agents, only nitrates and angiotensin-converting enzyme inhibitors have produced sustained hemodynamic improvement along with increased exercise tolerance in patients with CHF. Orally administered isosorbide dinitrate and topically applied nitroglycerin (NTG) ointment produce significant hemodynamic effects for as long as 4–8 hours but still require multiple daily dosing. The dose requirements and duration of effect of transdermal NTG in patients with CHF are not clearly established. In a first series of 8 patients with CHF, Jordan and colleagues[34] from Little Rock, Arkansas, gave transdermal NTG in incremental doses until

PA wedge pressure decreased ≥30% within 4 hours in 3 consecutive patients. Thus, the investigators found that a single dose of 60 mg/24 hours (120 cm²) was the minimal effective dose. The transdermal NTG or placebo was then given as a single application of 60 mg/24 hours in random double-blind fashion to 15 additional patients with CHF (8 received transdermal NTG, and 7 received placebo), and the hemodynamics were monitored up to 24 hours. After administration of transdermal NTG, the control PA wedge pressure of 22 mmHg decreased by 6 mmHg at 2 hours and reached maximal reduction at 8 mmHg at 4 hours. The reduction in PA wedge pressure remained significant through 12 hours but was no longer statistically significant by 18 hours after administration of the drug. Transdermal NTG also significantly reduced PA and RA pressures and pulmonary vascular resistance from 4 through 12 hours but did not affect systemic hemodynamics. No significant hemodynamic changes occurred after administration of placebo. Thus, transdermal NTG is an effective vasodilator in patients with CHF, but a dose ≥60 mg/24 hours is needed. Even with this dose, hemodynamic effects do not last beyond 18 hours, suggesting altered absorption or development of tolerance.

Elkayam and associates[35] from Los Angeles, California, studied the hemodynamic effect of a large dose of NTG (90 mg) given transdermally using a reservoir system in 10 patients with severe, long-standing CHF. Serial hemodynamic measurements over 24 hours revealed a mild decrease in mean PA wedge pressure. However, the change from baseline was significant only at 2 hours (19 ± 9 -vs- 27 ± 6 mmHg). Mean RA pressure decreased 1 hour after initiation of therapy, from 12 ± 7–8 ± 5 mmHg. However, the change from control was not statistically significant. No significant changes were noted in heart rate, mean BP, cardiac index, and systemic and pulmonary vascular resistance. Individual analysis of the effect of transdermal NTG on PA wedge pressure demonstrated a ≥20% reduction in 8 of 10 patients. However, persistent effect (>8 hours) was seen in only 4 patients. Removal of NTG patches at 24 hours did not result in hemodynamic rebound. Serum catecholamine levels and renin concentration did not change 2 and 24 hours after initiation of NTG therapy or after removal of NTG patches. Thus, a large dose (90 mg) of transdermal NTG using a reservoir system results in mild and mostly statistically insignificant hemodynamic effect in patients with chronic severe CHF. Although a reduction in PA wedge pressure is seen in most patients, rapid attenuation of this response is found in many patients and the effect only rarely lasts for 24 hours.

An editorial summarizing drug treatment of CHF appeared in the *British Heart Journal*.[36]

DIGITALIS AND WILLIAM WITHERING

On April 18, 1985, the Association of Physicians of Great Britain and Ireland and the British Cardiac Society held a joint meeting in Birmingham to commemorate the 200th anniversary of the publication of William Withering's, "An Account of the Foxglove." Other societies celebrated this bicentenary anniversary during 1985, and there were many articles on Withering and on digitalis. Several historic and modern pieces on digitalis were published in the September 1985 *British Heart Journal* including Krikler's historic piece on the "secret recipe" of "Old Mother Hutton" that provided Withering with the secret of digitalis (Fig. 8-3). The May 1985 issue of the *Journal of the American College of Cardiology Supplement* was devoted to digitalis. Burchell re-

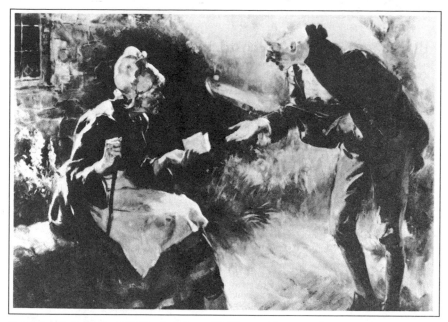

Fig. 8-3. Depiction by Will Meade Prince of William Withering exchanging golden sovereigns for the "secret recipe" held by "Old Mother Hutton." Reproduced with permission from the *British Heart Journal*, September, 1985.

viewed certain aspects of Withering's book in the June 28, 1985, *Journal of the American Medical Association*. The October 1985 issue of *The Journal of Clinical Pharmacology* was devoted entirely to historic and modern articles on digitalis.

References

1. WILSON JR, FINK L, MARIS J, FERRARO N, POWER-VANWART J, ELEFF S, CHANCE B: Evaluation of energy metabolism in skeletal muscle of patients with heart failure with gated phosphorus-31 nuclear magnetic resonance. Circulation 1985 (Jan); 71:57–62.

2. CHAKKO CS, GHEORGHIADE M: Ventricular arrhythmias in severe heart failure: incidence, significance, and effectiveness of antiarrhythmic therapy. Am Heart J 1985 (Mar); 109:497–504.

3. SOUFER R, WOHLGELERNTER D, VITA NA, AMUCHESTEGUI M, SOSTMAN D, BERGER HJ, ZARET BL: Intact systolic left ventricular function in clinical congestive heart failure. Am J Cardiol 1985 (Apr 1); 55:1032–1036.

4. SZLACHCIC J, MASSIE BM, KRAMER BL, TOPIC N, TUBAU J: Correlates and prognostic implication of exercise capacity in chronic congestive heart failure. Am J Cardiol 1985 (Apr 1); 55:1037–1042.

5. SHEN WF, ROUBIN GS, HIRASAWA K, CHOONG CYP, HUTTON BF, HARRIS PJ, FLETCHER PJ, KELLY DT: Left ventricular volume and ejection fraction response to exercise in chronic congestive heart failure: Difference between dilated cardiomyopathy and previous myocardial infarction. Am J Cardiol 1985 (Apr 1); 55:1027–1031.

6. FRANCIS GS, GOLDSMITH SR, ZIESCHE S, NAKAJIMA H, COHN JN: Relative attenuation of sympathetic drive during exercise in patients with congestive heart failure. J Am Coll Cardiol 1985 (Apr); 5:832–839.

7. WEBER KT, JANICKI JS: Lactate production during maximal and submaximal exercise in patients with chronic heart failure. J Am Coll Cardiol 1985 (Oct); 6:717–724.

8. FRANCIOSA JA, BAKER BJ, SETH L: Pulmonary versus systemic hemodynamics in determining exercise capacity of patients with chronic left ventricular failure. Am Heart J 1985 (Oct); 110:807–813.

9. ELKAYAM U, ROTH A, WEBER L, HSUEH W, NANNA M, FREIDENBERGER L, CHANDRARATNA AN, RAHIM-TOOLA SH: Isometric exercise in patients with chronic advanced heart failure: hemodynamic and neurohumoral evaluation. Circulation 1985 (Nov); 72:975–981.

10. MASSIE B, BOURASSA M, DIBIANCO R, HESS M, KONSTAM M, LIKOFF M, PACKER M: Long-term oral administration of amrinone for congestive heart failure: lack of efficacy in a multicenter controlled trial. Circulation 1985 (May); 71:963–971.

11. CHATTERJEE K, PARMLEY WW, COHN JN, LEVINE TB, AWAN NA, MASON DT, FAXON DP, CREAGER M, GAVRAS HP, FOUAD FM, TARAZI RC, HOLLENBERG NK, DZAU V, LEJEMTEL TH, SONNENBLICK EH, TURINI GA, BRUNNER HR: A cooperative multicenter study of captopril in congestive heart failure: hemodynamic effects and long-term response. Am Heart J 1985 (Aug); 110:439–447.

12. SHAW TRD, DUNCAN FM, WILLIAMS BC, CRICHTON E, THOMSON SA, DAVIS JRE, RADEMAKER M, EDWARDS CRW: Plasma free captopril concentrations during short and long term treatment with oral captopril for heart failure. Br Heart J 1985 (Aug); 54:160–165.

13. WILSON JR, FERRARO N: Effect of the renin-angiotensin system on limb circulation and metabolism during exercise in patients with heart failure. J Am Coll Cardiol 1985 (Sept); 6:556–563.

14. PACKER M, LEE WH, MEDINA N, YUSHAK M: Hemodynamic and clinical significance of the pulmonary vascular response to long-term captopril therapy in patients with severe chronic heart failure. J Am Coll Cardiol 1985 (Sept); 6:635–645.

15. KUBO SH, CODY RJ, LARAGH JH, PRIDA XE, ATLAS SA, YUAN Z, SEALEY JE: Immediate converting-enzyme inhibition with intravenous enalapril in chronic congestive heart failure. Am J Cardiol 1985 (Jan 1); 55:122–126.

16. FRANCIOSA JA, WILEN MM, JORDAN RA: Effects of enalapril, a new angiotensin-converting enzyme inhibitor, in a controlled trial in heart failure. J Am Coll Cardiol 1985 (Jan); 5:101–107.

17. CREAGER MA, MASSIE BM, FAXON DP, FRIEDMAN SD, KRAMER BL, WEINER DA, RYAN TJ, TOPIC N, MELIDOSSIAN CD: Acute and long-term effects of enalapril on the cardiovascular response to exercise and exercise tolerance in patients with congestive heart failure. J Am Coll Cardiol 1985 (July); 6:163–170.

18. PACKER M, MEDINA N, YUSHAK M, LEE WH: Usefulness of plasma renin activity in predicting hemodynamic and clinical responses and survival during long term converting enzyme inhibition in severe chronic heart failure: experience in 100 consecutive patients. Br Heart J 1985 (Sept); 54:298–304.

19. CLELAND JGF, DARGIE HJ, BALL SG, GILLEN G, HODSMAN GP, MORTON JJ, EAST BW, ROBERTSON I, FORD I, ROBERTSON JIS: Effects of enalapril in heart failure: a double blind study of effects on exercise performance, renal function, hormones, and metabolic state. Br Heart J 1985 (Sept); 54:305–312.

20. WEBSTER MWI, FITZPATRICK A, NICHOLLS G, IKRAM H, WELLS JE: Effect of enalapril on ventricular arrhythmias in congestive heart failure. Am J Cardiol 1985 (Sept 15); 56:566–569.

21. MCGRATH BP, ARNOLDA L, MATTHEWS PG, JACKSON B, JENNINGS G, KIAT H, JOHNSTON CI: Controlled trial of enalapril in congestive cardiac failure. Br Heart J 1985 (Oct); 54:405–414.

22. PACKER M, MEDINA N, YUSHAK M, LEE WH: Comparative effects of captopril and isosorbide dinitrate on pulmonary arteriolar resistance and right ventricular function in patients with severe left ventricular failure: results of a randomized crossover study. Am Heart J 1985 (June); 109:1293–1299.

23. MASKIN CS, OCKEN S, CHADWICK B, LEJEMTEL TH: Comparative systemic and renal effects of dopamine and angiotensin-converting enzyme inhibition with enalaprilat in patients with heart failure. Circulation 1985 (Oct); 72:846–852.

24. YOUNG JB, LEON CA, PRATT CM, SUAREZ JM, ARONOFF RD, ROBERTS R: Hemodynamic effects of an oral dopamine receptor agonist (fenoldopam) in patients with congestive heart failure. J Am Coll Cardiol 1985 (Oct); 6:792–796.

25. SIMONTON CA, CHATTERJEE K, CODY RJ, KUBO SH, LEONARD D, DALY P, RUTMAN H: Milrinone in congestive heart failure: acute and chronic hemodynamic and clinical evaluation. J Am Coll Cardiol 1985 (Aug); 6:453–459.

26. HOLMES JR, KUBO SH, CODY RJ, KLIGFIELD P: Milrinone in congestive heart failure: observations on ambulatory ventricular arrhythmias. Am Heart J 1985 (Oct); 110:800–806.

27. URETSKY BF, GENERALOVICH T, VERBALIS JG, VALDES AM, REDDY PS: MDL 17,043 therapy in severe congestive heart failure: characterization of the early and late hemodynamic, pharmacokinetic, hormonal and clinical response. J Am Coll Cardiol 1985 (June); 5:1414–1421.

28. AMIN DK, SHAH PK, HULSE S, SHELLOCK F: Comparative acute hemodynamic effects of intravenous sodium nitroprusside and MDL-17,043, a new inotropic drug with vasodilator effects, in refractory congestive heart failure. Am Heart J 1985 (May); 109:1006–1012.

29. AMIN DK, SHAH PK, SHELLOCK FG, HULSE S, BRANDON G, SPANGENBERG R, SWAN HJC: Comparative hemodynamic effects of intravenous dobutamine and MDL-17,043, a new cardioactive drug, in severe congestive heart failure. Am Heart J 1985 (Jan); 109:91–98.

30. LEJEMTEL TH, MASKIN CS, MANCINI D, SINOWAY L, FELD H, CHADWICH B: Systemic and regional hemodynamic effects of captopril and milrinone administered alone and concomitantly in patients with heart failure. Circulation 1985 (Aug); 72:364–369.

31. ELKAYAM U, WEBER L, MCKAY C, RAHIMTOOLA S: Spectrum of acute hemodynamic effects of nifedipine in severe congestive heart failure. Am J Cardiol 1985 (Sept 15); 56:560–566.

32. METTAUER B, ROULEAU J-L, BURGESS JH: Detrimental arrhythmogenic and sustained beneficial hemodynamic effects of oral salbutamol in patients with chronic congestive heart failure. Am Heart J 1985 (Apr); 109:840–847.

33. IMAIZUMI T, TAKESHITA A, ASHIHARA T, NAKAMURA M: The effects of sublingually administered nitroglycerin on forearm vascular resistance in patients with heart failure and in normal subjects. Circulation 1985 (Oct); 72:747–752.

34. JORDAN RA, SETH L, HENRY A, WILEN MM, FRANCIOSA JA: Dose requirements and hemodynamic effects of transdermal nitroglycerin compared with placebo in patients with congestive heart failure. Circulation 1985 (May); 71:980–986.

35. ELKAYAM U, ROTH A, HENRIQUEZ B, WEBER L, TONNEMACHER D, RAHIMTOOLA SH: Hemodynamic and hormonal effects of high-dose transdermal nitroglycerin in patients with chronic congestive heart failure. Am J Cardiol 1985 (Sept 15); 56:555–559.

36. DOLLERY CT, CORR L: Drug treatment of heart failure. Br Heart J 1985 (Sept); 54:234–242.

9

Miscellaneous Topics

PERICARDIAL HEART DISEASE

Primary acute pericardial disease

Permanyer-Miralda and associates[1] from Barcelona, Spain, studied 231 patients with primary acute pericardial disease (acute pericarditis or tamponade presenting without an apparent cause) according to the following protocol: general clinical and laboratory studies (stage I), pericardiocentesis (stage II), pericardial biopsy (stage III) and blind antituberculous therapy (stage IV). In 32 patients (14%) a specific etiologic diagnosis was obtained (13 with neoplasia, 9 with tuberculosis, 4 with collagen vascular disease, 2 with toxoplasmosis, 2 with purulent pericarditis and 2 with viral pericarditis). Diagnostic pericardiocentesis (32 patients) was performed when clinical activity and effusion persisted for >1 week or when purulent pericarditis was suspected, whereas therapeutic pericardiocentesis (44 patients) was performed to treat tamponade; their diagnostic yield was 6 and 29%, respectively. Diagnostic biopsy (20 patients) was carried out when illness persisted for >3 weeks, whereas therapeutic biopsy was performed whenever pericardiocentesis failed to relieve tamponade; their diagnostic yield was 5 and 54%, respectively. The diagnostic yield difference between diagnostic and therapeutic procedures was significant; in contrast, the global diagnostic yield of pericardiocentesis (19%) and biopsy (22%) was similar. At the end of follow-up (1–76 months; mean, 31 ± 20), no patient in whom a diagnosis of idiopathic pericarditis had been made showed signs of pericardial disease. It was concluded that a diagnostic procedure is not warranted as a routine method, a choice between therapeutic pericardiocentesis and biopsy is circumstantial and must be individualized, and only through a systematic approach can a substantial diagnostic yield be reached in primary acute pericardial disease.

Magnetic resonance imaging in constriction

Soulen and associates[2] from San Francisco, California, performed gated magnetic resonance imaging (MRI) in 5 patients with suspected constrictive pericardial disease using a superconducting magnet operating at 0.35 Tesla. Results were compared with those of echo and hemodynamic measurements in all patients, with chest films in 5, computed tomography in 2 and with histologic findings in 3. Pericardial thickness was >5 mm in 4 patients and 5 mm in 1 patient. Absence of MRI signal from the thickened pericardium was observed with extensive calcific deposits, and increased intensity of the thickened pericardium was associated with inflammatory disease. Dilation of the right atrium, venae cavae, and hepatic veins and RV narrowing was observed in all patients. The ventricular septum was straight in all patients. MRI allows both measurement of pericardial thickness and depicts internal cardiac anatomy without exposure to radiation or use of contrast medium. Satisfactory imaging with a large field of view can be performed in the presence of lung disease, thoracic deformity, or surgical "hardware"—conditions that limit echo and computed tomography. The inherently 3-D data permit imaging in any plane without loss of resolution. Thus, MRI appears to be the noninvasive method of choice for the diagnosis of constrictive pericardial disease.

Echo guided pericardiocentesis

Pericardiocentesis guided by 2-D echo has been used at the Mayo Clinic since April 1980. The 2-D examination localizes the pericardial fluid. Callahan and associates[3] from Rochester, Minnesota, reviewed their experiences in 132 consecutive 2-D echo directed pericardiocentesis performed between April 1980 and March 1984. They made particular note of the place on the body wall closest to the fluid. An entry track that permits puncture of the pericardial sac without damage to any vital structure is then selected for the pericardiocentesis needle. The volume of fluid obtained in 132 pericardiocenteses in 117 patients by this technique ranged from 75–1,700 ml (mean, 650). Seventy percent of the taps were done for therapy, 21% for diagnosis, and 9% for both therapy and diagnosis. A Teflon-sheathed intracath needle was used to complete 80% of the pericardiocenteses. In the other 20%, a large catheter was secondarily introduced and connected to a closed drainage system. There were no deaths related to the procedure. One symptomatic pneumothorax occurred. There were 3 minor complications. Two-D echo imaging of the heart and pericardial fluid permits a safe and effective means of performing pericardiocentesis.

Pericardiectomy for constriction

The records of 231 patients who underwent operation for constrictive pericarditis at the Mayo Clinic from 1936–1982 were reviewed and reported by McCaughan and colleagues[4] from Rochester, Minnesota. All had hemodynamically significant pericardial constriction preoperatively and pericardial disease was confirmed at operation. Pericardiectomy was performed through a left anterior lateral thoracotomy (34%), a median sternotomy (27%), a U-incision (21%), or a bilateral anterior thoracotomy (18%). Postoperatively, 28% of patients had evidence of low cardiac output. Seventy percent of the 32 deaths within 30 days of operation were due to low cardiac output. Operative risk was significantly related to preoperative disability (1% for class I or II, 10% for class III, and 46% for class IV). Long-term survival excluding operative mortality was not significantly influenced by the disability class preoperatively, the operative approach, or the development of low cardiac output in the immediate postoperative period. At the end of the follow-up interval, there were 141 patients in whom functional capacity could be assessed and 140 were class I or II. The authors recommended early pericardiectomy when pericardial constriction is diagnosed, and they recommended use of the left anterolateral thoracotomy as preferable for most patients. Discriminators for patients who survived pericardiectomy -vs- those who did not related to preoperative hemodynamic data. Differences in RV end-diastolic pressure and mean RA pressure reached statistical significance when the 2 groups were compared (RA pressure 24 mmHg for those who died -vs- 18 mmHg for those who survived). There was no significant difference in operative mortality related to pericardial calcium or to low voltage QRS complexes on ECG. Of 36 patients who survived early postoperative low cardiac output, 23 required augmentation of atrial filling pressures to improve poor hemodynamic condition. In 11 other patients additional inotropic drugs were necessary and in 2 patients intra-aortic balloon counterpulsation was used for 6 days in 1 and for 10 days in the other, and both survived.

CARDIOVASCULAR EFFECTS OF EXERCISE

Athletic heart syndrome

Huston and associates[5] from Irvine and Los Angeles, California, reviewed previous publications on the athletes' heart, a normal physiologic response to repetitive exercise. Tables 9-1 and 9-2 tabulate the reported observations. In the isotonic athlete, the size of the LV and RV cavities increase with a proportional increase in septal and free wall thicknesses. Hence, the LV mass is increased. The left atrium may be dilated and even thick walled. The EF and myocardial contratility remain unchanged. Stroke volume increases as training progresses. In the isometric athlete, septal and free wall thicknesses increase with little or no increase in LV end-diastolic diameter. LV mass increases but only in the same degree as lean body mass. Although information on atrial adaptation is lacking, no change has been shown to occur in contractility or EF. Stroke volume increases only in relation to any bradycardia

TABLE 9-1. *Heart rate and frequency of cardiac events on ambulatory monitoring of athletes and nonathletes. Reproduced with permission from Huston et al.*[5]

	CONTROLS	ATHLETES
Average lowest heart rate (beats/min)	45.4	37.7
Average highest heart rate (beats/min)	137.3	124.5
Sinus pauses of >2.0 sec (% of subjects)	5.7	37.1
First-degree AV block (% of subjects)	14.3	37.1
Second-degree atrioventricular block (% of subjects)		
Mobitz I	5.7	22.9
Mobitz II	0	8.6
Junctional rhythm (% of subjects)	0	20
VPC (% of subjects)	43	33
>5 premature ventricular systoles/hr	5.7	0
Runs of ventricular tachycardia (% of subjects)	5.7	0

TABLE 9-2. *Echo changes in isotonic and isometric athletes.* Reproduced with permission from Huston et al.[5]

	ISOTONIC	ISOMETRIC
LV end-diastolic diameter	↑	↑, no △
LV end-diastolic diameter per m² or per kg	↑	no △
LV end-systolic diameter	↑, ↓, no △	↑, ↓, no △
LV end-diastolic volume	↑	no △
LV posterior-wall thickness	↑	↑
LV mass	↑	↑
LV mass, per m² or per kg	↑	no △
Interventricular septal thickness	↑	↑
Interventricular-septum/posterior-wall ratio	↑, no △	↑, no △
RV diameter	↑	—
LA diameter	↑	—
EF	no △	no △
Cardiac output (resting)	no △	no △
Stroke volume	↑	↑, no △
Velocity of circumferential fiber shortening	↑, ↓, no △	no △

*↑ denotes increase, ↓ decrease, and no △ no change.

that may develop. Many athletic endeavors are a combination of isometric and isotonic work and thus may produce a combination of morphologic patterns.

Cardiovascular evaluation of the athlete

The focus of the 16th Bethesda Conference was the athlete with an underlying primary cardiovascular abnormality, and its goal was to arrive at a consensus for prudent recommendations regarding the eligibility of such athletes for competition. Before convening of this conference, no formal guidelines were available for this purpose and such recommendations to athletes were based largely on the intuition of the individual physician. The participants in this conference tried to determine which cardiovascular abnormalities and their severity would place the athlete at risk for sudden death, life-threatening cardiovascular alterations, or disease progression. This report by Mitchell and coworkers[6] is the best available on this subject.

Driscoll[7] from Rochester, Minnesota, also reviewed the various causes of sudden death in athletes and general guidelines in evaluating the athlete for potential cardiovascular disorders.

Runners

Although long-term isotonic exercise training is known to reduce resting heart rate and increase LV end-diastolic volume, it is unclear whether the increased LV output during exercise is related simply to the larger resting end-diastolic volume that persists during exercise, or whether further increases in LV volume occur. To determine the changes in LV volume and their time course during exercise, Crawford and investigators[8] from San Antonio, Texas, studied 30 runners. LV end-diastolic and end-systolic volumes were measured from biapical 2-D echo recorded during graded upright bicycle exercise. Although the absolute volume measurements were lower by echo, EF was not significantly different and the directional changes in volume during exercise were comparable. In the runners, resting LV end-diastolic volume measurements by echo correlated with their maximum bicycle exercise endurance times. LV end-diastolic volume, stroke volume, and EF increased during exercise with the most marked changes occurring in the first half of exercise. Systolic BP/end-systolic volume also increased during exercise, but the largest change occurred during the second half of exercise. LV volumes were larger in the 12 competitive runners compared with the 18 noncompetitive runners: resting end-diastolic volume 130 -vs- 87 ml, respectively. During exercise, the competitive runners had a larger increase in end-diastolic volume. Therefore highly trained competitive marathon runners make greater use of the less energy-consuming Frank-Starling mechanism to accomplish high levels of isotonic exercise performance compared with less well-trained runners.

Swimmers and weight lifters

Colan and coworkers[9] from Boston, Massachusetts, and Chicago, Illinois, studied LV hypertrophy in elite athletes to determine whether there is associated diastolic dysfunction. Echo indexes of early LV diastolic function in highly trained athletes were compared with those in age-matched normal volunteers. The athletes selected for study included: 11 swimmers with a pattern of myocardial hypertrophy and normal wall thickness to dimension ratio and 11 weight lifters whose wall thickness to dimension ratio was increased. Peak rates of LV dimension increase and wall thinning in swimmers and weight lifters were greater than in control volunteers despite significantly greater LV wall thickness and mass in the athletes. The increase in diastolic function indices was associated with greater ventricular size and systolic performance. Normalization of the peak rate of dimension increase for end-diastolic dimension and adjustments for the peak rate of wall thinning for fractional systolic thickening eliminated any differences between the two groups that were studied. These data indicate that diastolic function is normal in athletes with considerable physiologic hypertrophy. This is in contrast to findings in patients with hypertrophy associated with LV pressure or volume overload. These data suggest that factors other than or in addition to hypertrophy may alter LV segmental diastolic function in these patients.

Endurance training

Landry and associates[10] from Quebec, Canada, studied the sensitivity of cardiac structures to endurance training. To evaluate variability in adaptation, 20 sedentary subjects and 10 pairs of monozygotic twins were submitted to a 20-week endurance training program. Maximal oxygen (O_2) uptake increased significantly in both groups: 11 ml $O_2/kg/min^{-1}$, or 30%, in the sedentary group and 6 ml $O_2/kg/min^{-1}$, or 13%, in the monozygotic twins. Statistically significant increases in LV diameter, posterior wall and septal thicknesses, and LV end-diastolic volume and LV mass were observed in the sedentary subjects, but not in the monozygotic twins. The investigators demonstrated that after training, twin pairs differed more from each other than at the start. Concomitantly, within-pair resemblance was greater after training than before. Results indicate that cardiac dimensions are amenable to significant modifications under controlled endurance training conditions and furthermore that the extent and variability of the response of cardiac structures to training are perhaps genotype dependent.

Endurance athletes

Hauser and associates[11] from Royal Oak, Michigan, studied 12 highly trained male endurance athletes and 12 normally active matched control subjects by 2-D and M-mode echo to evaluate changes in the right- and left-sided heart chambers associated with intense aerobic training. Maximal oxygen uptake, a measure of cardiovascular fitness, ranged from 62–83 ml/kg/min in the athletes and from 33–49 ml/kg/min in the control subjects. The athletes had significantly greater LV wall thickness, LV chamber area, LA area, RV chamber area, RV wall thickness, and RA area. Proportionality of cardiac chamber enlargement in the athletes was shown by similar ratios of both RV to LV areas and RA to LA areas in the 2 groups. LV contractility was not significantly different between groups. Cardiac enlargement in endurance athletes enables a greater stroke volume for the performance of sustained, intense exercise; hypertrophy of the chamber walls normalizes wall stress. These changes occur symmetrically in both right and left cardiac chambers in the endurance athlete, reflecting bilateral hemodynamic loading. The symmetry of the endurance athlete's cardiac enlargement differs from most pathologic conditions, which have heterogeneous effects on specific cardiac chambers.

KAWASAKI DISEASE

Features of coronary disease

Nakanishi and associates[12] from Tokyo, Japan, described clinical, hemodynamic and angiographic features of obstructive CAD (≥90% diameter reduction) in 30 patients with Kawasaki disease. The mean age at the onset of Kawasaki disease was 2.9 ± 1.9 years and that at cardiac catheterization was 6.3 ± 2.8 years. Obstructive lesions were observed in the right coronary artery in 12 patients (group 1), in the LAD in 6 (group 2), in both right coronary artery and LAD in 10 (group 3), and in the LM coronary artery in 4 (group 4). Twenty-two patients (73%) had cardiac symptoms, including AMI in 10 (33%). Cardiac symptoms were observed in 41% in group 1, 100% in group 2, 80% in group 3, and 100% in group 4. LV end-diastolic pressure, end-diastolic volume, and EF were abnormal in 32% of the patients in group 1, a frequency less than that in other groups (83% in group 2, 78% in group 3, and 100% in group 4). Fifty percent had MR and 73% had LV wall motion abnormalities. No patient in groups 1 or 2 has died, but 8 of 14 patients in groups 3 and 4 have died. These observations indicate that coronary obstruction owing to Kawasaki disease can cause depressed LV function, MR, and LV wall motion abnormalities in children. Clinical and hemodynamic features of right coronary obstruction (isolated) are relatively benign compared with those of left coronary obstruction (isolated or combined with right obstruction).

Ventricular function

The long-term effects of Kawasaki disease on cardiac function were evaluated in 67 patients by Anderson and associates[13] from Cincinnati, Ohio. Serial M-mode echoes were obtained at the time of the initial diagnosis, 1–3 months, at 3–12 months, and at >12 months after the diagnosis. LV and LA dimensions, shortening fraction, LV and RV systolic time interval ratios, and computer analysis of digitized echoes of the LV chamber and posterior wall were obtained. The LA and LV dimensions were abnormal in half of the patients throughout the study periods. The shortening fraction was abnormal initially but became normal by the end of 3 months. The peak rates of emptying of the left ventricle and thickening of the posterior wall were significantly reduced in all evaluation periods. In addition, the peak rate of diastolic thinning of the posterior wall was reduced, although the peak rate of filling remained normal. Finally, >30% of patients studied beyond 12 months had a prolonged major filling and thinning period. There was no difference between patients with or without coronary artery aneurysms. All other systolic and diastolic phase intervals and rates of changes were normal. Contrary to previously published reports, it was concluded that patients with Kawasaki disease who do not have demonstrable CAD, exhibit abnormalities of cardiac chamber size and function long after their acute illness.

Nakano and associates[14] from Shizuoka, Japan, performed coronary angiograms in 75 children with Kawasaki disease examined within 3 months of the onset of illness. Ages ranged from 5 months to 12 years (mean, 2.8 years). Twenty-five patients had no significant coronary abnormalities and 14 had minimal enlargement with a maximum coronary diameter of ≤4 mm. In addition, there were 22 patients with moderate dilation of coronary arteries with maximum diameter of 4–8 mm, 7 patients with giant aneurysms of >8 mm, and 7 patients with stenotic lesions with or without AMI. Patients with giant aneurysms or stenotic lesions had a mildly depressed EF. Calculation of E_{max} using echo and pressure measurements before and after afterload reduction showed a marked decrease in estimated contractile state in patients with giant aneurysms or stenotic lesions. Follow-up study in 22 patients showed an improvement in the E_{max} measurements in patients with lesions that regressed to minimal enlargement (≤4 mm), whereas E_{max} tended to remain the same in patients with more severe lesions that did not regress.

Salicylate treatment

Koren and associates[15] from Toronto, Canada, compared the efficacy of high dose salicylates in reducing coronary artery involvement in Kawasaki disease in 36 children who received acetylsalicylic acid (ASA), 80–180 mg/kg/day, and in 18 who did not receive high dose ASA during the febrile phase of the disease and whose fever was controlled mainly with acetaminophen. The 2 groups were comparable with respect to age and body weight. In the ASA-treated group, the dose was adjusted to meet the therapeutic serum concentration range. There were significantly more cases of coronary involvement in the nontreated group (50%) than in the salicylate-treated group (17%) and of coronary aneurysms (39 -vs- 3%). During the febrile phase of the disease, salicylate serum concentrations achieved with a given dose were on the average 2-fold lower than during the nonfebrile phase, owing to impaired absorption of ASA. It is suggested that despite the difficulty in achieving therapeutic serum concentrations of salicylate during the febrile phase of Kawasaki disease with a dose as high as 100 mg/kg/day, this dose is potentially capable of preventing the associated CAD.

This article was followed by an editorial entitled, "Kawasaki Syndrome: Still a Mystery After 20 Years," by Bell.[16]

Aortocoronary bypass grafting

Suzuki and associates[17] from Osaka, Japan, reported on 6 children who underwent CABG for progressive coronary arterial obstruction due to Kawasaki disease. These patients were part of a study of 1,000 patients with a history of Kawasaki disease studied in Osaka. Coronary arterial lesions were detected in 246 of 1,000, and all have been monitored with serial coronary arteriography to determine prognosis. Occlusion, segmental stenosis, or critical stenosis were noted in 47 of 246 (19%) with 19 of 246 (7.7%) having a history of AMI. During this follow-up, 6 patients have come to successful CABG because of either progressive occlusive lesions of multiple arteries or significant narrowing associated with chest pain and abnormal exercise test or thallium perfusion defects. The investigators proposed that CABG should be used in patients after Kawasaki disease only if the progression of coronary lesions has been documented by serial angiogram, redistribution of a perfusion defect has been detected on delayed thallium imaging, and no coronary arterial lesions distal to these prospective graft sites have been detected. When these 3 conditions are satisfied, they further suggest that at least 1 of the following conditions must apply: localized stenosis in the LM progressing to critical stenosis, occlusion of ≥2 arteries, collateral vessels connecting to the peripheral portion of an occluded artery arise from the peripheral part of a vessel with progressive localized stenosis, or progressive localized stenosis or critical stenosis has developed in the LAD in addition to significant stenosis in the right coronary artery. Fortunately, most children with Kawasaki disease do not develop coronary abnormalities and those who do generally improve. There remain, however, a few children, such as documented in this study, who develop large aneurysms with subsequent development of significant stenosis, usually at the site of the inlet or outlet of the aneurysm.

TAKAYASU'S ARTERITIS

Hall and associates[18] from Rochester, Minnesota, reviewed findings in 32 patients in whom Takayasu arteritis was diagnosed at the Mayo Clinic between January 1, 1971, and December 31, 1983. Only patients whose angiographic findings were unequivocal were included in the study. Of the 32 patients, 26 were female, 23 were North American whites, 4 were Mexicans, 3 were Orientals, 1 was a Native American, and 1 was of Middle Eastern origin. Diagnosis was often delayed for long periods of time, with a median delay of 18 months. Patients had both nonvascular symptoms (arthralgias in 56%, fever in 44%, weight loss in 38%) and symptoms of vascular stenosis, such as arm claudication (47%) and systemic hypertension due to renal artery stenosis (41%). All patients had either multiple vascular bruits (94%) or absent pulsès (50%). Laboratory findings included anemia (44%) and elevations of erythrocyte sedimentation rate (78%). Almost all patients had multiple sites of arterial involvement documented by angiogram with various combinations of stenosis, luminal irregularity, and aneurysm formation. Response to corticosteroid treatment was usually very good, with dramatic improvement in nonvascular symptoms and return of pulses in 8 of the 16 patients with absent pulses before treatment. Five-year survival rate from time of diagnosis was 94%. Twelve patients underwent surgical procedures involving the carotid arteries (5 cases), subclavian artery (4 cases), and renal arteries (3 cases). Three aneurysms were resected: 1 had AVR for severe AR and 2 patients underwent PTCA. Pathologic changes were restricted to the media and adventitial layers of the vessel wall and were indistinguishable from those of giant cell or temporal arteritis. Takayasu arteritis is not restricted to any one racial group and is readily treatable with corticosteroids and surgical vascular reconstruction.

CARDIOVASCULAR FINDINGS IN THE ELDERLY

Intensity of cardiac sounds

Reddy and associates[19] from Pittsburgh, Pennsylvania, measured the absolute intensity of the first (S_1), third (S_3), and fourth (S_4) heart sounds (in mmHg) and the relative intensity of S_4 compared with S_1 in 146 normal persons aged 8–91 years using an infinite time constant, calibrated pressure mechanocardiograph applied to the chest wall with a loading pressure of 400 mmHg. The absolute intensity of S_1 and S_3 decreases with age, but the absolute intensity of S_4 does not increase with age. Therefore, the relative intensity of S_4 compared with S_1 increases with age. This finding may explain the increased frequency of S_4 in qualitative phonocardiograms in older persons.

ECG findings

Rajala and associates[20] from Tampere, Finland, evaluated the ECGs of 559 persons, 82% of the total population ≥85 years of age in the city of Tampere in 1977 and 1978 using the classification of the modified Minnesota code. The relative 5-year survival rates matched by age and sex were calculated for subjects with various ECG findings. Of the 559 persons, 391 (70%) died during the follow-up period. The lowest mortality rate was observed in those with no codable change or with minor abnormality in the ECG. ECG abnormalities suggestive of CAD were associated with significantly increased mortality. The greatest mortality rate was found in subjects with AF or first degree AV block. No increased risk of death was associated with left or right BBB, supraventricular premature contractions, or VPC.

Rajala and associates[21] from Tampere, Finland, surveyed in 1977 and 1978 674 persons aged ≥85 years living in 1 city in Finland; 559 persons (83%) were examined. ECG findings, classified according to the Minnesota code, were compared with reported cardiac symptoms, clinical CHF, clinical CAD, and relative cardiac volume on chest radiograph. ECG items had a poor association with cardiac symptoms. ST-segment depression, T-wave inversion, VPCs, and AF were related statistically highly significantly to clinical CHF, as were ST-segment depression and T-wave inversion to clinical CAD. High left R waves, VPC, and AF showed a significant association with cardiac enlargement (>500 m/m^2) and pulmonary congestion in chest radiographs.

Ventricular function

Nixon and associates[22] from Dallas, Texas, examined the effects of increasing and decreasing cardiac preload by 15% on the LV performance of 11 carefully screened normal subjects aged 61–73 years. Comparisons were made with 11 subjects aged 21–28 years. Two-D echoes were obtained before and at the termination of 5° of head-down tilt for 90 minutes and at the termination of graded lower body negative pressure to −40 mmHg. Heart rate and BP were unchanged after physiologic interventions. Changes in LV end-diastolic and stroke volumes were similar but of a smaller magnitude in the older subjects compared with changes in younger subjects. When LV end-diastolic volumes obtained at each extreme of preload variation were compared, the range of mean change was less in the older (23 ml, 26%) than in the younger subjects (31 ml, 41%). Control LV end-diastolic and end-systolic volumes were greater in the older subjects. This study shows that despite larger control LV volumes, alterations in preload produce changes in the LV end-diastolic and stroke volumes of these older subjects that conform to the normal LV function curve, but that these responses are diminished compared with changes in younger subjects, suggesting an age-related change in diastolic stiffness.

ECHO STUDIES

Determining LV mass and volume

Byrd and colleagues[23] from San Francisco, California, evaluated 84 normal adults to determine the ability of 2-D echo to measure LV mass accurately and the volume mass ratio. In this study, a modified Simpson's rule algorithm was used to calculate ventricular volumes from orthogonal to 2- and 4-chamber apical views. LV mass was calculated using an algorithm based on a model of the LV as a truncated ellipsoid. In this study, LV volumes and LV mass values were larger in normal men than in women (mean, 148 -vs- 108 g, respectively). Volume/mass ratios were constant at end-diastole and end-systole. These data suggest that 2-D echo may be used to define normal LV mass and the volume/mass ratio.

In obesity

Since few data have been reported regarding the influence of duration of obesity on cardiac performance, Nakajima and coworkers[24] from Osaka, Japan studied the performance of the left ventricle in 35 obese patients by means of noninvasive methods, including echo, carotid arterial pulse tracing, and phonocardiography. Patients were divided into 2 groups according to the duration of obesity: group 1 included patients who had been obese for <15 years, and group 2 comprised patients who had been obese for >15 years. There were no differences in the degree of obesity and cellularity of adipose tissue between the 2 groups. LV dimension and wall thickness, stroke volume, and cardiac output were significantly greater in both groups of obese patients than in nonobese control subjects. Group 2 had a significantly increased end-diastolic dimension index (calculated as end-diastolic dimension/cube root of body surface area), stroke index, and radius/wall thickness ratio of the left ventricle compared with group 1. Multiple regression analysis showed that end-diastolic dimension index, stroke index, and radius/wall thickness ratio correlated significantly with the duration of obesity. The investigators concluded that alterations of cardiac performance in obese patients with LV enlargement and wall thickening is attributed not only to the excess of body weight, but also to the duration of obesity.

In anorexia nervosa

The effects of reduction of LV muscle mass to subnormal levels on cardiac mechanics and afterload have not been fully characterized in man. Therefore, St. John Sutton and coworkers[25] from Philadelphia, Pennsylvania, investigated the effects of reduction of LV mass on cavity geometry, afterload, pump function, and exercise performance in 17 patients with anorexia nervosa and 10 age- and sex-matched normal subjects. LV mass index determined by 2-D echo was significantly lower than that in normal subjects (53 -vs- 79 g/m^2). LV end-diastolic and end-systolic volume indexes also were reduced in patients with anorexia nervosa compared with normal subjects (49 -vs- 65 ml/m^2; 14 -vs- 19 ml/m^2). Despite the reduction in LV mass and volume indexes, LV chamber architecture, mass/volume ratio, and short/long LV axis ratio were normal. LV afterload assessed as end-systolic meridional and circumferential wall stress was normal. EF, percent fractional shortening, and the relation between end-systolic wall stress and EF were all within normal limits. In 7 patients restudied after a 15–20% weight gain, LV mass and volume indexes increased significantly, but end-systolic wall stress and EF did not change. Ten patients with anorexia nervosa and resting heart rate and systolic BP significantly lower than control values underwent treadmill testing. Exercise duration, peak heart rate, peak systolic BP, and peak oxygen consumption were all significantly lower than normal. The hypotensive effect of fasting resulted in an initial decrease in afterload, which was the stimulus for reduction in LV mass. The LV remodeling associated with the mass reduction occurred in such a way that: 1) orthogonal, meridional, and circumferential wall stresses were normalized; 2) normal chamber shape and architecture were maintained; and 3) chamber function and stress-shortening relations were preserved. Thus down-regulation of LV mass per se, like up-regulation, is not associated with abnormal LV function.

In habitual alcoholics with and without hepatic cirrhosis

Dancy and associates[26] from London, UK, performed M-mode echo recordings of the left ventricle in 33 patients with alcoholic hepatic disease, 26 patients with various nonalcoholic hepatic diseases, and in 18 nonalcoholic control subjects. Groups were well matched for age and overall nutritional status (as assessed by anthropometry) and no subject studied had cardiorespiratory symptoms. Alcoholics had significantly increased LV free wall thickness and LV cavity dimension at end diastole. Multiple regression analysis of the data identified alcohol abuse as the most important variable affecting end-diastole, and this relation could not be explained by differences in age, sex, overall nutrition, cigarette smoking, thiamine status (total blood thiamine and thiamine pyrophosphate concentration), presence of hepatic disease, or severity of hepatic disease (cirrhotic -vs- noncirrhotic). The increase in LV free wall thickness was not significantly related to alcohol abuse. These results suggest that chronic alcohol abuse is an important independent risk factor for cardiac dilation, and that increase in end-diastole may be an early marker of alcoholic cardiomyopathy.

In systemic lupus erythematosus

Klinkhoff and associates[27] from Vancouver, Canada, studied prospectively clinical and echo findings in 47 patients with systemic lupus erythematosus (SLE) and in 46 age- and sex-matched controls. Pericardial abnormalities were identified in 10 patients with SLE and in no controls. Excluding MVP, valvular abnormalities were identified in 10 patients with SLE (21%) and in 3 controls (7%). In the patients with SLE, abnormalities included mitral valve leaflet thickening in 6, aortic valve thickening in 5, and mitral anular calcium in 2. The presence of valvular abnormalities correlated with duration but not with severity of SLE. The finding of systolic murmurs in 17 of 47 patients with SLE did not correlate with echo evidence of valvular disease. In 6 patients with SLE, valvular abnormalities detected by 2-D echo were not seen on M-mode echo.

Detecting incomplete mitral leaflet closure

The echo pattern of incomplete mitral leaflet closure (IMLC) is reported to be present in about 90% of patients with AMI and new onset of MR. To determine the significance of this echo sign, Kinney and Frangi[28] from Miami, Florida, retrieved all echoes containing this abnormality from a file of 1,200 consecutive echoes: 73 echoes manifested IMLC. These investigators also studied 52 patients without IMLC, but who were matched with the IMLC group with respect to a range of LV diameters at end-diastole and fractional shortening. The following was found in the control group: fewer wall motion abnormalities per patient, less frequent mitral "B bumps," and a smaller LV end-diastolic dimension. By logistic regression, the variable most important to the probability of having IMLC was the presence of mitral valve "B bumps." It was concluded that: 1) elevated LV filling pressure is associated with IMLC; and 2) IMLC is not specific for the subset of patients with papillary muscle dysfunction due to AMI. Rather, IMLC is commonly seen in association with dilated, usually ischemic cardiomyopathy.

Review of Doppler echo

Nishimura and associates[29] from Rochester, Minnesota, reviewed Doppler echo. They emphasized that Doppler echo has the capacity of measuring normal and abnormal velocities of blood flow noninvasively and that this procedure allows noninvasive quantitation of stenotic valve gradients, intracardiac pressures, and blood flow and semiquantitative assessment of valvular regurgitant lesions. This is a superb review article on Doppler echo.

CARDIAC CATHETERIZATION

As an outpatient

Klinke and associates[30] from Edmonton, Canada, reviewed the results of cardiac catheterization at their hospital when performed as an outpatient procedure. All cardiac catheterizations performed over a 66-month period was analyzed. A total of 3,071 outpatient cardiac catheterizations (83% of all cardiac catheterizations) were performed. The percutaneous femoral technique was used in 98% of the procedures. Most patients (79%) had both right- and left-sided cardiac catheterization and coronary angiography, which showed significant CAD (70%). Only 14% of the study results were normal. Thirty-four patients (1%) had major complications, including 4 deaths (0.13%). Seventy patients (2%) were admitted for observation only. More than 96% of all patients did not have a major complication and were discharged the same day. Thus, outpatient cardiac catheterization can be performed safely, with a potential reduction in hospital costs and better utilization of medical beds.

Return of transseptal approach

O'Keefe and associates[31] from Rochester, Minnesota, stressed that the use of the transseptal approach for catheterization at their institution had increased since 1980. The transseptal technique was used most commonly in adult patients with AS. They emphasized that recent innovations in equipment and refinement of the transseptal technique rendered it a safer procedure than was reported in the 1960s. Because fewer complications with this technique occur in patients in whom the transseptal procedure is done by physicians with extensive experience with this technique, the investigators recommended that the procedure be restricted to high volume cardiac catheterization laboratories that are equipped with biplane fluoroscopy.

Fick -vs- indicator dilution for cardiac output

Hillis and associates[32] from Dallas, Texas, performed a study to assess the relation between Fick and indicator dilution measurements of cardiac output in a large number of subjects and to evaluate this relation in patients with a low cardiac output, a high cardiac output, and left-sided cardiac regurgitation. In 808 patients (428 men, 380 women; mean age, 50 ± 11), cardiac output was measured by Fick and either thermodilution (right atrium to pulmonary artery) or indocyanine green dye (PA to systemic artery) within 10 minutes of each other. There was excellent agreement between Fick and both thermodilution and dye. The difference between Fick and indicator dilution measurements was 9 ± 9%; it was ≤10% in 67% and ≤20% in 91% of patients. The disparity between Fick and indicator dilution measurements was increased in patients with a low cardiac output (<2 L/min/m^2) (difference, 14 ± 11%) and those with AR or MR (difference, 13 ± 11%). In these groups, the disparity between Fick and thermodilution measurements was not exaggerated, but the disparity between Fick and dye measurements was greater. Thus, although there is excellent agreement between Fick and both thermodilution and dye measurements of cardiac output, thermodilution is preferable to dye in patients with a low cardiac output and those with AR or MR.

PHARMACOLOGIC TOPICS

Caffeine

Onrot and associates[33] from Nashville, Tennessee, investigated caffeine as a potential pressor agent in the treatment of orthostatic hypotension in persons with autonomic failure. Since such persons have relatively fixed sympathetic and renin system activity, the investigators reasoned that a caffeine-induced increase in BP without activation of these systems might suggest other mechanisms for this pressor effect. Thus, they examined the effects of caffeine and meals on BP and heart rate in 12 patients with autonomic failure. The influence of caffeine on plasma norepinephrine, epinephrine, and renin activity was also studied. Caffeine, 250 mg, increased BP by 12/6 mmHg, from 129 ± 25/78 ± 12 (mean ± SD) to a maximum of 141 ± 30/84 ± 16 mmHg at 45 minutes, but did not change heart rate, levels of norepinephrine or epinephrine, or plasma renin activity. BP decreased by 28/18 mmHg after a standardized meal, from 133 ± 32/80 ± 15 to a minimum of 105 ± 21/62 ± 12 mmHg at 60 minutes. After pretreatment with

250 mg of caffeine, the standardized meal induced a decrease of only 11/10 mmHg, from $140 \pm 33/79 \pm 7$–$129 \pm 31/69 \pm 13$ mmHg at 60 minutes. After long-term administration of caffeine (250 mg/day for 7 days) in 5 patients, postprandial BP remained higher after caffeine than after placebo. The investigators concluded that caffeine is a pressor agent and attenuates postprandial hypotension in autonomic failure and that this effect is not primarily due to elevations in sympathoadrenal activity or activation of the renin-angiotensin system. Caffeine may be useful in the treatment of orthostatic hypotension due to autonomic failure, especially in the postprandial state.

Alcohol

Although the prevailing view has been that alcohol intoxication causes depression of myocardial contractility, studies of acute hemodynamic effects of ethanol in normal subjects have yielded conflicting results, probably as a result of different study designs and use of clinical variables of varying validity as to cardiac function. Kelbaek and associates[34] from Herlev, Denmark, studied 6 healthy men aged 23–30 years by RNA at rest and at 2 submaximal exercise levels in the upright position during increasing alcohol intoxication. At light intoxication (serum ethanol 23 mmol/L), the median value of LVEF at rest decreased by 5%. At heavy intoxication (serum ethanol 45 mmol/L), the median LVEF decreased at rest by 11% and during 75% submaximal exercise, by 6%; heart rate at rest increased (median 81 -vs- 62 beats/min), and systolic BP decreased during 50% submaximal exercise (median 145 -vs- 163 mmHg). No significant changes of plasma epinephrine concentrations were recorded, whereas plasma norepinephrine concentrations were increased by 24% at rest during light intoxication and by 30–38% during heavy intoxication. No changes of LVEF and plasma catecholamine levels were recorded after ingestion of isovolumic, isocaloric drinks compared with values obtained before intake. Thus, influences of ingestion per se and repeated investigations of LV function were excluded. These findings suggest that in healthy subjects alcohol intoxication causes a dose-dependent impairment of cardiac contractility. Compensatory mechanisms may account for a reduced influence during exercise.

Platelets, prostaglandins, and stress

Platelets are believed to play a role in the pathogenesis of atherosclerosis and of the vascular obstruction that causes the acute complications of CAD. Since specific behavioral patterns appear to be related to the development of CAD and since emotional stress may predispose an individual to acute cardiovascular ischemia, Levine and colleagues[35] from San Antonio, Texas, hypothesized that platelet activation by catecholamines might be involved in these events. To study emotional stress, plasma samples were obtained from 61 senior medical residents immediately before they were to speak in public. There were significant increases in the plasma concentrations of the platelet-secreted proteins platelet factor 4 and β-thromboglobulin and epinephrine and norepinephrine immediately before speaking, which demonstrates that platelet activation and secretion occur in association with this type of emotional stress. Four trials were carried out to study the mechanism for this observed platelet secretion: 1) phenoxybenzamine; 2) propranolol; 3) aspirin (650 mg); and 4) aspirin (80 mg) were given several hours before the public speaking engagement. Neither phenoxybenzamine nor propranolol in doses that blocked the hemodynamic effects of α_1- and β_1-adrenergic stimulation modified platelet secretion. Aspirin also did not block platelet secretion, which suggests that platelets were not being stimulated through a cyclooxygenase-dependent pathway. This study provides direct evidence of platelet secretion in vivo in association with emotional stress and underscores the potential importance of platelet activation and secretion in the acute events that occur in patients with vascular disease.

Serneri and associates[36] from Florence, Italy, evaluated prostaglandin biosynthesis by the heart in 21 patients undergoing cardiac catheterization and coronary angiography for congenital or acquired heart diseases other than CAD. Prostacyclin (as 6-keto-PGF$_{1\alpha}$), PGE$_2$, PGF$_{2\alpha}$ and TXA$_2$ (as TXB$_2$) were measured by specific radioimmunoassay in blood from coronary sinus, aorta, and a peripheral vein under resting conditions and after cold pressor test (CPT). PGF$_{2\alpha}$ was always undetectable. In resting conditions, no significant differences in plasma 6-keto-PGF$_{1\alpha}$ or TXB$_2$ concentrations were found among coronary sinus, aorta, and peripheral venous blood and no transcardiac gradient existed (mean, $+0.4 \pm 1.2$ pg/ml for 6-keto-PGF$_{1\alpha}$, $+0.1 \pm 0.6$ pg/ml for PGE$_2$, and -0.4 ± 9.9 pg/ml for TXB$_2$). CPT was able to induce a significant increase in 6-keto-PGF$_{1\alpha}$ and PGE$_2$ concentrations in blood from the different sampling sites and a significant transcardiac gradient was found after CPT: $+11.6 \pm 7.4$ pg/ml for 6-keto-PGF$_{1\alpha}$ (p <0.01) and $+5.2 \pm 3.6$ pg/ml for PGE$_2$. TXB$_2$ levels significantly increased in peripheral venous blood (from 18 ± 6–29 ± 20 pg/ml), but they did not increase either in coronary sinus (from 22 ± 10–23 ± 10 pg/ml) or in aorta (from 22 ± 5–19 ± 7 pg/ml). These results indicate that cardiocoronary prostacyclin and PGE$_2$ synthesis is inappreciable under resting conditions but it becomes remarkable after sympathetic stimulation. On the contrary, no TXA$_2$ cardiocoronary biosynthesis seems to occur in patients free of CAD.

Calcium channel blockers—a review

Winniford and Hillis[37] from Dallas, Texas, reviewed the usefulness of verapamil, nifedipine, and diltiazem as therapy for tachyarrhythmias, systemic hypertension, pulmonary hypertension, CHF, Raynaud's phenomenon and disease, HC, Prinzmetal's variant angina, angina pectoris of effort, and angina pectoris at rest. The investigators pointed out that these pharmacologic agents differ markedly in their clinical utility. Verapamil is extremely effective in patients with supraventricular tachyarrhythmias, HC, and various anginal syndromes, but it appears to be ineffective or possibly even deleterious in patients with pulmonary hypertension, CHF of any cause, and Raynaud's phenomenon or disease. Nifedipine exerts a powerful vasodilatory effect and, as a result, is efficacious in patients with systemic or pulmonary hypertension, CHF, and Raynaud's phenomenon or disease. It is also beneficial in patients with various kinds of angina, especially when it is administered concomitantly with a β-adrenergic blocker. It is totally ineffective as an antiarrhythmic agent, but it is largely untested in patients with systemic or pulmonary hypertension, Raynaud's disease, and HC.

PRIMARY PULMONARY HYPERTENSION

Morphologic findings

Bjornsson and Edwards[38] from Rochester, Minnesota, described pulmonary histopathologic findings in 80 patients with a clinical diagnosis of primary pulmonary hypertension (PPH). The 80 cases included 73 autopsies, 6 open lung biopsy specimens, and 1 patient with both biopsy and autopsy tissue. (The clinical features of these patients were reported in *Circulation* 70:580–587, 1984.) Of the 80 cases, 45 (56%) had thromboembolic disease, 22 (28%) had plexogenic arteriopathy, and the remaining 13 (16%) had pulmonary veno-occulsive disease, primary medial hypertrophy, primary pulmonary arteritis, or changes consistent with pulmonary venous hypertension. The mean age was 16 years for primary pulmonary arteritis, 21–34 years for plexogenic pulmonary arteriopathy, primary medial hypertrophy, and pulmonary veno-occlusive disease, and 41 and 45 years for thromboembolic disease and pulmonary venous hypertension, respectively. In all forms except pulmonary veno-occlusive disease and apparent pulmonary venous hypertension, female patients were involved twice as often as male patients. With the exception of apparent pulmonary venous hypertension, patients with plexogenic pulmonary arteriopathy had the longest survival (63 months). Sudden death, however, occurred most frequently in patients with plexogenic disease (45%) and occurred 2.5 times as often in this group as in patients with thromboembolic disease. Among the 80 cases, the most frequent histopathologic lesions were medial hypertrophy, intimal proliferation and fibrosis, fibrinoid degeneration and necrosis, and thrombosis. Thrombi were commonly observed and may have developed in situ or by embolization; they were often rich in platelets when they occurred in small pulmonary vessels.

Spontaneous hemodynamic variability

The PA pressure and resistance at rest have been noted to vary spontaneously in patients with primary pulmonary hypertension (PPH). To evaluate this variation, Rich and associates[39] from Chicago, Illinois, measured hourly for 6 consecutive hours the heart rate, systemic and PA pressures, cardiac output, systemic and pulmonary revascular resistance in 12 patients (8 women, 4 men; aged 43 ± 13 years). After these baseline measurements, the patients were tested with hydralazine and nifedipine therapy. Spontaneous variability in pulmonary pressures and resistances occurred in each patient, with the amount of variation (coefficient of variation) in PA pressure averaging 8% and in total pulmonary resistance 13% over the 6 hours. The patients with the most variability in mean PA pressure also had the most variability in cardiac output. Variability also correlated with the severity of the disease, as the patients with the highest total pulmonary resistances also had the most variation for that factor. The amount of variability did not correlate, however, with the acute response to either hydralazine or nifedipine administration. Based on the average coefficients of variation in these 12 patients, estimates were obtained of the percent change needed for an observed change to be attributed to a drug effect with 95% confidence. From these estimates, it was projected that for a single patient, a mean change in pulmonary resistance of 36% or a mean change in PA pressure of 22% would be required to attribute the changes to a drug effect. Thus, spontaneous hemodynamic variability is a common phenomenon in patients with PPH and may account for substantial changes in PA pressure and pulmonary resistance at rest.

Therapy

Although short- and long-term hemodynamic effects of vasodilators in patients with PPH have been studied, the effect on survival remains unknown. Rich and coworkers[40] from Chicago, Illinois, measured the short-term response to nifedipine and hydralazine in 23 patients with primary pulmonary hypertension (PPH) and followed their clinical course over 2 years. A favorable drug response, defined as a decrease in the pulmonary vascular resistance in ≥20%, occurred in 18 patients (78%). Half of the patients who had a favorable short-term response were treated with long-term vasodilator therapy. Their clinical course was compared with that of responders who were not treated and with that of the nonresponders. Of the responders who were treated, 2 improved, 4 had no change, and 3 died; of the responders who were not treated, 1 improved, 3 had no change, and 5 died. Using stepwise Cox regression, the investigators evaluated age, sex, functional class on entry, PA pressure, pulmonary vascular resistance, and short-term drug response as predictors of survival and found only functional class and a favorable short-term drug response to be significant predictors. There was no difference in survival between the responders who were treated and those who were not. Thus, the investigators concluded that the ability to respond to short-term nifedipine or hydralazine therapy predicts longer survival for patients with PPH, but placing patients with a favorable short-term response on long-term vasodilator therapy does not affect the overall outcome.

In patients with PPH the administration of a vasodilating drug is often used to test pulmonary vasoreactivity. Hydralazine has been used as a test drug, but because of its long duration of action, there is a risk of sustained systemic arterial hypotension in patients with a fixed pulmonary vascular resistance. Groves and colleagues[41] from Denver, Colorado, Dallas, Texas, and Research Triangle Park, North Carolina, compared the acute hemodynamic effects of intravenous prostacyclin, a potent, short-acting vasodilator, with the effects of oral or intravenous hydralazine. Both prostacyclin and hydralazine increased cardiac output and decreased systemic pressure without changing PA pressure in 7 patients with PPH. The average decrease in total pulmonary resistance with prostacyclin ($-46\% \pm 5\%$) was more than that with hydralazine ($-32\% \pm 6\%$). The respective decreases in total systemic resistance were $-50 \pm 4\%$ -vs- $-43\% \pm 6\%$. The percent changes in individual responses to the 2 agents were correlated for PA pressure, systemic arterial pressure, total pulmonary resistance, and total systemic resistance. It was concluded that the pulmonary hemodynamic effects of prostacyclin resembled those of hydralazine. Prostacyclin may predict the acute pulmonary hemodynamic effects of hydralazine in PPH and because of its prompt, brief action may provide greater patient safety.

CARDIOVASCULAR SURGICAL TOPICS

Routine preoperative exercise testing before major noncardiac surgery

In patients about to undergo major noncardiac surgery under general anesthesia, specific clinical features are associated with an increased risk of postoperative death or cardiovascular complications. The most important of these risk factors is AMI within the previous 6 months. Other factors with an adverse prognostic impact include AS, decompensated CHF, preoperative arrhythmias, age >70 years, and emergency rather than elective surgery. Goldman et al devised an index of perioperative cardiac risk that is based on a weighted score determined by the risk factors present in each patient. Exercise test results were not included in their classic paper. Recently, Cutler et al reported a remarkable correlation between the results of preoperative exercise testing and the occurrence of postoperative cardiac complications in patients undergoing peripheral vascular surgery. Carliner and associates[42] from Baltimore, Maryland, carried out in 200 patients >40 years old and who were scheduled for elective major noncardiac surgery under general anesthesia a prospective study of preoperative exercise testing. The exercise test response was ECG positive in 32 patients (16%) (2 patients had a markedly positive test), equivocal in 11 patients (5.5%), and negative in 157 patients (78.5%). The patients were followed with a serial pre- and postoperative ECG and determinations of serum creatine kinase (CK) and CK-MB. Six patients (3%) had primary endpoints: 3 (1.5%) died postoperatively and 3 had definite postoperative AMI. Secondary endpoints of suspected postoperative myocardial ischemia or injury diagnosed by ECG or elevation in CK-MB levels occurred in 27 patients (14%). Endpoint events were more common in patients aged ≥70 years. Endpoint events also were more common in patients with an abnormal (positive or equivocal) preoperative exercise test response than in those with a negative response (27 -vs- 14%); however, preoperative exercise results were not statistically significant independent predictors of cardiac risk. Using multivariate analysis, the only statistically significant independent predictor of risk was the preoperative ECG. Endpoint events were more common in patients with an abnormal than in those with a normal ECG (23 -vs- 7%). Because the results of exercise testing do not appear to add substantially to the risk separation provided by the ECG at rest, exercise testing is not recommended as a routine preoperative method for assessing perioperative risk in older patients who are being evaluated before major elective noncardiac surgery under general anesthesia.

Therapy of mediastinitis

Trouillet and associates[43] from Paris, France, treated 19 critically ill adults with acute mediastinitis after cardiac surgery with granulated sugar, either directly (11 patients) or after failure of continuous irrigation (8 patients). Mediastinal tissue cultures were positive in 18 patients. Packing the mediastinal cavity with granulated sugar every 3 or 4 hours resulted in near-complete debridement of the wound and rapid formation of granulation tissue in all patients and sterilization of the wound after an average of 8 days. Dressings were easy and painless to change. Five (26%) patients died before discharge, but none because of wound complications. The rest were discharged on average 54 days (range, 29–120) after initial debridement of the wound; 11 underwent secondary surgical closure of the wound and in 3 the wound healed by granulation tissue formation alone. No recurrence of sternal infection had occurred after a mean follow-up of 8 months (range, 3–17).

CARDIAC AND/OR PULMONARY TRANSPLANTATION

Greenberg and associates[44] from Pittsburgh, Pennsylvania, evaluated long-term hemodynamic results in cardiac transplant patients treated with cyclosporine and prednisone. Nineteen patients were studied by cardiac catheterization and endomyocardial biopsy 13 ± 3 months after transplantation. Immunosuppression consisted of 6 ± 4 mg/kg/day cyclosporine and 20 ± 8 mg/day prednisone. Eighteen patients were asymptomatic but had developed postoperative systemic hypertension (17 on antihypertensive therapy). These patients were compared with a normotensive control group of 18 patients without cardiovascular disease. Significant differences were found in heart rate; RA, PA, PA wedge, systemic and pulmonary vascular resistance; and end-diastolic volume index and LVEF. The most frequent hemodynamic abnormalities included an elevated arterial pressure in 10 patients (56%), an elevated LV end-diastolic pressure in 6 patients (33%), and a reduced EF in 5 patients (28%). Hemodynamic abnormalities tended to resolve or improve in the 5 patients restudied 2 years after transplantation. There was no significant relation between fibrosis or inflammation on endomyocardial biopsy and hemodynamic abnormalities. It was concluded that mild to moderate hemodynamic abnormalities are common in asymptomatic cardiac transplant patients receiving cyclosporine and prednisone.

From March 1970 through December 1983, 40 orthotopic heart transplantation procedures were performed by Fuller and associates from Tucson, Arizona, at the University of Arizona Health Services Center.[45] Pulmonary infection with Legionnaire's disease agent (Legionella pneumophila) was documented by either culture or fluorescent antibody staining in 8 patients (20%). The primary symptom of pulmonary infection was fever occasionally associated with pleuritic chest pain, dyspnea, dry cough, or chills. Four patients had fever as the only symptom. Diagnosis was confirmed by transtracheal aspiration or direct percutaneous needle aspiration of the lesion. Treatment of each patient consisted of intravenous erythromycin (4 g/day). Patients with severe disease or those slow to respond also were treated with oral rifampin (600 mg/day). Although initial fevers disappeared rapidly after therapy was begun, radiographic clearing was delayed to an average of 1 month after presentation of the lesions. In all patients oral erythromycin was continued for 6–12 months. In 2 patients, symptoms recurred shortly after the treatment was changed from intravenous to oral erythromycin. Reinstituting intravenous therapy successfully eliminated symptoms. There were no deaths due to Legionnaire's disease.

The clinical heart-lung transplant program commenced at Stanford in 1981, and during the first 3.5 years of the program, 23 transplants have been carried out in 22 patients with severe pulmonary vascular disease by Dawkins and coworkers[46] from Stanford, California. Actuarial survival curves predict 1- and 2-year survival rate of 71 and 57%, respectively, for all patients (Fig. 9-1). As a result of increasing experience, the early mortality of 26% has been

Fig. 9-1. Actuarial survival curves for all patients undergoing heart-lung transplantation (△) compared with those for patients undergoing simple heart transplantation during the same period (●). Reproduced with permission from Dawkins et al.[46]

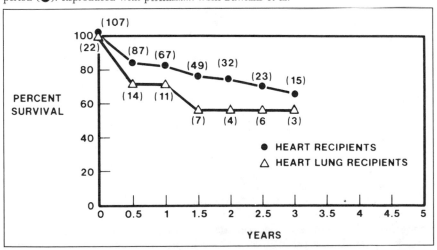

PERCENT SURVIVAL

● HEART RECIPIENTS
△ HEART LUNG RECIPIENTS

YEARS

reduced, with only 1 death occurring in the last 8 patients; prior cardiac surgery was a contributing factor in 3 of the 6 patients having early deaths. Two late deaths occurred 14 and 15 months after operation. One patient died suddenly as a result of an AMI, and the other patient died because of respiratory failure. At autopsy, both patients had severe proliferative coronary atherosclerosis with obliterative bronchiolitis affecting the lungs. An additional patient required a retransplant for obliterative bronchiolitis 37 months after the initial procedure, and he too was found to have severe CAD. Hemodynamics and LV function were normal in patients studied 1 and 2 years after undergoing the transplantation procedure. Thus, the early mortality and morbidity of combined heart and lung transplantation has been significantly reduced, but the long-term complications, particularly graft atherosclerosis and obliterative bronchiolitis, are yet to be fully controlled.

Brooks and associates[47] from Palo Alto and Stanford, California, reviewed infectious complications in 14 patients who received heart-lung transplants at Stanford University Medical Center from March 1981 to November 1983. Twenty-nine infections occurred in 12 patients: 18 bacterial, 9 viral, and 2 fungal. Sixteen (89%) of the bacterial infections occurred in the lung. Because of frequent colonization of the lower respiratory tract, the specificity of transtracheal aspiration and bronchoscopy was low. Empiric broad-spectrum antibiotic therapy was usually successful, and no patient died of bacterial infection. Cytomegalovirus infection occurred in 6 and herpes simplex virus infection in 3 patients. Two patients had invasive candidiasis at necropsy.

Yousem and associates[48] from Stanford, California, described morphologic pulmonary findings in patients who had either pulmonary biopsy or autopsy after total heart-lung transplantation at Stanford from 1980 until 1985. Of the 21 patients having combined heart-lung transplantation at Stanford, almost 80% survived beyond the immediate postoperative period, with the longest survivor greater than 3.5 years. Five patients died in the perioperative or immediate postoperative period and 11 returned to normal lives with essentially normal pulmonary function. In the remaining 5 allograft recipients recurrent respiratory infections and progressive obstructive airway disease developed, with superimposed restrictive deficits in 3 of them. Two open lung biopsies, 2 autopsies, and 1 retransplantation were performed in these 5 recipients. Morphologically, these 5 allograft recipients showed extensive bronchiolitis obliterans, interstitial and pleural fibrosis, and accelerated arterial and venous arteriosclerosis. Thus, bronchiolitis obliterans may prove to be a significant complication of heart-lung transplantation.

Bailey and associates[49] from Loma Linda, California, described the first case of cardiac xenotransplantation in a neonate. The recipient, who had aortic valve atresia, survived 20 days after the transplantation. Necropsy disclosed that the cardiac graft showed only traces of cell-mediated rejection. Transplant failure appeared to have resulted from a progressive, potentially avoidable humoral response, unmodified by immunosuppression. These investigators concluded that cardiac allotransplantation and selective baboon to human xenotransplantation deserve further exploration as investigational therapy for neborns with aortic valve atresia.

This article was followed by 2 editorials, the first entitled "Ethical Issues Raised by Research Involving Xenografts," and the second a statement of the Council on Scientific Affairs of the American Medical Association and entitled, "Xenografts." The latter report summarizes the published experience with animal and human xenografts to date and discusses the mechanism of xenograft rejection. The report concludes that the process of xenograft rejection qualitatively resembles allograft rejection, involving both cellular and humoral immune mechanisms, but differs quantitatively, depending on the genetic disparity between donor and recipient. Relative beneficial effects of various immunosuppression regimens, including cyclosporine on xenograft survival in donor recipient models with varying genetic disparity, have not yet been studied.

Jonasson and Hardy[50] from Chicago, Illinois, and New York City concluded the following: "What Dr. Bailey has demonstrated, however, in this remarkable experiment with Baby Fae is that orthotopic heart transplantation is technically feasible in the newborn, that even the strong cell-mediated immune response expected in a xenograft can be successfully suppressed with cyclosporine, and that a xenograft might serve as a most suitable short-term support for the circulation of a newborn with fatal congenital heart disease until a human heart donor can be found."

UNCATEGORIZABLE

Asymptomatic myocardial ischemia in diabetes mellitus

The reported higher frequency of painless AMI in diabetic patients suggests that asymptomatic transient myocardial ischemia may also be frequent in patients with diabetes mellitus. To explore this possibility, 51 patients with diabetes mellitus, aged 43–71 years (mean, 56 ± 8), 70 nondiabetic patients with CAD (mean age, 55 ± 5 years), and 40 nondiabetic patients without overt CAD (age, 54 ± 9) were evaluated in an investigation performed by Chiariello and associates[51] from Naples, Italy. Thirty-eight of the 51 diabetic patients (75%) had evidence of associated CAD and 19 (37%) had evidence of previous AMI. All patients underwent continuous 24-hour ambulatory ECG monitoring. In 18 of 51 diabetic patients, 93 episodes (73% of the total) of asymptomatic ST-segment changes were recorded; the total number of symptomatic episodes was 36, and they were observed in 7 patients (27%). Forty-eight (60%) asymptomatic and 32 symptomatic episodes of significant ST changes were found in nondiabetic patients with CAD. When patients with previous AMI were examined separately, asymptomatic episodes of significant ST changes were observed in 10 of 19 diabetic patients and in 5 of 25 nondiabetic patients with CAD. In an additional 28 diabetic patients who underwent exercise stress test, 15 had an abnormal ECG response; however, only 5 of them (33%) were symptomatic. This study suggests that the frequency of transitory myocardial ischemia, as assessed by ambulatory ECG monitoring and exercise stress test, is higher in diabetic patients than in nondiabetic control patients with CAD.

Cardiac problems in pregnancy—review

Sullivan and Ramanathan[52] from Memphis, Tennessee, superbly reviewed hemodynamic effects of pregnancy and the effect of pregnancy on the various cardiac conditions and how to manage various cardiac diseases during pregnancy (Table 9-3).

The king of hearts

Roberts and Podolak[53] from Bethesda, Maryland, described certain clinical and morphologic features in 23 patients in whom the heart at necropsy

TABLE 9-3. *Use of cardiovascular drugs during pregnancy. Reproduced with permission from Sullivan and Ramanathan.*[52]

AGENT	POTENTIAL PROBLEM
β-adrenergic receptor blockers	Uterine contraction, fetal bradycardia
Calcium blocking agents	Hypotension, cardiac failure
Digitalis	None known
Disopyramide	Uterine contraction
Diuretics	Fetal growth retardation
Heparin	Prematurity, stillbirth
Lidocaine	None known
Phenytoin	Birth defects
Quinidine, procainamide	None known
Warfarin	Teratogenic effects, hemorrhage

weighed ≥1,000 g (mean, 1,106). The heart weight/body weight ratio ranged from 1.2–2.7 (normal, 0.40). The 23 patients were derived from examination of the hearts of 7,671 patients with various cardiovascular disorders over a 25-year period. The massive cardiomegaly was the result of AR in 14 patients (61%): isolated in 8, associated with MR in 4, and with VSD in 2. Three others (13%) had combined AS and AR and 1 patient (4%) had MS and MR and mild AS. Four patients (17%) had HC and 1 patient (4%) had VSD with MS. They were 20–64 years old (mean, 42) and 21 (91%) were men. Four patients at necropsy had ≥1 major coronary artery narrowed >75% in cross-sectional area by atherosclerotic plaques, and only 4 patients had grossly visible LV scars, 2 of whom had insignificant coronary narrowing. Examination of an ECG in 17 of the 23 patients disclosed that Sokolow-Lyon criteria for LV hypertrophy was achieved in only 12 patients (71%) and Romhilt-Holt QRS voltage criteria faired even worse. Total 12-lead QRS voltage was >175 mm (10 mm = 1 mV) in 16 patients (94%) and it was >250 mm in 13 patients (76%). Total 12-lead QRS voltage in 17 patients ranged from 140–601 mm (mean, 323). Measurement of the sum of the 12-lead QRS voltage may be quite useful in diagnosing LV hypertrophy by ECG.

Pulmonary veno-occlusive disease

Pulmonary veno-occlusive disease was first described in 1934 but given its present name by Heath in 1966. It is an uncommon condition. Wagenvoort and associates[54] from Amsterdam, The Netherlands, collected 57 cases from a review of previous publications, not including a series of 43 cases briefly reported without detailed information by Dail in 1978. To the 57 cases, Wagenvoort and associates added 10 that had not been published previously. Of the total 67 patients, 40 were male and 27 female. They ranged in age from 11 days to 67 years; 20 patients were in the first decade of life, with 7 younger than 1 year of age at the time of death. The male predominance applied to adults only. Of the 30 patients <16 years of age, 15 were boys and 15 were girls; of the 37 adults, the male/female ratio was approximately 2/1. Pulmonary veno-occlusive disease differs from primary plexogenic arteriopathy in which boys and girls are affected equally, but in adults a pronounced female predominance is seen. Changes in the PAs in pulmonary veno-occlusive disease have attracted little attention compared with the attention given the veins. Medial hypertrophy is usually present. The investigators found that the arterial intimal alterations were often as severe as those in the veins. They found the PA intimal changes to occur in one-half of the 26 patients they studied histologically and morphometrically. They attributed both the arterial intimal changes and the venus changes to organization of thrombi.

Articles in United States cardiology journals in 1984

Several peer-review journals devoted exclusively to cardiology are published in the United States. Although the types of articles and the authors of (and reviewers for) the articles in the various American cardiologic journals are similar, the numbers of articles and pages utilized for them in the various journals are quite different. This article by Roberts[55] from Bethesda, Maryland, summarized the results of counting the numbers of editorial (nonadvertising) pages published and the types of articles published during 1984 in the *American Heart Journal*, the *American Journal of Cardiology*, *Circulation*, and the *Journal of the American College of Cardiology*. Analysis of the quantity of contents in the 4 major cardiologic journals for 1984 disclosed a total of 13,550 published editorial (nonadvertising) pages, including 11,377 pages (84%) in the regular issues (Table 9-4), 1,415 pages (10%) in the supplemental symposia issues, and 758 pages (6%) in supplemental issues for abstracts. Included in these 13,550 pages were 2,134 articles (1,878 [89%] being articles in the regular issues; 256 articles [11%] in the symposia issues) and 2,477 abstracts. In conclusion, this analysis shows that cardiologic journals use their page space differently. This analysis also discloses that some types of articles are neglected. Systemic hypertension is the world's most common

TABLE 9-4. *Comparison of the regular issues of the four major United States cardiovascular journals for 1984.*

	A	B	C	D
No. of pages (average/month)	2571 (214)	3403 (284)	3413 (201)	2990 (249)
For articles (pages/article)				
(average/month)	2392 (5,13)(199)	3077 (4.12)(256)	2252 (7.66)(188)	2682 (7.23)(224)
For letters (No.)(No. with replies)	21 (21)(14)	36 (80)(30)	0	30 (31)(21)
For staff, editorial board	10	15	18	39
For contents in brief	56	31	26	25
For contents with abstracts	0	145	0	98
For society news	0	0	77	15
For books	6	3	0	3
For volume indexes	56	69	30	62
For information for authors	24	15	4	28
For others	4	12	6	8
No. of articles (average/month)	466 (39)	747 (62)	294 (25)	371 (31)
Coronary heart disease	98 (21.0%)	140 (18.7%)	65 (22.1%)	80 (21.6%)
Arrhythmias and conduction				
disturbances	55 (11.8%)	76 (10.2%)	37 (12.6%)	46 (12.4%)
Systemic hypertension	9 (1.9%)	19 (2.5%)	11 (3.7%)	4 (1.1%)
Congestive heart failure	5 (1.1%)	16 (2.1%)	12 (4.1%)	10 (2.7%)
Valvular heart disease	18 (3.9%)	37 (5.0%)	11 (3.7%)	29 (7.8%)
Cardiomyopathy	7 (1.5%)	18 (2.4%)	9 (3.1%)	8 (2.2%)
Pericardial heart disease	1 (0.2%)	3 (0.4%)	2 (0.7%)	1 (0.3%)
Congenital heart disease	13 (2.8%)	47 (6.3%)	24 (8.2%)	38 (10.2%)
Cardiovascular pharmacology	9 (1.9%)	10 (1.3%)	4 (1.4%)	5 (1.3%)
Miscellaneous	24 (5.2%)	28 (3.7%)	20 (6.8%)	16 (4.3%)
Methods	10 (2.1%)	31 (4.1%)	10 (3.4%)	21 (5.7%)
Experimental studies	33 (7.1%)	64 (8.6%)	66 (22.4%)	50 (13.5%)
Editorials and point of view	18 (3.9%)	28 (3.7%)	22 (7.5%)	18 (4.9%)
Brief reports	166 (35.6%)	204 (27.3%)	0	44 (11.8%)
Historical studies	0	11 (1.5%)	1 (0.3%)	1 (0.3%)
From-the-Editor column	0	15 (2.0%)	0	0

cardiovascular condition. Yet only 2% of the 1,878 articles published in the regular issues of the 4 journals concerned this subject. This analysis of the 4 journals for 1 year is entirely a quantitative one. It concerns the quantity and type of content in each journal, not the quality of the content. Quality is another issue. It is less objective and more difficult to discuss numerically.

References

1. PERMANYER-MIRALDA G, SAGRISTA-SAULEDA J, SOLER-SOLER J: Primary acute pericardial disease: a prospective series of 231 consecutive patients. Am J Cardiol 1985 (Oct 1); 56:623–630.
2. SOULEN RL, STARK DD, HIGGINS CB: Magnetic resonance imaging of constrictive pericardial disease. Am J Cardiol 1985 (Feb 1); 55:480–484.
3. CALLAHAN JA, SEWARD JB, NISHIMURA RA, MILLER FA, REEDER GS, SHUB C, CALLAHAN MJ, SCHATTENBERG TT, TAJIK AJ: Two-dimensional echocardiographically guided pericardiocentesis: experience in 117 consecutive patients. Am J Cardiol 1985 (Feb 1); 55:476–479.
4. MCCAUGHAN BC, SCHAFF HV, PIEHLER JM, DANIELSON GK, ORSZULAK TA, PUGA FJ, PLUTH JR, CONNOLLY DC, McGOON DC: Early and late results of pericardiectomy for constrictive pericarditis. J Thorac Cardiovasc Surg 1985 (Mar); 89:340–350.
5. HUSTON TP, PUFFER JC, RODNEY WM: The athletic heart syndrome. N Engl J Med 1985 (July 4); 313:24–32.
6. MITCHELL JH, MARON BJ, EPSTEIN SE: 16th Bethesda Conference: cardiovascular abnormalities in the athlete: recommendations regarding eligibility for competition. J Am Coll Cardiol 1985 (Dec); 6:1189–1190.
7. DRISCOLL DJ: Cardiovascular evaluation of the child and adolescent before participation in sports. Mayo Clin Proc 1985 (Dec); 60:867–873.
8. CRAWFORD MH, PETRU MD, RABINOWITZ C: Effect of isotonic exercise training on left ventricular volume during upright exercise. Circulation 1985 (Dec); 72:1237–1243.
9. COLAN SD, SANDERS SP, MACPHERSON D, BOROW KM: Left ventricular diastolic function in elite athletes with physiologic cardiac hypertrophy. J Am Coll Cardiol 1985 (Sept); 6:545–549.
10. LANDRY F, BOUCHARD C, DUMESNIL J: Cardiac dimension changes with endurance training: indications of a genotype dependency. JAMA 1985 (July 5); 254:77–80.
11. HAUSER AM, DRESSENDORFER RH, VOS M, HASHIMOTO T, GORDON S, TIMMIS GC: Symmetric cardiac enlargement in highly trained endurance athletes: a two-dimensional echocardiographic study. Am Heart J 1985 (May); 109:1038–1044.
12. NAKANISHI T, TAKAO A, NAKAZAWA M, ENDO M, NIWA K, TAKAHASHI Y: Mucocutaneous lymph node syndrome: clinical, hemodynamic and angiographic features of coronary obstructive disease. Am J Cardiol 1985 (Mar 1); 55:662–668.
13. ANDERSON TM, MEYER RA, KAPLAN S: Long-term echocardiographic evaluation of cardiac size and function in patients with Kawasaki disease. Am Heart J 1985 (July); 110:107–115.
14. NAKANO H, UEDA K, SLATO A, NOGIMA K: Left ventricular systolic function in children with coronary arterial lesions following Kawasaki disease. Heart Vessels 1985; 1:89–93.
15. KOREN G, ROSE V, LAVI S, ROWE R: Probable efficacy of high-dose salicylates in reducing coronary involvement in Kawasaki disease. JAMA 1985 (Aug 9); 254:767–769.
16. BELL DM: Kawasaki syndrome: Still a mystery after 20 years (editorial). JAMA 1985 (Aug 9); 254:801.
17. SUZUKI A, KAMIYA T, ONO Y, TAKAHASI N, NAITO Y, KOU Y: Indication of aortocoronary by-pass for coronary arterial obstruction due to Kawasaki disease. Heart Vessels 1985; 1:94–100.
18. HALL S, BARR W, LIE JT, STANSON AW, KAZMIER FJ, HUNDER GG: Takayasu arteritis: a study of 32 North American patients. Medicine (Baltimore) 1985; 64:89–99.
19. REDDY PS, HAIDET K, MENO F: Relation of intensity of cardiac sounds to age. Am J Cardiol 1985 (May 1); 55:1383–1388.
20. RAJALA S, HAAVISTO M, KALTIALA K, MATTILA K: ECG findings and survival in very old people. Eur Heart J 1985 (Mar); 6:247–252.
21. RAJALA SA, GEIGER UKM, HAAVISTO MV, KALTIALA KS, MATTILA KJ: Electrocardiogram, clinical findings and chest x-ray in persons aged 85 years or older. Am J Cardiol 1985 (Apr 1); 55:1175–1178.

22. NIXON JV, HALLMARK H, PAGE K, RAVEN PR, MITCHELL JH: Ventricular performance in human hearts aged 61 to 73 years. Am J Cardiol 1985 (Dec 1); 56:932–937.

23. BYRD BF, WAHR D, WANG YS, BOUCHARD A, SCHILLER NB: Left ventricular mass and volume/mass ratio determined by two-dimensional echocardiography in normal adults. J Am Coll Cardiol 1985 (Nov); 6:1021–1025.

24. NAKAJIMA T, FUJIOKA S, TOKUNAGA K, HIROBE K, MATSUZAWA Y, TARUI S: Noninvasive study of left ventricular performance in obese patients: influence of duration of obesity. Circulation 1985 (Mar); 71:481–486.

25. ST. JOHN SUTTON MG, PLAPPERT T, CROSBY L, DOUGLAS P, MULLEN J, REICHEK N: Effects of reduced left ventricular mass on chamber architecture, load, and function: a study of anorexia nervosa. Circulation 1985 (Nov); 72:991–1000.

26. DANCY M, LEECH G, BLAND JM, GAITONDE MK, MAXWELL JD: Preclinical left ventricular abnormalities in alcoholics are independent of nutritional status, cirrhosis, and cigarette smoking. Lancet 1985 (May 18); 1:1122–1124.

27. KLINKHOFF AV, THOMPSON CR, REID GD, TOMLINSON CW: M-mode and two-dimensional echocardiographic abnormalities in systemic lupus erythematosus. JAMA 1985 (June 14); 253:3273–3277.

28. KINNEY EL, FRANGI MJ: Value of two-dimensional echocardiographic detection of incomplete mitral leaflet closure. Am Heart J 1985 (Jan); 109·87–90.

29. NISHIMURA RA, MILLER FA, CALLAHAN MJ, BENASSI RC, SEWARD JB, TAJIK AJ: Doppler echocardiography: theory, instrumentation, technique, and application. Mayo Clin Proc 1985 (May); 60:321–343.

30. KLINKE WP, KUBAC G, TALIBI T, LEE SJK: Safety of outpatient cardiac catheterizations. Am J Cardiol 1985 (Oct 1); 56:639–641.

31. O'KEEFE JH, VLIETSTRA RE, HANLEY PC, SEWARD JB: Revival of the transseptal approach for catheterization of the left atrium and ventricle. Mayo Clin Proc 1985 (Nov); 60:790–795.

32. HILLIS LD, FIRTH BG, WINNIFORD MD: Analysis of factors affecting the variability of Fick versus indicator dilution measurements of cardiac output. Am J Cardiol 1985 (Nov 1); 56:764–768.

33. ONROT J, GOLDBERG MR, BIAGGIONI I, HOLLISTER AS, KINCAID D, ROBERTSON D: Hemodynamic and humoral effects of caffeine in autonomic failure: therapeutic implications for postprandial hypotension. N Engl J Med 1985 (Aug 29); 313:549–554.

34. KELBAEK H, GJORUP T, BRYNJOLF I, CHRISTENSEN NJ, GODTFREDSEN J, VESTERGAARD B: Acute effects of alcohol on left ventricular function in healthy subjects at rest and during upright exercise. Am J Cardiol 1985 (Jan 1); 55:164–167.

35. LEVINE SP, TOWELL BL, SUAREZ AM, KNIERIEM LK, HARRIS MM, GEORGE JN: Platelet activation and secretion associated with emotional stress. Circulation 1985 (June); 71;1129–1134.

36. SERNERI GGN, GENSINI GF, ABBATE R, PRISCO D, ROGASI PG, CASTELLANI S, CASOLO GC, MATUCCI M, FANTINI F, DI DONATO M, DABIZZI RP: Spontaneous and cold pressor test-induced prostaglandin biosynthesis by human heart. Am Heart J 1985 (July); 110:50–55.

37. WINNIFORD MD, HILLIS LD: Calcium antagonists in patients with cardiovascular disease. Medicine (Baltimore) 1985 (Jan); 64:61–73.

38. BJORNSSON J, EDWARDS WD: Primary pulmonary hypertension: A histopathologic study of 80 cases. Mayo Clin Proc 1985 (Jan); 60:16–25.

39. RICH S, D'ALONZO GE, DANTZKER DR, LEVY PS: Magnitude and implications of spontaneous hemodynamic variability in primary pulmonary hypertension. Am J Cardiol 1985 (Jan 1); 55:159–163.

40. RICH S, BRUNDAGE BH, LEVY PS: The effect of vasodilator therapy on the clinical outcome of patients with primary pulmonary hypertension. Circulation 1985 (June); 71:1191–1196.

41. GROVES BM, RUBIN LJ, FROSOLONO MF, CATO AE, REEVES JT: A comparison of the acute hemodynamic effects of prostacyclin and hydralazine in primary pulmonary hypertension. Am Heart J 1985 (Dec); 110:1200–1204.

42. CARLINER NH, FISHER ML, PLOTNICK GD, GARBART H, RAPOPORT A, KELEMEN MH, MORAN GW, GADACZ T, PETERS RW: Routine preoperative exercise testing in patients undergoing major noncardiac surgery. Am J Cardiol 1985 (July 1); 56:51–58.

43. TROUILLET JL, FAGON JY, DOMART Y, CHASTRE J, PIERRE J, GIBERT C: Use of granulated sugar in treatment of open mediastinitis after cardiac surgery. Lancet 1985 (July 27); 2:180–184.

44. GREENBERG ML, URETSKY BF, REDDY S, BERNSTEIN RL, GRIFFITH BP, HARDESTY RL, THOMPSON ME, BAHNSON HT: Long-term hemodynamic follow-up of cardiac transplant patients treated with cyclosporine and prednisone. Circulation 1985 (Mar); 71:487–494.

45. FULLER J, LEVINSON MM, KLINE JR, COPELAND J: Legionnaires' disease after heart transplantation. Ann Thorac Surg 1985 (Apr); 39:308–311.

46. DAWKINS KD, JAMIESON SW, HUNT SA, BALDWIN JC, BURKE CM, MORRIS A, BILLINGHAM ME, THEODORE J, OVER PE, STINSON ED, SHUMWAY NE: Long-term results, hemodynamics, and complications after combined heart and lung transplantation. Circulation 1985 (May); 71:919–926.

47. BROOKS RG, HOFFLIN JM, JAMIESON SW, STINSON EB, REMINGTON JS: Infectious complications in heart-lung transplant recipients. Am J Med 1985 (Oct); 79:412–422.

48. YOUSEM SA, BURKE CM, BILLINGHAM ME: Pathologic pulmonary alterations in long-term human heart-lung transplantation. Hum Pathol 1985 (Sept); 16:911–923.

49. BAILEY LL, NEHLSEN-CANNARELLA SL, CONCEPCION W, JOLLEY WB: Baboon-to-human cardiac xenotransplantation in a neonate. JAMA 1985 (Dec 20); 254:3321–3329.

50. JONASSON O, MARDY MA: The case of Baby Fae. JAMA 1985 (Dec 20); 254:3358–3359.

51. CHIARIELLO M, INDOLFI C, COTECCHIA MR, SIFOLA C, ROMANO M, CONDORELLI M: Asymptomatic transient ST changes during ambulatory ECG monitoring in diabetic patients. Am Heart J 1985 (Sept); 110:529–534.

52. SULLIVAN JM, RAMANATHAN KB: Management of medical problems in pregnancy—severe cardiac disease. N Engl J Med 1985 (Aug 1); 313:304–309.

53. ROBERTS WC, PODOLAK MJ: The king of hearts: analysis of 23 patients with hearts weighing 1,000 grams or more. Am J Cardiol 1985 (Feb 1); 55:485–494.

54. WAGENVOORT CA, WAGENVOORT N, TAKAHASHI T: Pulmonary veno-occlusive disease: Involvement of pulmonary arteries and review of the literature. Hum Pathol 1985 (Oct); 16:1033–1041.

55. ROBERTS WC: Analysis of page utilization and types of articles published in four major American cardiology journals in 1985. Int J Cardiol 1985 (Aug); 8:353–360.

Author Index

Abate D, 222
Abbate R, 56, 401
Abben R, 15
Abbott RD, 117, 118, 193, 194
Abdulali SA, 289, 342
Aberg A, 131, 133
Abrahamsen AM, 160, 162
Abrams J, 199
Acampora D, 141, 142, 143
Acheson A, 230, 231
Adamec R, 22
Adams D, 27, 286
Adams PC, 213
Adgey AAJ, 156
Agarwal JR, 41
Agarwal KC, 354
Agatston AS, 285
Agranat O, 16
Ahnve S, 44, 145, 146, 147, 148, 150, 151
Aker UT, 2, 87
Akers MS, 12
Akhras F, 6
Akhtar M, 201
Alban J, 78
Albers JJ, 34, 35
Albin G, 239
Alderson PO, 12
Alexander S, 278
Algom M, 278
Allen BJ, 222
Allen HD, 331, 353
Allen J, 199
Allen M, 351
Allen PD, 116

Allen R, 269
Allen WM, 290
Allin D, 199
Allred E, 306
Allred EN, 281
Almazan A, 275
Almendral JM, 233
Als AV, 57
Al-Yusuf AR, 149
Amato JJ, 354
Ambrose JA, 54, 121
Ambrosioni E, 222
Ameisen O, 5, 53
Amery A, 262, 263, 264
Amin DK, 379
Amodeo C, 252
Amon RW, 65
Amparo EG, 128
Amsterdam EA, 217
Amuchestegui M, 368
Anastasiou-Nana M, 219
Anderson HV, 80, 85, 90
Anderson J, 199
Anderson JL, 219, 318
Anderson RH, 347, 352, 359
Anderson S, 199
Anderson TM, 392
Andresen D, 164
Antillon JR, 354
Antman EM, 66, 240
Aoshima M, 355
Appel AS, 33
Appel GB, 33
Appelbaum D, 173
Araujo L, 59
Arce J, 320
Arensman FW, 345

Aretz HT, 313
Armstron K, 226
Armstrong BE, 356
Armstrong MA, 24
Arnold AER, 88
Arnolda L, 376
Arntzenius AC, 39
Aroesty JM, 57
Aronoff RD, 377
Aronow WS, 117
Artinano E, 307
Arvan S, 125, 136
Ashihara T, 381
Ashram NE, 68
Askenazi J, 317
Athearn MW, 92, 93
Atlas SA, 371
Attar M, 165
Atwood JE, 226
Aucoin RA, 100
Aueron FM, 103
Austin J, 306
Averill DB, 55
Awan NA, 371
Aylmer AP, 261

Baaijens H, 154
Baardman T, 148
Bacharach SL, 79, 326
Badger RS, 60
Badillo P, 136
Baer F, 171
Baer L, 250
Baerman JM, 201, 205
Bahl V, 281, 282
Bahnson HT, 404
Bailar JC, 47

Bailey KR, 40
Bailey LL, 406
Bailey-Hoffman G, 269
Baird RJ, 261
Baker BJ, 221, 370
Bakkeren JAJM, 47
Balady GJ, 8
Balakumaran K, 14, 88
Baldwin JC, 300, 301,
    302, 305, 405
Ball SG, 375
Bandura A, 181
Bar F, 179
Barber JM, 160
Barboriak JJ, 251
Bardy GH, 242
Bargeron LM Jr, 332, 354,
    358
Barnaby PF, 159
Barnard RJ, 40
Barnay C, 215
Barr W, 394
Barr WK, 65, 315
Barrett-Connor E, 29, 32
Barry WH, 15
Barth JD, 39
Bartholomew M, 318
Bass TA, 319
Batchelder JE, 104
Bateman TM, 101
Bates ER, 103
Batsford WP, 205, 213
Battler A, 16
Batty JW, 168
Baumgartner W, 101, 102
Baur HR, 49
Baxley WA, 120
Becher H, 174
Beck W, 165
Becker LC, 126, 177
Beckers C, 2, 167, 170
Beder SD, 232
Bedynek JL, 4
Beekman R, 349, 350
Beelen A, 148
Been M, 288
Beerman LB, 335
Behar VS, 21, 22, 23, 94
Behrendt D, 349, 350
Belardinelli L, 197
Belhassen B, 324
Bell DM, 393
Bell J, 327
Beller GA, 19, 134
Bello L, 275
Bellocci F, 155
Bellotti P, 142, 144, 321
Belvins RD, 211
Bemis CE, 279
Benassi RC, 398

Benditt DG, 192, 196, 220
Benhorin J, 6, 124
Benson DW Jr, 192, 196,
    220
Berdoff RL, 301
Berenfeld D, 68, 324
Berenson GS, 33
Berger HJ, 368
Berger M, 301
Berger WE, 181
Berglund B, 48
Bergstrand R, 131, 133
Berman DS, 12, 124, 134
Bernard R, 177
Berne RM, 197
Bernhard A, 345
Bernstein L, 120
Bernstein RL, 404
Berra K, 181
Bershad S, 40
Bertaccini P, 222
Bertolasi CA, 217
Besozzi MY, 8
Bethge K-P, 164
Betocchi S, 325
Bhandari AK, 153, 235
Bharati S, 236
BHAT Research Group,
    158
Bhatia S, 240, 241
Bhatnagar D, 261
Bhatnagar SK, 149
Biaggioni I, 399
Biamino G, 171
Biello DR, 165
Bigger JT Jr, 157, 234
Billingham ME, 405, 406
Bini RM, 354
Bink-Boelkens MTE, 345
Bink-Boukens M, 193
Bircks W, 347
Birkenhager W, 262, 263,
    264
Bjelke E, 37
Bjorkholm M, 35
Bjornsson J, 401
Black HR, 235
Blackman MS, 342
Blackstone EH, 358
Blair SN, 43, 44, 256
Blanchot P, 215
Bland JM, 397
Blandford RL, 115
Blanke H, 169
Blankenhorn DH, 38
Blanski L, 199
Blaufox D, 270
Bleifeld W, 174, 177
Block PC, 82, 96
Blomback M, 178

Blomqvist CG, 58
Bloomfield P, 100
Blum CB, 33
Blum R, 67
Blumhardt R, 159
Boccadamo R, 227
Boden WE, 66, 139
Boehnert MT, 202
Boers GHJ, 47
Bohn D, 317
Boissel J-P, 164
Bolson EL, 60, 168
Boncheck LI, 278
Bonow RO, 79, 295, 320,
    325, 326
Borer J, 173
Borer JS, 5, 53, 279
Borkon A, 101, 102
Boros S, 196
Borow KM, 346, 353, 391
Bortolotti U, 359
Bory M, 177
Bos RJ, 148
Bosch X, 68, 88, 119, 149
Bosschieter EB, 35, 36, 37
Bott-Silverman C, 55
Botvinick EH, 80, 101,
    128, 322
Bouchard A, 149, 396
Bouchard C, 391
Boucher CA, 9, 10, 11,
    82, 96
Bough EW, 66
Bourassa MG, 3, 77, 81,
    88, 92, 93, 153, 371,
    372, 374
Bourke G, 38
Bove AA, 89, 180
Bove EL, 342
Bower R, 234
Boyan CP, 232
Boyle DMCC, 160
Boyle RM, 97
Braat SH, 4
Bracchetti D, 222
Brady PM, 195
Branch LG, 46
Brand A, 346
Brand DA, 141, 142, 143
Brand FN, 193, 194
Brandon G, 379
Brandt PW, 159
Brasseur LA, 2, 167
Brauman A, 278
Braun S, 68
Braunstein GD, 101
Braunsteiner H, 31
Braunwald E, 115, 116,
    173
Brawn WJ, 361

Bredlau CE, 3, 83, 84, 90
Breier C, 31
Bren GB, 121
Bresnahan D, 135, 317
Bresnahan DR, 54, 285, 288
Bresnahan JF, 89, 180, 285, 288
Breuer HWM, 300
Brewer HB, 40
Brewster DC, 11
Brin KP, 177
Brinker JA, 168, 177
Bristow D, 297
Bristow JD, 297
Brixko P, 262, 263, 264
Brodsky MA, 222
Brooks HL, 91, 278
Brooks N, 98
Brooks RG, 406
Brooks-Brunn JA, 178
Broudy D, 297
Brower RW, 139, 148, 177
Brown BG, 60, 97
Brown JW, 344, 348
Brown KA, 9
Brown MA, 159
Brown MS, 29, 31
Brown R, 195
Brown WV, 40
Brugada P, 4, 196, 197, 204, 230
Bruggemann T, 171
Brundage BH, 402
Brunner HR, 371
Bruschke VG, 39
Brush JE, 141, 142, 143
Brymer JF, 78
Brynjolf I, 400
Bucheleres G, 236
Buckingham TA, 191, 192
Buckley MJ, 308, 309
Buda AJ, 297
Bugiardini R, 72
Buis B, 39
Buja LM, 119, 172
Bulkley BH, 168, 177
Bull C, 332, 333, 334
Bulpitt C, 262, 263, 264
Burgess JH, 71, 381
Burgess N, 305
Burggraf GW, 237
Burkart F, 72
Burke CM, 405, 406
Burke GL, 33
Burn CS, 321
Bush CP, 354
Butler B, 214, 219
Butman S, 321
Butman SM, 45

Buttrick PM, 123
Buxton AE, 212, 233
Byington R, 158
Byrd BF, 322, 396
Byrd RC, 297
Byrum CJ, 342

Cabanoglu A, 348
Cain ME, 200
Cairns JA, 70, 71
Calderwood SB, 309
Caldwell JH, 168, 229
Caldwell RL, 344
Califf L, 140
Califf RM, 21, 22, 23, 140, 141, 149
Callaghnan J, 213
Callahan JA, 388
Callahan MJ, 388, 398
Camargo CA, 35
Camm AJ, 201
Campbell DB, 306
Campbell NPS, 156
Campbell RM, 193
Campbell RW, 202
Campbell RWF, 213
Campion B, 194
Cannon RO, 320
Cannon RO III, 325
Cantelli I, 222
Capone G, 55
Capone RJ, 203
Carabello BA, 125
Carey EL, 215
Carey JS, 97
Carim Y, 281
Carleen E, 235
Carliner NH, 404
Carmichael MJ, 358
Carnegie A, 257
Carpenter MA, 358
Carroll JD, 94
Carvalho A, 135
Carvalho MR, 348
Case J, 269
Case NB, 122
Case RB, 122
Cashion WR, 165
Casolo GC, 56, 401
Cass Principal Investigators and Associates, 95, 96
Cassidy DM, 233
Castaneda AR, 343, 355, 362
Castellani S, 401
Castelli WP, 39, 46
Castle H, 270
Cato AE, 403

Cercek B, 173, 174
Chadda K, 199, 202
Chadwick B, 377, 380
Chairella F, 142, 144
Chaitman BR, 3, 67, 87
Chakko CS, 367
Chalmer B, 141, 142, 143
Chance B, 367
Chandra N, 177
Chandran P, 227
Chandraratna PAN, 126, 370
Channer KS, 50
Chapman PD, 216
Charalmbopoulos C, 353
Charap MH, 58
Charbonnier B, 177
Chastre J, 404
Chatterjee K, 128, 322, 371, 378
Chawla SK, 273
Cheitlin M, 297
Cheitlin MD, 297
Chen CC, 303
Chengot M, 285
Chenzbraun A, 124
Cherkaoui O, 3
Chesebro JH, 89, 137, 173, 180
Chesler DA, 82
Cheymol G, 215
Chiang BN, 303
Chiarella F, 321
Chiariello M, 407
Chien S, 33
Chierchia S, 59, 72
Childs J, 269
Chin AJ, 343
Chino M, 170
Choong CYP, 296, 369
Christakis GT, 261
Christensen NJ, 400
Christiansen C, 140
CiSciascio G, 87
Claes J, 29, 30
Clancy KF, 279
Clark RE, 295
Clayden AD, 289
Cleland JGF, 375
Clement D, 262, 263, 264
Clements JP, 21
Clinton JE, 240
Cobanoglu A, 339, 347
Cobb FR, 149
Cobb LA, 229
Cody DV, 154
Cody RJ, 374, 378
Cohen JD, 269
Cohen LS, 173
Cohen M, 169, 259

Cohen MH, 232
Cohen MV, 293
Cohn JN, 369, 371
Cohn LA, 281, 306
Cohn LH, 281, 306
Co-investigators, 173
Cokkinos DV, 324
Col J, 167, 170
Colan SD, 327, 338, 346, 353, 391
Colavita PG, 214
Colditz GA, 46
Coleman E, 149
Coleman RE, 327
Collen D, 177
Collins D, 145, 146, 147, 150, 151
Collins JJ, 281, 306
Collins R, 179
Colombo A, 45
Colvin EV, 354
Come PC, 139
Commerford PJ, 165
Concepcion W, 406
Condorelli M, 407
Conetta DA, 319
Conklin CM, 101
Connolly DC, 16, 18, 129, 130, 131, 132, 388
Connor WE, 36
Conroy RM, 1, 42
Consensus Conference, 25, 26
Conti CR, 55, 66
Conway N, 136
Cook EF, 235
Cooley DA, 199, 278, 345, 349, 356
Cooper AA, 134
Cooper GR, 27
Cooper Jr. GN, 180
Cooperating Investigators from the Milis Study Group, 116
Copans H, 290
Copehaver GL, 64
Copel JA, 351
Copeland J, 405
Corbelli J, 104
Corbett JR, 12, 69, 119, 172
Corcos T, 77, 81, 88
Corr L, 382
Corr PB, 200
Cortina A, 121
Coryell KG, 351
Cosgrove DM, 99
Costa RK, 348
Costanzo-Nordin MR, 316
Cotecchia MR, 407

Coulander CD, 35, 36, 37
Coumel P, 215
Council on Scientific Affairs, 238
Cousineau D, 71
Covitz W, 236
Cowan LD, 29, 32
Cowley MH, 87
Cowley MJ, 82, 83
Cox J, 200
Craddock GB, 19, 134
Crampton RS, 235
Cran G, 160
Crawford MH, 65, 315, 390
Crawley JCW, 11
Crea F, 72, 164
Creager M, 371
Creager MA, 374
Crean PA, 53, 67, 119, 164
Cremer KF, 64
Cremieux AC, 299
Cresanta JL, 33
Crichton E, 373
Criley JM, 322, 323
Criqui MH, 29, 32
Croft CH, 69
Crosby L, 396
Crowley DC, 193, 254, 346
Crupi G, 344
Cueto-Garcia L, 326
Cukingnan RA, 97
Cumberland D, 91
Cummins RO, 231
Curb JD, 37
Currie PJ, 10, 285, 288
Curry PVL, 227, 228
Curtius JM, 300
Czeisler CA, 115, 116

Dabestani A, 321
Dabizzi RP, 56, 401
Dae M, 80
Dae MW, 101
D'Agostino R, 300, 301, 302
D'Alba P, 117
Dalen J, 173
D'Alonzo GE, 402
Daly L, 1, 38, 42
Daly P, 71, 378
D'Ambra MN, 308
Dancy M, 201, 397
Dangoisse V, 81
Daniel WG, 293, 294
Daniels W, 4

Danielson GK, 200, 280, 340, 352, 357, 360, 361, 388
Dannenberg AL, 117, 118
Dantzker DR, 402
Dargie HJ, 375
Darling RC, 11
Dash H, 64
David GK, 137
David PR, 77, 81, 88
Davies G, 72, 164
Davis JC, 211
Davis JL, 54
Davis JRE, 373
Davis K, 122
Davis KB, 91, 95, 96, 166, 167, 168
Davis RC, 4
Davison R, 135
Dawkins K, 305
Dawkins KD, 405
Day PJ, 291
De Bono DP, 177, 288
De Coster P, 2
De Feyter PJ, 89
De Koning H, 137
De Schaepdryver A, 262, 263, 264
De Zwaan C, 171, 179
Deal BJ, 195, 343
Deanfield J, 164, 333, 343
Debanne SM, 151, 153
Debono DP, 177
Debuitleir M, 201
Debusk RF, 181
Dec GW, 313
DeCastro CM, 13
Decoster PM, 167, 170
Defaie U, 178
Defeyter PJ, 85
Dekker A, 338
Del Negro AA, 180
Del Torso S, 360
Delclos G, 203
Deligonul U, 87
Dellborg M, 138
Dell'Italia LJ, 159
Demorizi NM, 288
Denes P, 155, 241
Denker S, 201
Dennies AR, 154
DePace NL, 279
DeRouen T, 97
Deruyttere M, 262, 263, 264
Dervan JP, 99
Desoyza N, 221
Desvigne-Nickens P, 173
Detre KM, 82, 83
Detry JMR, 167, 170

Detry JR, 2
Deverall PB, 227, 228, 347
Devereux RB, 279
Di Donato M, 56, 401
Di Donato RM, 361
DiBianco R, 199, 371, 372, 374
DiCarlo L, 201, 205, 211
Dick M, 254
Dick M II, 193
Didge HT, 174
Dilsizian V, 326
DiMarco JP, 153, 197
Dincer B, 2
Dinh H, 221
Dirschinger J, 63
Discigil KF, 206
DiSesa V, 306
Disesa VJ, 281
Distante A, 54, 74
Dobmeyer DJ, 276
Dodge HT, 60, 168, 173
Doherty JU, 212, 233
Dolgin M, 287, 289
Dollery C, 262, 263, 264
Dollery CT, 382
Domart Y, 404
Domenicucci S, 142, 144
Donaldson DR, 97
Dongas J, 201
Doorey AJ, 81
Dougherty AH, 216
Douglas JS, 83, 84, 85, 90
Douglas P, 396
Dove JT, 104
Doyle TP, 278
Drake CE, 276
Drayer JIM, 259
Dreifus L, 236
Drewinski GR, 261
Dressendorfer RH, 392
Drexel H, 31
Driscoll DJ, 314, 340, 390
Dubner SJ, 217
Duff HJ, 215, 222
Dulk K, 196
Dumesnil J, 391
Dumoulin P, 215
Duncan FM, 373
Duncan JJ, 256
Duncan JM, 349
Dunn HM, 156
Dunn RF, 120
Dunnigan A, 192, 220
Dunnigan AN, 196
Dunning AJ, 137, 157, 177
Dupras G, 3
Duran CG, 307

Duster MC, 345
Dwyer EM, 93
Dzau V, 371

Eagle KA, 235
Easley K, 99
East BW, 375
Echt DS, 218, 226
Edelmann B, 169
Editorial, 260, 262, 263
Edlund A, 48
Edward DW, 340
Edwards BS, 301
Edwards CRW, 260, 373
Edwards JE, 273, 283, 284, 285, 301
Edwards M, 117
Edwards WD, 283, 299, 326, 333, 334, 335, 336, 337, 352, 361, 401
Effert S, 169
Eichhorn P, 83
Eichler HG, 165
Eiho S, 56
Eisenberg MS, 231
Eisenberg PR, 123, 165
Eitel DR, 240
Elayda MA, 13
Elcff S, 367
Elencwajg BD, 217
Elkayam U, 370, 380, 382
Ellenbogen KA, 214
Ellis H, 278
Ellis SG, 299
Ellison CR, 38
Ellison RC, 38
El-Sherif N, 259
Elveback LR, 16, 18, 129, 130, 131, 132
Elwood JH, 160
Emura M, 167
Enderlein MA, 351
Endo M, 392
Eng A, 54
Engelmeier RS, 316, 318
Engler RL, 226
Ensminger S, 64
Entwisle G, 270
Epstein M, 281
Epstein SE, 295, 320, 325, 390
Erbel R, 177
Erikssen J, 335
Espiner EA, 257
Esterbrooks DJ, 181
Estes M, 216
Estruch MT, 277
Etienne F, 117
Evans AE, 160

Evans-Bell T, 211
Ewart CK, 181
Ewels CJ, 89
Ezri MD, 241

Fagard R, 262, 263, 264
Faggian G, 359
Fagon JY, 404
Faitel K, 211
Falcone RA, 233
Falk RH, 240
Fallon JT, 313
Falvo-Gerard L, 269
Fantini F, 56, 401
Farr JE, 256
Farrell B, 59
Favrot L, 199
Faxon DP, 371, 374
Fayerweather WE, 130
Fedor J, 94
Fee HJ, 97
Feit A, 259
Feld G, 217, 224
Feld H, 380
Felder SD, 233
Feldman RL, 55, 64, 66, 67
Feldt RH, 340
Ferguson D, 242
Ferguson RK, 261
Fernandez-Aviles, 275
Ferrario CM, 55
Ferraro N, 367, 373
Ferrick A, 155
Ferrick KJ, 157, 234
Feyter PJ, 89
Fiebig R, 174
Fifer MA, 116, 346
Figulla HR, 314, 315
Filho EF, 348
Filipchuk N, 119
Filipchuk NG, 12
Finberg S, 252
Fine G, 290
Fines P, 3
Fink L, 367
Finnie KJ, 70, 71
Fiore AC, 348
Fioretti P, 139, 148
Firth BG, 399
Fischer DR, 335
Fishbein MC, 290
Fisher JD, 155, 223, 233
Fisher LD, 91
Fisher ML, 126, 404
Fisher R, 127
FitzGerald GA, 48
Fitzpatrick A, 376
Flaherty JT, 62, 177

Flammang D, 215
Fleischmajer R, 40
Fleiss JL, 157
Fletcher PJ, 296, 369
Fletcher RD, 253, 254, 257
Flint CJ, 331
Floras JS, 258
Flores BT, 212
Flowers D, 206, 209, 214, 215, 219, 221
Flowers NC, 276
Force T, 100
Ford I, 375
Forette F, 262, 263, 264
Forman MB, 132
Forte J, 262, 263, 264
Fortuin NJ, 253
Foster ED, 91
Foster JR, 225
Fouad FM, 371
Fowler B, 47
Fox KM, 52, 64
Franciosa JA, 135, 221, 370, 375, 381
Francis CK, 173
Francis GS, 369
Francis MJ, 203
Franco I, 104
Frangi MJ, 398
Frank R, 215
Franklin R, 333
Frazier OH, 278
Frederick TM, 79
Freed MD, 355
Freedman B, 72
Freedman DS, 33
Freedman MH, 327
Freedman SB, 120
Freedom R, 346
Freeman AP, 127
Freidenberger L, 370
Freis ED, 257
Freis EDD, 254
Fremes SE, 261
French JW, 341
Fricker FJ, 335
Friedman GD, 24
Friedman PL, 15
Friedman SD, 374
Friedrich T, 122
Friesinger GC, 132
Fritz JK, 122, 166, 167
Froelicher V, 98
Froelicher VF, 44
Froggatt GM, 70, 71
Frohlich ED, 249, 260, 270
Frosolono MF, 403
Frottier J, 299

Frumin H, 211
Frye RL, 92, 93, 280
Fujii T, 77
Fujioka S, 396
Fuller J, 405
Fulton KL, 69, 73, 76
Furberg C, 179
Furberg CD, 269
Fuster V, 54, 121, 137, 305
Fyfe DA, 361
Fyhrquist F, 250

Gabliani GI, 12, 73, 76, 119
Gadacz T, 404
Gahrton G, 35
Gaitonde MK, 397
Galan K, 104
Gallagher J, 200, 242
Gallery CA, 60
Gallino A, 49
Gallo I, 307
Gallucci V, 359
Gander MP, 83
Ganesh B, 289
Gang ES, 220, 277
Gangadharan V, 171
Ganz P, 15
Ganz W, 124, 173, 174
Garan H, 206, 216
Garay SC, 34
Garbart H, 404
Garcia E, 13
Garcia EJ, 275
Garcia-Dorado A, 275
Garcia-Dorado D, 275
Garcia-Satue E, 307
Gardin JM, 321
Gardner T, 101, 102
Garfein OB, 93
Garnic JD, 15
Garrison RJ, 46
Garson A Jr, 193, 195, 199
Gash AK, 125
Gavish A, 6
Gavras HP, 371
Gay JA, 253
Gay WA, 47
Geary GG, 159
Geboers J, 29, 30
Gee DS, 297
Geibel A, 317
Geiger UKM, 395
Gelman JS, 67
Geltman EM, 165
Generalovich T, 379
Gensini GF, 56, 401

Gensini GG, 166
Gent M, 70, 71
George JN, 400
German LD, 214, 242
Gersh BJ, 92, 93, 103, 200
Gerstenblith G, 177
Gertz EW, 5
Gessman LJ, 288
Gettes LS, 225
Gheorghiade M, 367
Ghisla RP, 331
Gibert C, 299, 404
Gibson RS, 19, 134
Gidding SS, 254, 349, 350
Gilbert EM, 318
Gilboa Y, 278
Giles RW, 127
Gillen G, 375
Gillespie JA, 147
Gillespie MJ, 91, 95, 96
Gillette PC, 195, 199, 345
Gilpin E, 145, 146, 147, 148, 150, 151
Ginsberg HN, 40
Ginzton LE, 277
Girod DA, 344, 347
Gittenberger De Groot A, 338
Gjorup T, 400
Glasgow GA, 321
Gliklich J, 234
Glomset JA, 36
Go M, 4, 5
Godtfredsen J, 400
Goede LV, 97
Goel I, 93
Golbus M, 351
Gold HK, 116
Gold RJM, 351
Goldberg E, 301
Goldberg HL, 5
Goldberg MR, 399
Goldberg RJ, 191, 192, 203
Goldberg S, 99
Goldberg SJ, 331, 353
Goldberger AL, 146, 147
Goldhaber SZ, 179
Goldman L, 235
Goldman ME, 305
Goldschlager N, 240, 241
Goldsmith SR, 369
Goldstein J, 299
Goldstein JL, 29, 31
Goldstein NG, 252
Goldstein RL, 100
Goldstein S, 78, 158, 230, 231, 290
Golik A, 278
Gomez A, 275

Gonzalez J, 199
Goodwin JF, 325
Gordon HJ, 145
Gordon S, 171, 392
Gorlin R, 54
Gosselin AJ, 92, 93
Gotsman MS, 173
Gott V, 101, 102
Gottdiener J, 257
Gottdiener JS, 253, 254, 320
Gottlieb S, 124, 214
Gottlieb SH, 177, 277
Gottlieb SO, 168, 177
Gowers J, 237, 238
Gradman AH, 205
Graham I, 38
Grande P, 140
Grant G, 206
Gray RJ, 101
Grayboys TB, 199
Grazi S, 150
Green CE, 180
Green MS, 27
Green MV, 79, 326
Green SJ, 290
Green TP, 220
Greenberg BH, 297
Greenberg E, 242
Greenberg H, 93
Greenberg MA, 123
Greenberg ML, 197, 404
Greenspan AM, 195, 206, 209, 211, 218, 220
Gregg RE, 40
Greipp PR, 326
Grendahl H, 232
Greuntzig AR, 83, 84, 90
Griffin JC, 226
Griffin MR, 299
Griffith BP, 404
Griffith LSC, 207, 212, 213, 216, 231
Grimm RH Jr, 19, 269
Grogan EW, 233
Grose RM, 123
Grosgogeat Y, 215
Grossman W, 57, 116, 169
Grottum P, 160, 161
Groves BM, 403
Gruchow HW, 251
Gruentzig AR, 80, 82, 83, 85
Grundy SM, 30
Grunkemeier GL, 339, 347, 348
Guarnieri T, 196, 198
Guerci AD, 177
Guiney TE, 10

Guiteras Val P, 77
Gundersen T, 160, 162
Gunnar RM, 318
Gurland B, 269
Guthaner DF, 145
Guzman PA, 168

Haavisto M, 395
Haavisto MV, 395
Hadjimiltiades S, 279
Haeberli A, 49
Hagan RD, 256
Haggerty JJ, 103
Hagler DJ, 285, 288, 333, 334, 335, 336, 337, 352
Haidet K, 395
Haimowitz A, 301
Haines DE, 134
Hakki A-H, 2, 19, 20, 126, 127, 279
Halim MA, 98
Hall DG, 341
Hall MH, 290
Hall RJ, 13
Hall S, 394
Hallman GL, 349
Hallmark H, 395
Hallstrom AP, 229
Hamaker WR, 104
Hamdy R, 262, 263, 264
Hamer A, 277
Hammill SC, 200
Hampton EM, 219
Hamsten A, 178
Handler CE, 147
Hanley PC, 399
Hannon DW, 331
Hansen RM, 101
Hanson P, 8
Hanson TP, 301
Harada Y, 354
Harbrecht JJ, 181
Hardesty RL, 404
Hargrove WC, 227, 229
Harken AH, 227, 229
Harlan LC, 252
Harlan WR, 252
Harper M, 87
Harper RW, 10
Harrell FE Jr, 21, 22, 23
Harrington JT, 257
Harris F, 217
Harris MM, 400
Harris PJ, 296, 369
Harris WS, 36
Harsha DW, 33
Hartnell GG, 16
Hartwell TD, 116
Har-Zahav Y, 16

Hashida Y, 352
Hashimoto A, 354
Hashimoto T, 392
Hasin Y, 173
Haskell WL, 34, 181
Hassan MO, 258
Hassan Z, 291
Hattner RS, 80
Haufe M, 194
Hauser AM, 392
Hauser AW, 171
Hausmann D, 293, 294
Haverich A, 305
Haworth SG, 338
Hayashi H, 71, 354
Hayashi T, 170
Hayes DL, 239, 357
Heikkila K, 252
Heine DL, 216
Heintzen P, 345
Heintzen PH, 338
Heiss G, 27
Held P, 138
Helfant RH, 41
Heller B, 40
Heller GV, 57
Heller JA, 257
Heller SS, 122
Helmrich SP, 117
Hemberger JA, 77
Hendrickson J, 217, 224
Heng MK, 217
Henkel TW, 261
Henling CE, 356
Hennekens CH, 46, 179
Henning H, 145, 146, 147, 148, 150, 151
Henriquez R, 382
Henry A, 381
Henry JF, 262, 263, 264
Henry WL, 222, 321
Herman MV, 99
Hernandez J, 87
Herndon SP, 341
Herold M, 31
Herre JM, 226
Hess M, 371, 372, 374
Hess OM, 94
Hesslein PS, 193
Hettleman BD, 327
Heuch I, 37
Heupler FA, 55
Heyndrickx GR, 85
Hickey AJ, 274
Hickey N, 1, 38, 42
Higginbotham MB, 149
Higgins CB, 128, 322, 388
Hildner F, 285
Hilgard J, 241
Hilgenberg AD, 308

Hill JA, 55, 66
Hillis LD, 68, 69, 73, 76, 173, 399, 401
Hindman MC, 21, 22, 23
Hirasawa K, 369
Hirobe K, 396
Hiroki T, 58
Hirsh PD, 87
Hirzel HO, 83, 94
Hlatky MA, 141
Ho G, 291
Ho SWG, 6
Hobson CE, 309
Hochreiter C, 279
Hodgson JM, 103
Hodsden JE, 276
Hodsman GP, 375
Hoeg JM, 40
Hofflin JM, 406
Hoffman JR, 124
Hofling B, 49, 50, 51, 52
Hofmann T, 317
Hoit B, 145, 146
Holder DA, 70, 71
Hollenberg M, 4, 5
Hollenberg NK, 371
Hollister AS, 399
Hollman J, 104
Holman BL, 66
Holmes DR, 103, 180, 200, 239
Holmes DR Jr, 54, 89, 357
Holmes J, 67
Holmes JR, 378
Holt DW, 213
Holt J, 121
Holt PM, 227, 228
Holtzman R, 259
Hood WP, 120, 293, 294
Hopkins J, 65, 216
Hopkins RA, 356
Hordof HA, 193
Horneffer P, 101, 102
Horowitz L, 199
Horowitz LN, 195, 206, 209, 211, 218, 220, 223
Hoshino S, 344
Houle S, 261
Houston D, 252
Hsieh AM, 317
H-Sievers H, 345
Hsu L, 148
Hsu TL, 303
Hsueh W, 370
Huang DX, 29, 30
Hubbard JD, 40, 352
Huberty J, 80
Hugenholtz PG, 14, 85, 88, 89, 139, 148
Huhmann W, 177

Huikuri HV, 96
Hulley SB, 269
Hulse S, 379
Humen DP, 69
Hunder GG, 394
Hung J, 3
Hunt JD, 203
Hunt SA, 405
Hunter H, 223
Hunter S, 202, 353
Hurwitz A, 157
Hurwitz RA, 344
Huston TP, 389, 390
Hutton BF, 296, 369
Huttunen JK, 25
Hysing J, 232

Igarashi E, 124
Ikram H, 257, 376
Illingworth DR, 36
Ilstrup DM, 78, 273, 274
Imai Y, 344, 354
Imaizumi T, 381
Inada M, 135
Indolfi C, 407
Ingwall JS, 116
Inkeles S, 40
Insel H, 87
Insel PA, 240
Intarachot V, 217
Ionescu MI, 342
The IPPSH Collaborative Group, 262, 266, 267
Ischinger T, 87
Isenberg HS, 236
Ishida M, 167
Ishihara K, 354
Iskandrian AS, 19, 20, 126, 127, 279
Ivanov J, 261
Iwasaka T, 135

Jablonsky G, 70, 71
Jackson B, 376
Jackson G, 6
Jaffe AS, 116, 119, 123, 156, 165
Jahrmarker H, 194
Jaillon P, 215
James MA, 50, 62
Jamieson SW, 300, 301, 302, 305, 405, 406
Janicki JS, 369
Jansen DE, 12, 119
Jaski B, 85
Jedeiken R, 358
Jee LD, 259
Jenkins AC, 261

Jenkins D, 100
Jenkins JM, 193
Jennings G, 376
Jensen D, 98
Jeresaty RM, 273
Jewitt DE, 67
Johannessen KA, 159, 160, 161
Johannessen K-A, 163
Johansson S, 131, 133
Johnson A, 261
Johnson AM, 136
Johnson LL, 12
Johnson RA, 21, 22, 23, 313
Johnson SM, 73, 76
Johnston CI, 376
Johnston DL, 69
Jolley WB, 406
Jonas RA, 355, 362
Jonasson O, 407
Jones JV, 258
Jones M, 295
Jones TK, 341
Joob AW, 358
Joossens JV, 29, 30, 262, 263, 264
Jordan RA, 375, 381
Josa M, 100
Josephon MA, 65
Josephson MA, 216
Josephson ME, 212, 227, 229, 233
Joyal M, 64
Juaneda E, 338
Julresd TR, 340
Juni JE, 297
Just H, 317

Kafka H, 237
Kaijser L, 48
Kaiser GC, 91, 92, 93
Kaiser H, 169
Kajiwara N, 170
Kalff V, 10, 360
Kaltiala K, 395
Kambara H, 170
Kamikawa T, 71
Kamiya T, 394
Kammatsuse K, 170
Kan G, 137
Kanaya M, 354
Kane-Marsch S, 19, 20
Kannel WB, 43, 44, 117, 118, 193, 194, 236
Kanter KR, 359
Kaplan K, 135
Kaplan NM, 254, 257
Kaplan S, 331, 392

Kappagoda T, 148
Kappenberger L, 83
Kaprio J, 252
Karchmer AW, 309
Kardon MB, 260
Karlson KE, 180
Karpawich PP, 354
Karsch KR, 169
Kaski JC, 59, 72
Kasper W, 317
Kass EH, 39
Kassirer JP, 257
Katayama K, 77
Kates RE, 219
Katz AI, 254, 255
Katz C, 202
Katz RJ, 121
Kaufman DW, 117
Kaul S, 10, 216
Kavey RW, 342
Kawabori I, 341
Kawada M, 354
Kawai C, 56, 170
Kawanishi D, 126
Kay HR, 195, 206, 209, 211
Kay PH, 339
Kazmier FJ, 137, 394
Keane JF, 193, 195, 281, 282
Keats AS, 356
Keefe D, 219, 221
Keelan MH, 278
Keelan MH Jr, 91
Keenan DJM, 136
Keenan RL, 232
Kekwick CA, 237, 238
Kelbaek H, 400
Kelemen MH, 404
Kelly DT, 120, 296, 369
Kelly E, 206
Kelly ME, 104
Kelly MJ, 10, 145, 360
Kelsey SF, 82, 83
Kempen-Voogd N, 39
Kemper AJ, 100
Kennedy EE, 213
Kennedy GT, 65
Kennedy HL, 2, 87, 191, 192, 282, 284
Kennedy JW, 122, 166, 167, 168
Kennedy LJ, 191, 192
Kenny J, 67
Kent KM, 79, 82, 83, 89, 180
Kereiakes DJ, 86
Keren A, 124, 145
Keren G, 324
Kerin NZ, 211

Kern MJ, 65
Kertes PJ, 3
Kesteloot H, 29, 30
Kevaney J, 38
Khaja F, 78, 290
Khalilullah M, 281, 282
Khandelwal PD, 250
Kher A, 215
Khuri SF, 100
Kiat H, 376
Kienzle MG, 233
Kiess M, 10, 96
Kiff P, 67
Killen DA, 104
Killip T, 92, 93, 95, 96
Kim D, 145
Kim SG, 155, 223, 233
Kincaid D, 399
King H, 344, 348
King ML, 287, 289
King SB III, 83, 84, 85, 90
Kingma H, 4
Kinney CD, 156
Kinney EL, 398
Kinney JL, 252
Kiowski W, 72
Kirklin JK, 358
Kirklin JW, 332, 358
Kisslo J, 242, 286
Kisslo JA, 327
Kitano M, 355
Kjekshus J, 160, 161
Klatsky AL, 24
Kleijer WJ, 47
Kleikamp G, 347
Klein HO, 281
Klein LW, 41
Klein MD, 100
Klein MS, 165
Kleinman CS, 351
Kligfield P, 5, 53, 279, 378
Kline JR, 405
Klinke WP, 398
Klinkhoff AV, 397
Kloppenborg PWC, 47
Knapp E, 31
Knapp HR, 48
Knatterud G, 173
Knieriem LK, 400
Knill JR, 261
Kobayashi A, 71
Kobrin I, 260
Kodama K, 170
Kohchi K, 58
Kohno M, 77
Kohtoku S, 77
Kolodgie FD, 132
Konstam M, 371, 372, 374

Kooijman CJ, 14
Kopelman HA, 132
Koplin JR, 261
Koren G, 173, 393
Korfer R, 347
Korhonen UR, 96
Korr KS, 66
Koskenvuo M, 252
Koster RW, 157
Kostuk WJ, 69, 70, 71
Kotler MN, 1, 2, 93
Kotlewski A, 153
Kou Y, 394
Kousch D, 269
Koyanagi H, 354
Krafchek J, 286
Krajcer Z, 324
Kramer BL, 297, 368, 374
Kramer H, 279
Kramer JB, 200
Kramer MF, 116
Kramer-Fox R, 279
Krauss XH, 179
Krayenbuehl HP, 94
Kremer P, 174
Kremers M, 58
Kreutzer GO, 355
Kreuzer H, 314, 315
Krikler DM, 325
Krishnamurthy G, 297
Krol RB, 201, 205
Kromhout D, 35, 36, 37, 39
Kron IL, 153, 358
Krone RJ, 147
Kronmal RA, 27, 91, 92, 93
Kubac G, 398
Kübler W, 81
Kubo SH, 374, 378
Kuller LH, 229
Kumlin T, 25
Kumpeng V, 352
Kunis CL, 33
Kunis R, 93
Kurland LT, 299
Kurnik PB, 175
Kurosawa H, 344
Kushi LH, 38
Kusukawa R, 77, 128
Kuwahara M, 56
Kvam D, 216
Kveselis DA, 346
Kyle RA, 326
Kyoku I, 355

L'Abbate A, 54, 74
Labovitz AJ, 2, 282, 284, 308

Labresh KA, 291
Laddu A, 199
Lahiri A, 11
Lakatos E, 295
Lakier JB, 290
Laks MM, 277
Lal R, 216
Lally EV, 291
Lam C, 252
Lam J, 3, 67
Lam R, 290
Landa B, 202
Landis JR, 230, 231, 252
Landry F, 391
Lang P, 362
Lange PE, 338
Langford H, 270
Langinvainio H, 252
Laniado S, 68, 324
Lanzer P, 322
Lapeyre AC III, 137
Laragh JH, 250, 374
LaRaia PJ, 308
Laramee P, 173, 174
Larosa JC, 32, 33
Lasher JC, 159
Laskarzewski P, 29, 32
Lattanzi F, 54
Lauer M, 351
Laureano R, 56
Lavi S, 393
Le NA, 40
Le Winter M, 150, 151
Leachman RD, 324
Lee CN, 357
Lee DCS, 313
Lee KL, 21, 22, 23, 141
Lee NH, 117
Lee R, 199
Lee RG, 165
Lee SJK, 398
Lee WH, 373, 375, 377
Leech G, 397
LeFree MT, 103
Legrand V, 103
Lehmann MH, 201
Lehtonen A, 258
Leiboff RL, 121
Leidenius R, 250
Leier CV, 276
Leighton R, 230, 231
Leimgruber PP, 80, 83,
    84, 85, 90
Leitner E, 171
LeJemtel TH, 371, 377,
    380
Lenfant C, 28
Lennane RJ, 177
Lenox C, 352
Lenox CC, 335

Leon CA, 203, 377
Leon L, 205
Leon MB, 320
Leonard D, 378
Leonetti G, 262, 263, 264
Lerman BB, 153, 197
Lesch M, 317
Lesoway R, 69
Lesperance J, 3
Lev M, 236
Levin DC, 15
Levin RI, 58
Levine HD, 125
Levine JH, 196, 198
Levine S, 89
Levine SP, 400
Levine TB, 371
Levinson MM, 405
Levite HA, 123
Levy PS, 402
Levy RI, 41, 42, 43
Lew AS, 124, 173, 174
Lew H, 181
Lew RA, 38
Lewin A, 270
LeWinter M, 145, 146,
    147, 226
Lewis AB, 313
Lewis JF, 79
Lewis JM, 79, 165
Lewis JW, 307
Lewis SA, 87
Lewis SE, 12, 116, 119
Liao T-K, 340
Liberthson RR, 323
Lichey J, 122
Lichtlen PR, 293, 294
Lidell C, 224
Lie JT, 394
Liem B, 205
Light A, 135
Likoff M, 371, 372, 374
Lim J, 13
Lim YL, 10, 82
Lima JAC, 276
Lima SD, 276
Lin SG, 62
Lincoln C, 344, 353, 359
Linderer T, 171
Lindheimer MD, 254, 255
Lindsay G, 351
Lipnick RJ, 46
Lippman SM, 277
Lipscomb K, 58, 317
Lipton MJ, 128, 322
Lisch HJ, 31
Little WC, 315
Litwak R, 305
Liu P, 10, 96
Livelli F Jr, 234

Livesay JJ, 349
Livi U, 359
Llewellyn MP, 177
Lloyd EA, 165
Lnage P, 345
Locati E, 235
Lock JE, 281, 282
Loge D, 297
Lombardi F, 210
Lombardo M, 150
Lonn E, 124
Loogen F, 300
Loop FD, 99
Lorell BH, 116, 346
Lotan C, 173
Lotto A, 150
Lovejoy FH, 202
Lowenstein E, 323
Lown B, 210, 214
Lown D, 157
Lozy M, 38
Lperfido F, 155
Lubsen J, 177, 179
Luck JC, 226
Ludbrook P, 173, 175
Luderitz B, 198
Ludwig W, 19
Luig H, 314, 315
Lund-Johansen P, 262,
    263, 264
Luria MH, 151, 153
Luria MY, 173
Lurie PR, 313
Lutz JR, 219, 318
Lytle BW, 99

Mabin TA, 89, 165
Macartney FJ, 333, 352
MacCosbe P, 199
MacDonald RG, 55
Macfarlane D, 38
MacGregor GA, 250
Mackay A, 288
MacKenzie G, 156
MacMahon SW, 274
MacMillan JP, 13
MacMillan RM, 288
MacPherson D, 391
Maddahi J, 12, 124, 134
Madonik MM, 261
Madsen EB, 148
Magee P, 98
Magee T, 99
Magilligan DJ Jr, 307
Magovern JA, 306
Magro SA, 226
Maher MB, 40
Mahler SA, 203

Mahmud R, 201
Mahoney LT, 351
Mahony L, 344
Mair DD, 357
Maisel AS, 145, 146, 147, 150, 151, 226, 240
Malagold M, 169
Malcolm AD, 278
Malergue MC, 299
Malhotra H, 250
Malone P, 211
Mancini D, 380
Mancini GBJ, 103
Mandel WJ, 220, 277
Mandke NV, 354
Mangan KF, 253
Mann DE, 226
Mann DL, 226
Manners JM, 136
Manolio T, 101, 102
Mansfield PB, 341
Manyari D, 222
Manz M, 198
Manzoli U, 155
Maranhao V, 288
Marbey ML, 354
Marchand E, 153
Marchant PR, 115
Marchlinski FE, 212, 227, 233
Marcus B, 281
Mardy MA, 407
Maresh CM, 181
Maris J, 367
Mark DB, 21, 22, 23
Markandu ND, 250
Markis JE, 169, 173
Maron BJ, 253, 295, 320, 321, 326, 390
Maroto E, 275
Martin RD, 202
Martins JB, 232
Marx GR, 331, 353
Marzilli M, 78
Marzuk PM, 256
Maseri A, 59, 72, 164
Masini M, 54
Maskin CS, 377, 380
Mason DT, 371
Mason J, 235
Mason JW, 218
Massie B, 5, 297, 368, 371, 372, 374
Massumi GA, 13
Mata LA, 77, 88
Mathey DG, 168, 174, 177
Mathur D, 250
Mathur VS, 13
Matloff JM, 101, 290
Matoba Y, 167

Matos JA, 155, 223, 233
Matsuda M, 77, 128
Matsuda Y, 77, 128
Matsuzawa Y, 396
Matthay MA, 101
Matthews PG, 376
Matthews RA, 335
Mattila K, 395
Mattila S, 25
Matucci M, 401
Mauritson DR, 73, 76
Maxwell JD, 397
Maynard C, 122, 166, 167, 168
Mazuz M, 232
Mazzari M, 155
Mazzucco A, 359
McAllister RG, 225
McAuley BJ, 86
McAuley DB, 86
McCabe CH, 8, 91
McCans JL, 53
McCaughan BC, 340, 388
McComb JM, 156
McCornish MJ, 6
McCormick JR, 91
McDaniel HG, 57
McDonald M, 269
McDonald R, 269
McGill E, 269
McGoon DC, 280, 340, 361, 388
McGoon MD, 72, 73, 74, 75, 273, 274, 360
McGovern B, 206
McGrath BP, 376
McGrath LB, 332, 354, 358
McHenry P, 236
McIlmoyle EL, 160
McIntosh CL, 295
McKay C, 380
McKay RG, 57
McKee DC, 103
McKenna W, 343
McKenna WJ, 325
McKinnis RA, 149
Mclanahan S, 39
McLaran C, 200
McLaughlin PR, 261
McNamara DG, 199, 345
McNamara MT, 128, 322
McNamara PM, 236
McNamee P, 11
McPherson CA, 205, 213
Mead RH, 219
Medical Research Council Working Party, 262, 265, 266
Medina EO, 128

Medina N, 373, 375, 377
Medina R, 1
Medvedowsky J-L, 215
Mee RBB, 361
Megidish R, 324
Mehmel HC, 81
Mehta SR, 250
Meijler FL, 128
Meinertz T, 317
Meister SG, 55
Melendez LJ, 70, 71
Melidossian CD, 374
Melin JA, 2, 167, 170
Meltzer RS, 137
Mendelzon R, 217
Menlove RL, 318
Meno F, 395
Mentzer RM, 358
Merab JP, 157
Meran DO, 59
Merians DR, 34
Messerli FH, 260
Metsarinne K, 250
Mettauer B, 71, 381
Metzdorff MT, 339, 348
Meyer B, 55
Meyer H, 347
Meyer J, 177
Meyer RA, 331, 392
Meyers J, 44
The Miami Trial Research Group, 163
Michael JR, 196, 198
Michel PL, 177
Michels HR, 177
Michels VV, 314
Mickle DAG, 261
Mickle P, 69
Miettinen TA, 25
Mikell FL, 104
Milis Study Group, 115, 116
Miller AB, 319
Miller DC, 300, 301, 302, 305, 341
Miller DR, 117
Miller FA, 273, 274, 314, 388, 398
Miller HI, 324
Miller JM, 227, 229
Miller JP, 147
Miller NH, 181
Milliken JA, 237
Mills J, 313
Milner PG, 231
Mindich BP, 305
Mintz GS, 1, 2, 93, 195
Missell L, 36
Misserli FH, 252
Mitchell JH, 390, 395

Mitchell LB, 222
Mitchell RS, 300, 301, 302, 305
Mitsudo K, 170
Miura D, 214, 215, 219, 221
Miura T, 77
Miwa H, 170
Miyazaki S, 56
Mochtar B, 88
Mock MB, 92, 93, 103
Mockus L, 64
Mockus LJ, 52
Moise A, 23, 149
Molteni A, 317
Molthan M, 236
Mongiardo R, 155
Monro JL, 136
Monteferrante JC, 99
Montenero AS, 155
Moorehead C, 346, 349, 350
Moorman JR, 327
Morady F, 201, 205, 211, 235
Morales MA, 54, 74
Moran GW, 404
Moran JF, 316
Morgan JP, 139
Morganroth J, 1, 195, 199, 206, 211, 223, 225
Moris C, 121
Morissette D, 68
Moritani K, 77, 128
Morley AR, 213
Morris A, 405
Morris J, 120
Morris KG, 149
Morris S, 236
Morse JR, 70
Morton JJ, 375
Moscarelli E, 74
Moses HW, 104
Moss AJ, 122, 147, 235
Mosseri M, 173
Motulsky HJ, 240
Moulijn AC, 137
Moussa MAA, 149
Mudd G, 2
Mudd SH, 47
Mueller HS, 123, 173
Muesing RA, 32, 33
Muhlbaier L, 94
Muhlberger V, 31
Mukharji J, 58
Mulcahy R, 1, 38, 42
Mullen J, 396
Muller JE, 115, 116
Müller-Brand J, 72
Mullin SM, 82, 83

Multi-Center Post-Infarction Research Group, 122
Multiple Risk Factor Intervention Trial Research Group, 4, 268, 269
Mundth ED, 279
Muraoka R, 355
Murchison J, 288
Murphy ML, 221
Murray IPC, 127
Myers MG, 70, 71
Myers WO, 91, 92, 93
Myking OL, 163
Myler RK, 87

Naccarella F, 222
Naccarelli GV, 216
Nademanee K, 217, 224
Naessens J, 326
Nagle F, 8
Naito Y, 394
Nakae S, 354
Nakajima H, 369
Nakajima T, 396
Nakamura M, 381
Nakanishi T, 392
Nakano H, 355, 393
Nakao S, 139
Nakazawa M, 344, 354, 392
Nanas JN, 219
Nanna M, 370
Narayan A, 196
Narula O, 199
Nath HP, 120
Nathan DG, 327
National Institutes of Health Consensus Development Conference Statement,
Naukkarinen V, 25
Neaton JD, 19, 269
Neches WH, 193, 335
Nehlsen-Cannarella SL, 406
Nellessen U, 293, 294
Nelson DL, 80
Nelson JG, 282, 284
Nestico PF, 279
Nesto RW, 66, 70
Neufeld HN, 16
Neumann A, 353
Neumann P, 169
Neuspiel DR, 229
Neustein HB, 313
Newman G, 94
Nicholas J, 160

Nicholls G, 376
Nicholls MG, 257
Nicod P, 12
Nieger M, 314, 315
Nielsen A, 140
Nielsen AP, 226
Nieminski KE, 99
Nigam S, 122
Niles N, 279
Nimalasuriya A, 126
Nishimura RA, 180, 273, 274, 388, 398
Nistal F, 307
Nitzberg WD, 120
Niwa K, 392
Nixon JV, 395
Nobuyoshi M, 58, 170
Nogima K, 393
Nolan SP, 358
Nomoto S, 355
Nonogi H, 56
Nordrehaug JE, 159, 160, 161, 163
Norris RM, 159
Norwood WI, 343
Notargiacomo A, 257
Nowak J, 48
Nygaard TW, 134

Oakley CM, 325
Oakley D, 91
Obeid A, 275
O'Callaghan WG, 214
Ocken S, 377
O'Connell JB, 316, 318
O'Connell JW, 80
O'Donnell J, 236
Oelert H, 293, 294
O'Fallon WM, 299
Offord KP, 326
O'Gallagher D, 215
Ogawa A, 135
Ogawa H, 77, 128
Oglesby ME, 256
Oh JK, 78, 357
O'Hara MJ, 11
Okada RD, 9, 10, 11, 82, 96
O'Keefe JH, 399
Okereke OUJ, 278
Okin PM, 5, 53
Okuda H, 344
Oldham HN, 356
Olinger GN, 91, 278
Olivieri N, 327
Olley PM, 346
Olsen EGJ, 314
Olshansky B, 232

Olson HG, 45
Olson LJ, 283
O'Malley K, 262, 263, 264
Ong LY, 290
Onnasch DW, 338
Ono Y, 394
Onoyama H, 135
Onrot J, 399
Opie LH, 165, 259
Oppenheimer, 338
Oren A, 261
Orishimo TF, 229
Ornish D, 39
O'Rourke RA, 65, 159
Orszulak TA, 89, 280, 388
Ortiz E, 333
Osbakken M, 9
Osborn MJ, 200, 360
Oseran DS, 220, 277
O'Shea E, 275
Oshima M, 11
Oshrain C, 225
Osman MI, 151, 153
Ostrow HG, 325
Ott DA, 199
Otterstad JE, 335
Ouyang P, 177
Oyer PE, 226, 300, 301, 302, 305, 405

Pachinger O, 81
Pacifico AD, 354, 358
Packer DL, 327
Packer M, 371, 372, 373, 374, 375, 377
Padfield PL, 260
Padmanabhan VT, 290
Page K, 395
Painvin GA, 278
Palacios IF, 313
Pallas RS, 180
Pallides S, 353
Palma S, 217
Palmeri ST, 140, 149
Palmieri M, 222
Palombo C, 74
Pamelia FX, 19
Pan CW, 303
Panidis IP, 1, 2, 93
Pantopoulos D, 227
Papademetriou V, 254, 257
Papouchado M, 50, 62
Parenzan L, 344
Parisi AF, 100
Park SC, 335
Parker C, 115, 116

Parker JO, 59
Parker M, 135
Parkey RW, 12, 116, 119, 172
Parmley WW, 371
Parnell BM, 16
Participants in the Coronary Artery Surgery Study, 92, 93
Partinen M, 252
Partridge JB, 97
Parungao RF, 117
Passamani ER, 82, 83, 91, 95, 96, 115, 116, 173
Paterniti JR, 40
Patrono C, 48
Paul O, 36
Pearle DL, 180
Pearson T, 101, 102
Pechacek LW, 278
Pedersen TR, 163, 164
Pelech A, 346
Pell S, 130
Pellegrino A, 347
Pelletier G, 149
Pelletier GB, 68, 119
Pembrook-Rogers D, 233
Penkoske PA, 278
Pennert K, 131, 133
Pennock JL, 306
Pepe AJ, 93
Pepine CJ, 55, 64, 66, 67
Pepper JR, 98
Perez J, 123
Perez-Davila V, 123
Permanyer-Miralda G, 387
Perry HM, 289
Petch J, 298
Peter T, 124, 220, 277
Peters J, 194, 254
Peters RW, 404
Peterson C, 35
Peterson E, 307
Peterson J, 209
Peterson MD, 283, 284, 285
Peterson RJ, 356
Petitti DB, 24
Peto R, 179
Petrie J, 262, 263, 264
Petru MA, 65
Petru MD, 390
Peyrieux J-C, 164
Pfisterer M, 72
Phelps J, 34
Philbin DM, 308
Phillips HR III, 21, 22, 23
Phillipson BE, 36
Picano E, 54, 74

Pichler M, 134
Picone AL, 295
Pidgeon J, 98
Piehler JM, 180, 280, 388
Pieper JA, 64
Pierce WS, 306
Pierre J, 404
Pillai R, 98, 344
Pinkernell BH, 93
Pinson CW, 339
Piters KM, 45
Pitt A, 10
Pitts DE, 178
Pizzarello RA, 290
Plappert T, 396
Platia EV, 207, 212, 213, 216, 231
Plaza LR, 59
Plotnick GD, 126, 404
Plucinski DA, 317
Pluth JR, 280, 388
Podolak MJ, 407
Podrid PA, 214
Podrid PJ, 210
Pohost GM, 9, 10, 11, 82, 96
Poirier J-M, 215
Polak JF, 66
Poliak SC, 40
Poliner LR, 79
Pollak SJ, 3
Poole WK, 115, 116
Pop T, 317
Popio KA, 103
Popp RL, 145, 299
Port SC, 11
Porter CB, 65
Porter CJ, 193, 200, 357, 360
Ports TA, 80
Poser RF, 210
Posner B, 46
Powers ER, 173
Powers PL, 278
Power-Vanwart J, 367
Pozzoli M, 321
Pratt CM, 165, 203, 377
Price M, 257
Prida XE, 374
Pridie RB, 16
Priesnitz M, 122
Prieto-Granada J, 121
Primm K, 215
Prisco D, 56, 401
Probst P, 81
Propper R, 327
Proudfit WL, 13
Pryor DB, 21, 22, 23, 141
Przybylek J, 135
Puffer JC, 389, 390

Puga FJ, 340, 352, 357, 361, 388
Pyeritz RE, 276

Qaiyumi S, 291
Quinlan MF, 145
Quinones MA, 203
Qureshi SA, 98
Quyyumi AA, 52, 64

Raabe DS, 116
Rabinowitz B, 16
Rabinowitz C, 390
Rackley CE, 57, 180
Rad N, 318
Rademaker M, 373
Radford DJ, 298
Radford M, 286
Radichevich I, 250
Radley-Smith R, 345
Rae AP, 206, 209, 211, 218, 220
Raeder EA, 214
Raft D, 103
Raftery EB, 11
Rahimtoola SH, 27, 126, 153, 370, 380, 382
Rahlf G, 314, 315
Raizner AE, 79, 165, 168
Rajah SM, 97
Rajala S, 395
Ramanaden I, 148
Ramanathan KB, 407, 408
Ramos A, 217
Ramos RG, 171
Ramot Y, 278
Rankin J, 94
Rao A, 285
Rao AK, 173
Rao PS, 123
Rao RS, 97
Rapold HG, 81
Rapold HJ, 88
Rapoport A, 404
Raskin P, 257
Rath S, 16
Ratliff NB, 99
Rau G, 169
Raven PR, 395
Ray G, 11
Raynaud P, 177
Reddy PS, 379, 395
Reddy S, 404
Redish GA, 12, 119
Reece IJ, 278
Reed DM, 37
Reed GE, 99
Reed WA, 104

Reeder GS, 78, 89, 103, 180, 285, 288, 326, 388
Rees JR, 50
Reeves JT, 403
Reeves R, 120
Rehnqvist N, 224
Reiber JHC, 14, 39, 89
Reichek N, 396
Reid CL, 126
Reid GD, 397
Reid PR, 207, 212, 213, 216, 231
Reiffel JA, 234
Reisman S, 12
Reitano J, 287, 289
Reitz B, 101, 102
Reitz BA, 341
Rellas JS, 12
Relman AS, 177
Remington JS, 406
Remme PJ, 171
Remme WJ, 179
Ren J-F, 2, 93
Renkin J, 81, 170
Rennert G, 119
Rentrop KP, 169
Res J, 179
Res JCJ, 171
Reul GJ, 199
Revuelta JM, 307
Rheuban KS, 358
Ribner H, 135
Ribner HS, 317
Rice MJ, 352
Rich EC, 194
Rich S, 402
Richards DA, 154
Richez J, 22
Rickman FD, 165
Riemenschneider TA, 232
Rieur EC, 205
Rifkind BM, 27
Rigby ML, 332, 333, 334, 353, 359
Riley LJ Jr, 261
Riley MF, 139
Rinkenberger RL, 216
Ritchie JL, 122, 166, 167, 168, 229
Rittenhouse EA, 341
Ritter DG, 361
Ritter G, 230, 231
Rivera R, 180
Rizzoli G, 359
Roach RM, 283, 284, 285
Robert A, 2
Robert J, 77
Robert P, 3
Roberts R, 115, 116, 165, 173, 203, 377

Roberts WC, 103, 173, 291, 301, 303, 407, 409
Robertson D, 399
Robertson I, 375
Robertson JH, 242, 286
Robertson JIS, 375
Robertson R, 48
Robertson T, 115, 116
Robertson TL, 116
Robinson JC, 277
Robinson PJ, 333, 352
Robison AK, 175
Robles DE, 128
Rocchini AP, 193, 254, 346, 349, 350
Roden DM, 215
Rodney WM, 389, 390
Rodrigues E, 288
Rodriguez L, 173
Rogasi PG, 56, 401
Rogers WJ, 57, 120
Rokeach S, 120
Rolnitzky LM, 157
Romano M, 407
Romeo F, 72
Ronnevik PK, 160, 162
Rosati RA, 21, 22, 23, 141
Rose JS, 153
Rose V, 327, 351, 393
Rosenberg L, 117
Rosenfeld LE, 205, 213
Rosenthal A, 193, 254, 346, 349, 350
Rosenthal ME, 220, 277
Roses AD, 327
Rosing DR, 89, 295, 320, 325, 326
Rosman HS, 290
Rosner B, 39, 46
Rosoff MH, 293
Ross A, 173
Ross AM, 32, 33, 121
Ross DL, 154
Ross DN, 339
Ross EM, 303
Ross J Jr, 2, 93, 145, 146, 147, 148, 150, 151
Ross JK, 136
Rossall RE, 148
Rosseneu M, 29, 30
Rossi P, 87
Roth A, 370, 382
Roth JA, 97
Rothbart ST, 227
Rothrock DW, 36
Rotmensch H, 211
Rotmensch HH, 261
Rotstein Z, 16
Roubin GS, 80, 83, 84, 85, 90, 296, 369

Rouleau J, 71, 381
Rovai D, 74
Rowe RD, 346, 393
Rowland E, 343
Roy D, 119, 149, 153
Roy L, 48
Royal HD, 57
Rozenman Y, 173
Rubenfire M, 211
Rubin DA, 99
Rubin HS, 165
Rubin LJ, 403
Rubinstein A, 40
Rubler S, 287, 289
Rude RE, 116, 119, 172
Rudolph AM, 351
Rudolph W, 63
Ruffy R, 216
Ronnevik PK, 224
Ruskin JN, 191, 206, 216
Russell DW, 29, 31
Russell PA, 154
Russell RO, 57
Russo D, 21
Russo DJ, 21
Russo P, 347
Rutherford JD, 115, 116
Rutledge JC, 217
Rutman H, 378
Rutsch W, 177
Ryan TJ, 8, 91, 92, 93, 173, 374

Sabik J, 306
Sabiston D, 94
Sackett DL, 70, 71
Sacks FM, 30
Sadaniantz A, 139
Sagiv M, 8
Sagnella GA, 250
Sagrista-Sauleda J, 387
Sainiot AG, 299
Saito A, 355
Saito Y, 167
Saksena S, 227, 242
Sakurai T, 56
Salathia KS, 160
Sallan D, 327
Salter MCP, 97
Saltz-Rennert H, 119
Salzman C, 203
Samet P, 285
Samuels DA, 165
Sanders SP, 338, 343, 391
Sanford CF, 317
Santarelli P, 155
Santiago S, 252
Santinga JT, 297
Sapoznikov D, 173

Sareli P, 281
Sarna S, 25, 252
Sasayama S, 56
Satler LF, 180
Sato H, 170
Sauve MJ, 211
Sawatari K, 354
Sbressa C, 150
Scanlon PJ, 316, 318
Schaal SF, 276
Schaefer EJ, 41, 42, 43
Schaff HV, 92, 93, 103, 280, 357, 388
Schamroth CL, 281
Schartl M, 177
Schattenberg TT, 388
Schechtmann N, 80, 128
Schectman K, 123
Scheinman MM, 211, 235
Scheunemeyer T, 226
Schicha H, 169
Schick EC, 91
Schiller NB, 322, 396
Schlesselman SE, 32, 33
Schlumpf M, 83
Schmidt DH, 11
Schmidt P, 226
Schmidt PE, 178
Schmidt SB, 32, 33
Schmidt W, 169, 177
Schmouder RL, 252
Schnaper HW, 269
Schneider JA, 104
Schneider JF, 236
Schneider SP, 220
Schoenberger JA, 269
Schoenfeld MH, 206
Schofer J, 168, 174, 177
Schoonderwaldt HC, 47
Schork MA, 349
Schreiber J, 287, 289
Schreiber M, 49, 50, 51, 52
Schröder R, 164
Schroder R, 171
Schroeder JS, 77
Schwartz H, 121
Schwartz PJ, 150, 235
Schwarz FX, 81
Schwarzberg RJ, 12
Sclavo M, 139
Scott E, 67
Scott N, 150, 151
Scott WC, 305
Sealey BJ, 70, 71
Sealey JE, 374
Seals AA, 203
Sederholm M, 160, 161
Seelaus PA, 41
Segal BL, 211, 279

Seiden SW, 223
Seinfeld D, 155
Sekiguchi M, 170
Seldin DW, 12
Sellers D, 197
Sellers TD, 153
Selmon MR, 86
Selzer A, 120
Semenkovich CF, 156
Sementa A, 142, 144
Serneri GGN, 56, 401
Serruys PW, 14, 85, 88, 89, 171, 179
Serwer GA, 356
Seth L, 370, 381
Seward JB, 285, 288, 326, 333, 334, 335, 336, 337, 352, 388, 398, 399
Shackell M, 64
Shah PK, 124, 134, 173, 174, 379
Shah Y, 227
Shanks RG, 156, 160
Shapiro EP, 168, 177, 277
Shapiro M, 218
Shapiro S, 117
Shapiro WA, 235
Sharma AK, 361
Sharma B, 135
Sharma SC, 291
Sharom M, 164
Shaw DB, 237, 238
Shaw TRD, 373
Shechan DJ, 86
Shechan F, 122
Shechan FH, 168, 174
Sheffeld LT, 4
Shekelle RB, 36
Shellock F, 379
Shemin R, 116, 306
Shemin RJ, 281
Shen EN, 235
Shen WF, 296, 369
Sherez J, 324
Sherman LA, 123
Sherrid MV, 93
Sherry S, 178
Shimada I, 355
Shinebourne EA, 332, 333, 334, 353, 359
Shiraishi Y, 355
Shiroyama Y, 135
Shiu MF, 91
Shively B, 240
Shoen FJ, 309
Shore AC, 250
Shrivastava S, 281, 282
Shryock AM, 36
Shub C, 72, 73, 74, 75, 78, 273, 274, 388

Shumway NE, 300, 301, 305, 341, 405
Siart A, 293, 294
Siebold C, 194
Siegel R, 91, 278
Siegel RJ, 322, 323
Sifola C, 407
Silny J, 169
Silver MA, 301
Silverman NH, 351
Silverton NP, 91, 342
Simarro E, 121
Simmons M, 257
Simonin P, 22
Simonsen S, 335
Simonton CA, 378
Simoons ML, 14, 89, 139, 148, 171, 179
Simpfendorfer C, 104
Simpson JB, 86
Simpson RJ, 225
Singer J, 70, 71
Singh AK, 180
Singh B, 199
Singh BN, 65, 216, 217, 224, 259
Singh J, 199
Singh PN, 224
Sinoway L, 380
Sirowatka J, 19
Sjögren A, 224
Skalland L, 77
Skalsky E, 217
Sketch MH, 181
Slato A, 393
Sleight P, 258
Slymen DJ, 203
Slysh S, 99
Smallhorn J, 346
Smallpeice C, 227, 228
Smals AGH, 47
Smith A, 347
Smith DR, 289
Smith HC, 54, 89, 103, 180, 285, 288
Smith LDR, 353
Smith MS, 214
Smith P, 98
Smith RF, 132
Smith WM, 269
Smucker ML, 317
Snider AR, 254
Snider R, 193, 346
Sobel BE, 115, 116, 119, 123, 173, 175
Sobocinski KA, 251
Sokoloff NM, 206, 209, 211, 218, 220
Soler-Soler J, 387
Sollevi A, 48

Somberg J, 206, 209, 214, 215, 219, 221
Sondheimer HM, 342
Soni J, 201
Sonnenblick EH, 371
Sorensen SG, 318
Sostman D, 368
Soto B, 332
Soufer R, 368
Soulen RL, 388
Soward A, 10
Soward AI, 88
Sowers JR, 101
Spaet TH, 123
Spangenberg R, 379
Spann JF, 125
Speck SM, 168
Speizer FE, 46
Spicer RL, 193
Spielman SR, 195, 206, 209, 211, 218, 220
Spirito P, 142, 144, 321
Sprague MK, 191, 192
Sprecher DL, 40
Sridharan MR, 276
Srinivasan SR, 33
St. John Sutton MG, 396
Stadius ML, 122, 166, 167, 168
Stafford WJ, 298
Stajich J, 327
Stamler J, 36
Stamm SJ, 341
Stampfer MJ, 46, 179
Stanson AW, 394
Stanton BA, 100
Stare FJ, 38
Stark D, 322
Stark DD, 388
Starling L, 117
Starling MR, 159
Starr A, 339, 347, 348
Steck J, 199
Steele PM, 137
Steele PP, 225
Steinbeck G, 198
Stellin G, 359
Stemler J, 130
Stern A, 54
Stern AM, 193
Stern S, 6, 124
Stertzer SH, 87
Stevenson JG, 341
Stevenson WG, 230
Stewart DE, 257
Stewart JR, 171
Stine RA, 276
Stinson EB, 226, 300, 301, 302, 305, 406
Stinson ED, 405

Stolley PD, 117
Stone PH, 115, 116
Storey GCA, 213
Strain JE, 123
Strandberg T, 25
Strasser T, 262, 263, 264
Stratton JR, 168
Straub PW, 49
Strauss HW, 9, 11, 96
Strikwerda S, 39
Stringer JC, 275
Stryjer D, 278
Sturridge MF, 98
Suarez AM, 400
Suarez JM, 377
Subramanian R, 283
Subramanian VA, 47
Suchindran CM, 29, 32
Sudhof TC, 29, 31
Sugiura T, 135
Sugrue DD, 200
Sullivan JM, 407, 408
Sullivan M, 44, 98
Sunderland CO, 339, 347, 348
Superko R, 34
Sussman II, 123
Sutton GC, 64
Sutton TW, 115
Suzuki A, 394
Suzuki K, 167
Swan HJC, 12, 134, 379
Swedberg K, 138
Sweeney MS, 349
Swerdlow CD, 199, 209
Swinski LA, 309
Szlachcic J, 297, 368
Szpunar CA, 349, 350

Tack-Goldman, 47
Tadros SS, 261
Taeymans Y, 23, 68
Tajik AJ, 273, 274, 285, 288, 326, 333, 334, 335, 336, 337, 352, 388,
Takahashi M, 167, 313
Takahashi T, 408
Takahashi Y, 392
Takahasi N, 394
Takai A, 354
Takamoto T, 145
Takanashi Y, 344, 354
Takao A, 344, 392
Takebayashi S, 58
Takeshita A, 381
Takkunen JT, 96
Talano JV, 135

Talibi T, 398
Taliercio CP, 360
Tanaka KR, 277
Tanser PH, 70, 71
Tarazi RC, 371
Tarkoff DM, 287, 289
Tarui S, 396
Taylor CB, 34, 181
Taylor GJ, 104
Taylor PC, 99
Taylor RR, 6
Teasdale SJ, 261
Teichholz LE, 54
Teichman SL, 233
Teles de Mendonca J, 348
Teo KK, 148
Teply JF, 347
Terdiman R, 68
Theisen F, 194
Theisen K, 194
Theodore J, 405
Théroux P, 23, 68, 119, 149, 153
Thigpen T, 277
Thind GS, 261
Thomas D, 297
Thomas E, 236
Thomas FD, 342
Thompson CR, 397
Thompson DR, 115
Thompson ME, 404
Thompson PL, 145
Thompson RC, 323
Thompson TR, 196
Thomson SA, 373
Thyssen M, 300
Tiefenbrunn AJ, 175
Tietze U, 164
Tijssen JGP, 89
Tikkanc I, 250
Tilley B, 307
Tilsner V, 174
Tilton GD, 68
The TIMI Study Group, 175
Timmis GC, 166, 171, 392
Tokunaga K, 396
Tomlinson CW, 397
Tonnemacher D, 382
Toone E, 291
Topic N, 297, 368, 374
Topol EJ, 177, 253
Torres V, 206, 209, 214, 215, 219, 221
Tortolani AJ, 290
Tortoledo FA, 165
Tortoledo FE, 168
Tow DE, 100
Towell BL, 400

Traill TA, 253
Tramarin R, 321
Tran ZV, 34
Treese N, 317
Tresch DD, 91, 278
Trijbels FJM, 47
Trimble EL, 277
Troubaugh GB, 229
Trouillet JL, 404
Troup PJ, 91, 216
Trowitzsch E, 338
Trusso J, 218
Tsuji H, 135
Tubau J, 368
Tuomilehto J, 262, 263, 264
Turi ZG, 115, 116
Turina M, 94
Turini GA, 371
Turlapaty P, 199, 259
Turley K, 80
Tyler B, 130, 132
Tynan M, 347
Tyroler HA, 27
Tzivoni D, 6, 124

Uchida Y, 170
Uebis R, 169, 177
Ueda K, 355, 393
Ulene R, 126
Ulvenstam G, 131, 133
Umans V, 85
Underwood DA, 13
Upton SJ, 256
Upward J, 6
Uretsky BF, 379, 404
Urie PM, 145
Uther JB, 154

Vahanian A, 177
Val PG, 81
Valdes AM, 379
Valentine RP, 178
Valere PE, 299
Valty J, 215
Van Corler M, 137
Van De Kley GA, 177
Van De Werf F, 177
Van Den Brand M, 14, 85, 88, 89, 179
Van Der Velde EA, 39
Van Der Werf T, 128
Van Dorne D, 48
Van Eenige MJ, 171
Van Gent CM, 39
Van Hoogenhuyze DCA, 171
Van Tosh A, 301

Van Zetta AM, 205
Vanbutsele RJ, 2
Vandam LD, 232
Vander Salm TJ, 100
VanderBrug Medendorp S, 230, 231
Vandormael MG, 87
Vanhaecke J, 177
Vankoughnett KA, 59
Vanreet RE, 165
Varat MA, 125
Vargas FJ, 355
Varghese PJ, 121
Vasey C, 236
Vasu M, 230, 231
Veale D, 237, 238
Vecchio C, 142, 144, 321
Vedin A, 131, 133, 138
Veenbrink TWG, 128
Vega GL, 30
Veltri EP, 207, 212, 213
Venables AW, 360
Ventura HO, 252, 260
Verani MS, 79, 165, 168
Verbalis JG, 379
Verheugt FWA, 171, 179
Vermeer F, 171, 179
Verstraete M, 177
Vestergaard B, 400
Vetrovec GW, 87
Vilde JL, 299
Viquerat CE, 101
Virmani R, 132
Visser CA, 137
Vita NA, 368
Vitale DF, 79
Vitols S, 35
Vittecocq D, 299
Vlasses PH, 261
Vlietstra RE, 72, 73, 74, 75, 89, 103, 137, 180, 285, 288, 360, 399
Vogel M, 346
Vogel RA, 103
Vogt TM, 269
Vohringer H, 171
Vollset SE, 37
Von Arnim T, 49, 50, 51, 52
Von Der Lippe G, 160, 161, 163
Von Essen R, 169, 177
Von Leitner E-R, 164
Vonderlippe G, 159
Vos M, 392
Vranizan KM, 34, 35

Wackers FJ, 141, 142, 143
Wackers FJT, 21

Wagenvoort CA, 408
Wagenvoort N, 408
Wagner GS, 21, 22, 23, 140, 141
Wahl J, 259
Wahl JM, 126, 127
Wahr D, 396
Wahr DW, 80, 201
Waldecker B, 196, 230
Walden C, 29, 32
Waldhausen JA, 306
Waldo A, 199
Walker PR, 62
Walker SD, 77
Walker WE, 349
Wallace R, 29, 32
Waller BF, 103
Wallis J, 53
Wallsh E, 87
Walsh R, 318
Walsh RA, 65
Walsh WF, 127
Walter PF, 3
Wampler D, 345
Wanderman K, 119
Wang P, 234
Wang SP, 303
Wang T, 215
Wang YS, 396
Ward D, 201
Warin J-F, 215
Warner HF, 125
Waspe LE, 155, 223, 233
Wasserman AG, 32, 33, 121
Waternaux CM, 309
Waters DD, 23, 53, 67, 68, 77, 119, 149, 153
Watkins E, 278
Watkins L, 101, 102
Watkins WD, 308
Watson DA, 97
Watson DD, 19, 134
Watson RM, 320, 325
Waxman HL, 212
Webb CR, 206, 209, 211, 218, 220
Webber LS, 33
Weber KT, 369
Weber L, 370, 380, 382
Weber MA, 259
Webster MWI, 376
Wedel H, 131, 133
Wegscheider K, 122
Wei JY, 169
Weiner DA, 8, 374
Weinglass J, 58
Weinstein EM, 351
Weintraub R, 139
Weintraub WS, 41

Weisel RD, 261
Weisfeldt ML, 177
Weiskopf M, 101
Weiss AT, 124, 173
Weiss JL, 177, 276
Weitzman S, 119
Weksler BB, 47
Welber S, 173
Weld FM, 147
Wellens HJJ, 4, 196, 197, 204, 230
Wellons HA Jr, 104
Wells JE, 376
Weltman A, 34
Wennmalm A, 48
Wesley YE, 320
Westerhof PW, 128
Westveer DC, 171
Wetherbee JN, 91
Wheelan K, 172
Whistance T, 237, 238
White HD, 66
White RD, 140
Whitlock JA, 191, 192
Whitlow PL, 120
Whittington JR, 11
Whitworth HB, 90
Wiener-Kronish JP, 101
Wierman AM, 203
Wijns W, 2, 14, 85, 89
Wilcken DEL, 127, 274
Wilcosky T, 29, 32
Wilen MM, 375, 381
Wilhelmsen L, 131, 133
Wilhelmsson C, 131, 133
Wilkinson JL, 347
Wilkinson PR, 62
Willerson JT, 12, 115, 116, 119, 172
Willett WC, 46
Williams AJ, 252
Williams B, 262, 263, 264
Williams BC, 373
Williams DG, 314
Williams DO, 173
Williams GA, 282, 284, 308
Williams MA, 181
Williams OD, 27
Williams PT, 34, 35
Williams S, 221
Williams Van Hove E, 178
Wilson BH, 132
Wilson JR, 367, 373
Wilson P, 43, 44
Wilson PWF, 46
Wilson WR, 299
Wiman B, 178
Windhorst DM, 282

Winkle RA, 218, 219, 226
Winniford M, 172
Winniford MD, 68, 69, 73, 76, 399, 401
Winston SA, 211
Winters SL, 54
Wisneski JA, 5
Witchitz S, 299
Witkowski FX, 200
Woelfel A, 225
Wohlgelernter D, 368
Wolf NM, 55
Wolf PA, 193, 194
Wolfe C, 172
Wolfe CL, 12, 68, 119
Wolfe L, 327
Wolfe RA, 230, 231
Wolff M, 299
Wolfgang TC, 87
Wong BYS, 157
Wong M, 97
Wood DL, 200, 326
Wood PD, 34, 35
Woods PD, 34
Woosley RL, 215
Wren C, 202
Wright C, 64
Wright CM, 52
Wright JEC, 98
Wu D, 153
Wyeth R, 135
Wyndham CRC, 226
Wynn J, 221
Wynne J, 66
Wyse DG, 222
Wyse RKH, 333

Yacone L, 126, 127
Yacoub MH, 98, 345
Yakirevich VS, 342
Yale C, 217
Yamashita T, 71
Yamazaki N, 71
Yaney SF, 4
Yang XS, 29, 30
Yanowitz G, 318
Yasue H, 170
Yasuno M, 167
Yates AK, 227, 228
Yeoh CB, 93
Yli-Uotila RJ, 224
Yokota M, 355
Young AA, 154
Young JB, 165, 203, 377
Yousem SA, 406
Yuan Z, 374
Yushak M, 373, 375, 377
Yusuf S, 179

Zadrozny JH, 125
Zalewski A, 99
Zangl W, 81
Zappa P, 150
Zaret BL, 173, 368
Zaza A, 150

Zech LA, 40
Zehender M, 196, 230, 317
Zhao HX, 341
Ziesche S, 369
Zimmerman J, 234

Zimmerman M, 22
Zoll PM, 240
Zoll RH, 240
Zoltick JM, 4
Zuberbuhler Jr, 335

Subject Index

Acebutolol, in hypertension, 258–59

Acute myocardial infarction. *See* Myocardial infarction, acute

Adenosine, in supraventricular tachycardia, 197

Adrenal gland, after CABG, 101–3

Adventitial inflammation, in angina, 58

Age
  AMI in elderly, 117
  cardiomyopathy in elderly, 253
  cardiovascular findings in elderly, 395–96
    cardiac sounds, 395
    ECG findings, 395
    ventricular function, 395

Alcohol, 400
  in atrial fibrillation, 194
  blood lipids and, 35
  CAD and, 46
  hypertension and, 250–51

Amiodarone
  in angina pectoris, 72
  in atrial fibrillation, 195
  in hypertrophic cardiomyopathy, 325
  in supraventricular tachycardia, 197–98
  in ventricular arrhythmias, 211–14, 217–18

Amrinone, in CHF, 371

Amyloidosis, 326–27

Anesthesia
  cardiac arrest during, 232
  risk of, 323–24

Aneurysm, of coronary artery, 16

Angina pectoris, 50–72
  adventitial inflammation in, 58
  air embolism -vs- spasm, 55–56
  amiodarone in, 72
  angiographic findings in, 54–55
  anxiety and, 50
  arm exercise in, 8
  aspirin and sulfinpyrazone in, 70

beta blockers in, 67–70
calcium blockers in, 67–70
  and nitrates, 70
captopril in, 71
coenzyme Q_{10} in, 71–72
depression and, 50
diltiazem in, 64–69
dipyridamole-echo test, 54
exercise
  ST/HR slope and LV function, 53
  testing and, 58
  tolerance of, 53
hemodynamic responses to, 55
isosorbide dinitrate in, 59–62, 70
labetalol in, 64
molsidomine, 63–64
nicardipine in, 67
nifedipine in, 66–70
nisoldipine, 67
nitroglycerin in, 59–63
  transdermal, 62–63
pacing induced, 56–58
therapy
  effect on exercise test, 58
  effect of medical training on, 58–59
  review, 72
thromboxane release, 56
unstable, PTCA for, 88–89

Angina pectoris, variant
  coronary collaterals, 77
  diltiazem in, 77
  echo findings in, 74–77
  hyperventilation and cold pressor test, 72–73
  PTCA and, 77–78
  ventricular ectopic activity, 73–74

Angiography, in angina, 54–55
  See also Radionuclide angiography

Angioplasty. *See* Percutaneous transluminal coronary angioplasty

Angiotensin converting enzyme inhibitors, in hypertension, 260–61
Antianginal drugs
  acebutolol, 258–59
  bepridil, 214
  diltiazem, 64–69, 77
  nicardipine, 67
  nifedipine, 66–70
  nitroglycerin, 59, 62–63
  propranolol, 67–70
Anticoagulants, after AMI, 159
Antihypertensive drugs, 254–70
Aortic regurgitation, 290–98
  and hydrops, 351
Aortic valve replacement (AVR), 305–6
Aortic valve stenosis, 283–90
  LV mechanics in, 353
Apolipoproteins, predictors of CAD, 32
Arrhythmias
  See also Supraventricular tachycardia
  atrial fibrillation/flutter
    alcohol related, 194
    amiodarone treatment, 195
    diltiazem treatment, 194
    in infants and children, 192–193
    lone, 193
  after CABG, 99
  causing syncope, 232
  in healthy individuals, 191
  after Mustard repair of TGA, 345
Arterial switch operation, in TGA, 359–60
Aspirin
  in angina pectoris, 70
  after CABG, 97–98
  in Kawasaki disease, 393
Atenolol
  in hypertension, 258–60
  in mitral stenosis, 281
Athletes, study of, 389–92
Atresia, pulmonic valve, 338–40
Atrial fibrillation/flutter, 192–95
Atrial natriuretic peptide, 249–50
Atrial septal defect, 331–32
Atrioventricular block, 237–38
Atrioventricular canal defect, 332

Balloon dilation during PTCA, 80–81
Bendroflumethiazide, 263, 265
Bepridil, in ventricular arrhythmias, 214

Beta blockers
  in AMI, 159–64
  in angina pectoris, 67–70
  effect during exercise, 6–7
  in hypertension, 258–60
Bethesda Conference, 390
Biofeedback, in hypertension, 256
Bioprostheses
  Ionescu-Shiley, 307–8
  porcine, 307
Blalock-Taussig shunt, 354
Bundle branch block (BBB), 236–37

Caffeine, effects of, 399–400
  See also Coffee
Calcium channel blockers
  in AMI, 67–70
  in variant angina, 72
  review of, 401
Cancer, blood lipids and, 35
Captopril
  in angina pectoris, 71
  in CHF, 371–74, 377, 380
  in hypertension, 260–61
Cardiac amyloidosis, 326–27
Cardiac arrest,
  CABG after nonfatal, 91–92
  during ambulatory ECG recording, 231
  during anesthesia, 232
  out-of-hospital, nonfatal, 229–30
  prehospital resuscitation, 231–32
  prognosis after resuscitation, in young persons, 229
Cardiac output, Fick measurement for, 399
Cardiac surgery, 403–4
Cardiac transplantation, 404–7
Cardiac valve replacement, 305–9
Cardiology journals
  comparison of, 409–10
Cardiomyopathies
  hypertrophic, 320–26
    amiodarone in, 325
    anesthetic risk, 323–24
    apical variety, 324
    comparison of ventricular emptying and outflow gradient, 322–23
    diastolic abnormalities, 321–22
    Doppler flow study, 320–21
    echo observations in, 321–22
    in elderly, 253
    frequency of epicardial CAD, 324–25

in hypertension, 253
myocardial ischemia, 320
nifedipine, 325–26
verapamil in, 326
idiopathic dilated, 313–319
correlation of ultrastructure to
function, 314
digoxin on, 317
effect of Valsalva maneuver,
315
endomyocardial biopsy, 313
familial aggregation, 314–15
hydralazine in, 317
metoprolol therapy, 318–19
nifedipine in, 319
prevalence in England, 314
prognosis, 36, 316–17
programmed electrical stimulation, 317
relation to acute myocarditis,
313–14
myotonic muscular dystrophy,
327
noncardiac structure and, 327
thalassemia major, 327
Cardiopulmonary shunt, 356
Cardiovascular surgery
exercise testing before, 403
mediastinitis therapy, 404
See also Surgery
Cardioverters
and defibrillators, 226
See also Pacemakers and cardioverters; Pacing
Catheterization
Fick -vs- indicator dilution for
cardiac output, 399
as an outpatient, 398
transseptal approach, 399
Chlorthalidone, in hypertension,
268–69
Cholesterol
and coffee drinking, 24–25
See also Lipid levels
Cigarette smoking
AMI and, 117
CAD and, 41–42
hypertension and, 250
Coenzyme Q_{10}, 71–72
Coffee
and blood lipids, 34–35
CAD and, 45–46
and cholesterol, 24–25
Cold pressor test, in variant
angina pectoris, 72–73
Congenital heart disease, 331–62
aortic isthmic coarctation repair,
347–51
atrial septal defect (ASD), 331–
32

spontaneous closure in
infancy, 331–32
transatrial velocity by
Doppler, 331
atrioventricular canal defect, 332
effect of Down's syndrome on,
332
left AV valve replacement, 332
LV outflow obstruction, 346–47
aortic valve stenosis, 346
subaortic stenosis, 346–47
pediatric conditions, 351–54
absent right superior vena
cava, 352
aortic valve regurgitation and
hydrops, 351
criss-cross heart, 352–53
LV function and Fontan operation, 354
LV mechanics in AS and
coarctation, 353
newborn transitional circulation, 351
in offspring of affected
parents, 351–52
PA pressure by Doppler, 353
straddling AV valve, 352
subaortic stenosis and VSD,
353
pediatric cardiac surgery, 354–
62
anomalous pulmonary venous
repair, 355
arterial switch operation, 359–
60
AV connection repair, 358
baffle obstruction after
Mustard operation, 358–59
Blalock-Taussig shunt, 354
cardiopulmonary shunt, 356
double-outlet right ventricle
operation, 359
Ebstein's anomaly, 357
Fontan operation, 360–61
mitral valve double-orifice
repair, 357–58
normothermic caval inflow
occlusion, 355–56
pulmonary venous stenosis
repair, 354
repair without transfusions,
356–57
single ventricle with subaortic
stenosis repair, 362
truncus arteriosus repair, 361–
62
ventricular function after
Fontan, 360
pulmonic valve atresia, 338–40
pulmonic valve stenosis, 338

tetralogy of Fallot, 340–43
  with absent pulmonic valve,
    340–41
  electrophysiologic findings
    after repair, 343
  operative repair, 341–43
transposition of the great
  arteries (TGA), 343–45
  arrhythmia after Mustard
    repair, 345
  arterial switch operation, 345
  Mustard-type repair, 344–45
  tricuspid valve, 343–44
  ventricular function after
    repair, 344
ventricular septal defect (VSD),
  333–38
  with aneurysm, 335–37
  isolated, 335
  localized by Doppler and
    echo, 333–34
  pulmonary arterial develop-
    ment, 338
  standardized nomenclature,
    333
Congestive heart failure (CHF),
  367–83
  digitalis and William Withering,
    382–83
  exercise and, 368–71
  fatigue and, 367
  LV function intact, 368
  treatment,
    amrinone, 371
    captopril, 371–74
      -vs- isosorbide dinitrite, 377
      -vs- milrinone, 380
    dobutamine -vs- enalaprilat,
      377
    enalapril, 374–76
    fenoldopam, 377
    isosorbide dinitrate, 377
    MDL 17,043, 379–80
    milrinone, 378, 380
    nifedipine, 380
    nitroglycerin
      sublingual, 381
      transdermal, 381–82
    salbutamol, 381
  ventricular arrhythmia, 367–68
Coronary angioplasty. See Percutaneous transluminal coronary
  angioplasty
Coronary artery bypass grafting
  (CABG), 91–103
  adrenal gland function after,
    101–3
  AMI after, 99
  for AMI, 180
  arrhythmia after, 99

aspirin and dipyridamole after,
  97–98
cardiac arrest, nonfatal, 91–92
compared with PTCA, 103–5
effect of exercise on, 98
effect on exercise-induced ventricular arrhythmias, 96
effect on hospital readmissions,
  100–1
effect of platelet-inhibiting drugs
  on, 97–98
endarterectomy and, 99
factors determining long-term
  survival, 91
fate of preoperative defect on
  exercise imaging, 96–97
graft material compared, 99
in Kawasaki disease, 394
LV function and, 93–96
after mitral valve replacement,
  306
multiple operations, 98–99
narrowing of graft, 103
in older persons, 92–93
pericardial effusion after, 101
stroke after, 101
unstable angina after, 99–100
Coronary Artery Surgery Study
  (CASS), 91, 95–96
Coronary artery disease, 1–105
  See also Angina pectoris; Coro-
    nary artery bypass grafting;
    Coronary narrowing
  alcohol and, 46
  apolipoproteins as predictors, 32
  cigarette smoking and, 41–42
  coffee and, 45–46
  detection of, 1–16
    aneurysm, 16
    coronary arteries, status of, 13
    coronary collaterals, 13–14
    echo, value of, 1–2
    ectasia, 16
    exercise testing, 4–9
    family history, value of, 1
    MRFIT, 4–5
    potentials, late, 3–4
    radionuclide studies, 9–13
      gated blood pool scans, 12–
        13
      thallium-201 scans, 9–12
    statistical analysis of noninva-
      sive tests, 23
    transstenotic coronary pres-
      sure gradient, 14–16
    Valsalva maneuver, 2
  estrogens and, 46–47
  homocystinuria, 47
  hypertrophic cardiomyopathy,
    324–25

lipid levels in, 25–41
obesity and, 44–45
physical activity and, 42–44
potentials, late, 3–4, 22–23
prognosis
  by exercise thallium-201, 19–21
  by jeopardy score, 21–22
  by leukocyte count, 19
  by myocardial ischemia, 16–19
  by ventricular late potentials, 22–23
risk factors in, 24–25
Coronary artery occlusion, PTCA for, 85–87
Coronary heart disease. *See* Coronary artery disease
Coronary narrowing
  in CAD, 23–24
  exercise and, 53
  of graft, 103
Creatine, release after PTCA, 78
Creatine kinase, 115, 116–17
  as risk indicator, 139–41
  and streptokinase, 169
Cyclosporine, in transplantation, 404–5

Deferoxamine, in thalassemia major, 327
Diabetes mellitus
  and AMI, 119–20
  and myocardial ischemia, 407
Diet
  blood lipids and, 35–39
  fish in, 35–38
  Pritikin, 40–41
Digitalis
  in AMI, 157–59
  Withering and, 382–83
Digoxin
  and cardioversion, 226
  in idiopathic dilated cardiomyopathy, 317
Diltiazem
  in angina pectoris, 64–69, 77
  in atrial fibrillation, 194
  after PTCA, 81–82
  in variant angina pectoris, 77
Dipyridamole
  after CABG, 97–98
  and echo test, 54
Disopyramide, in ventricular arrhythmias, 222
Diuretics in hypertension, 257–58
Dobutamine
  in AMI, -vs- nitroprusside, 159
  in CHF, 377

Doppler echo
  See also Echocardiography
  in atrial septal defect, 331
  evaluation of cardiac valves, 308
  in hypertrophic cardiomyopathy, 320–21
  PA pressure, 353
  review of, 398
  in valve replacement, 308
  in ventricular septal defect, 333–34
Down's syndrome and AV canal defect, 332
Drug therapy, effect of platelet-inhibiting, on CABG, 97–98

Ebstein's anomaly, 357
Echocardiography
  See also Doppler echo
  in alcoholics, 397
  in anorexia nervosa, 396–97
  for detecting CAD, 1–2
  in diagnosing amyloidosis, 326–27
  and dipyridamole test, 54
  findings in families with the Marfan syndrome, 303–5
  in hypertrophic cardiomyopathy, 321–22
  for LV function, 93–94
  of LV mass and volume, 396
  mitral leaflet closure, incomplete, 98
  M-mode for pericardial effusion, 135
  in obesity, 396
  in systemic lupus erythematosus, 397–98
  for variant angina pectoris, 74–77
  in ventricular septal defect, 333–34
Elderly. *See* Age
Electrocardiography (ECG)
  changes during PTCA, 78–79
  in diagnosing AMI, 124–25, 169
  in valvular heart disease, 291–92
Electrophysiologic studies
  in diagnosing AMI, 125–26
  for tetralogy of Fallot, 343
  for ventricular arrhythmias, 209, 213
Embolism, air, 55–56
Enalapril
  in CHF, 374–76
  in hypertension, 260–61
Enalaprilat, in CHF, 377
Encainide, 215

Endarterectomy, 98
Endocardial resection, 227–29
Esmolol, -vs- propranolol in supra-
    ventricular tachycardia, 199
Estrogen, CAD and, 46–47
European Infarction Study Group,
    164
European Working Party on Hyper-
    tension in the Elderly
    (EWPHE), 262–64
Exercise
    in AMI, 181–82
    in angina, 53
    blood lipids and, 34
    after CABG, 98
    cardiovascular effects, 389–92
        athletic heart syndrome, 389–
            90
        endurance athletes, 392
        evaluation of athletes, 390
        runners, 390–91
        swimmers, 391
        weight lifters, 391
    in CHF, 368–71
    coronary narrowing and, 53
    in hypertension, 256–58
Exercise-induced disorders, ventric-
    ular arrhythmias, 96
Exercise testing
    in angina pectoris, 58
    in CAD, 4–9
    before surgery, 403

Family history, as risk factor for
    CAD, 1
Fenoldopam in CHF, 377
Fibrinopeptide A, in AMI, 123–24
Fick measurement of cardiac
    output, 399
Flecainide, in ventricular arrhyth-
    mias, 215–17
Fontan procedure, echo after,
    LV function and, 354, 360
    permanent pacing after, 360–61

Heart
    criss-cross, 352–53
    size of, 407–8
Heart disease. See Cardiac and
    Coronary headings; Myocar-
    dial heart disease; Valvular
    heart disease; and names of
    specific diseases and condi-
    tions, e.g., Angina pectoris,
    Congenital heart disease
Hemodynamic responses in
    angina, 55

Homocystinuria, 47
Hydralazine
    in idiopathic dilated cardiomy-
        opathy, 317
    in primary pulmonary hyperten-
        sion, 402–3
Hydrochlorothiazide, 257–58, 261,
    263, 268
Hypertension, 249–70
    alcohol and, 250–51
    angiotensin converting enzyme
        inhibitors, 260–61
    atenolol in, 258–60
    atrial natriuretic peptide and,
        249–50
    cardiomyopathy, in elderly, 253
    chlorthalidone in, 268–69
    cigarette smoking and, 250
    enalapril, 260–61
    hypertrophic cardiomyopathy
        and, 253
    lead and, 252
    LV diastolic function in, 254
    Osler's maneuver and pseu-
        dohypertension, 252–53
    pregnancy and, 254
    RV wall thickness on, 255
    sleep apnea syndrome and, 252
    snoring and, 252
    treatment, 254–270
        acebutolol, 258–59
        angiotension converting
            enzyme inhibitors, 260–61
        atenolol, 258–60
        bendroflumethiazide, 263,
            265
        beta-blockers, 258–60
        biofeedback, 256
        captopril, 260–61
        chlorthalidone, 268–69
        clinical trials, 261–70
        diuretics, 257–58
        enalapril, 260–61
        exercise, aerobic, 256–57
        hydrochlorothiazide, 257–58,
            261, 263, 268
        labetalol, 259–60
        methyldopa, 261, 263
        metoprolol, 258
        nitroglycerin, 261–62
        nitroprusside, 261–62
        nondrug, 254–57
        oxprenolol, 263
        pindolol, 258
        potassium, 257
        propranolol, 258, 259, 261,
            263
        triamterene, 263
Hypertension Detection Follow-up
    Program (HDFP), 270

Infarction. *See* Myocardial infarction, acute
International Prospective Primary Prevention Study (IPPPS), 262–63, 266–68
Ionescu-Shiley bioprosthesis, 307–8
Ischemia. *See* Myocardial ischemia
Isosorbide dinitrate
  in angina pectoris, 59–62, 70
  in CHF, 377
Isotretinoin, for blood lipids, 40

Jatene repair of TGA, 344
Jeopardy score for CAD, 21–22

Kawasaki disease, 392–94
  CABG in, 394
  coronary disease in, 392
  salicylate treatment, 393
  ventricular function, 392–93

Labetalol
  in angina pectoris, 64
  in hypertension, 259–260
Lead, in blood, and hypertension, 252
Left ventricular function/dysfunction
  after AMI, 121–22
  and CABG, 79, 93–96
  in CHF, 368
  echo studies, 93–94
  and Fontan operation, 354
  in hypertension, 254
  outflow obstruction, 346–47
  valves and, 295–96
Legionnaire's disease, in transplantation, 405
Leukocytes, as prognostic factor, 19
Lidocaine, in AMI, 156–57
Lipid levels,
  alcohol and, 35
  beta blockers and, 258
  CAD and, 31–32
  cancer and, 35
  in China, 29
  coronary score and, 31–32
  diets and, 35–39
  education program, 28
  effect of coffee on, 31–35
  exercise and, 34
  isotretinoin and, 40
  LDL receptor gene, 28
  neomycin for, 40
  in nephrotic syndrome, 33
  niacin for, 40

obesity and, 33–34
predictor of CAD, 32
recommendations for reducing, 26–27
Research Clinics Program Prevelance Study, 27–28
review of, 41
treatment, 39–40
triglycerides, 29–31
value of lowering, 25–27
Lipid Research Clinics Primary Prevention Trials, 28
Lorcainide, in ventricular arrhythmias, 218–20

Magnetic resonance imaging
  in AMI, 128
  in hypertrophic cardiomyopathy, 322
Marfan syndrome, cardiac abnormalities in families, 303–5
MDL 17,043 in CHF, 379–80
Medical Research Council (MRC) trial, 262–63, 265
Mediastinitis, 404
Methyldopa, in hypertension, 261, 263
Metoprolol
  in AMI, 160–61, 163
  in hypertension, 258
  in idiopathic dilated cardiomyopathy, 318–19
Mexiletine, in ventricular arrhythmias, 217–18
MIAMI Trial Research Group, 163
Milrinone, in CHF, 378, 380
Mitral anular calcium, 282
Mitral regurgitation, 279–281
Mitral stenosis, 281–82
Mitral valve
  double-orifice repair, 357–58
  See also Valvular heart disease
Mitral valve prolapse, 273–79
Mitral valve replacement (MVR), 306, 308–9
  CABG after, 306
M-mode echo. *See* Echocardiography
Molsidomine, in angina pectoris, 63–64
Morphine, in AMI, 156
Multiple Risk Factor Intervention Trial (MRFIT), 4–5, 19, 268–69
Mustard operation for TGA, 344–45, 358–59
Myocardial heart disease, 313–27
  cardiac amyloidosis, 326–27
  See also Cardiomyopathies; Myocardial infarction, acute

Myocardial infarction, acute, 115–81
  age and, 117
  angina pectoris and, 128–29
  anticoagulants after, 159
  after CABG, 99, 118–19
  cigarette smoking and, 117
  coagulation problems, 122–24
  complications, 131–39
    atrial fibrillation, 135
    free wall rupture, 138–39
    LV aneurysm, 136–38
    LV thrombus, 135
    papillary muscle rupture, 139
    pericardial effusion, 135
    recurrence, 131
    RV dysfunction, 132–35
    ventricular septal rupture, 138–139
  coronary collaterals, 120–21
  creatine kinase, 116
  diabetes and, 119–20
  diagnosis of
    angiographic indications, 128
    criteria for, 116–17
    ECG observations, 124–25
    echo observations, 125–26
      compared with RNA, 127–28
    magnetic resonance imaging, 128
    RNA observations, 126–27
  infarct size, 119–20
  LV function, 121–22
  outcome, 129–30
    in the employed, 130–31
  prognostic indexes, 139–56
    creatine kinase level, 139–41
    ECG, initial, 141
    echo, 149
      -vs- cineangiography, 145
      exercise testing, 147–49
      infarct extension, 146–47
      location of infarction, 145
      LV ejection fraction, 145
      LV thrombus, 142–45
      programmed ventricular stimulation, 153–56
      radionuclide angiography, 149–50
      ST segment depression, 141–42
      type A behavior, 141
      ventricular arrhythmia, 150–52
  silent infarction, 117–18
  time to pain onset, 115
  treatment, 156–82
    anticoagulants, 159
    beta blockers, 159–64

    CABG, 180
    calcium channel blockers, 164–65
    digitalis, 157–59
    dobutamine, 159
    exercise, 181
    home -vs- group rehabilitation, 180–81
    lidocaine, 156–57
    morphine, 156
    nitroprusside, 159
    PTCA with and without thrombolysis, 180
    thrombolysis
      intracoronary, 165–71
        -vs- intravenous, 178–80
      intravenous, 171–78
    type A behavior and, 122
Myocardial ischemia
  chest pain and, 50–53
  in diabetes, 407
  hypertrophic cardiomyopathy and, 320
  as prognostic factor, 16–19
  silent, 49

N-acetylprocainamide, 221
Neomycin, for blood lipids, 40
Nephrotic syndrome, blood lipids and, 33
Niacin, for blood lipids, 40
Nicardipine, in angina pectoris, 67
Nifedipine
  in AMI, 165
  in angina pectoris, 66–70
  in CHF, 380
  in hypertrophic cardiomyopathy, 325–26
  in primary pulmonary hypertension, 402–3
Nisoldipine, in angina pectoris, 67
Nitrates, in angina pectoris, 59–62, 70
Nitroglycerin
  in AMI, 166
  in angina pectoris, 59, 62–63
  in CHF, 381–82
  in hypertension, 261–62
  during PTCA, 81
Nitroprusside
  in AMI, -vs- dobutamine, 159
  in hypertension, 261–62
Norlorcainide, 218–20
Nuclear magnetic resonance. See Magnetic resonance imaging

Obesity
  blood lipids and, 33–34

CAD and, 44–45
echo studies, 396
Osler's maneuver and pseudohypertension, 252–53
Oxprenolol
in AMI, 164
in hypertension, 263

Pacemakers and cardioverters,
238–42
guidelines for implanting, 238–
39
Pacing
external, 240
inducing angina, 56–58
inducing arrhythmia, 196
transesophageal, 196–97
Pediatric cardiology. *See* Congenital
heart disease
Percutaneous transluminal coronary angioplasty (PTCA), 78–
91
angina and, 77
comparison with CABG, 103–5
coronary perfusion, 80
creatine release after, 78
diltiazem after, 81–82
ECG changes during, 78
effect of intimal dissection, 90
of LM coronary artery, 87
LV performance on, 79
of multiple coronary arteries,
87–88
on myocardial perfusion, 80
nitroglycerin during, 81
with previous coronary thrombosis, 89
producing acute coronary occlusion, 91
restenosis after, 89–90
results, 82–85
for total coronary artery occlusion, 85–87
for unstable angina, 88–89
for variant angina, 77–78
Pericardial effusion, after CABG,
101
Pericardial heart disease, 387–89
acute, 387
echo-guided pericardiocentesis,
388
magnetic resonance imaging in,
388
pericardiectomy for, 388–89
Physical activity
See also Exercise listings
CAD and, 42–44

Pindolol, in hypertension, 258
Plasminogen activator, 175–78
Platelets
inhibitors, 47–49
effect on CABG, 97–98
prostaglandins, stress, and,
400–1
Potassium
concentrations after timolol,
160
in hypertension, 257
Potentials, late
as prognostic factor for CAD,
22–23
value of, in CAD, 3–4
Prednisone, in transplantation,
404–5
Pregnancy
cardiac problems in, 407
hypertension and, 254
Pritikin, Nathan, 40–41
Procainamide, in ventricular
arrhythmias, 217–22, 224–25
Programmed electrical stimulation, 204–10, 211–12, 215–16,
218–19, 221, 226
in idiopathic dilated cardiomyopathy, 317
Propafenone
in supraventricular tachycardia,
198
in ventricular arrhythmias, 221–
22
Propranolol, 10
in AMI, 159–60
in angina pectoris, 67–70
in hypertension, 258–59, 261,
263
-vs- esmolol in supraventricular
tachycardia, 199
Prostacyclin
aspirin and, 47–48
in primary pulmonary hypertension, 403
Prostaglandins
in AMI, 122–23
CAD and, 47–49
platelets, stress, and, 400–1
Prostheses. *See* Bioprostheses; Valvular heart disease
Pseudohypertension, Osler's
maneuver and, 252–53
Psychologic factors
angina and, 50
in cardiac arrhythmia, 202
type A behavior, 122, 141
Pulmonary hypertension, primary,
401–3
Pulmonary veno-occlusive disease,
408–9

Quinidine, in ventricular arrhythmias, 218, 221–25

Radionuclide angiography (RNA)
  in diagnosing AMI, 149–50
  in diagnosing CAD, 9–13
Research Clinics Program Prevalence Study, 27–28
Right ventricle
  double-outlet, 359
  wall thickness in hypertension, 255

Salbutamol, in CHF, 381
Septal defects, echo for, 333–34
Senning repair of TGA, 344
Sinus node dysfunction, pacing for, 239–40
Sleep apnea syndrome, and hypertension, 252
Smoking. See Cigarette smoking
Snoring, and hypertension, 252
Sotalol, 224–25
Statistical analyses, for noninvasive tests, 2–3
Stenoses, 14–15
  mitral, 281–82
  pulmonic, 338, 354
  subaortic, 362
  thallium-201 testing, 9–10, 12, 19–21
  transstenotic pressure gradient, 14–16
ST/HR slope and LV function, 53
St. Jude Medical prosthesis, 306–7
Streptokinase, in AMI, 135, 165–80
Stress, platelets, prostaglandins, and, 400–1
Stroke, after CABG, 101
Sulfinpyrazone, in angina pectoris, 70
Supraventricular tachycardia
  adenosine in, 197
  amiodarone in, 197–98
  esmolol -vs- propranolol, 199
  natural history, 195
  pacing and, 196
  propafenone in, 198
  surgical ablation, 199–201
  theophylline in, 196
  transesophageal pacing, 196–97
  verapamil in, 198–99
Surgery
  See also Cardiac surgery; Cardiovascular surgery; Coronary artery bypass grafting; Congenital heart disease: Pediatric cardiac surgery; Percutaneous

transluminal coronary angioplasty
  for supraventricular tachycardia, 199–201
  tetralogy of Fallot, 340–43
  transplantation, 404–5
Syncope, 232–35
  from arrhythmias, 232
  unexplained, 232–33
Systemic lupus erythematosus, 397–98
Systolic Hypertension in the Elderly Program (SHEP), 269–70

Tachycardia
  See Supraventricular tachycardia
Tetralogy of Fallot, 340–43
Thalassemia major, 327
Takayasu's arteritis, 394–95
Technetium scintigraphy, 172–73
Thallium testing, 9–12, 19–21
  after CABG, 96–97
  after PTCA, 89
Theophylline, and tachycardia, 196
Thrombolysis in Myocardial Infarction (TIMI) study, 175–77
Thrombolysis
  intracoronary, 165–71
  -vs- intravenous, 178–80
  intravenous, 171–78
Thrombosis, before PTCA, 89
Thromboxane
  in angina, 56
  in CAD, 47
  in diagnosis of AMI, 122–23
  release in angina, 56
Tiapamil, in AMI, 165
Timolol, in AMI, 160, 162–64
Tocainide, for ventricular arrhythmias, 226
Transplantation, 404–5
Transposition of great arteries (TGA), 343–46
  arrhythmia after Mustard repair, 345
  arterial switch for, 359–60
  Jatene repair, 344
  Mustard-type repair, 344–45
  Senning repair, 344
  tricuspid valve, 343–44
  ventricular function after repair, 344
Treadmill testing, 4–8
Triamterene, 263
Tricuspid valve, 300–1
  TGA and, 343–44

Tricyclic antidepressant drugs, arrhythmia and, 202–3
Truncus arteriosus repair, 361–62

Urokinase, in AMI, 170–71, 174–75, 178–80

Valsalva maneuver
  effects on LV function, 2
  in idiopathic dilated cardiomyopathy, 315
Valvular heart disease, 273–309
  aortic regurgitation, 290–98
    ankylosing spondylitis, 291
    carcinoid syndrome, 303
    ECG findings, 291–92
    E-point septal separation, 292–93
    exercise ejection fraction response, 296–98
    idiopathic etiology, 290–91
    LV end-systolic dimension, 293–95
    LV function, on operative result, 295–96
  aortic valve anatomy, normal, 301–2
  aortic valve stenosis, 283–90
    angina and coronary arterial narrowing, 290
    coronary luminal diameter, 289–90
    echo-determined
      prosthetic valve size, 288
      severity, 284–87
    H-V conduction, 288–89
    morphologic features of valves, 283
  cardiac valve replacement, 305–9
    anatomic analysis, 309
    bioprostheses
      Ionescu-Shiley, 307–8
      porcine, 307
    Doppler evaluation of, 308
    mitral, 306
      right-sided failure after, 308–9
    St. Jude Medical prosthesis, 306–7
  infective endocarditis, 298–300
  Marfan syndrome, in families, 303–5
  mitral anular calcium, 282–83
  mitral regurgitation, 279–81
    forward ejection fraction, 279
    secondary to ruptured chordae tendineae, 280–81

ventricular arrhythmias, 279–80
  value of pulmonary arterial V wave,
mitral stenosis, 281–82
  atenolol on exercise capacity, 281
  open mitral valve reconstruction, 281–82
  percutaneous catheter mitral commissurotomy, 281
mitral valve
  echo evaluation after operation, 305
  morphology, 301
mitral valve prolapse, 273–79
  with atrial flutter, 276
  in drug addicts, 275
  hyperthyroidism, 278
  infective endocarditis prophylaxis, 274–75
  long-term follow-up, 273
  operative therapy, 278–79
  pregnancy and, 277
  relation to LV size in the Marfan syndrome, 276
  ruptured chordae tendineae and, 273–74
  secondary to RV enlargement, 275–76
  sickle cell anemia, 277–78
  with WPW syndrome, 276–77
tricuspid valve disease, 300–1
Ventricular arrhythmias, 191–229
  See also Arrhythmias, ventricular
  amiodarone, 211–14, 217–18
  antiarrhythmic drug efficacy, 209
  bepridil, 214
  CABG for, 96
  cardioversion
    defibrillation and, 226
    induced, 226
  CHF and, 367–68
  diagnosis, 201–2
  disopyramide, 222
  electrophysiologic testing, 209, 213
  encainide, 215
  endocardial resection, 227–29
  exercise induced, CABG for, 96
  flecainide, 215–17
  Holter monitoring, 211–13
    -vs- electrophysiologic study, 209
  lorcainide, 218–20
  LV endocardial resection, 227–29
  mexiletine, 217–18
  N-acetylprocainamide, 221

norlorcainide, 218–20
pacemakers, 196–97, 226–27
procainamide, 217–22, 224–25
programmed electrical stimula-
    tion, 204–12, 215–16, 218–19,
    221, 226
propafenone, 221–22
psychologic factors and, 202
quinidine, 218, 221–25
sotalol, 224–25
spontaneous variability, 203–4
tocainide, 226
tricyclic antidepressant drugs
    and, 202–3
verapamil, 198–99, 225
Ventricular ectopic activity, in
    variant angina pectoris, 73–74
Ventricular function assessment
    after Fontan, 360
    in Kawasaki disease, 362–63
    after TGA repair, 344

Ventricular septal defect, 333–38
    with aneurysm, 325
    isolated, 335
    localized by Doppler and echo,
        333–34
    pulmonary artery development,
        338
    standardized nomenclature, 333
Verapamil
    in AMI, 164–5
    in angina pectoris, 69–70
    in hypertrophic cardiomyopathy,
        326
    in supraventricular tachycardia,
        198–99
    in ventricular arrhythmis, 198–
        99, 225

Withering, William, 382–83
Wolff-Parkinson-White (WPW)
    syndrome, 276–77